ELSEVIER

evolve

To access your Student Resources, visit the web address below:

http://evolve.elsevier.com/Buck/CCS/

- **Study Tips**
  Thoughts and advice from the author to help medical coding students.
- **Medical Coding in the News**
  The latest developments in the world of coding, updated frequently.
- **WebLinks**
  Links to places of interest on the web specific to your needs.
- **Links to Related Products**
  See what else Elsevier has to offer in your specific field of interest.

AF718862

2005

CCS CODING EXAM REVIEW

The Certification Step

2005

CCS CODING EXAM REVIEW

The Certification Step

Carol J. Buck, MS, CPC, CPC-H
Program Director, Retired
Medical Secretary Programs
Northwest Technical College
East Grand Forks, Minnesota

Chief Reviewer
Judy Trueblood-Hatcher, CCS, CPC, CPC-H
Coding Instructor
Baylor University Medical Center at Dallas
Dallas, Texas

ELSEVIER
SAUNDERS

ELSEVIER
SAUNDERS

11830 Westline Industrial Drive
St. Louis, Missouri 63146

CCS Coding Exam Review 2005: The Certification Step 1-4160-2396-8
Copyright © 2005, Elsevier Inc. All rights reserved.

No part of this publication may be reproduced or transmitted in any form or by any means, electronic or mechanical, including photocopying, recording, or any information storage and retrieval system, without permission in writing from the publisher. Permissions may be sought directly from Elsevier's Health Sciences Rights Department in Philadelphia, PA, USA: phone (+1) 215 238 7869, fax: (+1) 215 238 2239, e-mail: healthpermissions@elsevier.com. You may also complete your request on-line via the Elsevier homepage (http://www.elsevier.com), by selecting "Customer Support" and then "Obtaining Permissions".

NOTICE

Medical Coding is an ever-changing field. Standard safety precautions must be followed, but as new research and clinical experience broaden our knowledge, changes in treatment and drug therapy may become necessary or appropriate. Readers are advised to check the most current product information provided by the manufacturer of each drug to be administered to verify the recommended dose, the method and duration of administration, and contraindications. It is the responsibility of the licensed prescriber, relying on experience and knowledge of the patient, to determine dosages and the best treatment for each individual patient. Neither the publisher nor the author assumes any liability for any injury and/or damage to persons or property arising from this publication.

CPT codes are copyright of the American Medical Association. CPT only © 2004. *Current Procedural Terminology, 2005, Professional Edition,* American Medical Association. All rights reserved.

Although for mechanical reasons all pages of this publication are perforated, only those pages imprinted with an Elsevier Inc. copyright notice are intended for removal.

International Standard Book Number 1-4160-2396-8

Senior Acquisitions Editor: Susan Cole
Developmental Editor: Beth LoGiudice
Publishing Services Manager: Pat Joiner
Senior Project Manager: David Stein
Senior Designer: Kathi Gosche

Printed in United States of America
Last digit is the print number: 9 8 7 6 5 4 3 2 1

Working together to grow libraries in developing countries

www.elsevier.com | www.bookaid.org | www.sabre.org

ELSEVIER BOOK AID International Sabre Foundation

Dedication

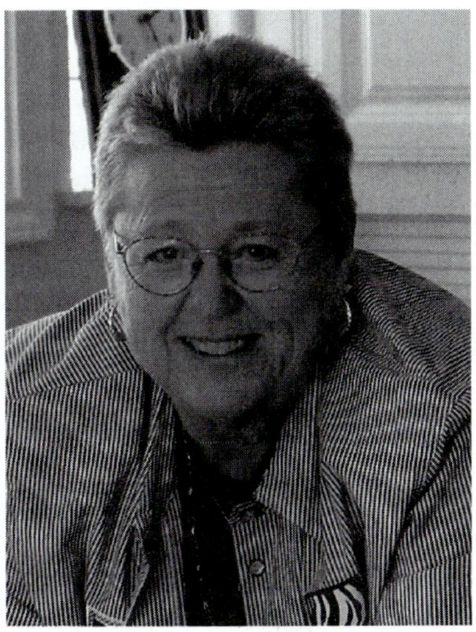

To coding instructors,
who each day strive to enhance the lives
of their students and provide the next generation
of knowledgeable medical coders.

Carol J. Buck

Acknowledgments

There are so many, many people that participated in the development of this text and only through the effort of all the team members has it been possible to publish this text. **Jackie Grass**, who lent her technical coding knowledge and enthusiasm to this project and whose willingness to always step in to help bring each project in on time is the most valuable ability. **Jody Klitz**, who spent endless hours ensuring this material was correct. **Marilyn Rasmussen**, who provided her coding skills to this task with great determination. **Sue Moe**, whose exceptional knowledge of medical terminology, anatomy, and pathophysiology improved the material greatly. **Cyndi Stahl**, whose great determination, sense of adventure, and willingness to go into unknown territory was the greatest help. **Judy Trueblood-Hatcher** who has been a steady guiding presence through the development of the text and who never failed to keep the faith during the journey.

Sally Schrefer, Executive Vice President, Nursing and Health Professions, who possesses great listening skills and the ability to ensure the publication of high-quality educational materials. **Andrew Allen**, Publishing Director, Health Professions, who sees the bigger picture and shares the vision. **Susan Cole**, Senior Acquisitions Editor, who guided this project to completion with her steady hand. **Beth LoGiudice**, Developmental Editor, who has performed minor miracles daily during the development of this text. **David Stein**, Senior Project Manager, and **David Rushing**, Producer, who both ensured that we all completed our work on time. The employees of Elsevier have participated in the publication of this text and demonstrated the highest levels of professionalism and competence.

Preface

Thank you for purchasing *CCS Coding Exam Review 2005: The Certification Step*, the latest guide to the CCS certification exam. This 2005 edition has been carefully reviewed and updated with the latest content, making it the most current guide for your review. The author and publishers have made every effort to equip you with skills and tools you will need to succeed on the exam. To this end, the *CCS Coding Exam Review 2005* presents essential information about all health care coding systems and anatomy and terminology, as well as sample exams for practice, both in print and on CD-ROM. No other review guide on the market brings together such thorough coverage of all necessary exam material in one source.

ORGANIZATION OF THIS TEXTBOOK

Following a basic outline approach, this textbook takes a practical approach to assisting you with your exam preparations. The text is divided into four units—Anatomy, Terminology, and Pathophysiology; Reimbursement Issues; Overview of CPT, ICD-9-CM and HCPCS Coding; and Coding Challenge—and there are seven appendices for your reference. Additionally, there is a bound-in CD-ROM with a Practice Exam to help your progress.

Unit I, Anatomy, Terminology, and Pathophysiology
Covers all the essential body systems and terms you'll need to get certified. Organized by body systems, the sections also include illustrations to review each major anatomical area and quizzes to check your understanding and recall.

84 UNITI Anatomy, Terminology, and Pathophysiology

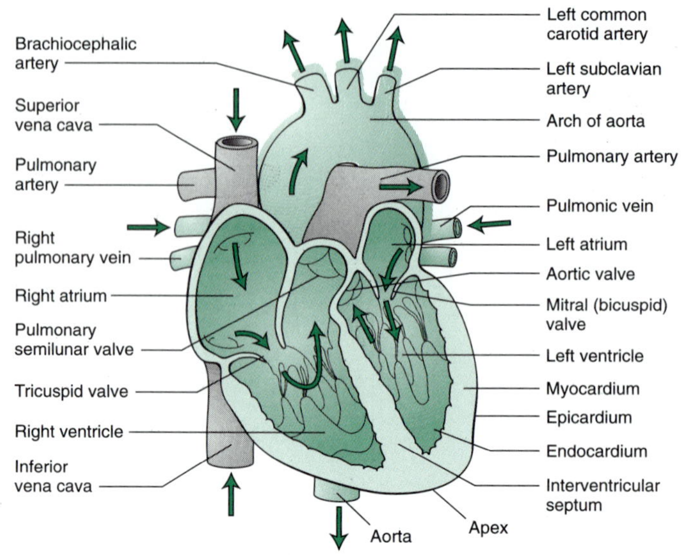

Figue 1-18 Intemal view of the heart.

Parietal pericardium: outermost covering
Visceral pericardium: innermost (epicardium)
Pericardial cavity: contains fluid

Unit II, Reimbursement Issues
Provides a review of important insurance and billing information to help you review the connections between medical coding, insurance, billing, and reimbursement.

APC Payment Status Indicators (SI) (Figure 2-4)

Passthrough codes

Services, procedures, and/or supplies not included in APC package

Paid in addition to APC payment

Copyright © 2005, Elsevier Inc. All rights reserved.
CPT only © 2004. *Current Procedural Terminology, 2005, Professional Edition*, American Medical Association. All rights reserved.

Unit III, Overview of CPT, ICD-9-CM, and HCPCS Coding Contains comprehensive coverage of the different coding systems and their applications, making other references unnecessary! Simplified text and clear examples are the highlights of this unit, while illustrations are included to clarify difficult concepts.

Vascular Families Are Like a Tree

- Main branch—first order
- Second-order branch
- Third-order branch
- Brachiocephalic Vascular Family **(Figure 3-7)**

Report farthest extent of catheter placement in a vascular family

Embolectomy and Thrombectomy (34001-34490)

Embolus: Dislodged thrombus

Thrombus: Mass of material in vessel located in place of formation

May be removed by dissection or balloon

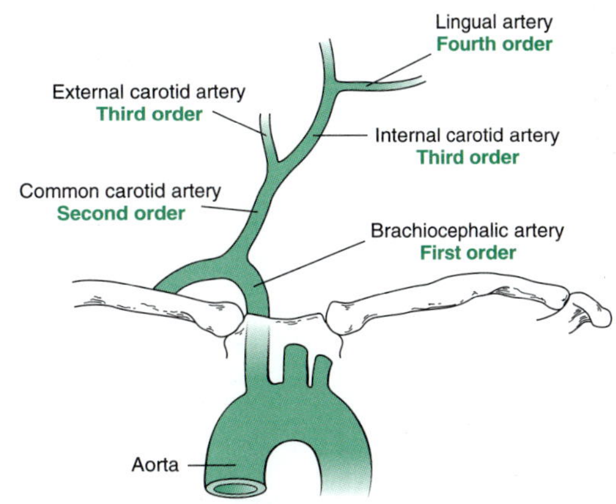

Figure 3-7 Brachiocephalic vascular family with first-, second-, third-, and fourth-order vessels.

Unit IV, Coding Challenge Contains a sample "final" exam with the same question types as the actual CCS exam, to be completed after your review.

PART 1

1. A 2-year-old child was brought to the outpatient radiology department at the hospital by his father for an ultrasound of child's heart. At the age of 10 months, he was diagnosed with a heart murmur due to ventricular septal defect. At age 11 months, the child developed congestive heart failure, and at that time the physician prescribed diuretics and digitalis.

745.4	Bulbus cordis anomalies and anomalies of cardiac septal closure, ventricular septal deviation
785.2	Symptoms involving cardiovascular system, undiagnosed cardiac murmurs
747.29	Other congenital anomalies of circulatory system, other anomalies of aorta, other congenital
779.8	Other specified conditions originating in the perinatal period, other specified conditions originating in the perinatal period

A. 745.4
B. 745.4, 785.2
C. 747.29, 745.4
D. 745.4, 779.29

About the CD-ROM

The companion CD-ROM included in the back of this review guide contains valuable software to assist you with your preparation for the CCS coding certification examination. It includes a timed and scored 81-question practice exam, modeled after the actual certification exam that contains two major sections, with the first section containing 60 multiple-choice questions and the second section containing 21 assign-the-code questions. The exam is designed to be taken twice—once as a pre-exam and once as a post-exam. The Pre-Exam must be completed at the start of your study, and the Post-Exam should be taken after your study is complete. By comparing the results of both exam modes, you can see your improvement after using the review guide.

Summary Screen

When using the program, the Summary screen serves as home base. Here you can find information relating to your progress and performance in different exam sections and subject areas. From this screen, you can choose an exam mode, submit an exam section, check your progress, or review your results.

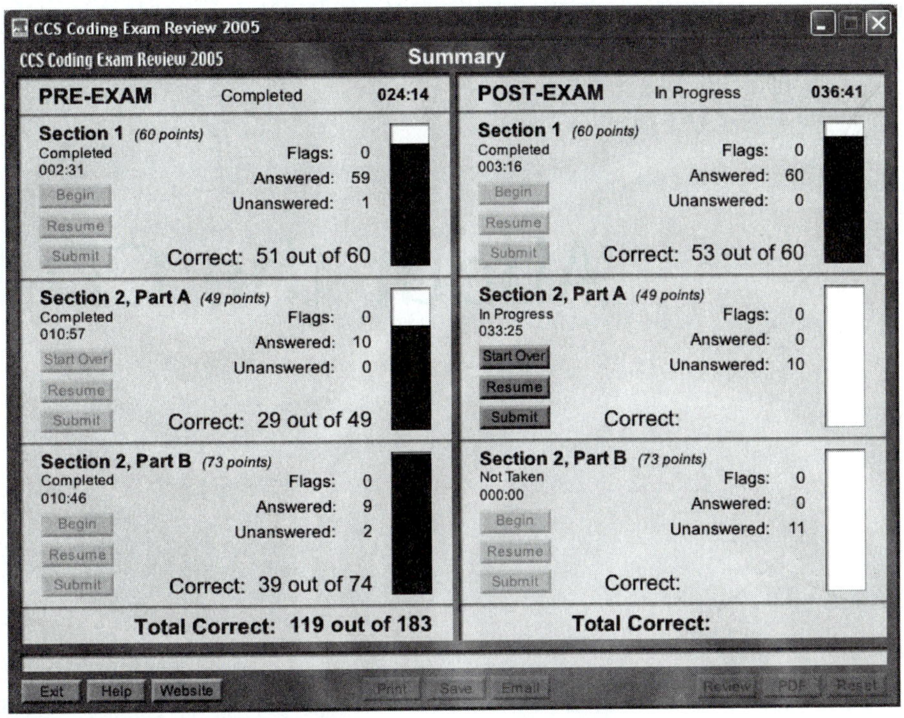

Summary screen.

In addition to displaying your scores for completed sections and tracking the total elapsed time, this screen also shows the answered, unanswered, and flagged questions in each subsection. You can return to the Summary screen at any point while taking or reviewing an exam, and all information related to your answers and position is saved.

Taking the Exam

Section 1 can be taken using the mouse by clicking the letter buttons to select answers and navigation buttons to move from question to question. You may also use the keyboard to type the letter that corresponds to the answer (A, B, C, D) and the left and right arrow keys to navigate. For Section 2, codes can be typed into the pop-up answer sheet as you read through the case, and your answers will be saved when you close the answer sheet. You can also make notes to the right of the answer area, which will also be saved if the answer sheet is closed.

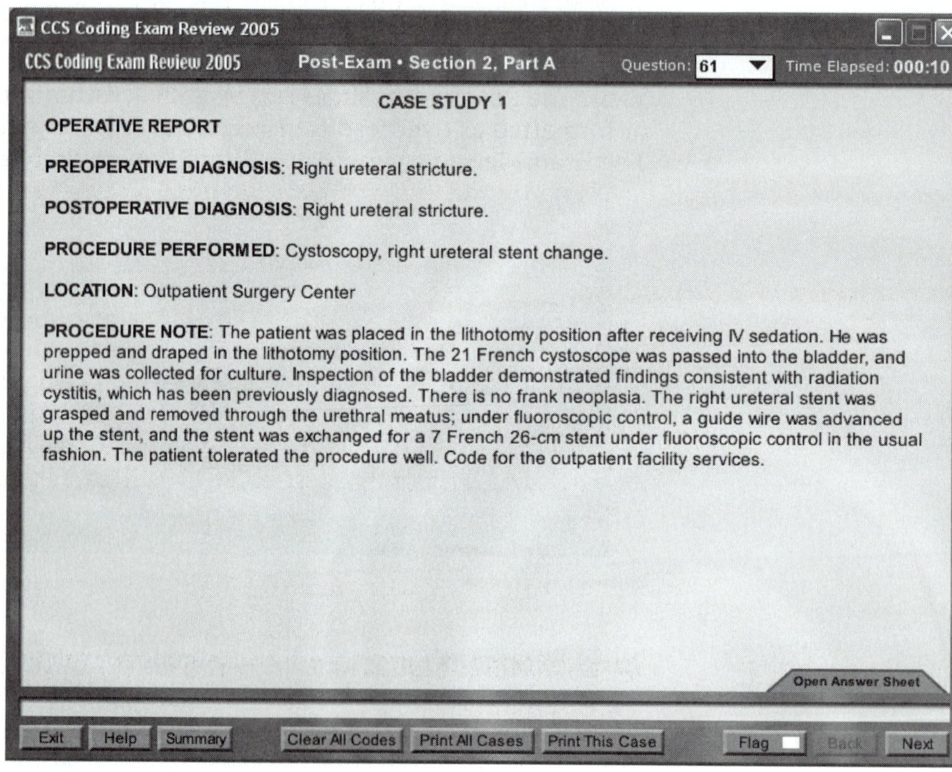

Section 2 Question Screen.

The Exam screen also displays the current question number, which doubles as a pull-down menu that allows you to jump to any question in the current section. An X mark next to a question number in that menu indicates unanswered and flagged questions. The Flag button at the bottom of the screen allows you to mark questions for later reference.

Reviewing Your Results

Once you have taken both exam modes, you have the option to review all the exam questions with rationales, even the ones you answered correctly. The correct answer is shown for each question, and a rationale is given for each answer option. You can also compare your results on the Pre- and Post-Exams by viewing the bar graph on the Summary Screen or printing out a score sheet.

Additional instructions and help files are included on the CD-ROM to assist you in using the software.

Supplemental Resources

However you decide to prepare for the certification exam, we have developed supplements designed to complement the *CCS Coding Exam Review 2005*. Each of these supplements has been developed with the needs of both students and instructors in mind.

Instructor's Curriculum Resource on CD-ROM

No matter what your level of teaching experience, this total-teaching solution will help you plan your lessons with ease, and the author has developed all the curriculum materials necessary to use the textbook in the classroom. Included in the printed material are all answers to the textbook and workbook exercises, a course calendar and syllabus, lesson plans, and ready-made tests for easy assessment. The CD-ROM includes all printed content, a comprehensive PowerPoint collection of the entire text, and a test bank in ExamView. The PowerPoint slides can be easily customized to support your lectures or formatted as overhead transparencies or handouts for student note-taking. The ExamView test generator will help you quickly and easily prepare quizzes and exams, and the test banks can be customized to your specific teaching methods.

Evolve Learning Resources

The Evolve companion website offers many resources that will extend your studies beyond the classroom. Related WebLinks and industry news offer you the opportunity to expand your knowledge base and stay current with this ever-changing field, and additional material is available for help and practice. Instructors can also download all materials available from the Instructor's Curriculum Resource, as well as content updates and industry news.

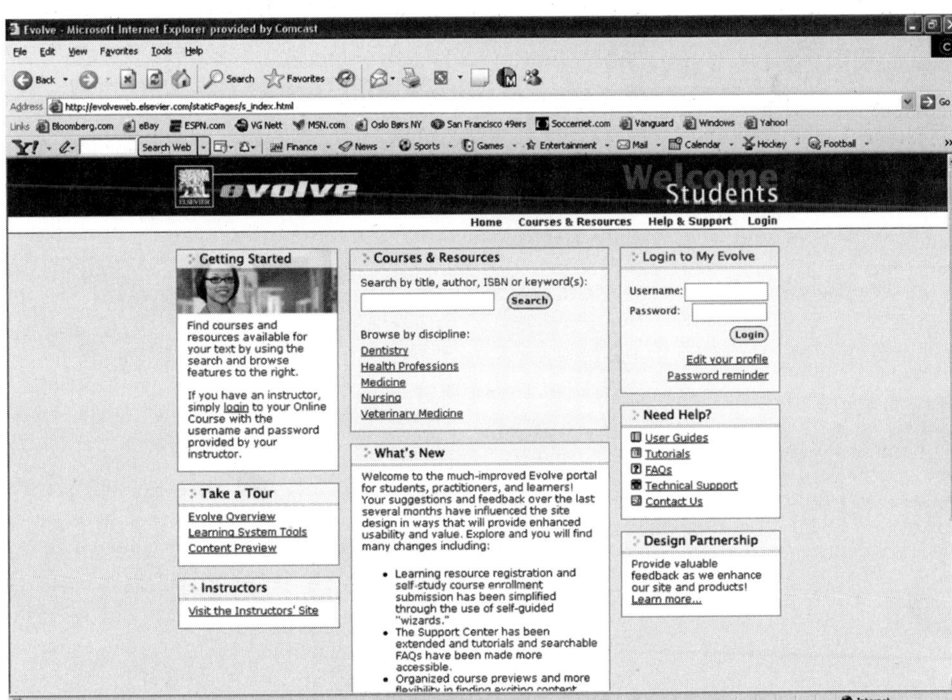

A Course Management System (CMS) is also available free to instructors who adopt this textbook. This web-based platform gives instructors yet another resource to facilitate learning and to make medical coding content accessible to students. In addition to the Evolve Learning Resources available to both faculty and students, there is an entire suite of tools available that allows for communication between instructors and students. Students can log on through the Evolve portal to take online quizzes, participate in threaded discussions, post assignments to instructors, or chat with other classmates, while instructors can use the online grade book to follow class progress.

To access this comprehensive online resource, simply go to the Evolve home page at http://evolve.elsevier.com and enter the user name and password provided by your instructor. If your instructor has not set up a Course Management System, you can still access the free Evolve Learning Resources at http://evolve.elsevier.com/Buck/CCS/.

Development of this Edition

This book would not have been possible without a team of educators and professionals, including practicing coders and technical consultants. The combined efforts of the team members have made this text an incredible learning tool.

THE TEAM

Lead Coding Specialist, **Jacqueline Grass**
Coding Specialist, **Jody Klitz**
Coding Specialist, **Marilyn Rasmussen**
Anatomy, Terminology, and Pathophysiology Specialist, **Sue Moe**

Technical Research Assistant
Cynthia Stahl, CPC, CCS-P
Reimbursement and Coding Specialist
Lebanon, Indiana

Chief Reviewer
Judy Trueblood-Hatcher, CCS, CPC, CPC-H
Coding Instructor
Baylor University Medical Center at Dallas
Dallas, Texas

Reviewers

Marie T. Conde, MPA, RHIT, CCS
Program Director and Instructor, HIT
City College of San Francisco
San Francisco, California

Jana Marie Hensche, RHIT
Inpatient Hospital Coder—Medical Revenue Systems
Austin Medical Center
Austin, Minnesota

Deanna D. Mandley, RHIT, CCS, CCS-P
President
D. Mandley & Associates
Stow, Ohio

Contents

Introduction

This review was developed to help you as you prepare for your certification examination. First, congratulations on your initiative. Preparing for a certification examination can seem like a daunting and formidable task. You have already taken the first and hardest step: You have made a commitment. Your steely determination and organizational skills are your best tools as you organize to complete this exciting journey successfully.

This text has been developed to serve as a tool in your preparation for the facility-based outpatient (facility-based) certification examination. There are two facility-based coding certifications: CCS (Certified Coding Specialist) and CPC-H (Certified Professional Coder—Hospital). The American Health Information Management Association (AHIMA) offers the CCS, and the American Academy of Professional Coders offers the CPC-H. Although the formats of the examinations are different, the commonality is that both assess your medical coding ability. Regardless of which examination you take, you will have to know how to assign medical codes to patient services and diagnoses. This textbook is focused on providing you with that coding practice as well as anatomy, terminology, reimbursement, and coding concepts in **preparation for the CCS**.

This text is divided into:

- Success Strategies
- Unit I: Anatomy, Terminology, and Pathophysiology
- Unit II: Reimbursement Issues
- Unit III: Overview of CPT, ICD-9-CM, and HCPCS Coding
- Unit IV: Coding Challenge
- Appendix A: Official Guidelines for Coding and Reporting
- Appendix B: Medical Terminology
- Appendix C: Combining Forms
- Appendix D: Prefixes
- Appendix E: Suffixes

Copyright © 2005, Elsevier Inc. All rights reserved.
CPT only © 2004. *Current Procedural Terminology, 2005, Professional Edition*, American Medical Association. All rights reserved.

- Appendix F: Abbreviations
    - Appendices B-F are combined lists of Medical Terminology, Combining Forms, Prefixes, and Suffixes used within Unit I, Anatomy and Terminology.
- Appendix G: Further Text References
- Appendix H: Pharmacology Review

The material in this review features the following:

- Comprehensive guide in outline format
- Photos and drawings to illustrate key points
- Practice Examination (CD)—60 questions and 21 case studies
- Final Examination (text)—60 questions and 21 case studies

My personal best wishes to you as you prepare for your certification. You can do this!

Carol J. Buck

Our goals can only be reached through a vehicle of a plan, in which we must fervently believe, and upon which we must vigorously act. There is no other route to success.
Stephen A. Brennen

Copyright © 2005, Elsevier Inc. All rights reserved.
CPT only © 2004. *Current Procedural Terminology, 2005, Professional Edition*, American Medical Association. All rights reserved.

Success Strategies

How do you prepare for a certification examination? The answers to that question are as varied as the persons preparing for a certification examination. Each person comes to the preparation with different educational, coding, and personal experiences. Therefore, each must develop a plan that meets his or her individual needs and preferences. Success Strategies will help you to develop your individual plan.

CERTIFICATION EXAMINATIONS

The CCS certification examination consists of Part I (60 multiple-choice questions) and Part II (21 medical records cases). The 60 multiple-choice questions cover documentation, CPT, ICD-9-CM, HCPCS, reimbursement, and data quality. The examination is administered over 6 hours (see pg. 9 for 2005 changes).

Date and Location

Although every journey begins with the first step, you have to know where you are going to make a plan to get there.

Choose the **date and location** for taking the certification examination. The certifying organizations' web sites contain detailed information about the examination sites and dates (www.ahima.org) as well as a great deal of specific information about the CCS. You can also contact AHIMA at the following address:

American Health Information Management Association
Attn: CCS Examination
233 North Michigan Avenue, Suite 2150
Chicago, IL 60601-5800
Telephone: 312-233-1100

Copyright © 2005, Elsevier Inc. All rights reserved.
CPT only © 2004. *Current Procedural Terminology, 2005, Professional Edition,* American Medical Association. All rights reserved.

After you have obtained the examination materials, read all the information carefully. Review all competencies outlined in the material to ensure that your study plan contains strategies to address each of these competencies.

The questions within this textbook are not the same questions that are in the certification examinations, but the skill and knowledge that you gain through analysis, coding, and recall will increase your ability to be successful on examination day.

AHIMA's coding examination information will indicate the coding specifics. For example, the levels of the evaluation and management key components (history, examination, and medical decision-making complexity) are stated in the certification questions so you will not be required to assign the levels.

MANAGING YOUR TIME

Role strain! That is what you get when you have so many different roles in your life and you cannot find time for all of them. Know that feeling? Are you a daughter/son, mother/father, wife/husband, student, friend, worker, volunteer, hobbyist? The list is endless. Each takes time from your schedule, and somehow you now need to fit into the role of successful learner. Because you have only 24 hours in your day, being a successful learner requires a time-balancing act. Maybe you will have to be satisfied with dust bunnies under your bed, dishes in your kitchen sink, or fewer visits with your friends. Whatever you have to do to juggle the time around to give yourself ample time to devote to this important task of examination preparation, you must do and make a plan for in advance; otherwise, life just takes over and you find you do not have adequate study time.

If you are planning a big event in your life—moving, a trip, and so on—think about postponing it until after the examination. Your focus right now has to be on yourself. Make your motto "It's All About Me!" Sounds self-centered, I know, and most likely very different from who you are, but just this once, you need to carve out the time you need to accomplish this important goal. This time is for yourself. Make it happen for yourself. Move everything you can out of the way, focus on this preparation, and give this preparation your best effort.

SCHEDULE

Each person has an individual learning style. The coding profession seems to attract those most influenced by logic and facts. The best way for a logical and factual person to learn is to problem-solve and apply the information. Hands-on practice is how you will build your skill and confidence for the examination.
Choose a location to be your Study Central.

Gather into Study Central the following study resources

- Certification information from www.ahima.org/certification
- CPT, current edition
- ICD-9-CM, current edition
- HCPCS, current edition
- Official Guidelines for Coding and Reporting (Appendix A)
- Medical dictionary
- Coding textbooks, professional journals, and magazines
- Terminology, anatomy, or pathology text, as needed
- See Appendix G for Further Text References

Make Study Central your special place where you can get away from all other responsibilities. Make it a quiet, calm getaway, even if it is a corner of your bedroom.

Copyright © 2005, Elsevier Inc. All rights reserved.
CPT only © 2004. *Current Procedural Terminology, 2005, Professional Edition,* American Medical Association. All rights reserved.

In this quiet place have a comfortable chair, adequate lighting, supplies, and sufficient desktop surface to use all your coding books. This is your place to focus all your attention on preparation for the examination, without distractions.

Plan your **schedule** from now until the certification examination using a calendar. Make weekly goals so that you have definite tasks to accomplish each week and you can check the tasks off—a great feeling of accomplishment comes from being able to check off a task. In this way, you can see your progress on your countdown to success.

Choose a specific **time** each day or several times a week when you are going to study, and mark them on your calendar. Make this commitment in writing. After each study session, you should check off that date on the calendar as a visual reminder that you are sticking to your plan and are one step closer to your goal.

You should plan your study time in advance, know what you are going to be studying the next session, and **be prepared** for that upcoming study session. This will greatly increase the amount of material you are able to cover during the session. At the end of each session, decide what you are going to study next session and ensure that you have all the material and references you will need readily available. At the end of each session, you should be ready for the next study session.

Your plan should include those areas where you know you will need improvement. For example, when is the last time you read, not referenced or reviewed, but really read, the CPT Anesthesia Guidelines? You probably do not code anesthesia services often, if ever, and as such are not familiar with the information in these guidelines. That is an area for improvement, and your plan should include a thorough reading of all the CPT section guidelines.

DO THIS BEFORE YOU BEGIN YOUR STUDY

Assess your strengths and weaknesses. By making this assessment, you will know where to concentrate your efforts and where to focus your study schedule. You know those areas where you already have strong skills and knowledge and will not need to spend as much time preparing in these areas. The **Practice Examination** is an 81-question examination that you can use as a tool to assess your current skill level. This examination should be taken before you begin your study and then again immediately after you have completed your entire study schedule. Do not analyze the questions by reviewing the rationales provided in the Practice Examination; rather, wait until after you have completed your studies and have taken this same examination a second time. If you review the rationales after the first time you take the examination, you will know the answers too well to provide a valid comparison between examinations. See Unit IV of this textbook for further directions on the Practice Examination.

After you have completed your course of study, take the Practice Examination again. You should plan to cover the examination in the same amount of time as will be given for the certification examination you are going to take. Compare your scores with those from the first time you took this examination. Note the areas where you did not demonstrate sufficient skills and knowledge.

Develop a **second plan** to improve the specific areas where you believe you need further study.

You are now ready to take the **Final Examination** that is located in this text. Take the examination in the same amount of time that will be allocated for the certification examination (6 hours). It is best if you complete this final in one sitting, thereby mimicking the actual examination. If your schedule does not allow for taking the examination in one sitting, plan to take it in several sessions, but always keep track of the time used to ensure that you take the examination in the same amount of time allowed for the official examination. Learning to work within the time allocated is part of the skill you are developing. Remember, the certification

Copyright © 2005, Elsevier Inc. All rights reserved.
CPT only © 2004. *Current Procedural Terminology, 2005, Professional Edition*, American Medical Association. All rights reserved.

examinations assess not only your coding knowledge but also your efficiency in completing the test within the allocated time.

USING THIS TEXT

Unit I is a review of the anatomy, terminology, and pathophysiology by organ systems designed to provide you with a quick review of that organ system. In addition, there is a list of combining forms, prefixes, suffixes, and abbreviations that are often used in that organ system. At the end of each organ system, there is a quiz that will give you an opportunity to assess your knowledge of anatomy/terminology and pathophysiology.

Unit II is a review of reimbursement issues and terminology. A quiz is located at the end of the unit to assess your knowledge.

Unit III is a review of CPT, HCPCS, and ICD-9-CM. The CPT and ICD-9-CM material follows the order of the manuals. There is no quiz at the end of this unit because you will be applying this material in the Practice Examination and in the Final Examination.

Unit IV contains the examinations. The Practice Examination is an 81-question examination located on the **CD** and is to be taken twice—once before you begin your study and the second time after you have completed your study. You should allow 6 hours (360 minutes) to complete the Practice Examination because this is the amount of time you will have for the certification review. The CD stores your score from your Practice Examination and compares the results from the first and second time you took the examination; therefore, you can see not only your score on each section but also the improvement from the first to the second examination. The Final Examination is also an 81-question, paper-and-pencil examination that is located in the text, and you should allow 6 hours (360 minutes) to complete the examination. Both examinations are divided into the following sections:

Section 1—60 Questions (See pg. 9 for 2005 examination changes.)

Medical Terminology

Anatomy

ICD-9-CM

HCPCS

Concepts of Coding and Reimbursement

Pathophysiology

Section 2—21 Case Studies (See pg. 9 for 2005 examination changes.)

Part 1: Outpatient records

Part 2: Inpatient records

There are many ways you could use this text. However you decide to prepare, you should take the examination before you begin your study to ensure that you develop a study plan that includes time and activities that will increase your knowledge in those areas where your test scores indicate areas of weakness. You could then take the units in the order in which they are presented, or you may want to review the anatomy/terminology and pathophysiology for a body system and then review the CPT material for that body system. There is no one set way to approach the use of this text because each individual will have a personal learning style and preferences that will direct how the material is used. Your skills may be very strong in one or

Copyright © 2005, Elsevier Inc. All rights reserved.
CPT only © 2004. *Current Procedural Terminology, 2005, Professional Edition,* American Medical Association. All rights reserved.

more coding or knowledge areas, and you will want to delete those areas from your individual study plan.

This text is not meant to be the only study source; rather, it is just one tool among many that you will use. For example, if your terminology skills need a complete overhaul, the brief overview in this text may not meet your needs. You may want to supplement this text with a terminology text and an in-depth study of terminology.

Appendices are a resource for you as you prepare your study plan.

Appendix A: Official Guidelines for Coding and Reporting is the rules for use of ICD-9-CM codes and will be referenced in Unit III during review of the use of ICD-9-CM codes.

Appendix B: Medical Terminology is a complete alphabetic list of all the medical terms listed in the Medical Terminology portion of the organ system reviews used in Unit I.

Appendix C: Combining Forms is a complete alphabetic list of the combining forms used in Unit I.

Appendix D: Prefixes is a complete alphabetic list of the prefixes used in Unit I.

Appendix E: Suffixes is a complete alphabetic list of the suffixes used in Unit I.

Appendix F: Abbreviations is a complete list of the abbreviations referenced in Unit I.

Appendix G: Further Text References is a list of texts that you may want to obtain to supplement your study plan.

Appendix H: Pharmacology Review

DAY BEFORE THE EXAMINATION

No cramming! Your study time is now over, and cramming the day before the test is not a good idea because it just increases your anxiety level. This day is your day to prepare yourself. Do some things that you enjoy. Take your mind off the examination. Pamper yourself: You deserve it.

Assemble pencils (No. 2), erasers, two forms of identification, CPT, ICD-9-CM (Volume 1, 2, and 3), HCPCS code books if necessary for your specific examination, medical dictionary, and examination admission ticket. Check the AHIMA web site for the specifics of what to bring to the examination site.

You cannot have excessive writing, sticky notes, labels, and so forth in your code books. Check the examination details to ensure that your books meet the specifications identified by the testing organization.

If allowed, take bottled water and snacks because the day is long.

Review the certification packet information one last time to ensure that you have all the required material.

Listen to the weather and traffic reports. Plan your route to the examination site. If it is in a new location, drive to the location before the big day.

Eat a light supper and get to bed early. Set the alarm in plenty of time to arrive at the site early. It is a good idea to have a friend or family member give you an early wake-up call to ensure that you do not oversleep.

DAY OF THE EXAMINATION

Wear comfortable clothes, and be prepared for any room temperature. A short-sleeved shirt with a sweater is a good plan. Dress in layers so you can ensure that you will be comfortable in any environment.

Copyright © 2005, Elsevier Inc. All rights reserved.
CPT only © 2004. *Current Procedural Terminology, 2005, Professional Edition*, American Medical Association. All rights reserved.

Take a watch with you.

Eat a good breakfast. Avoid caffeine because it initially stimulates you but will decrease your concentration in the long run.

Arrive early. The doors are locked to those who arrive late. This is a day to be **early**.

Ensure that you have the correct room for your examination. Often there are several examinations being administered at one time, so be certain you are in the correct room for your examination.

THE CERTIFICATION EXAMINATION

You are ready for this! You have planned your work and have worked your plan. Now it is time to reap the rewards for all that hard work.

Choose a good location in which to sit. Choose a location that will not get a lot of traffic from those leaving the room.

Place all your supplies on the table.

Someone will distribute the examination after the general directions have been given to the group.

Have faith in yourself, and visualize yourself being successful. Say to yourself, "You can do this" and then take several deep breaths before you begin to help relax you.

Quickly review the entire examination. Note the location of the halfway mark. This will help you to keep on schedule.

Some prefer to take the parts of the examination out of order, beginning with those questions about which they are most confident. Others prefer to start at the beginning and work through all questions in order. The approach that you use will depend on your individual test-taking style.

When you come to a question for which you are unsure of the answer, you may wish to skip over it and come back to all those ones you were unsure of at the end of the examination, depending on the time available. Or you may want to attempt each question and mark those you are unsure of so that you can return to them when you have finished the entire examination. Again, the approach you will use depends on your individual style. If you mark questions to return to and are using a scan sheet on which to enter your answers, be certain that you return and remove the erasure marks because these tests are machine-scanned and those stray pencil marks can give inaccurate responses. You will receive only your score, not the test or the answer sheet; if your stray pencil marks suggest inaccurate responses, you will have no way to fix those mistakes.

Read the directions. This may sound too simple, but many persons do not completely read the directions, only to find that the directions gave specific directions about what or what not to code on a certain case (for example, "code only this certain portion of the procedure"). Yet the choices for answers included the full coding of the case as a selection; if you did not read all the directions, you would choose the response with codes for all the items listed in the report. For example, the question may have directed you to code the service only, not the diagnosis, and yet one of the choices would be the correct service and diagnosis codes, which of course would be an incorrect answer based on the directions. So read all of the directions.

Your speed and accuracy are being tested. You do not have time to labor over each question for a long time if you intend to complete all the questions. Read the directions, read the question, put down your best assessment of the answer, and then move on to the next question. Place a light mark by the question about which you have doubts.

Words such as *always, every, never,* and *all* generally indicate broad terms that, with true/false questions, usually indicate a false question.

Copyright © 2005, Elsevier Inc. All rights reserved.
CPT only © 2004. *Current Procedural Terminology, 2005, Professional Edition*, American Medical Association. All rights reserved.

If you do not know the answer to the question, first try eliminating those that you know are incorrect and then select the answer that seems most likely to be correct.

Judge the time as you are moving through the examination. Keep assessing whether you are making sufficient progress or whether you can slow down or need to speed up.

Answer all questions. Even if you have to guess, at least fill in an answer. The best situation is that you answer all questions and have time left over to go back over the questions about which you are in doubt.

Erase all stray pencil marks on your test. Be neat with your work; neatness makes a difference when the machine scores your test.

Be certain to carefully complete the information sheet that accompanies the examination. This sheet will include your name, address, and other information that ensures that your test results are accurately recorded.

Use every minute of the test time, but it is not a good idea to begin second-guessing yourself. Do not return to those questions for which you did not have serious doubts about the correct answer. Usually, your first answer is the best.

When the time is finished, hand in your examination, and pat yourself on the back. You have done an excellent job! Now it is time to go get a good supper and a good night's sleep.

DAYS AFTER THE EXAMINATION

You will miss the preparation! Okay, maybe not miss it exactly, but your life will be different now without that constant preparation.

Relax and await the results in confidence. You have done your best. That is always good enough!

Be proud of yourself; this was no small undertaking, and you did it.

> *You measure the size of the accomplishment by the obstacles you had to overcome to reach your goal.*
>
> *Booker T. Washington*

COMPUTERIZED CERTIFICATION EXAMINATIONS (CCS AND CCS-P) BEGIN IN 2005 FOR AHIMA

A testing service has been contracted by AHIMA to administer the CCS and CCS-P examinations in a computer-based format. The paper/pencil certification examination will no longer be available as both certification examinations will be administered exclusively in the computer-based format. The applications for the CCS and CCS-P submitted after January 1, 2005 will be for the computer-based format, and computer-based testing will be offered starting May 2005.

The new computer-based tests will be 4 hours long and contain:

- The CCS contains **60 multiple choice questions** to be completed in 1 hour in addition to **6 inpatient cases** (ICD-9-CM Volumes 1, 2, and 3) and **7 outpatient cases** (ICD-9-CM Volumes 1, 2, and CPT) to be completed in 3 hours.
- The CCS-P contains **60 multiple choice questions** to be completed in 1 hour in addition to **16 outpatient cases** (ICD-9-CM Volumes 1, 2, CPT, and HCPCS) to be completed in 3 hours.

Historically the tests were administered only twice a year, but with this new computer-based approach, there will be more opportunities throughout the year to take the tests. Application to take the examination is made in the same way to AHIMA. Visit the AHIMA web site (www.ahima.org/certification) for the latest information on this new computer-based testing.

Copyright © 2005, Elsevier Inc. All rights reserved.
CPT only © 2004. *Current Procedural Terminology, 2005, Professional Edition*, American Medical Association. All rights reserved.

The number of questions in this text reflects the configuration of the test prior to the January 2005 change. The competencies for the test remain the same, only the number of questions/cases and the length of time to complete the CCS and CCS-P examination have changed. So, your preparation for the test will need to be the same.

Copyright © 2005, Elsevier Inc. All rights reserved.
CPT only © 2004. *Current Procedural Terminology, 2005, Professional Edition,* American Medical Association. All rights reserved.

UNIT I

Anatomy, Terminology, and Pathophysiology

INTEGUMENTARY SYSTEM

The skin and accessory organs (nails, hair, and glands)

Layers (Figure 1-1)

Epidermis: outermost layer

Basal layer, deepest region of epidermis (stratum germinativum)

Stratum corneum is the outermost layer of epidermis

Dermis: middle layer, also known as corium, meaning true skin

Two layers of stratum

Subcutaneous Tissue or Hypodermis: innermost layer contains fat tissue

Nails

- Keratin plates covering the dorsal surface of each finger and toe
- Lunula—semilunar or half-moon, white area at base of nail plate
- Cuticle, narrow band of epidermis at base and sides of nail
- Paronychium, soft tissue around nail border

Glands

- Sebaceous glands located in dermal layer
  Secrete sebum, which lubricates skin and hair
- Sweat glands (sudoriferous) originate in dermis (subcutaneous tissue, see Fig. 1-1 below) and extend up through epidermis
  Openings are pores

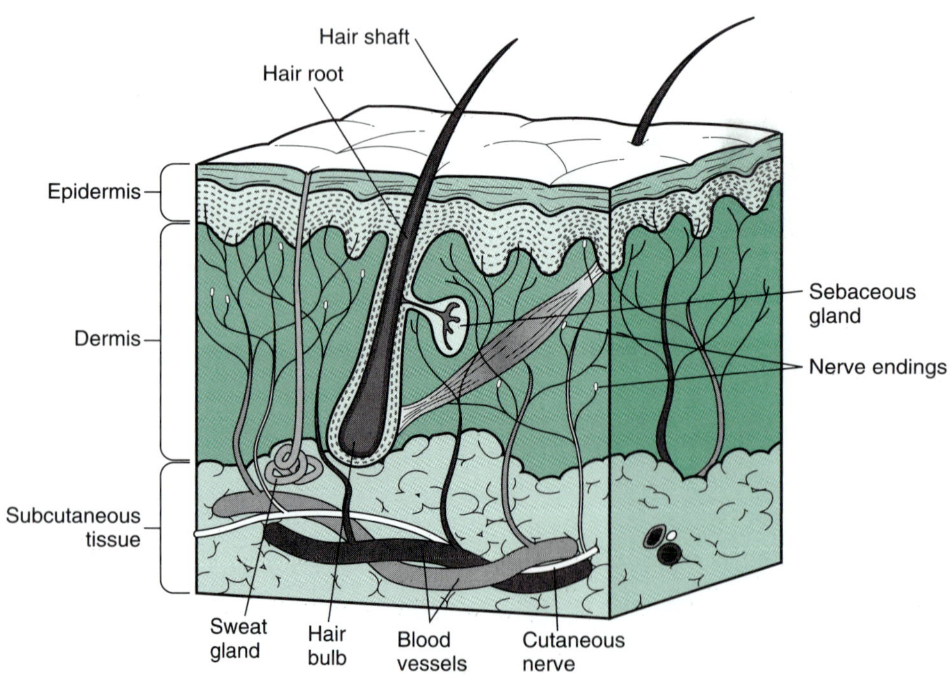

Figure 1-1 Integumentary system.

Copyright © 2005, Elsevier Inc. All rights reserved.
CPT only © 2004. *Current Procedural Terminology, 2005, Professional Edition,* American Medical Association. All rights reserved.

COMBINING FORMS

1. aden/o, adnen/o	in relationship to a gland
2. adip/o	fat
3. albin/o	white
4. aut/o	self
5. bi/o	life
6. cauter/o	burn
7. crypt/o	hidden
8. cutane/o	skin
9. cyan/o, cryan/o	blue
10. derm/o, dermat/o	skin
11. eosin/o	rosy
12. erythem/o	red
13. erythr/o	red
14. heter/o	different
15. hidr/o	sweat
16. ichthy/o	dry/scaly
17. jaund/o	yellow
18. kerat/o	hard
19. lip/o	fat
20. lute/o	yellow
21. melan/o	black
22. myc/o	fungus
23. necr/o	death
24. onych/o	nail
25. pachy/o	thick
26. pil/o	hair
27. poli/o	gray matter
28. rhytid/o	wrinkle
29. rube/o	red
30. seb/o	sebum/oil
31. staphyl/o	clusters
32. steat/o	fat
33. strept/o	twisted chain
34. trich/o	hair
35. ungu/o	nail

Copyright © 2005, Elsevier Inc. All rights reserved.
CPT only © 2004. *Current Procedural Terminology, 2005, Professional Edition*, American Medical Association. All rights reserved.

36. xanth/o	yellow
37. xer/o	dry

PREFIXES

1. epi-	on/upon
2. hyper-	over
3. hypo-	under
4. intra-	within
5. para-	beside
6. per-	through
7. peri-	surrounding
8. sub-	under

SUFFIXES

1. -coccus	spherical bacterium
2. -ectomy	removal
3. -ia	condition
4. -malacia	softening
5. -opsy	view of
6. -plasty	surgical repair
7. -rrhea	discharge
8. -tome	an instrument to cut
9. -tomy	to cut

MEDICAL ABBREVIATIONS

1. bx	biopsy
2. ca	cancer
3. derm	dermatology
4. I&D	incision and drainage
5. subcu, subq, SC, SQ	subcutaneous

MEDICAL TERMS

Absence	Without
Adipose	Fatty
Albinism	Lack of color pigment
Allograft	Homograft, same species graft
Alopecia	Condition in which hair falls out
Anhidrosis	Deficiency of sweat

Copyright © 2005, Elsevier Inc. All rights reserved.
CPT only © 2004. *Current Procedural Terminology, 2005, Professional Edition*, American Medical Association. All rights reserved.

Autograft	From patient's own body
Biopsy	Removal of a small piece of living tissue for diagnostic purposes
Causalgia	Burning pain
Collagen	Protein substance of skin
Debridement	Cleansing of or removal of dead tissue from a wound
Delayed flap	Pedicle of skin with blood supply that is separated from origin over time
Dermabrasion	Planing of the skin by means of sander, brush, or sandpaper
Dermatologist	Physician who treats conditions of the skin
Dermatoplasty	Surgical repair of skin
Electrocautery	Cauterization by means of heated instrument
Epidermolysis	Loosening of the epidermis
Epidermomycosis	Superficial fungal infection
Epithelium	Surface covering of internal and external organs of the body
Erythema	Redness of skin
Escharotomy	Surgical incision into necrotic (dead) tissue
Fissure	Cleft or groove
Free full-thickness graft	Graft of epidermis and dermis that is completely removed from donor area
Furuncle	Nodule in the skin caused by staphylococci entering through hair follicle
Homograft	Allograft, same species graft
Ichthyosis	Skin disorder characterized by scaling
Incise	To cut into
Island pedicle flap	Contains a single artery and vein that remains attached to origin temporarily or permanently
Leukoderma	Depigmentation of skin
Leukoplakia	White patch on mucous membrane
Lipocyte	Fat cell
Lipoma	Fatty tumor
Melanin	Dark pigment of skin
Melanoma	Tumor of epidermis, malignant and black in color
Mohs' surgery or Mohs' micrographic surgery	Removal of skin cancer in layers by a surgeon who also acts as a pathologist during surgery
Muscle flap	Transfer of muscle from origin to recipient site
Neurovascular flap	Contains artery, vein, and nerve
Pedicle	Tumor on a stem
Pilosebaceous	Pertains to hair follicles and sebaceous glands
Sebaceous gland	Secretes sebum
Seborrhea	Excess sebum secretion

Copyright © 2005, Elsevier Inc. All rights reserved.
CPT only © 2004. *Current Procedural Terminology, 2005, Professional Edition*, American Medical Association. All rights reserved.

Sebum	Oily substance
Split-thickness graft	All epidermis and some of dermis
Steatoma	Fat mass in sebaceous gland
Stratified	Layered
Stratum (strata)	Layer
Subungual	Beneath the nail
Xanthoma	Tumor composed of cells containing lipid material, yellow in color
Xenograft	Different species graft
Xeroderma	Dry, discolored, scaly skin

Copyright © 2005, Elsevier Inc. All rights reserved.
CPT only © 2004. *Current Procedural Terminology, 2005, Professional Edition,* American Medical Association. All rights reserved.

INTEGUMENTARY SYSTEM QUIZ

1. This is the outermost layer of the skin:
   a. basal
   b. dermis
   c. epidermis
   d. subcutaneous

2. Which of the following is NOT a part of the skin or accessory organs:
   a. hair
   b. sebaceous gland
   c. nail
   d. haversian

3. This prefix means beside:
   a. para-
   b. intra-
   c. per-
   d. epi-

4. This combining form means hair:
   a. xanth/o
   b. trich/o
   c. ichthy/o
   d. kerat/o

5. The lunula is the:
   a. narrow band of epidermis at the base of the nail
   b. opening of the pores
   c. outermost layer of epidermis
   d. white area at the base of the nail plate

6. The subcutaneous tissue is also known as:
   a. dermal
   b. adipose
   c. hypodermis
   d. stratum corneum

7. Which of the follow combining forms does not refer to a color:
   a. cyan/o
   b. jaund/o
   c. eosin/o
   d. pachy/o

8. This medical term means the surgical incision into dead tissue:
   a. onychomycosis
   b. escharotomy
   c. keratotomy
   d. curettage

Copyright © 2005, Elsevier Inc. All rights reserved.
CPT only © 2004. *Current Procedural Terminology, 2005, Professional Edition*, American Medical Association. All rights reserved.

9. This suffix means surgical repair:
   a. -opsy
   b. -rrhea
   c. -plasty
   d. -tome

10. The soft tissue around the nail border is the:
    a. cuticle
    b. lunula
    c. paronychium
    d. corium

A 261

Copyright © 2005, Elsevier Inc. All rights reserved.
CPT only © 2004. *Current Procedural Terminology, 2005, Professional Edition*, American Medical Association. All rights reserved.

INTEGUMENTARY SYSTEM—PATHOPHYSIOLOGY

Lesions and Other Abnormalities (Figure 1-2)

Macule

- Flat area of color change
- No elevation or depression

Example: flat moles (nevi), measles, freckles

Papule

- Solid elevation
- Less than 0.5 cm in diameter

Example: warts, lichen planus, elevated mole

Nodule

- Solid elevation 0.5 to 1 cm in diameter
- Extends deeper into dermis than papule

Example: lipoma

Pustule

- Elevated area
- Filled with purulent fluid

Example: pimple

Tumor

- Solid mass
- Larger than 1 cm

Example: hemangioma, neoplasm

Plaque

- Flat, elevated surface
- Equal or greater than 1.0 cm

Example: psoriasis, seborrheic keratoses

Wheal

- Type of plaque
- Results in transient edema in dermis

Example: insect bite, allergic reaction

Vesicle

- Small blister
- Fluid within or under epidermis

Example: herpes zoster (shingles), varicella (chickenpox)

Copyright © 2005, Elsevier Inc. All rights reserved.
CPT only © 2004. *Current Procedural Terminology, 2005, Professional Edition*, American Medical Association. All rights reserved.

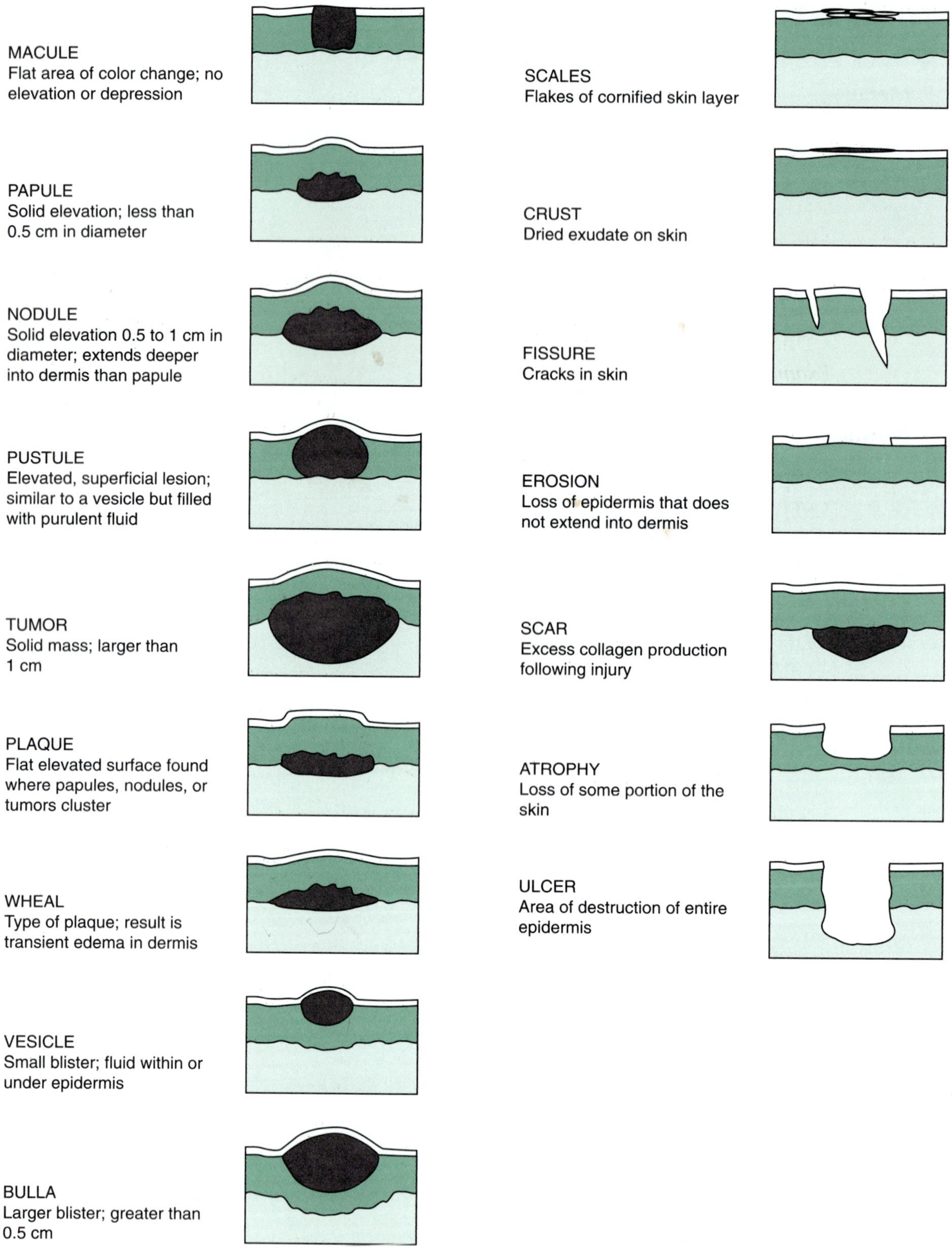

Figure 1-2 Lesions of the skin.

Copyright © 2005, Elsevier Inc. All rights reserved.
CPT only © 2004. *Current Procedural Terminology, 2005, Professional Edition*, American Medical Association. All rights reserved.

Bulla

- Large blister
- Greater than 0.5 cm

Example: blister

Scales

- Flakes of cornified skin layer

Example: dry skin

Crust

- Dried exudate on skin

Example: scab

Fissure

- Cracks in skin

Example: athlete's foot

Erosion

- Loss of epidermis
- Does not extend into the dermis

Example: varicella

Scar

- Excess collagen production following surgery or trauma

Example: healed surgical wound

Atrophy

- Loss of some portion of skin

Example: aged skin

- Not a lesion

Ulcer

- Area of destruction of entire epidermis

Example: ulcer on heel

Pressure Ulcer (Figure 1-3)

Result of pressure or force

- Occludes blood flow, causing ischemia
- Develops over bony prominence

Locations

- Coccygeal (end of spine, heel, or elbow)
- Sacral (between hips)

Copyright © 2005, Elsevier Inc. All rights reserved.
CPT only © 2004. *Current Procedural Terminology, 2005, Professional Edition*, American Medical Association. All rights reserved.

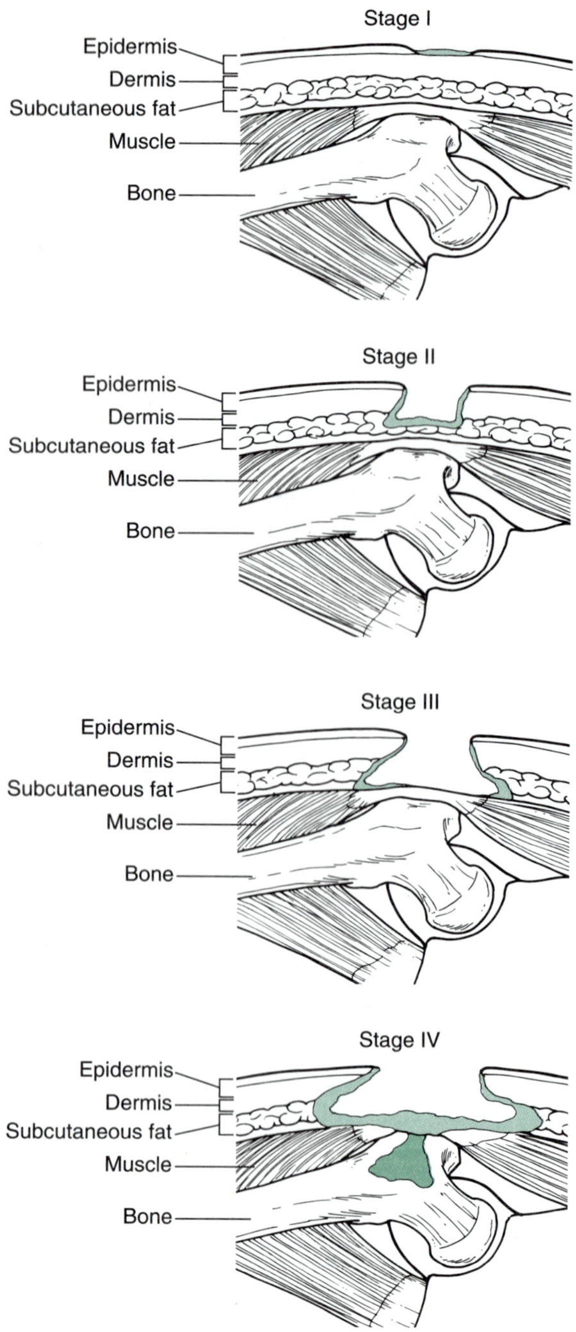

Figure 1-3 Stage I, II, III, and IV of pressure ulcers.

- Ischial (lower hip)
- Trochanteric (outer hip)

Staging or classification system

- Stage I: erythema of skin
- Stage II: partial loss of skin (epidermis or dermis)
- Stage III: full thickness loss of skin (up to but not through fascia)
- Stage IV: full thickness loss (extensive destruction and necrosis)

Deep ulcers may require surgical debridement

Copyright © 2005, Elsevier Inc. All rights reserved.
CPT only © 2004. *Current Procedural Terminology, 2005, Professional Edition*, American Medical Association. All rights reserved.

Keloids

- Sharply elevated, irregularly shaped scars that progressively enlarge
- Due to excessive collagen in corneum
- Result of tissue repair or trauma
- Familial tendency for formation

Inflammatory Disorders

Atopic dermatitis

Often caused by food allergy

Exogenous (external cause) includes:

- Irritant dermatitis
- Allergic contact dermatitis

Endogenous (internal cause) includes:

- Seborrheic dermatitis

Results in activation of

- Mast cells
- Eosinophils
- T lymphocytes
- Monocytes

Greater in those with family history of

- Asthma
- Dry skin
- Eczema
- Allergic rhinitis

Common in children and infants

Results in

- Chronic inflammation
- Scratching
- Erythema
- Thickened leathery skin (lichenification)
- Secondary *Staphylococcus aureus* infection

Treatment

- Topical steroid
- Antibiotic for secondary infection
- Antihistamines

Copyright © 2005, Elsevier Inc. All rights reserved.
CPT only © 2004. *Current Procedural Terminology, 2005, Professional Edition*, American Medical Association. All rights reserved.

Allergic contact dermatitis

Most common in infants and children

Hypersensitivity to sensitizing antigens

- Microorganisms
- Drugs
- Foreign proteins
- Chemicals
- Latex
- Metals
- Plants

Manifestations

- Scaling
- Lichenification (leathery, thickened skin)
- Erythema
- Itching (pruritus)
- Vesicular lesions
- Edema

Diagnosis and treatment

- Check medical history
- Patch test
- Avoidance of irritant
- Skin lubrication and hydration
- Steroids
    - Topical
    - Systemic
- Topical tacrolimus

Irritant contact dermatitis

Response to

- Chemical
- Exposure to irritant

Treatment

- Removal of irritant
- Topical agents

Stasis dermatitis

- Usually on the legs

Copyright © 2005, Elsevier Inc. All rights reserved.
CPT only © 2004. *Current Procedural Terminology, 2005, Professional Edition*, American Medical Association. All rights reserved.

Associated with

- Phlebitis
- Vascular trauma
- Varicosities

Progress

- Begins with erythema and pruritus
- Progresses to scaling, hyperpigmentation, petechia (small hemorrhagic areas)
- Lesion becomes ulcerated

Treatment

- Elevate legs
- Reduce standing
- No constricting clothes
- External compression
- Antibiotics for acute lesions
- Silver nitrate or Burow's solution for chronic lesions

Seborrheic dermatitis

Common chronic inflammation of the sebaceous glands

Periods of remission and exacerbation

Often of:

- Scalp (cradle cap in infants)
- Ears
- Eyelids
- Eyebrow
- Nose
- Axillae
- Chest
- Groin

Lesions are:

- Scaly (dry or greasy)
- White or yellowish
- Mildly pruritic

Treatment

- Mild cases
    - Soap/shampoo of
        - Coal tar
        - Sulfur
        - Salicylic acid
- More severe cases
    - Corticosteroid

Copyright © 2005, Elsevier Inc. All rights reserved.
CPT only © 2004. *Current Procedural Terminology, 2005, Professional Edition*, American Medical Association. All rights reserved.

Papulosquamous disorders

Conditions associated with

- Scales
- Papules
- Plaque
- Erythema

Three types

- Psoriasis
- Pityriasis
- Lichen planus

Psoriasis

Chronic, relapsing, proliferating disorder

Usually begins by age 20

Cause unknown, suggested to be:

- Genetic
- Immunologic
- Biochemical alterations
- Triggering agent

Commonly occurs on

- Face
- Scalp
- Elbows
- Knees

Results in

- Thickened dermis and epidermis
- Well-demarcated plaque
- Cell hyperproliferation
- Inflammation (pruritus)

Treatment

Only palliative (treatment of symptoms)

Mild cases

- Keratolytic agents
- Corticosteroids
- Emollients

Moderate cases

- Interleukin-2 inhibitors
- Ultraviolet light

Copyright © 2005, Elsevier Inc. All rights reserved.
CPT only © 2004. *Current Procedural Terminology, 2005, Professional Edition*, American Medical Association. All rights reserved.

- Coal tar
- Cyclosporin
- Vitamin D analogs

Severe cases

- Topical agents
- Corticosteroids
- Antimetabolic
- Hospitalization

Pityriasis rosea (p. Rosea)

Unknown cause

Self-limiting inflammatory disorder

Type of pityriasis

Occurs most often in young adults

Primary lesions

- Begin with herald patch
- 3 to 4 cm
- Salmon-pink colored
- Circular
- Well-defined lesions

Secondary lesions

- 14 to 21 days
- Trunk and upper extremities
- Oval lesions
- Severe itching

Diagnosis

May be confused with:

- Secondary syphilis
- Seborrheic dermatitis
- Psoriasis

Treatment

- Antihistamines
- Corticosteroids
- Ultraviolet light
- Sunlight

Lichen planus

Occurs on skin and mucous membranes

Unknown cause (idiopathic)

Copyright © 2005, Elsevier Inc. All rights reserved.
CPT only © 2004. *Current Procedural Terminology, 2005, Professional Edition*, American Medical Association. All rights reserved.

Autoimmune inflammatory disorder

Onset ages 30 to 70

Lesions

- Begin as pink lesions that turn into violet-colored pruritic papules
- Results in hyperpigmentation
- 2- to 10-mm flat lesions with central depression
- Last 12 to 18 months
- Tend to reoccur

Treatment

- Antihistamines
- Corticosteroids
    - Topical
    - Systemic

Acne vulgaris

Site of lesion is sebaceous (pilosebaceous) follicles

Primarily on face and upper trunk

Usually occur in patients between the ages of 12 and 25

Types

Noninflammatory acne
- Whiteheads
- Blackheads

Inflammatory acne
- Follicle walls rupture
- Sebum expels into dermis
- Inflammation begins

Cause is unknown

Treatment

- Topical
    - Antibiotics
    - Benzoyl peroxide
    - Tretinoin
- Systemic
    - Antibiotic
    - Hormones
    - Corticosteroids
    - Isotretinoin

Copyright © 2005, Elsevier Inc. All rights reserved.
CPT only © 2004. *Current Procedural Terminology, 2005, Professional Edition*, American Medical Association. All rights reserved.

Diaper dermatitis

- Variety of disorders

Results of:

- Urine
- Feces
- Plastic diaper cover
- Allergic reaction
- Secondary *Candida albicans* infection

Treatment

- Clean, dry area
- Expose to air
- Topical antifungal medications
- Topical steroids

Pruritus (itching)

- Symptom of skin disorder
- Can be localized or generalized

Causes

- Primary skin disorder
  Example: eczema or lice
- System disease
  Example: chronic renal failure
- Opiates

Treatment is for underlying condition

- Antihistamines
- Minor tranquilizers
- Application of emollients (lotions)
- Topical steroids

Skin Infections

Bacterial

Impetigo

Most common in infants and children

Usually on face and begins as small vesicles

Caused by primarily by Staphylococcus

Sometimes by group A beta-hemolytic *Streptococcus*

Copyright © 2005, Elsevier Inc. All rights reserved.
CPT only © 2004. *Current Procedural Terminology, 2005, Professional Edition,* American Medical Association. All rights reserved.

Treatment in mild cases

- Topical antibiotics
- Topical antiseptics

Treatment in moderate cases

- Systemic antibiotics
- Local compresses
- Analgesics

Cellulitis

Caused primarily by staphylococcus

Often secondary to an injury

Results in

- Erythema, usually of lower trunk and legs
- Fever
- Localized pain
- Lymphangitis

Treatment

- Systemic antibiotics
- Burow soaks for pain relief

Furuncles (boils)

Infected hair follicle

Usually caused by Staphylococcus

Developed boils drains pus and necrotic tissue

Squeezing spreads infection

Collection of furuncles that have merged is a carbuncle

Folliculitis

- Infection of hair follicles

Results in

- Erythema
- Pustules

Caused by

- Skin trauma, such as irritation or friction
- Poor hygiene
- Excessive skin moisture

Copyright © 2005, Elsevier Inc. All rights reserved.
CPT only © 2004. *Current Procedural Terminology, 2005, Professional Edition,* American Medical Association. All rights reserved.

Treatment

- Cleansing of area
- Topical antibiotics

Acute necrotizing fasciitis

Flesh-eating disease

- Virulent strain of gram-positive, group A beta-hemolytic streptococcus
- Mortality rate of over 40%

Caused by

- Skin trauma
- Skin infection

Areas secrete tissue-destroying enzyme, proteases

- Extreme inflammation and pain
- Rapidly increasing
- Dermal gangrene develops

Systemic toxicity may develop with

- Fever
- Disorientation
- Hypotension
- Tachycardia
- May lead to organ failure

Treatment

- Antimicrobial therapy
- Fluid replacement
- Removal of areas of infection

Viral

Herpes simplex (cold sores)

Caused by

- Herpes simplex virus type 1 (HSV-1)
  - Most common type
  - Results in fever blisters or cold sores on or near lips
- Herpes simplex virus type 2 (HSV-2)
  - Genital and oral type
  - Prominent sexually transmitted disease

Primary infections may show no symptoms (asymptomatic)

Virus remains in nerve tissue to later reactivate

Copyright © 2005, Elsevier Inc. All rights reserved.
CPT only © 2004. *Current Procedural Terminology, 2005, Professional Edition*, American Medical Association. All rights reserved.

Reactivation may be triggered by:

- Stress
- Common cold
- Exposure to sun

Presents with burning or tingling

Develops painful vesicles that rupture

- Causes spreading
- May cause secondary infection of the eye
    - Episode lasts several weeks
    - Treatment may include antiviral medication
        - No permanent cure exists

Herpes zoster (shingles)

Usually older adult

Caused by varicella-zoster virus (VZV)

- Virus was dormant and then reactivates
- Result of varicella or chickenpox, usually in childhood

Affects one cranial nerve or one dermatome (an area of skin served by one nerve or one side of the body)

Results in:

- Pain
- Rash (unilateral)
- Paresthesia (abnormal touch sensation, such as burning)

Course

- Several weeks
- Pain may continue even after lesion disappears

Treatment

- Clears spontaneously
- Antiviral medications provide symptomatic relief
- Sedatives
- Analgesic
- Antipruritics

Warts (verrucae)

Caused by human papillomavirus (HPV)

Numerous types of HPV

Spread by contact

Copyright © 2005, Elsevier Inc. All rights reserved.
CPT only © 2004. *Current Procedural Terminology, 2005, Professional Edition,* American Medical Association. All rights reserved.

Appear anywhere on body

Present with a grayish appearance

Variety of shapes and sizes

Plantar warts are located on pressure points of the body (such as feet; plantar means the bottom surface of the foot)

Painful when pressure is applied

Treatment

- Liquid nitrogen
- Topical keratolytics
- Laser
- Often persist even with treatment

Fungal (mycoses)

Usually superficial

Fungus lives off dead cells

Tinea

Superficial skin infections

Tinea capitis
- Infection of scalp
- Common in children
- Treatment with oral antifungal medication

Tinea corporis (ringworm)
- Infection of the body
- Presents as a red ring
- Produces burning sensation and pruritus
- Treatment with topical antifungal medication

Tinea pedis (athlete's foot)
- Involves feet and toes
- Produces pain, inflammation, fissures, and foul odor
- Treatment with topical antifungal medication

Tinea unguium (onychomycosis)
- Nail infection
  - Usually toenails
- Nail turns white then brown, thickens and cracks
- Spreads to other nails

Candidiasis

- Caused by *Candida albicans*
- Normally on mucous membranes of the gastrointestinal tract and vagina

Copyright © 2005, Elsevier Inc. All rights reserved.
CPT only © 2004. *Current Procedural Terminology, 2005, Professional Edition*, American Medical Association. All rights reserved.

- Poor health and certain conditions predispose individuals to overarching infection by candidiasis
  - Such as antibiotic therapy, which changes the balance of the normal flora in the body
- Treatment is topical or oral antifungal medications

Tumors of the Skin

Benign Tumors

Keratoses

Seborrheic keratoses

- Proliferation of basal cells
- Dark colored lesion
- Found on trunk and face

Actinic keratoses

- Pigmented, scaly patch
- Often caused by exposure to sun
- Often in fair-skinned individuals
- May develop into squamous cell carcinoma
- Treatment with cryosurgery (freezing area) or excision

Keratoacanthoma

- Occurs in hair follicles
- Usually in those over 60
- Often of face, neck, back of hands, and other locations exposed to the sun
- Resolve spontaneously or are excised

Moles (nevi)

- Located on any body part
- Various shapes and sizes
- May become malignant
  - Especially if located in area of continual irritation

Malignant Tumors

Squamous cell carcinoma

Similar to basal cell carcinoma

Most often appears in areas exposed to the sun

Rarely metastatic (spreading)

Easily treated with good prognosis

Basal cell carcinoma

Common type of skin cancer

Developed in deeper skin layers (basal cells) than squamous cell carcinoma

Copyright © 2005, Elsevier Inc. All rights reserved.
CPT only © 2004. *Current Procedural Terminology, 2005, Professional Edition*, American Medical Association. All rights reserved.

Often occurs with sun exposure in fair-skinned individuals

Easily treated with good prognosis

Malignant melanoma

Originates in cells that produce pigment (melanocytes) or a mole

Increased incident with

- Sun exposure
- Genetic predisposition

Often multicolored with irregular borders

Grow downward into tissues

Metastasize quickly

Treatment is removal with extensive border excision

Depending on extent, chemotherapy or radiation therapy may be used

Kaposi's sarcoma

Rare form of skin cancer

Associated with

- Human immunodeficiency virus (HIV)
- Acquired immunodeficiency syndrome (AIDS)

Herpes virus may be found in lesions

Cells originate from the endothelium in small blood vessels

Painful lesions develop rapidly, appearing as purple macules

Radiation and chemotherapy are common treatments

Copyright © 2005, Elsevier Inc. All rights reserved.
CPT only © 2004. *Current Procedural Terminology, 2005, Professional Edition*, American Medical Association. All rights reserved.

INTEGUMENTARY SYSTEM PATHOPHYSIOLOGY QUIZ

1. A pimple is an example of a:
   a. papule
   b. vesicle
   c. pustule
   d. nodule

2. A Stage III pressure ulcer involves:
   a. erythema of skin
   b. partial loss of epidermis and dermis
   c. full thickness loss of skin up to but not through fascia
   d. full thickness loss of skin with extensive destruction and necrosis

3. This type of dermatitis is often caused by food allergies and is common in children and infants.
   a. atopic
   b. irritant contact
   c. stasis
   d. seborrheic

4. Psoriasis, pityriasis, and lichen planus are three types of this disorder.
   a. dermatitis
   b. inflammatory
   c. acne
   d. papulosquamous

5. This condition begins with a herald spot.
   a. psoriasis
   b. pityriasis
   c. lichen planus
   d. dermatitis

6. This skin infection is caused by group A beta hemolytic streptococci, and the lesions appear as firm red spots with itching, burning, and tenderness.
   a. furuncles
   b. folliculitis
   c. erysipelas
   d. fasciitis

7. This type of herpes produces cold sores.
   a. herpes zoster
   b. shingles
   c. VZV
   d. herpes simplex

8. This condition is caused by the human papillomavirus.
   a. mycoses
   b. verrucae
   c. shingles
   d. folliculitis

Copyright © 2005, Elsevier Inc. All rights reserved.
CPT only © 2004. *Current Procedural Terminology, 2005, Professional Edition,* American Medical Association. All rights reserved.

9. This type of tumor occurs in the hair follicles.
   a. keratoses
   b. nevi
   c. Kaposi's
   d. keratoacanthoma

10. This type of superficial carcinoma is rarely metastatic.
    a. squamous cell
    b. basal cell
    c. melanoma
    d. Kaposi's sarcoma

Copyright © 2005, Elsevier Inc. All rights reserved.
CPT only © 2004. *Current Procedural Terminology, 2005, Professional Edition*, American Medical Association. All rights reserved.

MUSCULOSKELETAL SYSTEM

Skeletal System

- Comprises 206 bones, cartilage, and ligaments
- Provides organ protection, movement, framework, stores calcium, hematopoiesis (formation of blood cells)

Classification of Bones

Long bones (tubular)

- Length exceeds width of bone
- Broad at ends, such as the thigh, lower leg, upper arm, and lower arm

Short bones (cuboidal)

- Larger ends on short bones, such as the wrist and ankle

Flat

- Thin
- Cover body parts, such as the skull

Irregular

- Varied shapes, such as zygoma of face or vertebrae

Sesamoid

- Rounded
- Found near joint, such as the kneecap

Structure

Long Bones (Figure 1-4)

Diaphysis: shaft
Epiphysis: ends
- Articular cartilage covers epiphyses and serves as a cushion

Epiphyseal line or plate: growth plate that disappears when fully grown
Metaphysis: flared portion of bone near epiphyseal plate
Periosteum: outer covering
Cortical or compact bone: hard bone beneath periosteum mainly found in shaft
- Medullary cavity contains yellow marrow (fatty bone marrow)

Cancellous bones: spongy or trabecular
- Contains red bone marrow (blood cell development)

Two Skeletal Divisions

Axial (trunk)

Appendicular (appendages)

Axial Skeleton, 80

Skull (Figure 1-5)

Cranial

- Frontal (forehead)
- Parietal (sides and top)

Copyright © 2005, Elsevier Inc. All rights reserved.
CPT only © 2004. *Current Procedural Terminology, 2005, Professional Edition*, American Medical Association. All rights reserved.

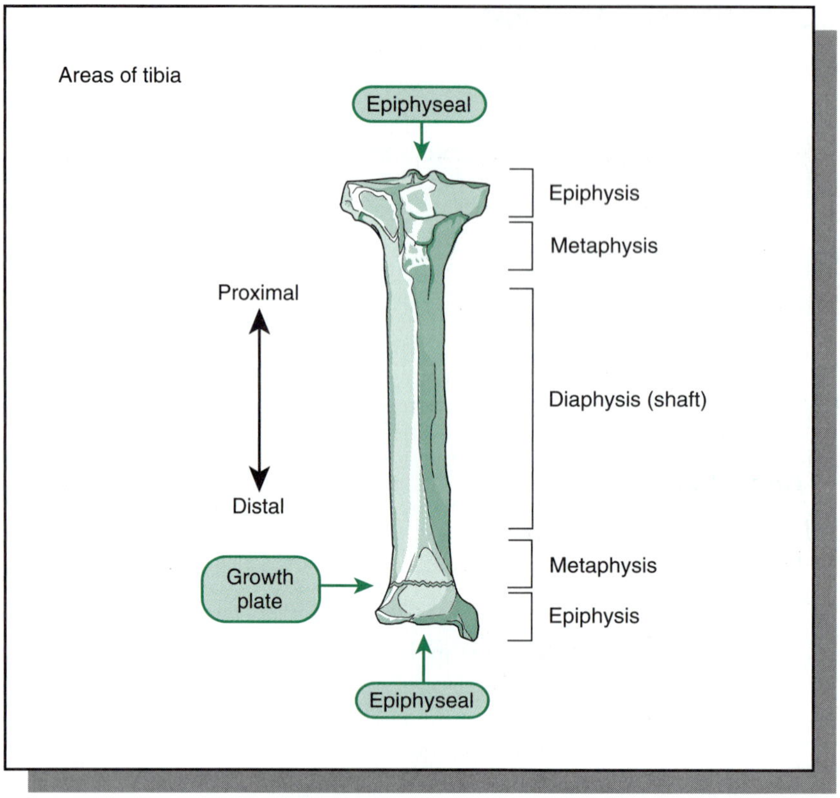

Figure 1-4 Structure of bones.

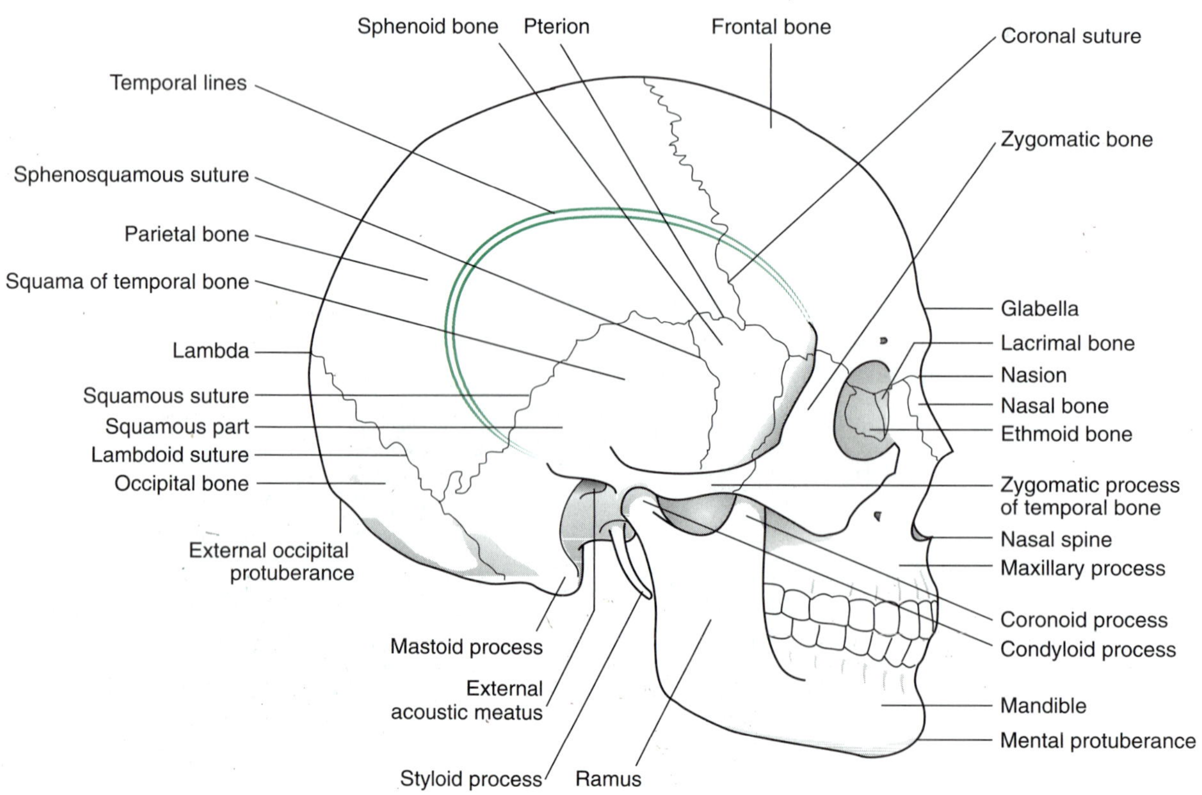

Figure 1-5 Lateral view of the skull.

Copyright © 2005, Elsevier Inc. All rights reserved.
CPT only © 2004. *Current Procedural Terminology, 2005, Professional Edition,* American Medical Association. All rights reserved.

- Temporal (lower sides)
- Occipital (posterior of cranium)
- Sphenoid (floor of cranium)
- Ethmoid (area between orbits and nasal cavity)
- Styloid process (below ear)
- Zygomatic process (cheek)

Ear bones (Figure 1-6)

- Malleus
- Incus
- Stapes

Face (Figure 1-7)

- Nasal (bridge of nose)
- Maxilla (upper jaw)
- Zygomatic (arch of cheekbone)
- Mandible (lower jawbone)
- Lacrimal (near orbits)
- Palate (separates oral and nasal cavities)
- Vomer (base, nasal septum)

Hyoid

- Supports tongue
- U shaped
- Attached by ligaments and muscles to larynx and skull

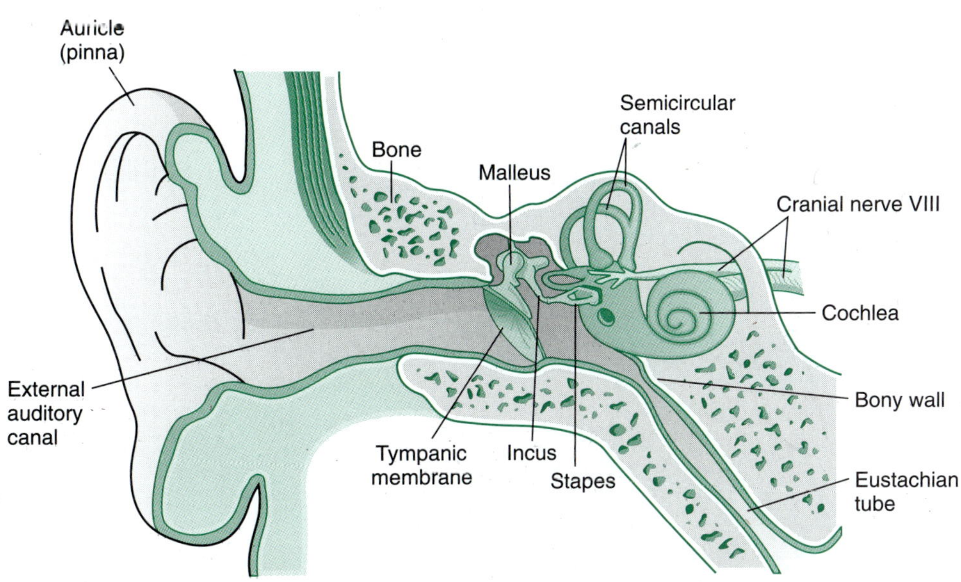

Figure 1-6 Structure of the ear and three divisions of external, middle, and inner ear.

Copyright © 2005, Elsevier Inc. All rights reserved.
CPT only © 2004. *Current Procedural Terminology, 2005, Professional Edition,* American Medical Association. All rights reserved.

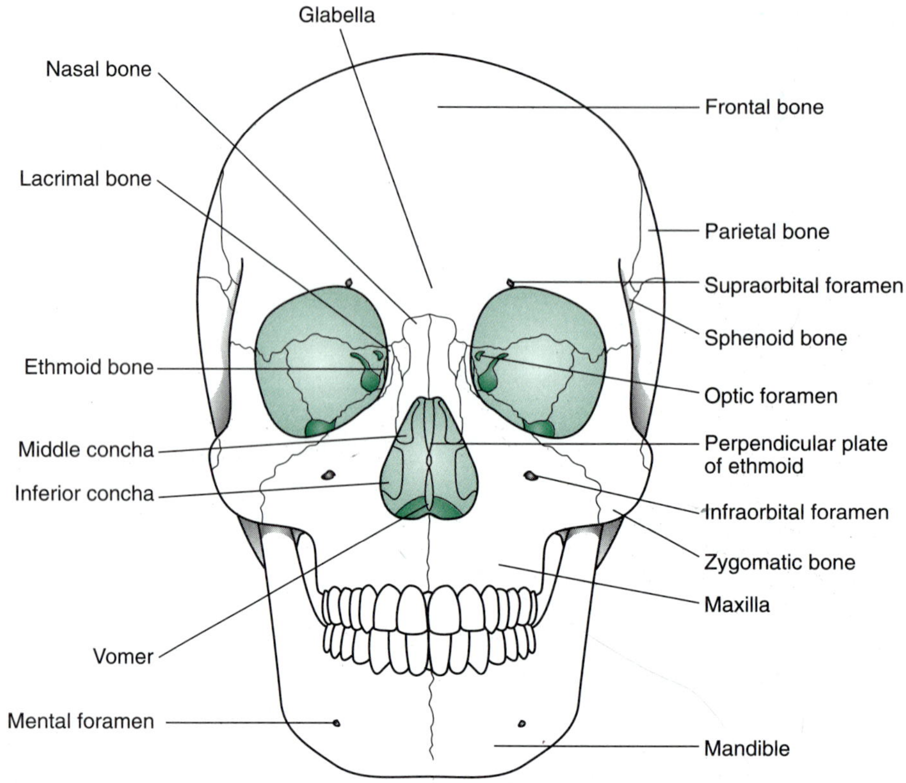

Figure 1-7 Frontal view of the skull.

Spine (Figure 1-8)

- Cervical vertebrae
  - C1-7
  - First atlas (C1)
  - Second axis (C2)
- Thoracic vertebrae (T1-12)
- Lumbar vertebrae (L1-5)
- Sacrum
- Coccyx

Thorax (Figure 1-9)

- Ribs, 12 pairs
  - True ribs, 1-7
  - False ribs, 8-10
  - Floating ribs, 11 and 12
- Sternum

Copyright © 2005, Elsevier Inc. All rights reserved.
CPT only © 2004. *Current Procedural Terminology, 2005, Professional Edition,* American Medical Association. All rights reserved.

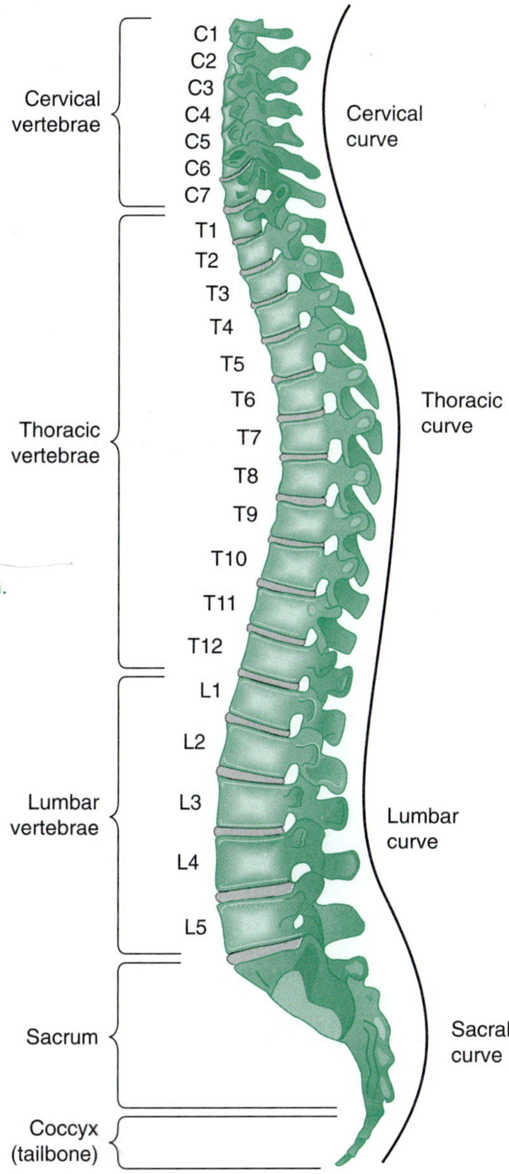

Figure 1-8 Anterior view of the vertebral column.

Appendicular Skeleton, 126 (Figure 1-10)

Lower extremities

Pelvis

Ilium (uppermost part) wing shaped

- Acetabulum, depression on lateral hip surface into which head of femur fits

Ischium (posterior part)

Pubis (anterior part)

Pubis symphysis (cartilage between pubic bones)

Femur (thighbone)

Trochanter (processes at neck of femur)

Head fits into the acetabulum

Copyright © 2005, Elsevier Inc. All rights reserved.
CPT only © 2004. *Current Procedural Terminology, 2005, Professional Edition,* American Medical Association. All rights reserved.

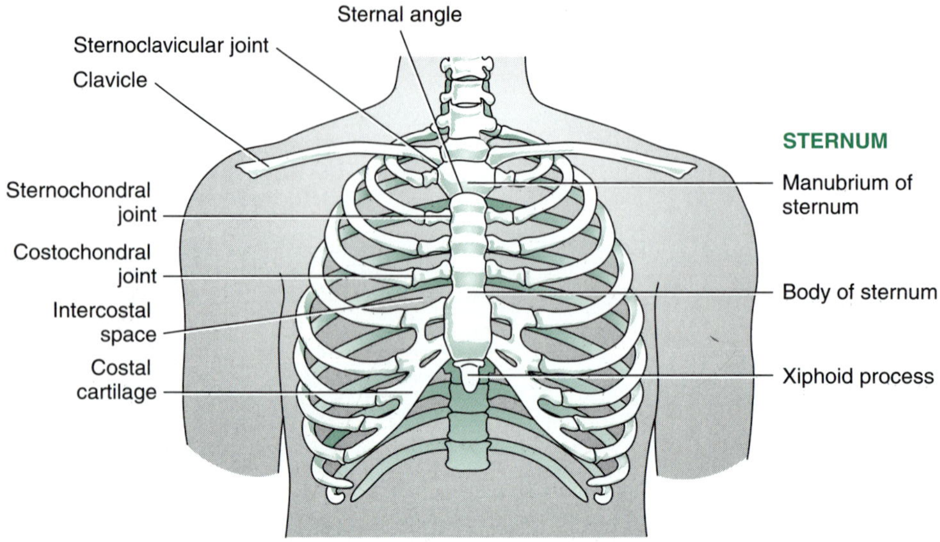

Figure 1-9 The thoracic cage.

Patella (kneecap)

Tibia (shinbone)

Fibula (smaller bone in lower leg)

Tarsus (ankle bone)

Calcaneus (heel bone)

Metatarsal (foot instep)

Phalanges (toes)

Lateral malleolus (lower part of fibula)

Medial malleolus (lower part of tibia)

Upper extremities

Clavicle (collarbone)

Scapula (shoulder blade)

Humerus (upper arm)

Radius (forearm, thumb side)

Ulna (forearm, little finger side)

Carpals (wrist)

Metacarpals (hand)

Phalanges (finger)

Olecranon (tip of elbow)

Joints (Articulations/Reticulations)

Condyle, rounded end of bone

Classified by degree of movement

Synarthrosis (immovable)

Example: joint between cranial bones

Copyright © 2005, Elsevier Inc. All rights reserved.
CPT only © 2004. *Current Procedural Terminology, 2005, Professional Edition*, American Medical Association. All rights reserved.

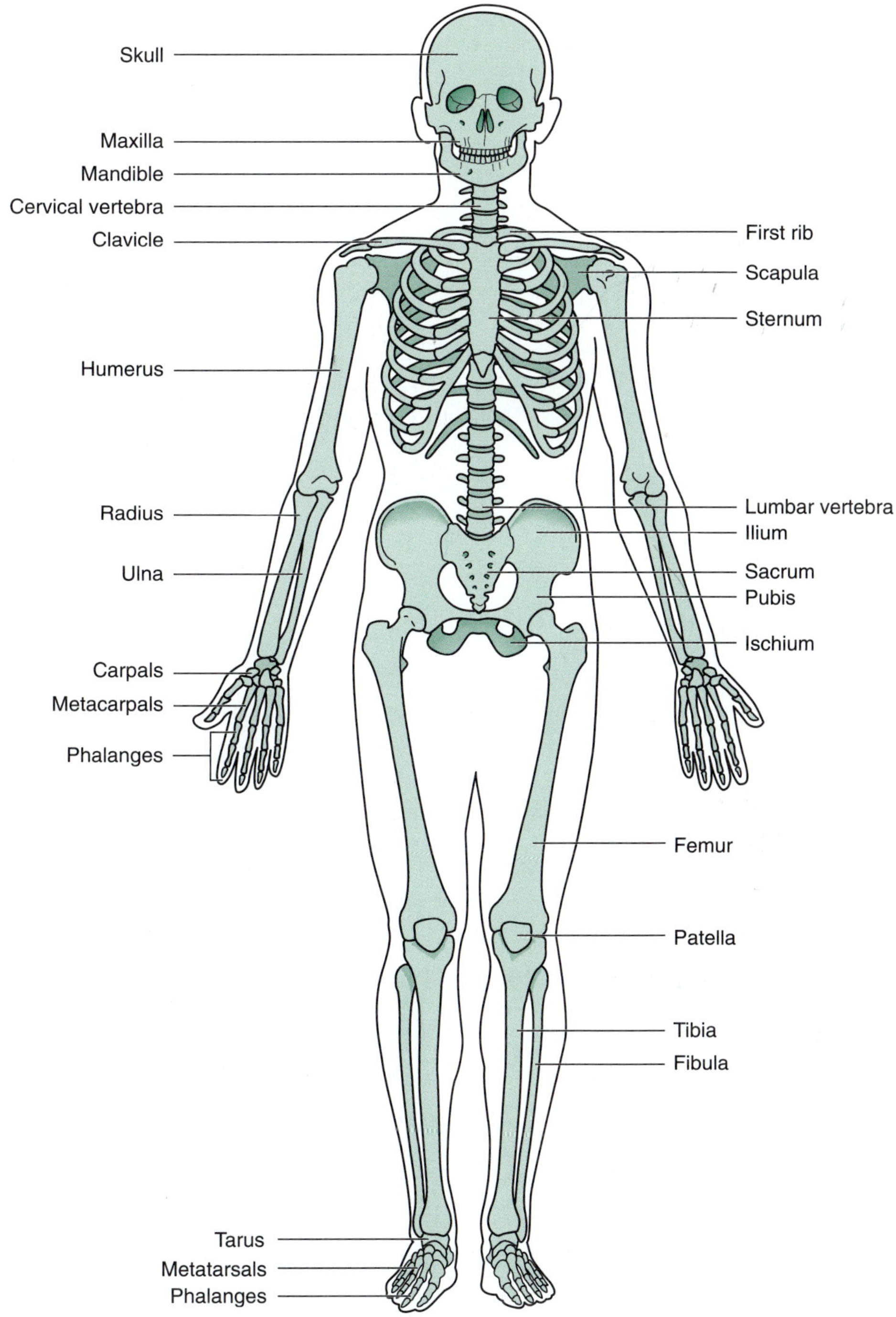

Figure 1-10 Skeletal system.

Amphiarthrosis (slightly movable)

Example: intervertebral (joint between bodies of the vertebra)

Diarthrosis (considerably movable)

Types, hinge or ball and socket

Example: elbow

Bursa, sac of synovial fluid located near joints

Copyright © 2005, Elsevier Inc. All rights reserved.
CPT only © 2004. *Current Procedural Terminology, 2005, Professional Edition*, American Medical Association. All rights reserved.

Muscular System

Functions

- Heat production
- Movement
- Posture
- Protection
- Shape

Muscle Tissue Types

Skeletal

Striated (cross stripes) (Figures 1-11 and 1-12)

Move body

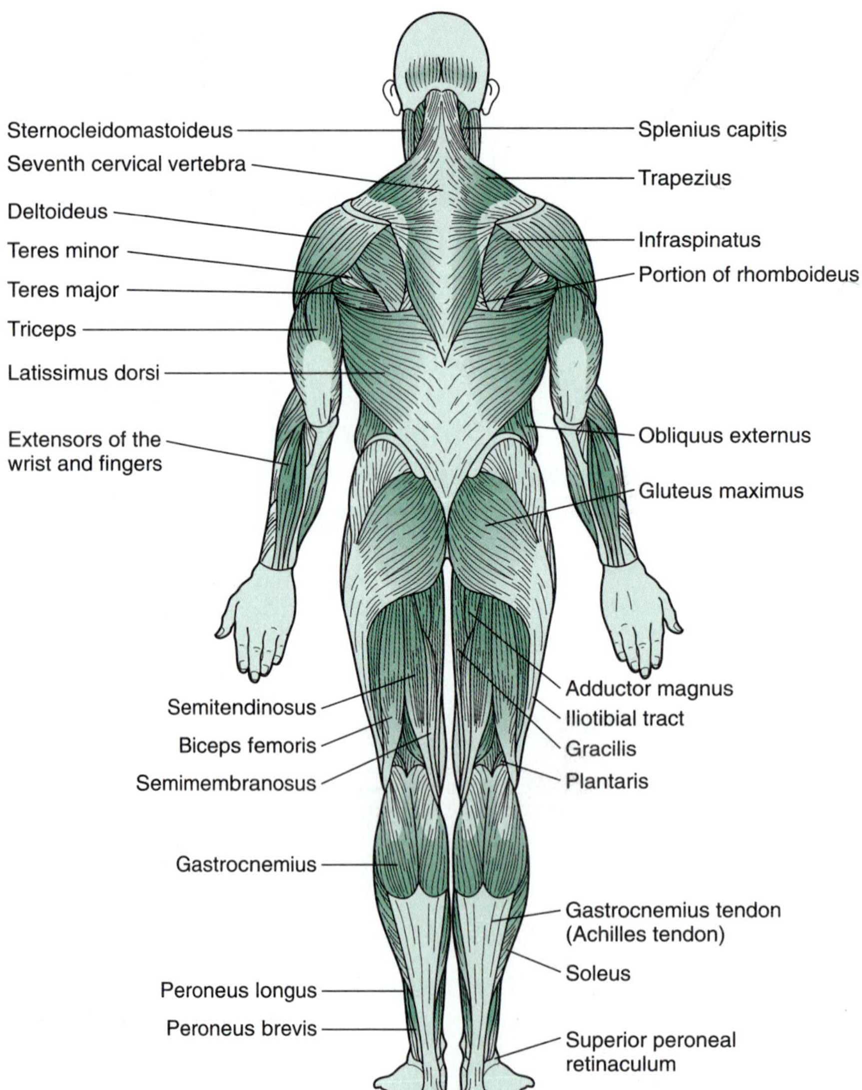

Figure 1-11 Muscular system, posterior view.

Copyright © 2005, Elsevier Inc. All rights reserved.
CPT only © 2004. *Current Procedural Terminology, 2005, Professional Edition,* American Medical Association. All rights reserved.

Voluntary

Attaches to bones

- Most attach to two bones with a joint in between
- Origin, point where muscle attaches to stationary bone
- Insertion, where muscle attaches to movable bone
- Body of muscle, main part of muscle

Cardiac/Heart Muscle

Striated

Involuntary

Moves blood by means of contractions

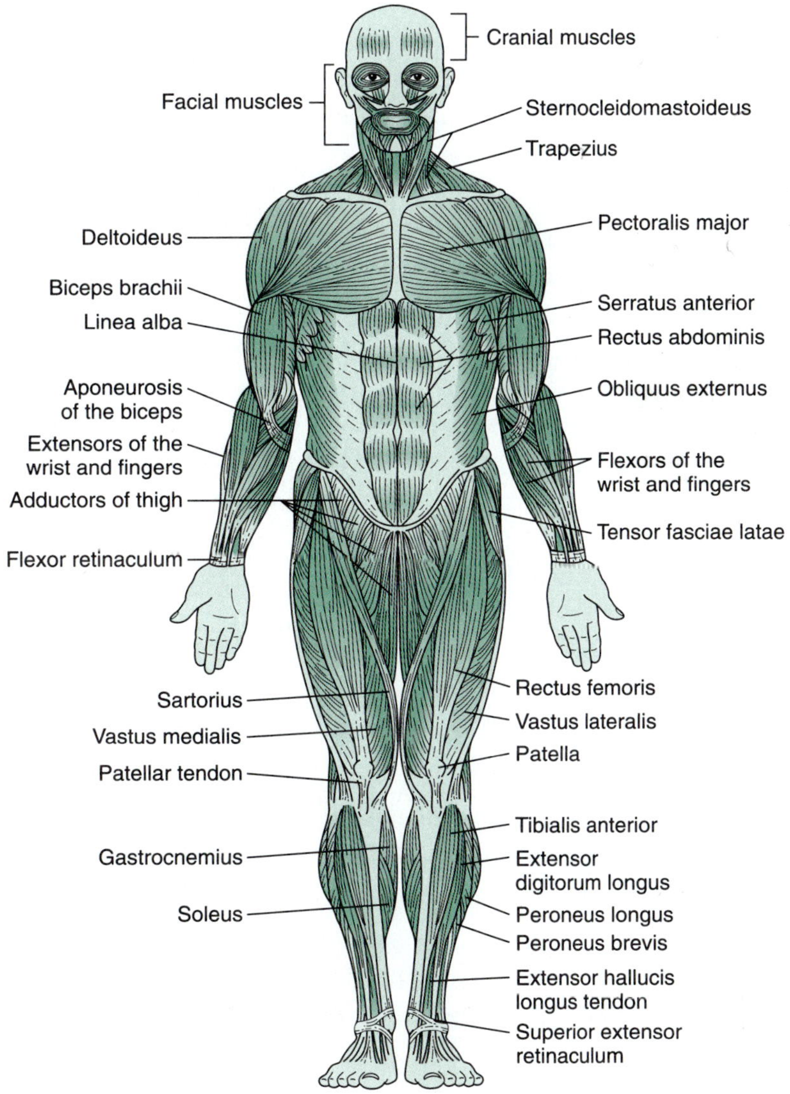

Figure 1-12 Muscular system, anterior view.

Copyright © 2005, Elsevier Inc. All rights reserved.
CPT only © 2004. *Current Procedural Terminology, 2005, Professional Edition*, American Medical Association. All rights reserved.

Smooth/Visceral

- Linings such as bowel, urethra, blood vessels
- Nonstriated
- Involuntary

Tendons Anchor Muscle to Bone

Ligaments Anchor Bones to Bones

Muscle Action

Muscle Capabilities

- Stretches
- Contracts
- Receives and responds to stimulus
- Returns to original shape and length

Muscle Movement

- Prime mover, responsible for movement
- Synergist, assists prime mover
- Antagonist, relaxes as prime mover and synergists contract, resulting in movement

Terms of Movement

- Flexion (bend)
- Extension (straighten)
- Abduction (away)
- Adduction (toward)
- Rotation (turn on axis)
- Circumduction (circular)
- Supination (upward)
- Pronation (downward)
- Hyperextension (overextension)
- Inversion (inward)
- Eversion (outward)

Names of Muscles

Head and Neck

Facial
- Orbicularis oris (opens mouth)
- Zygomaticus (elevates corners of mouth)
- Orbicularis oculi (opens and closes eyelid)

Mastication (chewing)
- Masseter (used to chew)
- Temporal (closes jaw)

Sternocleidomastoid (rotates head and neck)

Trapezius (extends head)

Copyright © 2005, Elsevier Inc. All rights reserved.
CPT only © 2004. *Current Procedural Terminology, 2005, Professional Edition*, American Medical Association. All rights reserved.

Upper Extremities

Biceps (flexes elbow)

Triceps brachii (extends elbow)

Deltoid (abducts upper arm)

Latissimus dorsi (extends upper arm)

Pectoralis major (flexes upper arm)

Trunk

External oblique (compresses abdomen)

Internal oblique (compresses abdomen)

Transversus abdominis (compresses abdomen)

Rectus abdominis (flexes trunk)

Respiratory

Diaphragm (separates thorax from abdomen)

Intercostal (between ribs)

Lower Extremities

Thigh

- Gluteus maximus (abducts thigh)
- Abductor brevis (abducts thigh)
- Iliopsoas (flexes thigh)

Hamstring (flexes lower leg)

Quadriceps (extends lower leg)

Sartorius (flexes and rotates leg)

Tibialis anterior (dorsiflexes foot)

Peroneus longus (everts foot)

Gastrocnemius (calf, with soleus flexes foot, also flexes knee)

Soleus (calf, flexes foot)

Achilles tendon (largest tendon)

COMBINING FORMS

1. acetabul/o	hip socket
2. ankyl/o	bent, fused
3. aponeur/o	tendon type
4. arthr/o	joint
5. burs/o	fluid-filled sac in a joint
6. calc/o, calci/o	calcium
7. carp/o	carpals (wrist bones)
8. chondr/o	cartilage

Copyright © 2005, Elsevier Inc. All rights reserved.
CPT only © 2004. *Current Procedural Terminology, 2005, Professional Edition*, American Medical Association. All rights reserved.

9. clavic/o, clavicul/o	clavicle (collar bone)
10. cost/o	rib
11. crani/o	cranium (skull)
12. disk/o	intervertebral disk
13. femor/o	thighbone
14. fibul/o	fibula
15. humer/o	humerus (upper arm bone)
16. ili/o	ilium (upper pelvic bone)
17. ischi/o	ischium (posterior pelvic bone)
18. kinesi/o	movement
19. kyph/o	hump
20. lamin/o	lamina
21. lord/o	curve
22. lumb/o	lower back
23. mandibul/o	mandible (lower jawbone)
24. maxill/o	maxilla (upper jawbone)
25. menisc/o	meniscus
26. menisci/o	meniscus
27. metacarp/o	metacarpals (hand)
28. metatars/o	metatarsals (foot)
29. myel/o	bone marrow
30. my/o, muscul/o	muscle
31. olecran/o	olecranon (elbow)
32. orth/o	straight
33. oste/o	bone
34. patell/o	patella (kneecap)
35. pelv/i	pelvis (hip)
36. petr/o	stone
37. phalang/o	phalanges (finger or toe)
38. pub/o	pubis
39. rachi/o	spine
40. radi/o	radius (lower arm)
41. sacr/o	sacrum
42. scapul/o	scapula (shoulder)
43. scoli/o	bent
44. spondyl/o	vertebra
45. stern/o	sternum (breast bone)

Copyright © 2005, Elsevier Inc. All rights reserved.
CPT only © 2004. *Current Procedural Terminology, 2005, Professional Edition,* American Medical Association. All rights reserved.

46. synovi/o	synovial membrane
47. tars/o	tarsal (ankle/foot)
48. ten/o	tendon
49. tend/o	tendon (connective tissue)
50. tendin/o	tendon (connective tissue)
51. tibi/o	shin bone
52. uln/o	ulna (lower arm bone)
53. vertebr/o	vertebra

PREFIXES

1. inter-	between
2. supra-	above
3. sym-	together
4. syn-	together

SUFFIXES

1. -asthenia	weakness
2. -blast	embryonic
3. -clast, -clasia, -clasis	break
4. -desis	fusion
5. -listhesis	slipping
6. -malacia	softening
7. -physis	to grow
8. -porosis	passage
9. -schisis	split
10. -tome	instrument that cuts
11. -tomy	incision

MEDICAL ABBREVIATIONS

1. ACL	anterior cruciate ligament
2. AKA	above-knee amputation
3. BKA	below-knee amputation
4. C1-C7	cervical vertebrae
5. CTS	carpal tunnel syndrome
6. fx	fracture
7. L1-L5	lumbar vertebrae
8. OA	osteoarthritis

Copyright © 2005, Elsevier Inc. All rights reserved.
CPT only © 2004. *Current Procedural Terminology, 2005, Professional Edition*, American Medical Association. All rights reserved.

9. RA	rheumatoid arthritis
10. T1-T12	thoracic vertebrae
11. TMJ	temporomandibular joint

MEDICAL TERMS

Arthrocentesis	Injection and/or aspiration of joint
Arthrodesis	Surgical immobilization of a joint
Arthrography	Radiography of joint
Arthroplasty	Reshaping or reconstruction of a joint
Arthroscopy	Use of scope to view inside joint
Arthrotomy	Incision into a joint
Articular	Pertains to a joint
Aspiration	Use of a needle and a syringe to withdraw fluid
Atrophy	Wasting away
Bunion	Hallux valgus, abnormal increase in size of metatarsal head that results in displacement of the great toe
Bursitis	Inflammation of bursa
Chondral	Referring to the cartilage
Closed fracture repair	Not surgically opened with/without manipulation and with/without traction
Closed treatment	Fracture site that is not surgically opened and visualized
Colles' fracture	Fracture at lower end of radius that displaces the bone posteriorly
Dislocation	Placement in a location other than the original location
Endoscopy	Inspection of body organs or cavities using a lighted scope that may be inserted through an existing opening or through a small incision
Fasciectomy	Removal of the band of fibrous tissue
Fissure	Groove
Fracture	Break in a bone
Ganglion	Knot
Internal/External fixation	Application of pins, wires, screws, placed externally or internally to immobilize a body part
Kyphosis	Humpback
Lamina	Flat plate
Ligament	Fibrous band of tissue that connects cartilage or bone
Lordosis	Anterior curve of spine
Lumbodynia	Pain in the lumbar area
Lysis	Releasing
Manipulation or reduction	Alignment of a fracture or joint dislocation to normal position

Copyright © 2005, Elsevier Inc. All rights reserved.
CPT only © 2004. *Current Procedural Terminology, 2005, Professional Edition,* American Medical Association. All rights reserved.

Open fracture repair	Surgical opening over or remote opening as access to a fracture site
Osteoarthritis	Degenerative condition of articular cartilage
Osteoclast	Absorbs or removes bone
Osteotomy	Cutting into bone
Percutaneous	Through the skin
Percutaneous fracture repair	Repair of a fracture by means of pins and wires inserted through the fracture site
Percutaneous skeletal fixation	Considered neither open nor closed; the fracture is not visualized, but fixation is placed across the fracture site under x-ray imaging
Reduction	Replacement to normal position
Scoliosis	Lateral curve of the spine
Skeletal traction	Application of pressure to bone by means of pins and/or wires inserted into the bone
Skin traction	Application of pressure to bone by means of tape applied to the skin
Spondylitis	Inflammation of vertebrae
Subluxation	Partial dislocation
Supination	Supine position
Synchondrosis	Union between two bones (connected by cartilage)
Tendon	Attaches a muscle to a bone
Tenodesis	Suturing of a tendon to a bone
Tenorrhaphy	Suture repair of tendon
Traction	Application of pressure to maintain normal alignment
Trocar needle	Needle with a tube on the end; used to puncture and withdraw fluid from a cavity

Copyright © 2005, Elsevier Inc. All rights reserved.
CPT only © 2004. *Current Procedural Terminology, 2005, Professional Edition*, American Medical Association. All rights reserved.

MUSCULOSKELETAL SYSTEM QUIZ

1. Tubular is another name for these bones:
   a. short
   b. long
   c. flat
   d. irregular

2. These bones are found near joints:
   a. irregular
   b. flat
   c. sesamoid
   d. broad

3. The zygoma is an example of this type of bone:
   a. irregular
   b. flat
   c. sesamoid
   d. broad

4. The diaphysis is this part of the bone:
   a. end
   b. surface
   c. shaft
   d. marrow

5. Which is NOT a part of the cranium:
   a. condyle
   b. sphenoid
   c. ethmoid
   d. parietal

6. This is NOT an ear bone:
   a. malleus
   b. stapes
   c. incus
   d. styloid

7. This term describes the growth plate:
   a. endosteum
   b. epiphyseal
   c. metaphysis
   d. periosteum

8. This is a depression on the lateral hip surface into which the head of the femur fits:
   a. ilium
   b. ischium
   c. patella
   d. acetabulum

Copyright © 2005, Elsevier Inc. All rights reserved.
CPT only © 2004. *Current Procedural Terminology, 2005, Professional Edition,* American Medical Association. All rights reserved.

9. The tip of the elbow is the:
   a. olecranon
   b. trapezium
   c. humerus
   d. tarsal

10. This term describes an immovable joint:
    a. amphiarthrosis
    b. diarthrosis
    c. synarthrosis
    d. ischium

Copyright © 2005, Elsevier Inc. All rights reserved.
CPT only © 2004. *Current Procedural Terminology, 2005, Professional Edition*, American Medical Association. All rights reserved.

MUSCULOSKELETAL SYSTEM—PATHOPHYSIOLOGY

Injuries

Fractures

Classification of fractures

Open/closed

- Open (compound): skin is broken
- Closed (simple): skin is not broken

Complete/incomplete

- Complete: bone is broken all the way through
  Example: oblique, linear, and transverse
- Incomplete: bone is not broken all the way through
  Example: greenstick, torus, stress, and transchondral

Treatment

- Reduction (realignment of bone fragments by manipulation)
- Immobilization (returns to normal alignment and holds in place)
- Traction (application of pulling force to hold bone in alignment)
  - Skeletal traction uses internal devices (pins, screws, wires, etc.) inserted into bone with ends sticking out through skin for attachment of traction device **(Figure 1-13)**
  - Skin traction is the use of strapping, elastic wrap, or tape attached to skin to which weights are attached **(Figure 1-14)**

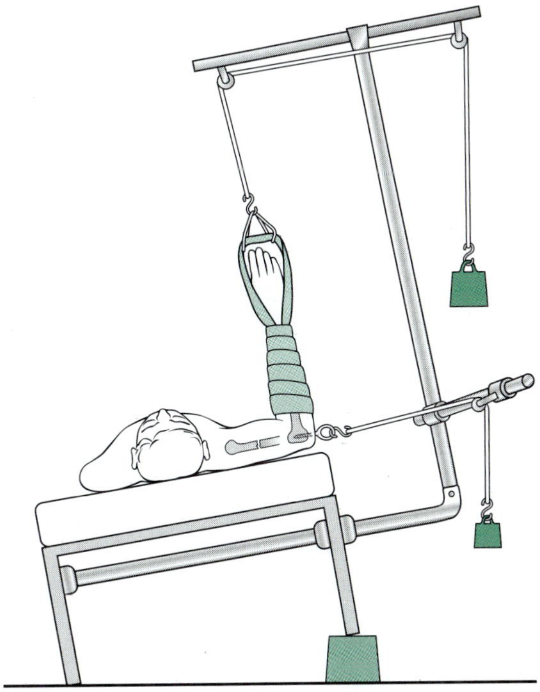

Figure 1-13 Skeletal traction uses the patient's bones to secure internal devices to which traction is attached.

Copyright © 2005, Elsevier Inc. All rights reserved.
CPT only © 2004. *Current Procedural Terminology, 2005, Professional Edition*, American Medical Association. All rights reserved.

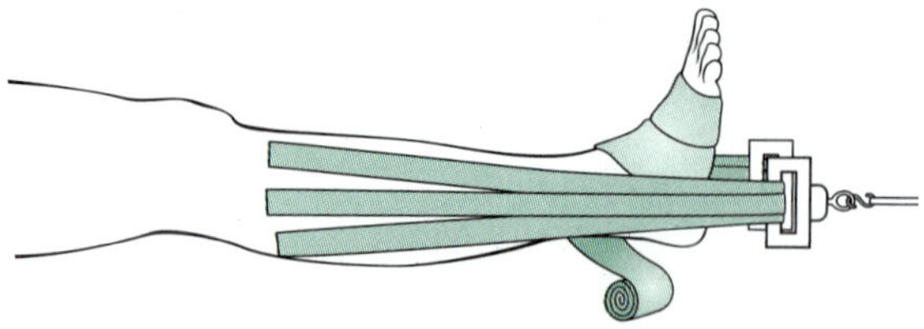

Figure 1-14 Skin traction utilizes strapping, wraps, or tape to which traction is attached.

Improper union

- Nonunion: failure of bone ends to grow together
- Malunion: incorrect alignment of bone ends
- Delayed union: union only after delay of many months

Dislocations

- Soft tissue damage usually caused by trauma
- May cause fracture of bone due to displacement
- Can result in nerve and tissue damage
- Treatment is reduction and immobilization

Sprains and strains

- Soft tissue damage usually caused by trauma to tendons and ligaments
- Strain partial tear of muscle or ligament
- Sprain results from overuse or overextension of a ligament

Bone Disorders

Osteomyelitis

Bone infection

Usually caused by bacteria

- Exogenous osteomyelitis is caused by bacteria that enter from outside the body
- Hematogenous osteomyelitis is from infection within the body

Osteoporosis

Common disorder in postmenopausal women
- Lower levels of calcium and phosphate

Decreased bone mass and density
- Fractures more common due to decrease in strength of bone

Treatment

- Increased intake of calcium and vitamin D
- Increased weight-bearing activity

Osteomalacia and rickets

Caused by vitamin D and phosphate deficiency

Copyright © 2005, Elsevier Inc. All rights reserved.
CPT only © 2004. *Current Procedural Terminology, 2005, Professional Edition*, American Medical Association. All rights reserved.

Osteitis deformans (Paget's disease)

Abnormal enlarging and softening of bone

Unknown cause

Treatment

- Increased intake of protein, calcium, and vitamin D

Spinal curvatures

- Lordosis: swayback
    - Inward curvature of the spine
- Kyphosis: humpback
    - Outward curvature of the spine
- Scoliosis
    - Lateral curvature of the spine

Spina bifida

Congenital abnormality in which vertebrae do not close correctly around the spine

Joint Disorders

Bursitis: inflammation of the bursa

Arthritis: inflammation of the joints

Osteoarthritis

This is degenerative or wear/tear arthritis

Chronic inflammation of joint

Increased pain on weight-bearing or movement

Affects weight-bearing joints

- Leads to loss of articular cartilage
- Sclerosis of bone
- Osteophytes (bone spurs)

Symptoms

- Pain and stiffness
- Crepitation (bone on bone creates characteristic grinding sound)

Classifications

- Primary (idiopathic)
    - No known cause
- Secondary
    - Associated with joint instability, joint stress, or congenital abnormalities

Copyright © 2005, Elsevier Inc. All rights reserved.
CPT only © 2004. *Current Procedural Terminology, 2005, Professional Edition*, American Medical Association. All rights reserved.

Treatment

- Symptomatic
- Arthroplasty

Rheumatoid arthritis (RA)

Inflammatory disease that is progressive

Systemic autoimmune disease

- Can invade arteries, lung, skin, and other organs with nodules

Affects small joints

- Destroys the synovial membrane, articular cartilage, and surrounding tissues

Leads to loss of function due to fixation and deformity

Treatment

- Symptomatic
- Arthroplasty

Infectious and septic arthritis

Infectious process

Usually affects single joint

Without antimicrobial intervention, permanent joint damage results

Gout (gouty arthritis)

Inflammatory arthritis

Often affects the joint of the great toe

Caused by excessive amounts of uric acid that crystallizes in connective tissue of joints

Leads to inflammation and destruction of joint

Ankylosing spondylitis (AS)

Inflammatory disease that is progressive

Affects vertebral joints

Leads to rigid spinal column and sacroiliac joints

Tendon, Muscle, and Ligament Disorders

Muscular dystrophy

Progressive degenerative muscle disorder

Most often affects boys

- Genetic predisposition

Copyright © 2005, Elsevier Inc. All rights reserved.
CPT only © 2004. *Current Procedural Terminology, 2005, Professional Edition*, American Medical Association. All rights reserved.

Primary fibromyalgia syndrome

Symptoms

- Generalized aching and pain
- Tender points
- Fatigue
- Depression

Usually appears in middle-aged women

Polymyositis

General muscle inflammation causing weakness

- With skin rash = dermatomyositis

Tumors

Bone tumors

Origin of bone tumors

- Osteogenic (bone cells)
- Chondrogenic (cartilage cell)
- Collagenic (fibrous tissue cell)
- Myelogenic (marrow cell)

Osteoma

- Benign
- Abnormal outgrowth of bone

Chondroblastoma

- Rare
- Usually benign

Osteosarcoma

- Malignant tumor of long bones
- Usually in young adults
- Typically causes bone pain

Multiple Myeloma

- Malignant
- Progressive and generally fatal
- Usually in those over 40

Chondrosarcoma

- Malignant cartilage tumor
- Usually in middle-aged and older individuals

Copyright © 2005, Elsevier Inc. All rights reserved.
CPT only © 2004. *Current Procedural Terminology, 2005, Professional Edition*, American Medical Association. All rights reserved.

- In late stages, symptoms include local swelling and pain
    - Worsens with time
- Surgical excision is usually treatment of choice

Muscle tumors

Rare

Rhabdomyosarcoma is an aggressive, invasive carcinoma with widespread metastasis

Copyright © 2005, Elsevier Inc. All rights reserved.
CPT only © 2004. *Current Procedural Terminology, 2005, Professional Edition*, American Medical Association. All rights reserved.

MUSCULOSKELETAL SYSTEM PATHOPHYSIOLOGY QUIZ

1. A compound fracture is also known as a(n):
   a. complete
   b. incomplete
   c. closed
   d. open

2. This is a common bone disorder in postmenopausal women resulting from lower levels of calcium and potassium.
   a. Paget's disease
   b. lordosis
   c. osteoporosis
   d. rheumatoid arthritis

3. This inflammatory disease is progressive and leads to a rigid spinal column.
   a. polymyositis
   b. ankylosing spondylitis
   c. primary fibromyalgia syndrome
   d. septic arthritis of the spine

4. This type of tumor arises from the bone cells.
   a. osteogenic
   b. chondrogenic
   c. collagenic
   d. myelogenic

5. This type of tumor is the most common type of malignant bone tumor that occurs in those over 40.
   a. rhabdomyosarcoma
   b. chondrosarcoma
   c. osteosarcoma
   d. multiple myeloma

6. A general muscle inflammation with an accompanying skin rash is:
   a. muscular dystrophy
   b. dermatologic arthritis
   c. ankylosing spondylitis
   d. dermatomyositis

7. A cartilage tumor that usually occurs in middle-aged and older individuals:
   a. chondrosarcoma
   b. osteosarcoma
   c. chondroblastoma
   d. rhabdomyosarcoma

8. The returning of the bone to normal alignment is
   a. immobilization
   b. traction
   c. reduction
   d. manipulation

Copyright © 2005, Elsevier Inc. All rights reserved.
CPT only © 2004. *Current Procedural Terminology, 2005, Professional Edition*, American Medical Association. All rights reserved.

9. The result of overuse or overextension of a ligament is
   a. strain
   b. sprain
   c. fracture
   d. displacement

10. Primary osteoarthritis is also known as
    a. secondary
    b. functional
    c. congenital
    d. idiopathic

Copyright © 2005, Elsevier Inc. All rights reserved.
CPT only © 2004. *Current Procedural Terminology, 2005, Professional Edition*, American Medical Association. All rights reserved.

RESPIRATORY SYSTEM

Supplies oxygen to body and helps clean body of waste

Two tracts (Figure 1-15)

Upper respiratory tract (nose, sinuses, pharynx, and larynx)

Lower respiratory tract (trachea, bronchial tree, and lungs)

Lined with specialized membranes

- Purifies air by trapping irritants
- Covered with cilia that move mucus upward

Upper Respiratory Tract (URT)

Nose

Sense of smell (olfactory)

Moistens and warms air

Nasal septum divides interior

Sinuses

Frontal

Ethmoidal

Maxillary

Sphenoidal

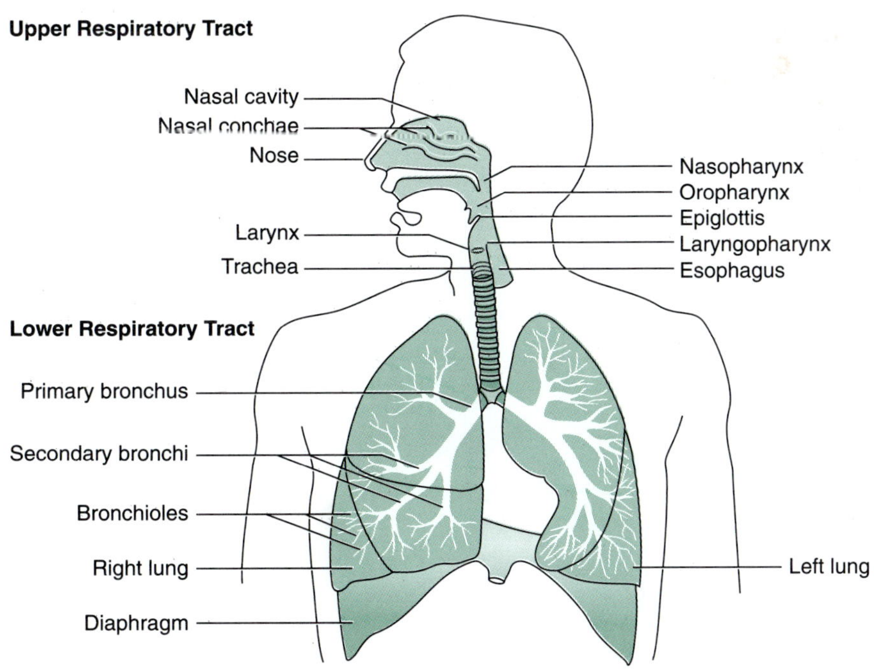

Figure 1-15 Upper and lower respiratory system.

Copyright © 2005, Elsevier Inc. All rights reserved.
CPT only © 2004. *Current Procedural Terminology, 2005, Professional Edition*, American Medical Association. All rights reserved.

Pharynx (Throat)

Passageway for both food and air

Nasopharynx contains adenoids

Oropharynx contains tonsils

Laryngopharynx leads to larynx

Larynx (Voice Box)

Contains vocal cords

Lower Respiratory Tract (LRT)

Trachea (Windpipe)

Mucus-lined tube with C-shaped cartilage rings to hold windpipe open

Air passageway

Bronchi

Trachea divides into branches—right branch and left branch

Branches divide into smaller bronchioles that are tipped with alveoli (air sacs that exchange gases)

Lungs

Covered by pleura

Cone-shaped organs

Base rests on diaphragm

Left lung contains two lobes

Right lung contains three lobes

Respiration

Inspiration—oxygen moves in

Expiration—carbon dioxide moves out

COMBINING FORMS

1. adenoid/o	adenoid
2. alveol/o	alveolus
3. atel/o	incomplete
4. bronch/o	bronchus
5. bronchi/o	bronchus
6. bronchiol/o	bronchiole
7. coni/o	dust
8. diaphragmat/o	diaphragm

Copyright © 2005, Elsevier Inc. All rights reserved.
CPT only © 2004. *Current Procedural Terminology, 2005, Professional Edition*, American Medical Association. All rights reserved.

9. epiglott/o	epiglottis
10. laryng/o	larynx
11. lob/o	lobe
12. muc/o	mucus
13. nas/o	nose
14. orth/o	straight
15. ox/i	oxygen
16. oxy/o	oxygen
17. pharyng/o	pharynx
18. phren/o	diaphragm
19. pleur/o	pleura
20. pneum/o	lung/air
21. pneumat/o	air
22. pneumon/o	lung/air
23. pulmon/o	lung
24. py/o	pus
25. rhin/o	nose
26. sept/o	septum
27. sinus/o	sinus
28. spir/o	breath
29. thorac/o	thorax
30. tonsill/o	tonsil
31. trache/o	trachea

PREFIXES

1. a-	not
2. an-	not
3. endo-	within
4. eu-	good
5. pan-	all
6. poly-	many

SUFFIXES

1. -algia	pain
2. -ar	pertaining to
3. -ary	pertaining to
4. -capnia	carbon dioxide

Copyright © 2005, Elsevier Inc. All rights reserved.
CPT only © 2004. *Current Procedural Terminology, 2005, Professional Edition*, American Medical Association. All rights reserved.

5. -centesis — puncture to remove
6. -dynia — pain
7. -eal — pertaining to
8. -ectasis — stretching
9. -emia — blood
10. -gram — record
11. -graph — recording instrument
12. -graphy — recording process
13. -itis — inflammation
14. -meter — measurement or instrument that measures
15. -metry — measurement of
16. -oxia — oxygen
17. -pexy — fixation
18. -phonia — sound
19. -pnea — breathing
20. -rrhage, -rrhagia — bursting of blood
21. -scopy — to examine
22. -spasm — contraction of muscle
23. -stenosis — blockage, narrowing
24. -stomy — opening
25. -thorax — chest
26. -tomy — cutting, incision

MEDICAL ABBREVIATIONS

1. ABG — arterial blood gas
2. AFB — acid-fast bacillus
3. ARDS — adult respiratory distress syndrome
4. BiPAP — bi-level positive airway pressure
5. COPD — chronic obstructive pulmonary disease
6. CPAP — continuous positive airway pressure
7. DLCO — diffuse capacity of lungs for carbon monoxide
8. FEF — forced expiratory flow
9. FEV_1 — forced expiratory volume in one second
10. FEV_1:FVC — ratio of forced expiratory volume in one second to forced vital capacity
11. FRC — functional residual capacity
12. FVC — forced vital capacity

Copyright © 2005, Elsevier Inc. All rights reserved.
CPT only © 2004. *Current Procedural Terminology, 2005, Professional Edition*, American Medical Association. All rights reserved.

13. HHN hand-held nebulizer
14. IPAP inspiratory positive airway pressure
15. IRDS infant respiratory distress syndrome
16. MDI metered dose inhaler
17. MVV maximum voluntary ventilation
18. PAWP pulmonary artery wedge pressure
19. PCWP pulmonary capillary wedge pressure
20. PEAP positive end-airway pressure
21. PEEP positive end-expiratory pressure
22. PFT pulmonary function test
23. PND paroxysmal nocturnal dyspnea
24. RDS respiratory distress syndrome
25. RV respiratory volume
26. RV:TLC ratio of respiratory volume to total lung capacity
27. TLC total lung capacity
28. TLV total lung volume
29. URI upper respiratory infection
30. V/Q ventilation/perfusion scan

MEDICAL TERMS

Ablation	Removal or destruction by cutting, chemicals, or electrocautery
Adenoidectomy	Removal of adenoids
Apnea	Cessation of breathing
Asphyxia	Lack of oxygen
Asthma	Shortage of breath caused by contraction of bronchi
Atelectasis	Incomplete expansion of lung, collapse
Auscultation	Listening to sounds, such as to lung sounds
Bacilli	Plural of bacillus, a rod-shaped bacteria
Bilobectomy	Surgical removal of two lobes of a lung
Bronchiole	Smaller division of bronchial tree
Bronchoplasty	Surgical repair of the bronchi
Bronchoscopy	Inspection of the bronchial tree using a bronchoscope
Catheter	Tube placed into the body to put fluid in or take fluid out
Cauterization	Destruction of tissue by the use of cautery
Cordectomy	Surgical removal of the vocal cord(s)
Crackle	Abnormal sound when breathing
Cyanosis	Bluish discoloration

Copyright © 2005, Elsevier Inc. All rights reserved.
CPT only © 2004. *Current Procedural Terminology, 2005, Professional Edition*, American Medical Association. All rights reserved.

Drainage	Free flow or withdrawal of fluids from a wound or cavity
Dysphonia	Speech impairment
Dyspnea	Shortage of breath, difficult breathing
Emphysema	Air accumulated in organ or tissue
Epiglottidectomy	Excision of the covering of the larynx
Epistaxis	Nose bleed
Glottis	True vocal cords
Hemoptysis	Bloody sputum
Intramural	Within the organ wall
Intubation	Insertion of a tube
Laryngeal web	Congenital abnormality of connective tissue between the vocal cords
Laryngectomy	Surgical removal of the larynx
Laryngoplasty	Surgical repair of the larynx
Laryngoscope	Fiberoptic scope used to view the inside of the larynx
Laryngoscopy	Direct visualization and examination of the interior of larynx with a laryngoscope
Laryngotomy	Incision into the larynx
Lavage	Washing out
Lobectomy	Surgical excision of a lobe of the lung
Nasal button	Synthetic circular disk used to cover a hole in the nasal septum
Orthopnea	Difficulty in breathing
Percussion	Tapping with sharp blows as a diagnostic technique
Pharyngolaryngectomy	Surgical removal of the pharynx and larynx
Pleura	Covers the lungs and lines the thoracic cavity
Pleurectomy	Surgical excision of the pleura
Pleuritis	Inflammation of the pleura
Pneumocentesis	Surgical puncturing of a lung to withdraw fluid
Pneumonolysis	Surgical separation of the lung from the chest wall to allow the lung to collapse
Pneumonotomy	Incision of the lung
Rales	Coarse sound on inspiration, also known as crackle
Rhinoplasty	Surgical repair of nose
Rhinorrhea	Nasal mucus discharge
Segmentectomy	Surgical removal of a portion of a lung
Septoplasty	Surgical repair of the nasal septum
Sinusotomy	Surgical incision into a sinus
Spirometry	Measuring breathing capacity

Copyright © 2005, Elsevier Inc. All rights reserved.
CPT only © 2004. *Current Procedural Terminology, 2005, Professional Edition*, American Medical Association. All rights reserved.

Tachypnea	Quick, shallow breathing
Thoracentesis	Surgical puncture of the thoracic cavity, usually using a needle, to remove fluids
Thoracoplasty	Surgical procedure that removes rib(s) and thereby allows the collapse of a lung
Thoracoscopy	Use of a lighted endoscope to view the pleural spaces and thoracic cavity or to perform surgical procedures
Thoracostomy	Surgical incision into the chest wall and insertion of a chest tube
Thoracotomy	Surgical incision into the chest wall
Total pneumonectomy	Surgical removal of an entire lung
Tracheostomy	Creation of an opening into the trachea
Tracheotomy	Incision into the trachea
Transtracheal	Across the trachea

Copyright © 2005, Elsevier Inc. All rights reserved.
CPT only © 2004. *Current Procedural Terminology, 2005, Professional Edition,* American Medical Association. All rights reserved.

RESPIRATORY SYSTEM QUIZ

1. This is NOT a part of the lower respiratory tract:
   a. trachea
   b. larynx
   c. bronchi
   d. lungs

2. Another name for the voice box is:
   a. oropharynx
   b. pharynx
   c. laryngopharynx
   d. larynx

3. This is the windpipe:
   a. pharynx
   b. larynx
   c. trachea
   d. sphenoid

4. The interior of the nose is divided by the:
   a. septum
   b. sphenoid
   c. oropharynx
   d. apical

5. This combining form means incomplete:
   a. atel/o
   b. alveol/o
   c. ox/i
   d. pneumat/o

6. This prefix means breathe:
   a. py/o
   b. lob/o
   c. spir/o
   d. pleur/o

7. This prefix means all:
   a. a-
   b. an-
   c. pan-
   d. poly-

8. This abbreviation refers to a syndrome that involves difficulty in breathing:
   a. ABG
   b. ARDS
   c. BiPAP
   d. FEF

Copyright © 2005, Elsevier Inc. All rights reserved.
CPT only © 2004. *Current Procedural Terminology, 2005, Professional Edition*, American Medical Association. All rights reserved.

9. This abbreviation refers to the amount of air the patient can expel from the lungs in one second:
   a. PFT
   b. PND
   c. RDS
   d. FEV_1

10. This suffix means breathing:
   a. -stenosis
   b. -spasm
   c. -pexy
   d. -pnea

Copyright © 2005, Elsevier Inc. All rights reserved.
CPT only © 2004. *Current Procedural Terminology, 2005, Professional Edition*, American Medical Association. All rights reserved.

RESPIRATORY SYSTEM—PATHOPHYSIOLOGY

Signs and Symptoms of Disorders

Dyspnea

- Difficult or painful breathing
- Increased respiratory effort

Hypoventilation

- Decreased alveolar ventilation

Hyperventilation

- Increased alveolar ventilation

Hemoptysis

- Bloody sputum

Hypoxia

- Reduced oxygenation of tissue cells

Cough

- Caused by irritant
- Protective reflex
- Acute cough is up to 3 weeks
- Chronic cough is over 3 weeks

Tachypnea

- Rapid breathing

Apnea

- Lack of breathing

Orthopnea

- Requiring sitting upright to facilitate breathing

Pulmonary Diseases and Disorders

Hypercapnia

- Increased carbon dioxide in arterial blood
- Decreased ability to breathe
- Can result in respiratory acidosis

Hypoxemia

- Reduced oxygenation of arterial blood

Copyright © 2005, Elsevier Inc. All rights reserved.
CPT only © 2004. *Current Procedural Terminology, 2005, Professional Edition*, American Medical Association. All rights reserved.

Acute respiratory failure

- Inadequate gas exchange
- Hypoxemia
- Can result from trauma or disease

Adult respiratory distress syndrome (ARDS)

- Acute injury to alveolocapillary membrane
- Results in edema and atelectasis
- In infants, infant respiratory distress syndrome (IRDS)

Pulmonary edema

- Accumulation of fluid in lung tissue
- Most common cause is heart disease

Aspiration

- Passage of fluid and solid particles into the lung
- Can cause severe pneumonitis
  - Localized inflammation of the lung

Atelectasis

Compression atelectasis

- Collapse of alveoli
- May be caused by external pressure on lung from abdominal distention, pleural effusion, or pneumothorax

Absorption atelectasis

- Most common type
- Mucus blocks airways
- Excess gas absorbed into alveoli cause collapse

Bronchiectasis

- Chronic, irreversible dilation of bronchi
- Example of various types
  - Capillary
  - Cystic
  - Follicular
  - Varicose

Respiratory acidosis

- Decreased level of pH

Bronchiolitis

- Inflammation of bronchioles
- Usually in children less than 2

Copyright © 2005, Elsevier Inc. All rights reserved.
CPT only © 2004. *Current Procedural Terminology, 2005, Professional Edition*, American Medical Association. All rights reserved.

- Viral infection (respiratory syncytial virus, or RSV)
- Example of various types
  - Constrictive
  - Proliferative
  - Obliterative

Pneumothorax

- Air collected in pleural cavity
- Can lead to lung collapse
- Spontaneous pneumothorax is spontaneous rupture of visceral pleura
- Secondary pneumothorax is a result of trauma to the chest

Pneumoconiosis

- Dust particles in the lung
  - Examples of dust: coal, asbestos, fiberglass

Empyema

Infectious pleural effusion

- Pus in pleural space
- May be a complication of pneumonia
- Treatment is that for pneumonia

Pulmonary embolism

- Air, tissue, or embolus occlusion
- Lodges in pulmonary artery or branch of artery
- Risk with congestive heart failure
- Most clots originate in leg veins

Cor pulmonale

- Hypertrophy or failure of right ventricle
- Result of lung, pulmonary vessels, or ch[illegible] disorders
- Acute is secondary to pulmon[illegible]
- Chronic is second[illegible]

Pleurisy (pleuritis)

- Inflammation [illegible]
- Often preceded [illegible]

Infectious disease

Upper respiratory infec[illegible]

- Acute inflammator[illegible] trachea and above

Examples:
  - Common cold
  - Croup

Copyright © 2005, Elsevier Inc. All rights reserved.
CPT only © 2004. *Current Procedural Terminology, 2005, Professional Edition,* American Medical Association. All rights reserved.

- Sinusitis
- Laryngitis

Lower respiratory infection (LRI)

Pneumonia

- Inflammation of the lungs with consolidation
- Categorized according to causative organism
- Can be caused by bacteria, protozoa, fungi, or virus

Examples:

- Lobar pneumonia
- Legionnaires' disease
- Bronchitis
- Bronchiolitis

Tuberculosis

- Communicable lung disease
- Caused by *Mycobacterium tuberculosis*

Chronic obstructive pulmonary disease (COPD)

Irreversible airway obstruction that decreases expiration

Includes

- Asthma
  - Bronchial spasms
  - Dyspnea
  - Wheezing
- Chronic bronchitis
  - Constant inflammation of bronchial tubes
- Emphysema
  - Loss of elasticity and enlargement of alveoli

Copyright © 2005, Elsevier Inc. All rights reserved.
CPT only © 2004. *Current Procedural Terminology, 2005, Professional Edition,* American Medical Association. All rights reserved.

RESPIRATORY SYSTEM PATHOPHYSIOLOGY QUIZ

1. Acute injury to the alveolocapillary membrane that results in edema and atelectasis:
   a. hypoxemia
   b. acute respiratory distress syndrome
   c. bronchiolitis
   c. pneumoconiosis

2. The condition in which pus is in the pleural space and is often a complication of pneumonia:
   a. empyema
   b. cor pulmonale
   c. pneumothorax
   d. atelectasis

3. The most common type of atelectasis is
   a. compression
   b. inflammation
   c. chronic
   d. absorption

4. This condition is a result of the accumulation of dust particles in the lung.
   a. pleurisy
   b. tuberculosis
   c. chronic obstructive pulmonary disease
   d. pneumoconiosis

5. An irreversible airway obstructive disease in which the symptoms are bronchial spasm, dyspnea, and wheezing:
   a. pleurisy
   b. empyema
   c. bronchiolitis
   d. asthma

6. Capillary, cystic, follicular, and varicose are examples of
   a. bronchiectasis
   b. cor pulmonale
   c. pneumothorax
   d. atelectasis

7. The condition in which there is a loss of elasticity and enlargement of alveoli:
   a. chronic bronchitis
   b. asthma
   c. emphysema
   d. empyema

8. The definition of a chronic cough is one that lasts for over this number of weeks:
   a. 2
   b. 3
   c. 4
   d. 5

Copyright © 2005, Elsevier Inc. All rights reserved.
CPT only © 2004. *Current Procedural Terminology, 2005, Professional Edition*, American Medical Association. All rights reserved.

9. A condition marked by an increase in the carbon dioxide in the arterial blood and decreased ability to breathe that can result in respiratory acidosis:
   a. hypercapnia
   b. hypoxemia
   c. acute respiratory failure
   d. pulmonary edema

10. This condition often follows a viral infection and occurs in children under 2 years of age. Examples of the various types of the condition are constrictive, proliferating, and obliterative.
    a. pneumoconiosis
    b. pulmonary edema
    c. bronchiolitis
    d. bronchiectasis

Copyright © 2005, Elsevier Inc. All rights reserved.
CPT only © 2004. *Current Procedural Terminology, 2005, Professional Edition,* American Medical Association. All rights reserved.

CARDIOVASCULAR SYSTEM

Consists of blood, blood vessels, and heart

Blood

Carries

Oxygen and nutrients to cells

Waste and carbon dioxide to kidneys, liver, and lungs

Hormones from endocrine system

Regulates

Temperature by circulating blood

Protection

White cells produce antibodies

Composed of Two Parts:

Liquid part (extracellular): plasma

Water 91%

Protein 1%, albumin, globulins, fibrinogen

2% ions, nutrients, waste products, gases, regulating substances

Formed part

- Leukocytes (WBCs)
    - Neutrophils
    - Lymphocytes
    - Monocytes
    - Eosinophils
    - Basophils
- Erythrocytes (RBCs)
- Platelets/thrombocytes

Vessels

Function

To carry nutrients and oxygen (blood)

Types

Arteries (Figure 1-16)

Inner layer, endothelium

Lead away from heart

Branches are arterioles

Copyright © 2005, Elsevier Inc. All rights reserved.
CPT only © 2004. *Current Procedural Terminology, 2005, Professional Edition*, American Medical Association. All rights reserved.

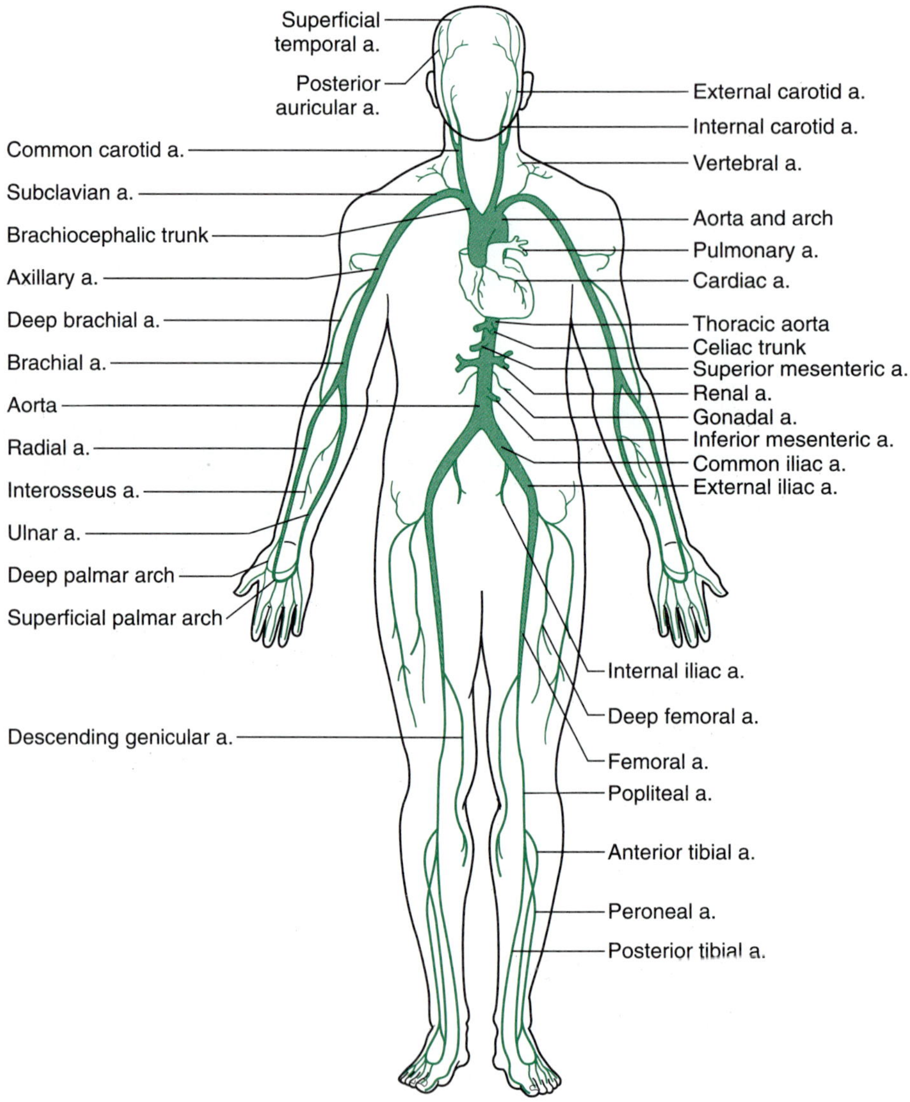

Figure 1-16 Arteries of the circulatory system.

Capillaries

Carry blood from arterioles to venules

Exchange vessels

Veins (Figure 1-17)

Carry blood to heart

Venules are small branches

Heart

Circulates blood

Four Chambers (Figure 1-18)

Two upper: right and left atria (singular atrium) receive blood

Two lower: right and left ventricles discharge blood (pump)

Copyright © 2005, Elsevier Inc. All rights reserved.
CPT only © 2004. *Current Procedural Terminology, 2005, Professional Edition*, American Medical Association. All rights reserved.

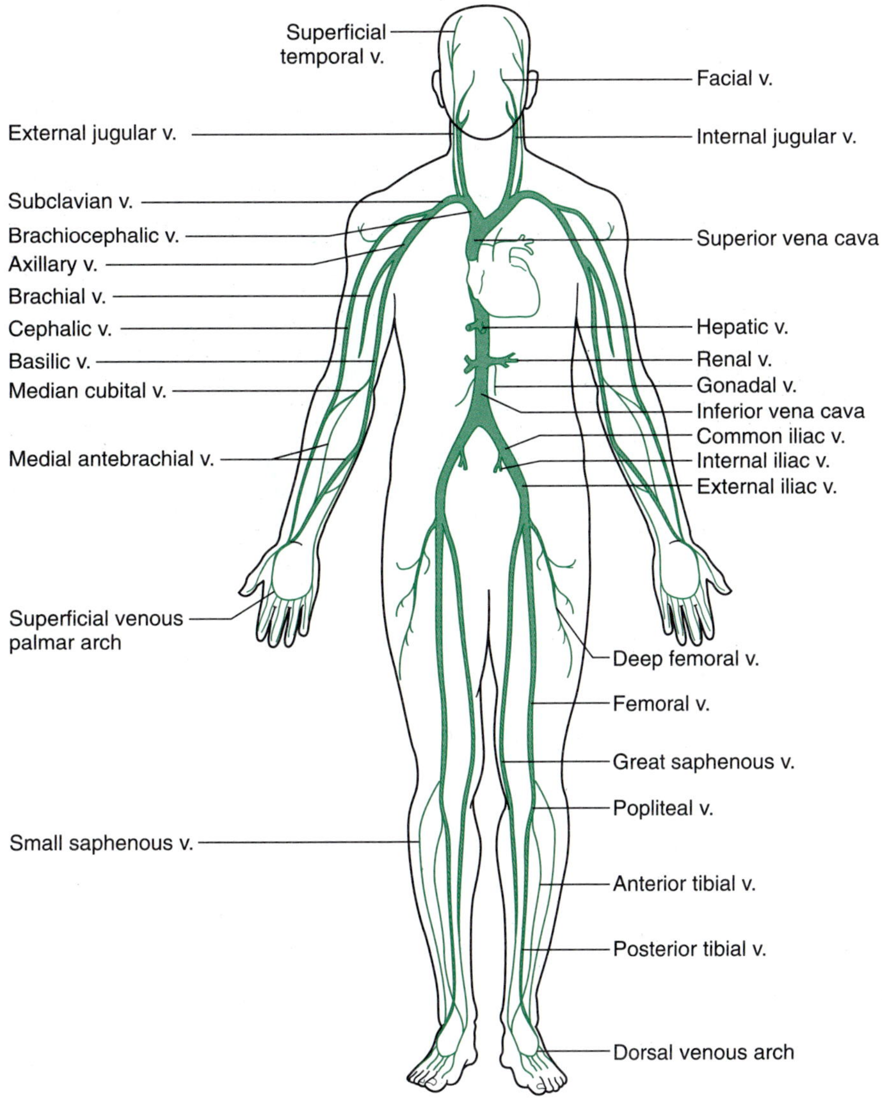

Figure 1-17 Veins of the circulatory system.

Chamber Walls

Composed of three layers

Endocardium: smooth inner layer
Myocardium: middle muscular layer
Epicardium: outer layer

Septa (Singular Septum)

Divide chambers

Interatrial septum: separates two upper chambers
Interventricular septum: separates two lower chambers

Pericardium

Sac that covers heart in two layers

Copyright © 2005, Elsevier Inc. All rights reserved.
CPT only © 2004. *Current Procedural Terminology, 2005, Professional Edition,* American Medical Association. All rights reserved.

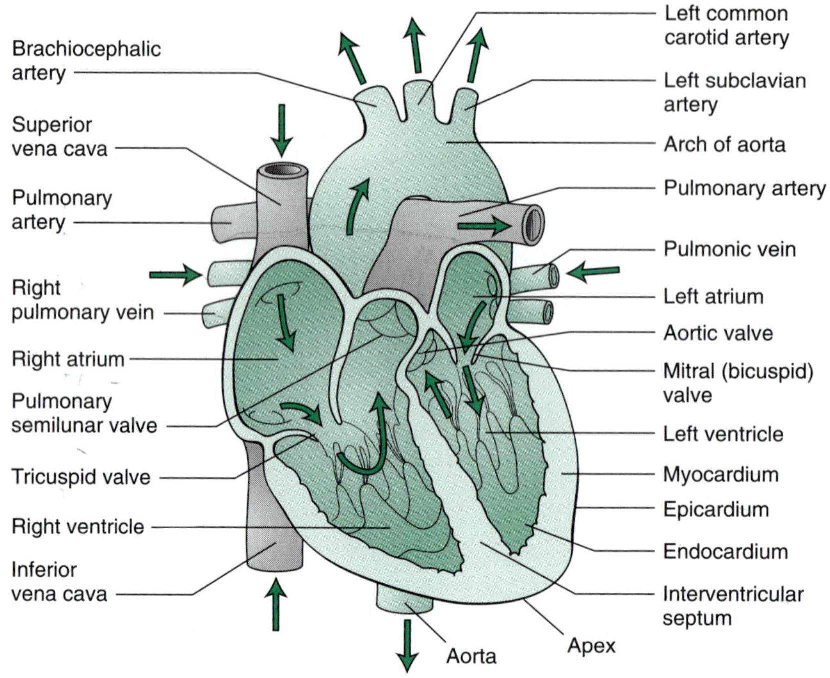

Figure 1-18 Internal view of the heart.

Parietal pericardium: outermost covering
Visceral pericardium: innermost (epicardium)
Pericardial cavity: contains fluid

Valves

Tricuspid: right atrium to right ventricle
Pulmonary: at entrance of pulmonary artery
Aortic: at entrance of aorta
Bicuspid (mitral): left atrium to left ventricle

Conduction System (Figure 1-19)

Sinoatrial node: SA node, nature's pacemaker, sends impulses to atrioventricular node
Atrioventricular node: AV node, located on interatrial septum and sends impulses to bundle of His
Bundle of His: divides into right and left bundle branches in septum
Purkinje fibers: in walls of ventricles

Heartbeat

Two Phases

Diastole: relaxation
Systole: contraction

COMBINING FORMS

1. angi/o — vessel
2. aort/o — aorta

Copyright © 2005, Elsevier Inc. All rights reserved.
CPT only © 2004. *Current Procedural Terminology, 2005, Professional Edition,* American Medical Association. All rights reserved.

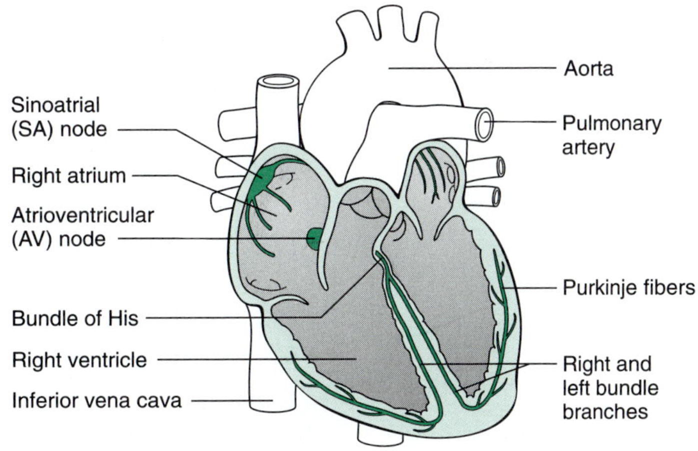

Figure 1-19 Electrical system of the heart.

3. ar/o, ather/o	plaque
4. arter/o	artery
5. arteri/o	artery
6. atri/o	atrium
7. brachi/o	arm
8. cardi/o	heart
9. cholester/o	cholesterol
10. coron/o	heart
11. cyan/o	blue
12. my/o, muscul/o	muscle
13. ox/o	oxygen
14. pericardi/o	pericardium
15. phleb/o	vein
16. sphygm/o	pulse
17. steth/o	chest
18. thromb/o	clot
19. valv/o	valve
20. valvul/o	valve
21. vascul/o	vessel
22. vas/o	vessel
23. ven/o	vein
24. ventricul/o	ventricle

PREFIXES

1. a-	not
2. an-	not

Copyright © 2005, Elsevier Inc. All rights reserved.
CPT only © 2004. *Current Procedural Terminology, 2005, Professional Edition*, American Medical Association. All rights reserved.

3. bi- two
4. brady- slow
5. de- lack of
6. dys- bad, difficult, painful
7. endo- in
8. hyper- over
9. hypo- under
10. inter- between
11. intra- within
12. meta- change
13. peri- surrounding
14. tachy- fast
15. tetra- four
16. tri- three

SUFFIXES

1. -dilation widening, expanding
2. -emia blood
3. -graphy recording process
4. -lysis separation
5. -megaly enlargement
6. -oma tumor
7. -osis condition
8. -plasty repair
9. -sclerosis hardening
10. -stenosis blockage, narrowing
11. -tomy cutting, incision

MEDICAL ABBREVIATIONS

1. ASCVD arteriosclerotic cardiovascular disease
2. ASD atrial septal defect
3. ASHD arteriosclerotic heart disease
4. AV atrioventricular
5. CABG coronary artery bypass graft
6. CHF congestive heart failure
7. CK creatine kinase
8. CPK creatine phosphokinase
9. CVI cerebrovascular insufficiency

Copyright © 2005, Elsevier Inc. All rights reserved.
CPT only © 2004. *Current Procedural Terminology, 2005, Professional Edition,* American Medical Association. All rights reserved.

10. DSE	dobutamine stress echocardiography
11. HCVD	hypertensive cardiovascular disease
12. LBBB	left bundle branch block
13. LVH	left ventricular hypertrophy
14. MAT	multifocal atrial tachycardia
15. MI	myocardial infarction
16. NSR	normal sinus rhythm
17. PAC	premature atrial contraction
18. PAT	paroxysmal atrial tachycardia
19. PST/PSVT	paroxysmal supraventricular tachycardia
20. PTCA	percutaneous transluminal coronary angioplasty
21. PVC	premature ventricular contraction
22. RBBB	right bundle branch block
23. RSR	regular sinus rhythm
24. RVH	right ventricular hypertrophy
25. SVT	supraventricular tachycardia
26. TEE	transesophageal echocardiography
27. TST	treadmill stress test

MEDICAL TERMS

Anastomosis	Surgical connection of two tubular structures, such as two pieces of the intestine
Aneurysm	Sac formed outside the vessel, artery, or heart
Angina	Sudden pain
Angiography	Radiography of the blood vessels
Angioplasty	Procedure in a vessel to dilate the vessel opening
Atherectomy	Removal of plaque by percutaneous method
Auscultation	Listening for sounds within the body
Bundle of His	Muscular cardiac fibers that provide the heart rhythm to the ventricles
Bypass	To go around
Cardiopulmonary	Refers to the heart and lungs
Cardiopulmonary bypass	Blood bypasses the heart through a heart-lung machine
Cardioverter-defibrillator	Surgically placed device that directs an electric shock to the heart to restore rhythm
Circumflex	A coronary artery that circles the heart
Cutdown	Incision into a vessel for placement of a catheter
Edema	Swelling due to abnormal fluid collection in the tissue spaces
Electrode	Lead attached to a generator that carries the electric current from the generator to the atria or ventricles

Copyright © 2005, Elsevier Inc. All rights reser
CPT only © 2004. *Current Procedural Terminology, 2005, Professional Edition*, American Medical Association. All rights rese

Electrophysiology	Study of the electrical system of the heart, including study of arrhythmias
Embolectomy	Removal of blockage (embolism) from vessel
Endarterectomy	Incision into an artery to remove inner lining
Epicardial	Over the heart
False aneurysm	Sac of clotted blood that has completely destroyed the vessel and is being contained by the tissue that surrounds the vessel
Fistula	Abnormal opening from one area to another area or to the outside of the body
Hematoma	Mass of blood that forms outside the vessel
Hemolysis	Breakdown of red blood cells
Hypoxemia	Low level of oxygen in the blood
Hypoxia	Low level of oxygen in the tissue
Intracardiac	Inside the heart
Invasive	Entering the body, breaking skin
Noninvasive	Not entering the body, not breaking skin
Nuclear cardiology	Diagnostic specialty that uses radiologic procedures to aid in diagnosis of cardiologic conditions
Order	Shows subordination of one thing to another; family or class
Pericardiocentesis	Procedure in which a surgeon withdraws fluid from the pericardial space by means of a needle inserted percutaneously
Pericardium	Membranous sac enclosing heart and ends of great vessels
Swan Ganz catheter	A catheter that measures pressure in the heart
Thoracostomy	Incision into the chest wall and insertion of a chest tube
Thromboendarterectomy	Procedure to remove plaque or clot formations from a vessel by percutaneous method
Transvenous	Through a vein

ed.
ved.
5, Elsevier Inc. All rights reserved.
04. *Current Procedural Terminology, 2005, Professional Edition,* American Medical Association. All rights reserved.

9. These are the chambers that receive blood:
   a. right and left ventricle
   b. left ventricle and right atrium
   c. right atrium and right ventricle
   d. right and left atria

10. This combining form means plaque:
    a. atri/o
    b. brachi/o
    c. cyan/o
    d. ather/o

ɔ, Elsevier Inc. All rights reserved.
ʋ4. *Current Procedural Terminology, 2005, Professional Edition*, American Medical Association. All rights reserved.

CARDIOVASCULAR SYSTEM—PATHOPHYSIOLOGY

Vascular Disorders

Coronary artery disease (CAD)/ischemic heart disease (IHD)

Thickening of the arterial intima (innermost layer) and accumulation of lipid

- Produces narrowing and stiffening of vessel

Location of lesions leads to various vascular disease

- Femoral and popliteal arteries = peripheral vascular disease
- Carotid arteries = stroke
- Aorta = aneurysmal disease
- Coronary arteries = ischemic heart disease or myocardial infarction

Result of decreased oxygen supply

Risk factors increased by:

- Age
- Family history of CAD
- Hyperlipidemia
- Low HDL-C (good cholesterol)
- Hypertension
- Cigarette smoking
- Diabetes mellitus
- Obesity, particularly abdominal

Ischemia

Deficiency of blood

- Often due to constriction or obstruction of blood vessel

Localized myocardial ischemia

- Oxygen demand in excess of ability of the vessel
- Presenting symptoms
  - Chest pain (angina pectoris)
  - Hypotension
  - Changes in ECG

Transient ischemia: Heart muscle begins to perform at a low level due to lack of oxygen (reversible ischemia)

Irreversible ischemia is when the heart muscle dies—necrosis (myocardial infarction)

- Prolonged ischemia of 30 minutes or more
- Reestablishment of blood flow reduces the residual necrosis
  - Thrombolytic agents to dissolve or split up thrombus
  - Primary percutaneous transluminal coronary angioplasty (PTCA)

Cardiac enzymes are released from the damaged cells

- Blood test reveals elevation of enzymes confirming myocardial infarction

Hypertension

Defined as 120/80 or greater

- **Figure 1-20** illustrates the new hypertension classifications

Copyright © 2005, Elsevier Inc. All rights reserved.
CPT only © 2004. *Current Procedural Terminology, 2005, Professional Edition,* American Medical Association. All rights reserved.

Classification of blood pressure for adults aged 18 years or older[1]

Category	Systolic (mm Hg)	Diastolic (mm Hg)
Normal	<130	<85
High Normal	130–139	85–89
Hypertension[2]		
Stage 1 (mild)	140–159	90–99
Stage 2 (moderate)	160–179	100–109
Stage 3 (severe)	≥180	≥110

[1] Not taking antihypertensive drugs and not acutely ill. When systolic and diastolic pressures fall into different categories, the higher category should be selected.

[2] Based on the average of two or more readings taken at each of two or more visits after an initial screening.

Figure 1-20 Classification of blood pressure.

Leading cause of death in United States due to damage to brain, heart, and kidneys

Cause is unknown in 95% of cases

Known as:

- Primary hypertension
- Essential hypertension

5% of cases are secondary to underlying disease

Increased resistance damages heart and blood vessels

- Retinal vascular changes are monitored to assess therapy and disease progression

Chronic hypertension often leads to end-stage renal disease

- Result of progressive sclerosis of renal vessels

Treatment

- Medications
  - ACE (angiotensin-converting enzyme) inhibitor
  - Alpha-adrenergic or beta-adrenergic receptor blocker
  - Diuretic
  - Calcium channel blocker
- Lifestyle changes

Hypotension

Abnormally low blood pressure

Types:

Orthostatic (postural) hypotension

- Fall in both systolic and diastolic arterial blood pressure on standing

Copyright © 2005, Elsevier Inc. All rights reserved.
CPT only © 2004. *Current Procedural Terminology, 2005, Professional Edition*, American Medical Association. All rights reserved.

- Associated with:
  - Dizziness
  - Blurred vision
  - Possibly fainting (syncope)
- Caused by insufficient blood flow through brain
- Can be acute (temporary) or chronic

Chronic orthostatic hypotension

- Secondary to a disease
- Such as:
  - Endocrine
  - Metabolic
  - Central nervous system disorders
- Idiopathic or primary
  - No known cause
- Treatment for secondary hypotension is for underlying disease correction

Aneurysm

Dilation of a vessel wall or cardiac chamber

- Danger is rupture of the aneurysm

Atherosclerosis is common cause

Arteriosclerosis and hypertension also common in persons with aneurysms

True aneurysm

- Involves all three layers of arterial wall
- Causes weakening in arterial wall

False aneurysm

- Usually result of trauma
- Also known as aneurysmal hematoma or pseudoaneurysm

Thrombus

Blood clot that remains attached to vessel wall and occludes the vessel

Dislodged thrombus is a thromboembolus

Caused by such conditions as the following:

- Trauma
- Infection
- Low blood pressure
- Obstruction
- Atherosclerosis

Risks that thrombus can

- Dislodge
- Grow to occlude blood flow

Copyright © 2005, Elsevier Inc. All rights reserved.
CPT only © 2004. *Current Procedural Terminology, 2005, Professional Edition*, American Medical Association. All rights reserved.

Pharmacologic treatment with anticoagulants

- Heparin
- Warfarin derivatives

Invasive intervention

- Balloon-tipped catheter to remove or compress thrombus

Thrombophlebitis caused by inflammation (phlebitis)

Caused by

- Trauma
- Infection
- Immobility

Commonly associated with:

- Endocarditis
- Rheumatic heart disease

Embolism

Mass that is present and circulating in the blood

Can be a(n):

- Air bubble
- Fat
- Bacterial
- Cancer cells
- Foreign substances
- Dislodged thrombus

Obstructs vessel

- Pulmonary emboli goes through the venous side or right side of the heart on the way to the pulmonary artery
- Systemic or arterial emboli originates in left side of the heart

  Associated with:
  - Myocardial infarction
  - Left-side heart failure
  - Endocarditis
  - Valvular disease
  - Dysrhythmias

Peripheral arterial disease

Thromboangiitis obliterans (Buerger disease)

- Occurs most often in young men who are heavy smokers
- Inflammatory disease of the peripheral arteries
- Involves small or medium arteries of feet

Copyright © 2005, Elsevier Inc. All rights reserved.
CPT only © 2004. *Current Procedural Terminology, 2005, Professional Edition*, American Medical Association. All rights reserved.

    - Sometimes involves hands
    - May necessitate amputation

Raynaud disease and phenomenon

- Spasms of small arteries of hands
    - Sometimes involves feet
- Fingertips thicken and nails become brittle
- Raynaud phenomenon is secondary to primary disease, such as:
    - Scleroderma
    - Pulmonary hypertension

Treatment of underlying condition

- No known origin or treatment
- Smoking aggravates the condition

Varicose veins

Blood pools in vessel

Tends to be progressive

Often in legs

Leads to:

- Swelling
- Fatigue
- Possible ulcerations

Heart Disorders

Congestive heart failure

- Can be left-side or right-side heart failure
- Heart cannot generate adequate output
- Acute onset often a result of acute myocardial ischemia

Congenital heart defects

- Valvular defects
- Tetralogy of Fallot
- Ventricular atrial septal defect

Infection and inflammation of the heart

Infective endocarditis

- Leads to destruction and permanent damage to heart valves
- Caused by bacteria (most common), virus, fungi, parasites
- Patients with heart defects or damage usually take antibacterial medication prior to invasive procedures

Pericarditis

- Inflammation of pericardium of heart

Copyright © 2005, Elsevier Inc. All rights reserved.
CPT only © 2004. *Current Procedural Terminology, 2005, Professional Edition*, American Medical Association. All rights reserved.

Rheumatic fever

- Involves all three layers of arterial wall
- Results in formation of scar tissue of the myocardium and heart valves
- In 10% of cases leads to rheumatic heart disease
- Family tendency to develop
- Begins as carditis (inflammation of heart)

Cardiac Dysrhythmias

Includes abnormal heart rate of

- Slow (bradyarrhythmia or bradycardia, <60 bpm)
- Fast (tachyarrhythmia or tachycardia, >100 bpm)
- Extrasystoles (intermittent additional heart contractions)
- Heart blocks (missed contractions)

May result from myocardial infarction or systemic abnormalities

Valvular heart disease

Valves are made of endocardial tissue

Endocardial damage can be congenital or acquired

Damage leads to stenosis and/or incompetence valve

Includes:

- Valvular stenosis creates increased resistance, resulting in increased pressure in cardiac chamber behind valve
- Valvular regurgitation is failure of valve leaflet to close tightly, allowing backflow of blood
  - Result of lesion that shrinks
  - Functional valvular regurgitation is a result of increased chamber size (cardiomegaly)

Stenosis

Aortic stenosis

- Caused by congenital malformation, degeneration, or rheumatoid arthritis
- Results in a decreased blood flow
- Symptoms are bradycardia and faint pulse
- May lead to heart murmur and hypertrophy

Mitral stenosis

- Impaired flow from left atrium to left ventricle
- Caused by rheumatic fever, bacterial infections
- Symptom is decreased cardiac output
- May lead to:
  - Pulmonary hypertension
  - Right ventricular heart failure
  - And/or edema

Copyright © 2005, Elsevier Inc. All rights reserved.
CPT only © 2004. *Current Procedural Terminology, 2005, Professional Edition*, American Medical Association. All rights reserved.

Regurgitation

Flow in the opposite direction from normal

Types

- Mitral regurgitation (MR): backflow of blood from left ventricle into left atrium
- Aortic regurgitation (AR): backflow of blood from aorta into the left ventricle
- Pulmonic regurgitation (PR): backflow of blood from pulmonary artery into right ventricle
- Tricuspid regurgitation (TR): backflow of blood from right ventricle into the right atrium
- Valvular regurgitation (VR): backflow of blood

Heart Wall Disorders

Acute pericarditis

Roughening and inflammation of pericardium (sac around heart)

Constrictive pericarditis (restrictive pericarditis)

Forms fibrous lesions that encase heart

- Compresses heart
- Reduces output

Pericardial effusion

Accumulation of fluid in pericardial cavity

Results in pressure on the heart

- Sudden development of pressure on the heart is tamponade

Cardiomyopathies

Myocardium = muscular walls of heart

Group of diseases that affect myocardium

Cause can be idiopathic (most common) or caused by an underlying condition

Types of cardiomyopathy

- Dilated cardiomyopathy (congestive cardiomyopathy)
  - Ventricular distention and impaired systolic function
- Hypertrophic cardiomyopathy
  - Cause is often hypertensive or valvular heart disease
  - Results in thickened interventricular septum (septum between the ventricle chambers)
- Restrictive cardiomyopathy
  - Myocardium becomes stiffened
  - Heart enlarges (cardiomegaly)
  - Dysrhythmias common
  - Caused by infiltrative diseases such as amyloidosis

Copyright © 2005, Elsevier Inc. All rights reserved.
CPT only © 2004. *Current Procedural Terminology, 2005, Professional Edition*, American Medical Association. All rights reserved.

CARDIOVASCULAR SYSTEM PATHOPHYSIOLOGY QUIZ

1. Lesion of the carotid artery may lead to
   a. heart attack
   b. stroke
   c. peripheral vascular disease
   d. ischemic heart disease

2. Blood pressure above this is considered hypertension:
   a. 120/80
   b. 130/70
   c. 140/90
   d. 110/70

3. Tachyarrhythmia or fast heart rate is that in excess of _______ bpm.
   a. 60
   b. 80
   c. 90
   d. 100

4. Angina pectoris is
   a. heart block
   b. heart murmur
   c. chest pain
   d. barrel chest

5. In this type of regurgitation there is a backflow of blood from the left ventricle into the left atrium.
   a. aortic
   b. pulmonic
   c. tricuspid
   d. mitral

6. In this type of heart wall disorder, fibrous lesions form and encase the heart.
   a. constrictive pericarditis
   b. acute pericarditis
   c. pericardial effusion
   d. cardiom

7. W wn cause"?
   a.
   b.
   c.
   d.

8. This myopathy.
   a. h
   b. va
   c. di
   d. res

Copyright © 2005, Elsevier Inc. All rights reserved.
CPT only © 2004. *Current Procedural Terminology, 2005, Professional Edition,* American Medical Association. All rights reserved.

9. This peripheral arterial disease most often occurs in young men who are heavy smokers.
   a. Buerger's
   b. Pick's
   c. Addison's
   d. Glasser's

10. This cardiomyopathy results in a thickened interventricular septum.
    a. restrictive
    b. congestive
    c. dilated
    d. hypertrophic

Copyright © 2005, Elsevier Inc. All rights reserved.
CPT only © 2004. *Current Procedural Terminology, 2005, Professional Edition*, American Medical Association. All rights reserved.

FEMALE GENITAL SYSTEM AND PREGNANCY

Terminology

Ovaries (pair): produce ova (single female gametes), ova: plural; ovum: singular (Figure 1-21)

Fallopian Tubes: (uterine tubes or oviducts): ducts from ovary to uterus

Uterus (womb): muscular organ that holds embryo

Three layers:

Endometrium: inner mucosa
Myometrium: middle layer/muscle
Perimetrium/Uterine serosa: outer layer
Cervix: lower narrow portion of uterus
Fundus: the upper rounded part of the uterus

Vagina: tube from uterus to outside of body

Vulva: external genitalia
Clitoris: erectile tissue
Labia majora: outer lips of vagina
Labia minora: inner lips of vagina
Bartholin's gland: glands on either side of vagina
Hymen: membrane that covers entrance to vagina

Perineum: area between anus and vaginal orifice

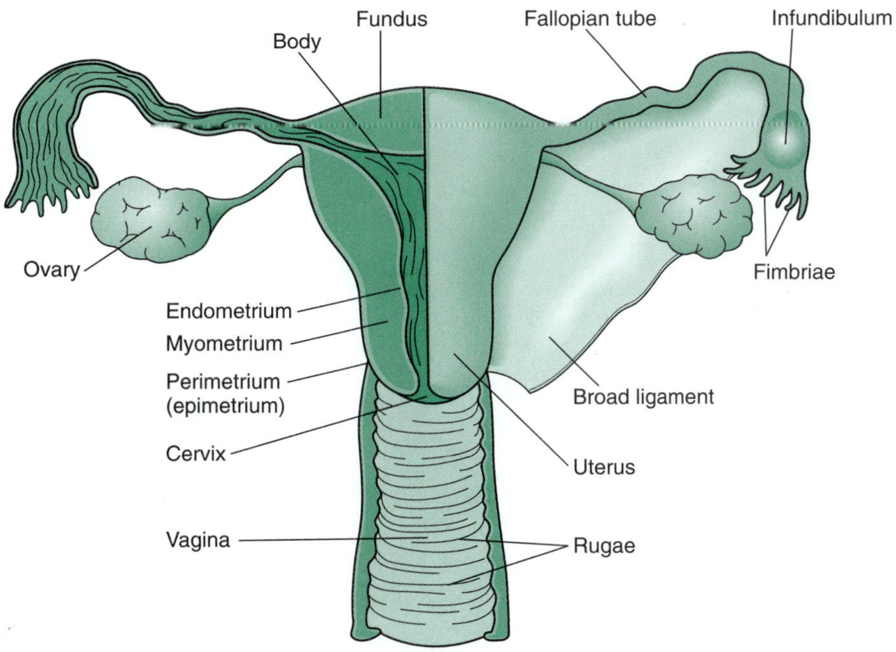

Figure 1-21 Female reproductive system.

Copyright © 2005, Elsevier Inc. All rights reserved.
CPT only © 2004. *Current Procedural Terminology, 2005, Professional Edition*, American Medical Association. All rights reserved.

Accessory Organs (Figure 1-22)

Breasts: mammary glands

Composed of glandular tissue containing milk glands/lactiferous ducts

In response to hormones, develop milk by means of lactiferous or milk ducts

Lactiferous ducts transfer milk to nipple

Nipple, surrounded by areola

Menstruation and Pregnancy

Proliferation Phase

Menstruation (Days 1–5): discharge of blood fluid containing endometrial cells, blood cells, and glandular secretions from endometrium
Endometrium repair (Days 6–12): begins by means of estrogen (hormone) and during which endometrium thickens and the ovum (egg) matures in graafian follicles

Secretory Phase

Ovulation (Days 13–14): occurs when the graafian follicles rupture and ovum travels down fallopian tube
Premenstruation (Days 15–28): a period of time in which graafian follicles fill with corpus luteum and secrete estrogen and progesterone to stimulate build up of uterine lining. If after 5 days no fertilization occurs, cycle repeats

Pregnancy

- Prenatal stage of development from fertilization to birth (39 weeks)
- Fertilized ovum or zygote develops in a double cavity: yolk sac (produces blood cells) and amniotic cavity (contains amniotic fluid)
- Embryo, fertilized ovum
- Fetus, unborn offspring, 9 weeks until birth

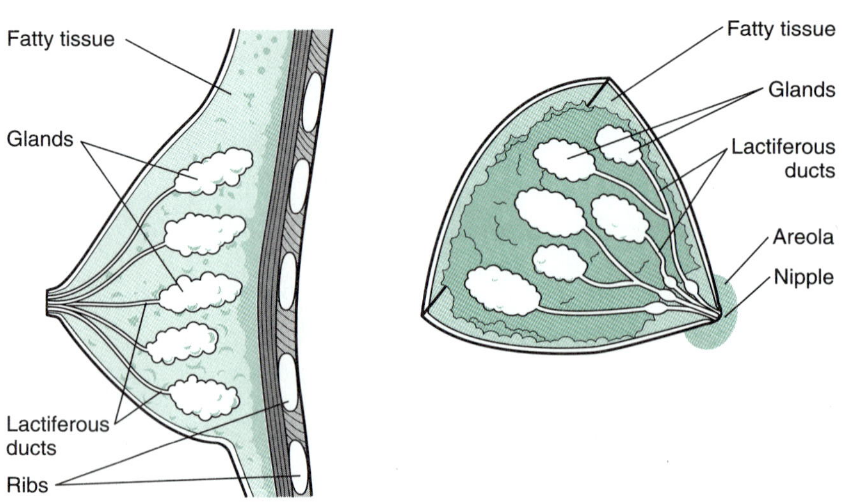

Figure 1-22 Breast structure.

Copyright © 2005, Elsevier Inc. All rights reserved.
CPT only © 2004. *Current Procedural Terminology, 2005, Professional Edition,* American Medical Association. All rights reserved.

Placenta Forms Within Uterine Wall and Produces Hormone—Human Chorionic Gonadotropin (HCG)

- HCG stimulates corpus luteum to produce estrogen and progesterone for several months
- Placenta then produces hormones
- Expelled after delivery (afterbirth)

Gestation, Approximately 266 Days

- 280 days used when calculating Estimated Date of Delivery (EDD) or that time from last menstrual period (LMP)
- Three trimesters

First	LMP-12 weeks
Second	13-27 weeks
Third	28 weeks-EDD

COMBINING FORMS

1. amni/o	amnion
2. arche/o	first
3. cephal/o	head
4. cervic/o	cervix
5. chori/o	chorion
6. colp/o	vagina
7. crypt/o	hidden
8. culd/o	cul-de-sac
9. episi/o	vulva
10. fet/o	fetus
11. galact/o	milk
12. gynec/o	female
13. gyn/o	female
14. hymen/o	hymen
15. hyster/o	uterus
16. lact/o	milk
17. lapar/o	abdominal wall
18. mamm/o	breast
19. mast/o	breast
20. men/o	menstruation, month
21. metr/o	uterus, measure
22. metri/o	uterus
23. my/o, muscul/o	muscle
24. nat/a	birth

Copyright © 2005, Elsevier Inc. All rights reserved.
CPT only © 2004. *Current Procedural Terminology, 2005, Professional Edition,* American Medical Association. All rights reserved.

25. nati/i birth
26. olig/o few
27. oo/o egg
28. oopho/o ovary
29. ov/o egg
30. ovari/o ovary
31. ovul/o ovulation
32. perine/o perineum
33. peritone/o peritoneum
34. salping/o uterine tube
35. top/o place
36. uter/o uterus
37. vagin/o vagina
38. vulv/o vulva

PREFIXES

1. ante- before
2. dys- painful
3. ecto- outside
4. endo- in
5. extra- outside
6. in- into
7. intra- within
8. multi- many
9. neo- new
10. nulli- none
11. nulti- none
12. post- after
13. primi- first
14. pseudo- false
15. retro- backwards
16. uni- one

SUFFIXES

1. -arche beginning
2. -cyesis pregnancy
3. -gravida pregnancy
4. -o/rrhexis rupture

Copyright © 2005, Elsevier Inc. All rights reserved.
CPT only © 2004. *Current Procedural Terminology, 2005, Professional Edition,* American Medical Association. All rights reserved.

5. -para woman who has given birth
6. -parous to bear
7. -rrhea discharge
8. -tocia labor
9. -version turning

MEDICAL ABBREVIATIONS

1. AFI amniotic fluid index
2. AGA appropriate for gestational age
3. ARM artificial rupture of membrane
4. BPD biparietal diameter
5. BPP biophysical profile
6. BV bacterial vaginosis
7. CHL crown-to-heel length
8. CNM certified nurse midwife
9. CPD cephalopelvic disproportion
10. CPP chronic pelvic pain
11. D&C dilation and curettage
12. D&E dilation and evacuation
13. DUB dysfunctional uterine bleeding
14. ECC endocervical curettage
15. EDC estimated date of confinement
16. EDD estimated date of delivery
17. EFM electronic fetal monitoring
18. EFW estimated fetal weight
19. EGA estimated gestational age
20. EMC endometrial curettage
21. ERT estrogen replacement therapy
22. FAS fetal alcohol syndrome
23. FHR fetal heart rate
24. FSH follicle-stimulating hormone
25. HPV human papillomavirus
26. HSG hysterosalpingogram
27. HSV herpes simplex virus
28. IVF in vitro fertilization
29. LEEP loop electrosurgical excision procedure
30. LGA large for gestational age

Copyright © 2005, Elsevier Inc. All rights reserved.
CPT only © 2004. *Current Procedural Terminology, 2005, Professional Edition,* American Medical Association. All rights reserved.

31. PID pelvic inflammatory disease
32. PROM premature rupture of membranes
33. SHG sonohysterogram
34. SROM spontaneous rupture of membrane
35. SUI stress urinary incontinence
36. TAH total abdominal hysterectomy
37. VBAC vaginal birth after cesarean

MEDICAL TERMS

Abortion	Termination of pregnancy
Amniocentesis	Percutaneous aspiration of amniotic fluid
Amniotic sac	Sac containing the fetus and amniotic fluid
Antepartum	Before childbirth
Cesarean	Surgical opening through abdominal wall for delivery
Chorionic villus sampling	CVS, biopsy of the outermost part of the placenta
Cordocentesis	Procedure to obtain a fetal blood sample; also called a percutaneous umbilical blood sampling
Curettage	Scraping of a cavity using a spoon-shaped instrument
Cystocele	Herniation of the bladder into the vagina
Delivery	Childbirth
Dilation	Expansion (of the cervix)
Ectopic	Pregnancy outside the uterus (i.e., in the fallopian tube)
Hysterectomy	Surgical removal of the uterus
Hysterorrhaphy	Suturing of the uterus
Hysteroscopy	Visualization of the canal and cavity of the uterus using a scope placed through the vagina
Introitus	Opening or entrance to the vagina from the uterus
Ligation	Binding or tying off, as in constricting the blood flow of a vessel or binding fallopian tubes for sterilization
Oophorectomy	Surgical removal of the ovary(ies)
Perineum	Area between the vulva and anus; also known as the pelvic floor
Placenta	A structure that connects the fetus and mother during pregnancy
Postpartum	After childbirth
Salpingectomy	Surgical removal of the uterine tube
Salpingostomy	Creation of a fistula into the uterine tube
Tocolysis	Repression of uterine contractions
Vesicovaginal fistula	Creation of a tube between the vagina and the bladder

Copyright © 2005, Elsevier Inc. All rights reserved.
CPT only © 2004. *Current Procedural Terminology, 2005, Professional Edition*, American Medical Association. All rights reserved.

FEMALE GENITAL SYSTEM AND PREGNANCY QUIZ

1. This is NOT one of the three layers of the uterus:
   a. perimetrium
   b. endometrium
   c. myometrium
   d. epimetrium

2. The lower portion of the uterus is the:
   a. cervix
   b. vagina
   c. perineum
   d. labia majora

3. The approximate gestation of a human fetus is:
   a. 266 days
   b. 276 days
   c. 290 days
   d. 292 days

4. The LMP is the:
   a. later maternity phase
   b. last menstrual period
   c. low metabolic pregnancy
   d. late menstruation phase

5. Name of the stage that describes the development of the fetus from fertilization to birth is the:
   a. postpartum
   b. antepartum
   c. prenatal
   d. natal

6. Which of the following correctly identifies the three trimesters of gestation:
   a. LMP-12 weeks, 13-27 weeks, 28-EDD
   b. LMP-14 weeks, 15-27 weeks, 28-EDD
   c. LMP-14 weeks, 15-28 weeks, 29-EDD
   d. LMP-11 weeks, 12-26 weeks, 27-EDD

7. Combining form means few:
   a. oopho/o
   b. olig/o
   c. nati/i
   d. top/o

8. Combining form means hidden:
   a. amni/o
   b. crypt/o
   c. chori/o
   d. fet/o

Copyright © 2005, Elsevier Inc. All rights reserved.
CPT only © 2004. *Current Procedural Terminology, 2005, Professional Edition*, American Medical Association. All rights reserved.

9. Suffix means the beginning:
   a. -cyesis
   b. -rrhea
   c. -arche
   d. -orrhexis

10. Prefix meaning within:
   a. ante-
   b. dys-
   c. ecto-
   d. endo-

Copyright © 2005, Elsevier Inc. All rights reserved.
CPT only © 2004. *Current Procedural Terminology, 2005, Professional Edition*, American Medical Association. All rights reserved.

FEMALE GENITAL SYSTEM AND PREGNANCY—PATHOPHYSIOLOGY

Menstrual and Hormonal Disorders

Dysmenorrhea

Painful menstruation

- Types are primary and secondary

Primary dysmenorrhea

- No underlying condition but begins with commencement of ovulation
- Cramping is caused by excess of prostaglandin
  - Causes contractions and ischemia
  - Develops 24 to 48 hours prior to menstruation
- Treatment
  - Nonsteroidal antiinflammatory agents
  - Progesterone

Secondary dysmenorrhea

- Caused by an underlying disorder, such as:
  - Polyps
  - Tumors
  - Endometriosis
  - Pelvic inflammatory disease
- Treatment
  - Directed at underlying disorder

Amenorrhea

Amenorrhea is the absence of menstruation

- Types are primary and secondary

Primary amenorrhea

- Menstruation has never occurred
- May be genetic disorder:
  - Turner's syndrome (ovaries do not function)

Secondary amenorrhea

- Cessation of menstruation
  - Individual has previously menstruated
  - Examples of causes:
    - Tumors
    - Stress
    - Eating disorders
    - Competitive sports participation

Copyright © 2005, Elsevier Inc. All rights reserved.
CPT only © 2004. *Current Procedural Terminology, 2005, Professional Edition*, American Medical Association. All rights reserved.

Dysfunctional uterine bleeding (DUB)

- Abnormal bleeding from the uterus
- Occurs when no organic cause can be identified

Abnormal menstruation types:

- Oligomenorrhea: in excess of 6 weeks between periods
- Polymenorrhea: less than 3 weeks between periods
- Metrorrhagia: bleeding between cycles
- Menorrhagia: increase in amount and duration of flow
- Hypomenorrhea: light or spotty flow
- Menometrorrhagia: irregular cycle with varying amounts and duration

Premenstrual syndrome (PMS)

Also known as premenstrual tension (PMT)

Occurs before onset of menses (luteal phase) and ends at onset of menses

Cluster of common symptoms, such as:

- Weight gain
- Breast tenderness
- Sleep disturbances
- Headache
- Irritability

Cause is unknown

Treatments vary depending on individual symptoms

Endometriosis

Endometrial tissue develops outside the uterus

Responses to hormone cycle

- Ectopic (out of place) endometrial tissue degenerates, sheds, and bleeds
- Causes irritation, inflammation, and pain
- Continued cycles produce fibrous tissue
    - Adhesions and obstructions can then form
    - Interferes with normal bodily function
    - For example, fallopian tube endometriosis may lead to obstructed tubes

Primary symptom is dysmenorrhea
- May also cause painful intercourse (dyspareunia)

Risks

- Increased risk for cancers of:
    - Breast
    - Ovaries
    - Non-Hodgkin lymphoma

Copyright © 2005, Elsevier Inc. All rights reserved.
CPT only © 2004. *Current Procedural Terminology, 2005, Professional Edition*, American Medical Association. All rights reserved.

Treatment includes

- Hormonal suppression
- Surgical removal of endometrial tissue
    - May require hysterectomy and BSO (bilateral salpingo-oophorectomy)

Infection, Inflammation, and Sexually Transmitted Diseases

Pelvic inflammatory disease (PID)

Infection of the reproductive tract

- Primarily ovaries and fallopian tubes
- Usually originates in cervix or vagina
    - Migrates up through the reproductive tract

Types

- Acute
- Chronic

Commonly forms adhesions and strictures

- May lead to infertility

Candidiasis

Yeast infection

- *Candida albicans (Monilia)*

Not sexually transmitted

Opportunistic infection that may follow

- Infection treated with antibiotics
- Period of reduced resistance
- Increased glucose or glycogen levels

Affects the mucous membranes

Produces a white, thick, curd-type discharge

Result may be dyspareunia and dysuria

Treatment

- Antifungal substances such as nystatin
- Identification and treatment of underlying condition

Chlamydia

Most common sexually transmitted disease (STD)

Cause

- Bacteria, chlamydia *(Chlamydia trachomatis)*

Symptoms

- Asymptomatic or mild discharge and dysuria

Copyright © 2005, Elsevier Inc. All rights reserved.
CPT only © 2004. *Current Procedural Terminology, 2005, Professional Edition*, American Medical Association. All rights reserved.

Treatment

- Antimicrobial

Genital herpes

Cause

- Virus, herpes simplex 2 (HSV-2)

Symptoms

- Ulcers and vesicles

Treatment

- Antiviral, manage outbreaks
- There is no cure for genital herpes

Genital warts

Cause

- Virus, human papillomavirus

Symptoms

- Polyps or grey lesions

Treatment

- Excision
- There is no cure for genital warts

Gonorrhea

Cause

- Bacteria, *Neisseria gonorrhoeae*
- Some strains are drug-resistant

Symptoms

- Dysuria
- Discharge

Treatment

- Antibacterial drugs

Syphilis

Cause

- Bacteria, *Treponema pallidum*

Copyright © 2005, Elsevier Inc. All rights reserved.
CPT only © 2004. *Current Procedural Terminology, 2005, Professional Edition*, American Medical Association. All rights reserved.

Symptoms

- Primary syphilis
    - Ulcer or chancre at site of entry
- Secondary syphilis
    - Headache
    - Fever
    - Rash

Treatment

- Penicillin

Trichomoniasis

Cause

- Protozoa, *Trichomonas vaginalis*

Symptoms

- Usually asymptomatic

Treatment

- Antimicrobial drugs

Benign Lesions

Leiomyomas

Well-defined, solid uterine tumor

Also known as:

- Uterine fibroids
- Fibromyoma
- Fibroma
- Myoma
- Fibroid

Classification is based on location of tumor within the uterine wall

- Submucous = beneath endometrium
- Subserous = beneath serosa
- Intramural = in muscle wall

Symptoms

- May be asymptomatic
- Abnormal uterine bleeding
- Pressure on nearby structures, such as bladder and rectum
- Constipation
- Pain
- Sensation of heaviness

Copyright © 2005, Elsevier Inc. All rights reserved.
CPT only © 2004. *Current Procedural Terminology, 2005, Professional Edition*, American Medical Association. All rights reserved.

Treatment

- Surgical excision of lesions
- Hysterectomy may be necessary

Adenomyosis

Within uterine myometrium

Symptoms

- Usually asymptomatic
- Abnormal menstrual bleeding
- Enlarged uterus

Treatment

- Symptomatic in mild cases
- Surgical in severe cases
  - Excision of adenomyosis or hysterectomy

Malignant Lesions

Carcinoma of the breast

Accessory of reproductive system

Most often develops in upper outer quadrant
- Due to location, often spread to lymph nodes
- May metastasize to lungs, brain, bone, liver, etc.

Majority arise from epithelial cells of ducts and lobules

Second most common cancer of women

Most are adenocarcinoma
- Invasive ductal carcinoma most common type
- Invasive lobular carcinoma second most common type

Increased risks

- Heredity
  - Especially history of mother or sister that developed breast cancer
  - Mutated breast cancer gene (BRCA-1)
  - Familial breast cancer syndrome associated with BRCA-2
- Lower socioeconomic status
- Residence in Western developed country
- Race
- History of proliferating breast disease
- Late menopause
- Obesity
- High alcohol intake
- Exposure to estrogen
- Nulliparity (no viable birth)

Copyright © 2005, Elsevier Inc. All rights reserved.
CPT only © 2004. *Current Procedural Terminology, 2005, Professional Edition*, American Medical Association. All rights reserved.

- Delay of first viable birth
- Radiation exposure

Symptoms

- Painless, hard nodule
  - Moves freely in early stages
  - Fixed in more advanced stages

Treatment

- Surgical
  - Lumpectomy
  - Mastectomy with or without axillary node
- Irradiation
- Chemotherapy
- Combination of above
- If neoplasm is responsive to hormone, hormone-blocking agents are administered

Carcinoma of the uterus (endometrial cancer)

Most frequent pelvic cancer

Usually postmenopausal

Associated with higher levels of estrogen

Increases risk

- Obesity
- Early menarche
- Delayed menopause
- Hypertension
- Diabetes mellitus
- Nulliparity (no viable births)
- Some types of colorectal cancer
- Oral contraceptives

Symptoms

- Abnormal, excessive uterine bleeding
- Postmenopausal bleeding
- No simple screening test available
  - Uterine cells may be aspirated for evaluation

Staging of endometrial, cervical, and ovarian malignancies

- I Confined to corpus
- II Involves corpus and cervix
- III Extends outside uterus but not outside true pelvis
- IV Extends outside the true pelvis or involves rectum or bladder

Copyright © 2005, Elsevier Inc. All rights reserved.
CPT only © 2004. *Current Procedural Terminology, 2005, Professional Edition*, American Medical Association. All rights reserved.

Treatment

- Pharmaceutical
- Surgical
- Irradiation
- Chemotherapy
- Combination of above

Carcinoma of the cervix

Routinely found on Papanicolaou smear

Dysplasia is an early change in cervical epithelium

Increases risks:

- Herpes simplex virus type 2 (HSV-2)
- Human papillomavirus (HPV)
- Young age of sexual activity
- Smoking
- Lower socioeconomic status

Symptoms

- Early stages asymptomatic
- Later stages
    - Bleeding
    - Discharge
- Biopsy is used to confirm

Treatment

- Pharmaceutical
- Surgical
- Irradiation
- Chemotherapy
- Combination of above

Carcinoma of the ovary

Cause is unknown

Increased risks

- Genetic factors
- Endocrine
    - Nulliparous
    - Early menarche
    - Late menopause
    - Non-breast feeding
    - Late first pregnancy
    - Postmenopausal estrogen replacement therapy (ERT)

Copyright © 2005, Elsevier Inc. All rights reserved.
CPT only © 2004. *Current Procedural Terminology, 2005, Professional Edition*, American Medical Association. All rights reserved.

Tumor categories

- Germ cell tumors
  - Arise from primitive germ cells, usually the testis and ovum
- Types
  - Germinoma
  - Yolk sac
  - Endodermal sinus tumor
  - Teratoma
  - Embryonal carcinoma
  - Polyembryoma
  - Gonadoblastoma
  - Some types of choriocarcinoma
- Categories
  - Dermoid cysts (benign)
  - Malignant tumors
  - Primitive malignant
    - Embryonic
    - Extraembryonic cells
- Epithelial tumors
  - Most common gynecologic cancer
- Gonadal stromal tumors
- Symptoms
  - Pelvic heaviness
  - Dysuria
  - Increased urinary frequency
  - Sometimes vaginal bleeding
- Treatment
  - Excision
  - Hysterectomy, including bilateral salpingo-oophorectomy with omentectomy (fold of peritoneum)
  - Chemotherapy
  - Radiation therapy
  - Combination of above

Carcinoma of the fallopian tubes

Primary fallopian tube tumors

- Rare
- Must be located within the tube to be considered primary
  - Adenocarcinoma most common primary tumor
- Most tumors are secondary

Symptoms

- Often asymptomatic
- Bleeding or discharge
- Irregular menstruation
- Pain

Copyright © 2005, Elsevier Inc. All rights reserved.
CPT only © 2004. *Current Procedural Terminology, 2005, Professional Edition*, American Medical Association. All rights reserved.

Treatment

- Hysterectomy, including bilateral salpingo-oophorectomy with any necessary omentectomy (fold of peritoneum)
- Chemotherapy
- Radiation therapy
- Combination of above

Carcinoma of the vulva

Usually squamous cell carcinoma (90%)

Increased risk with STDs

Symptoms

- Can be asymptomatic
- Pruritic valvular lesion

Treatment

- Radical vulvectomy with node dissection
- Wide local excision

Carcinoma of the vagina

Usually squamous cell carcinoma

Increased risk

- Human papillomavirus (HPV)
- Postmenopausal hysterectomy
- History of abnormal Pap
- History of other carcinomas

Symptoms

- Often asymptomatic
- Vaginal pain, discharge, or bleeding

Treatment

- Squamous cell—radiation
- Early tumors may be excised
- Vaginectomy
- Hysterectomy
- Lymph node dissection

Pregnancy

Placenta previa

Opening of the cervix is obstructed by displaced placenta

Copyright © 2005, Elsevier Inc. All rights reserved.
CPT only © 2004. *Current Procedural Terminology, 2005, Professional Edition,* American Medical Association. All rights reserved.

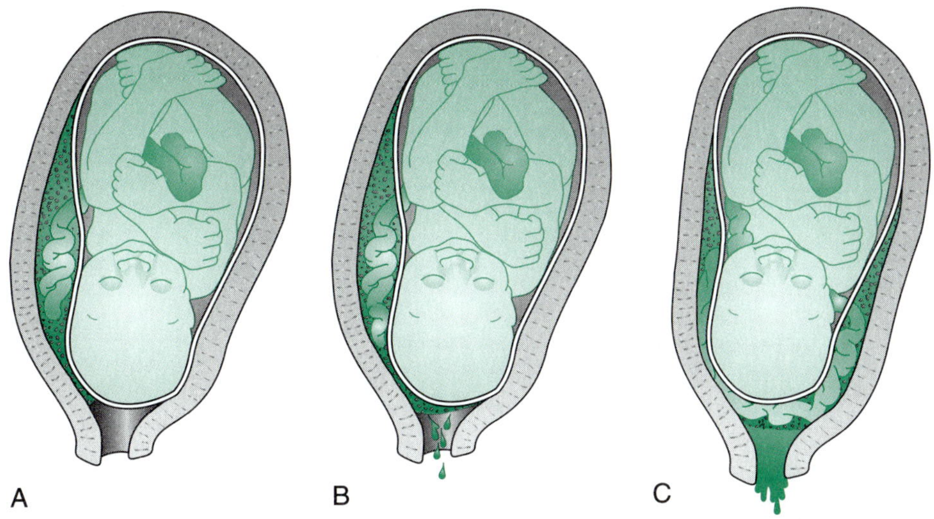

Figure 1-23 *A.* Marginal placenta previa. *B.* Partial placenta previa. *C.* Total placenta previa

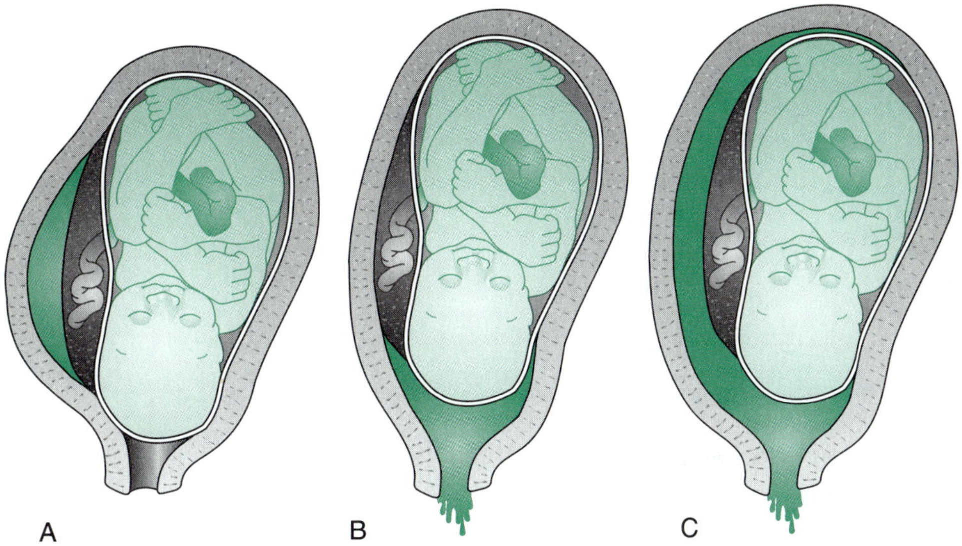

Figure 1-24 Abruptio placentae is classified according to the grade of separation of the placenta from the uterine wall. *A.* Mild separation in which hemorrhage is internal. *B.* Moderate separation in which there is external hemorrhage. *C.* Severe separation in which there is external hemorrhage and extreme separation.

Types (Figure 1-23)

- Marginal
- Partial
- Total

Abruptio placentae (Figure 1-24)

Premature separation of placenta from uterine wall

Eclampsia

Serious condition of pregnancy characterized by

- Hypertension
- Edema
- Proteinuria

Copyright © 2005, Elsevier Inc. All rights reserved.
CPT only © 2004. *Current Procedural Terminology, 2005, Professional Edition,* American Medical Association. All rights reserved.

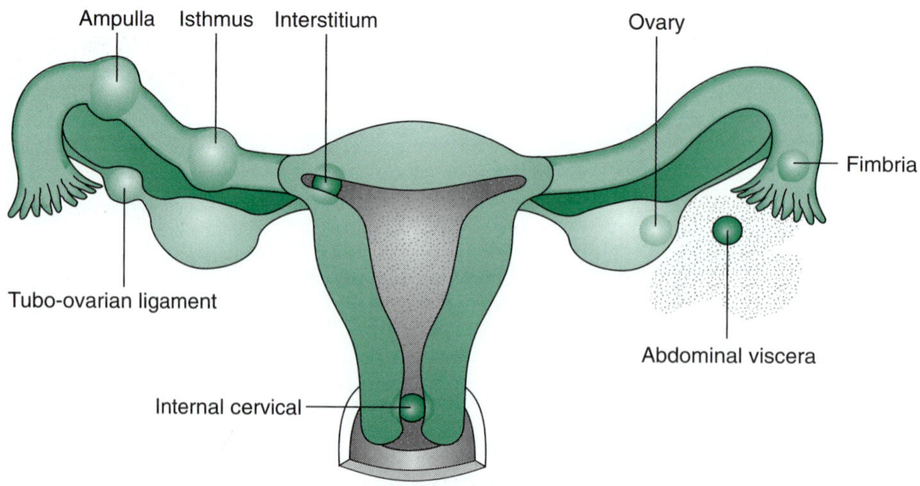

Figure 1-25 Ectopic pregnancy most often occurs in the fallopian tube. Pregnancy outside the uterus may end in life-threatening rupture.

Ectopic pregnancy (Figure 1-25)

Implantation of fertilized ovum outside uterus
- Often fallopian tubes

Hydatidiform mole

- Benign tumor of placenta
- Secretes hormone (chorionic gonadotropic hormone, CGH)
- Indicates positive pregnancy test

Malpositions and malpresentations (Figure 1-26)

- Breech
- Vertex
- Face
- Brow
- Shoulder

Abortion

Types

- Spontaneous
  - Miscarriage
  - Happens naturally
  - Uterus completely empties
- Incomplete
  - Uterus does not completely empty
  - Requires intervention to remove remaining fetal material
- Missed
  - Fetus dies naturally
  - Requires intervention to remove fetal material

Copyright © 2005, Elsevier Inc. All rights reserved.
CPT only © 2004. *Current Procedural Terminology, 2005, Professional Edition,* American Medical Association. All rights reserved.

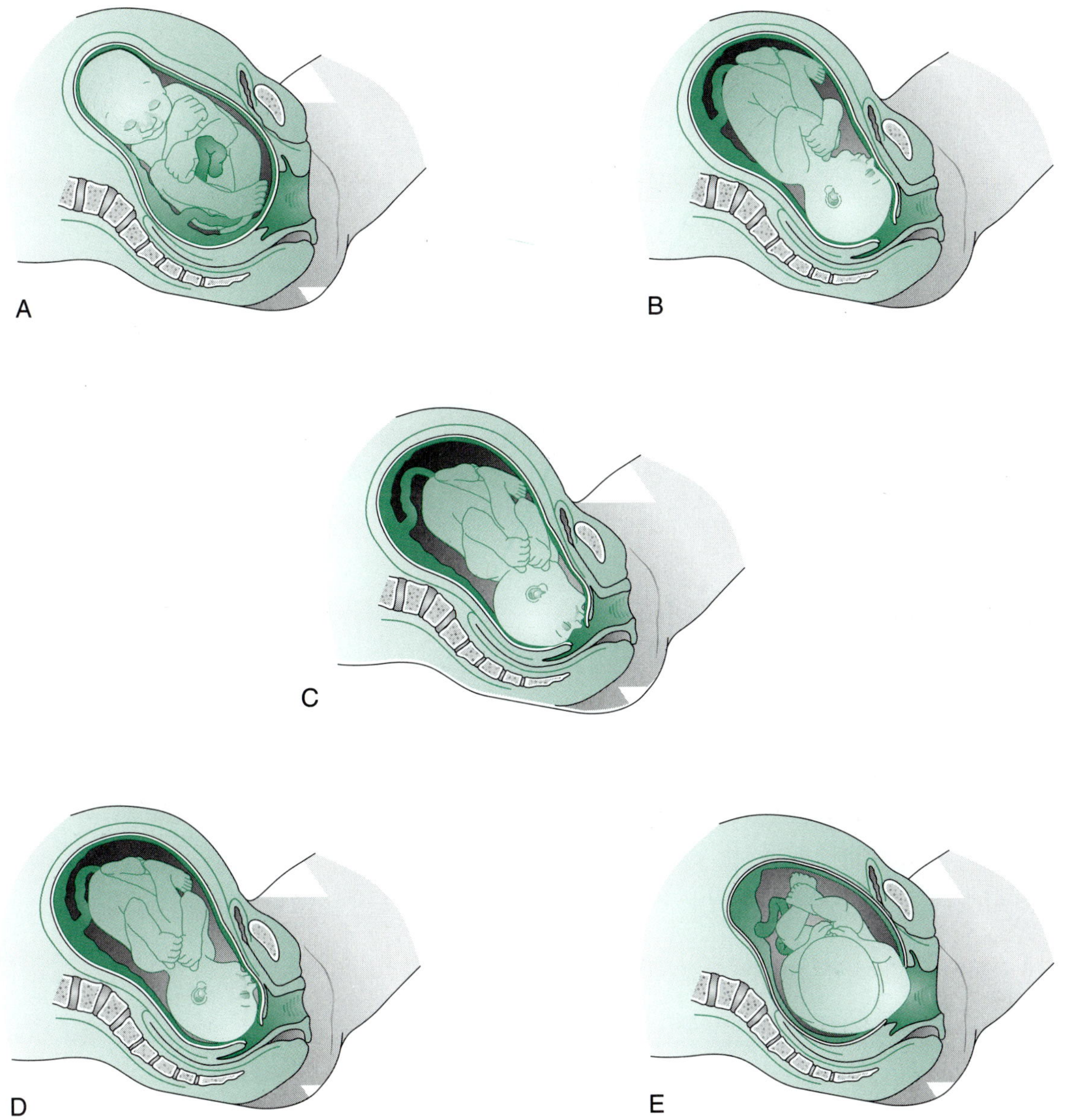

Figure 1-26 Five types of malposition and malpresentation of the fetus: *A.* Breech. *B.* Vertex. *C.* Face. *D.* Brow. *E.* Shoulder.

- Septic
  - Similar to missed
  - Has added complication of infection
  - Requires intervention to remove fetal material
  - Vigorous treatment of infection

Methods

- D&C
  - Dilation and curettage (scraping)
- Evacuation (suction)

Copyright © 2005, Elsevier Inc. All rights reserved.
CPT only © 2004. *Current Procedural Terminology, 2005, Professional Edition*, American Medical Association. All rights reserved.

- Intra-amniotic injections
  - Saline (salt) solution
- Vaginal suppositories
  - Such as prostaglandin

Copyright © 2005, Elsevier Inc. All rights reserved.
CPT only © 2004. *Current Procedural Terminology, 2005, Professional Edition*, American Medical Association. All rights reserved.

FEMALE GENITAL SYSTEM AND PREGNANCY PATHOPHYSIOLOGY QUIZ

1. The most common solution used for intra-amniotic injections is _______.
   a. prostaglandin
   b. saline
   c. estrogen
   d. chorionic gonadotropic hormone

2. This type of dysmenorrhea is treated with nonsteroidal antiinflammatory agents and progesterone.
   a. secondary
   b. constrictive
   c. periodic
   d. primary

3. In this type of amenorrhea there is a cessation of menstruation.
   a. secondary
   b. constrictive
   c. periodic
   d. primary

Match the abnormal menstruation type with the correct definition

4. oligomenorrhea _______ a. increased amount and duration of flow
5. metrorrhagia _______ b. bleeding between cycles
6. menorrhagia _______ c. in excess of 6 weeks

7. Increased risks of breast cancer, ovarian cancer, and non-Hodgkin lymphoma exist with this condition.
   a. endometriosis
   b. pelvic inflammatory disease
   c. sexually transmitted disease
   d. dysfunctional uterine bleeding

8. This benign lesion is also known as uterine fibroids.
   a. adenomyosis
   b. squamous cell
   c. leiomyoma
   d. extraembryonic cell primitive

9. Marginal, partial, and total are the types of this condition.
   a. abruptio placentae
   b. placenta previa
   c. ectopic pregnancy
   d. hydatidiform mole

10. Which of the following is NOT a malposition of fetus.
    a. breech
    b. shoulder
    c. back
    d. brow

Copyright © 2005, Elsevier Inc. All rights reserved.
CPT only © 2004. *Current Procedural Terminology, 2005, Professional Edition,* American Medical Association. All rights reserved.

MALE GENITAL SYSTEM

- Function, reproduction
- Structure, essential organs, and accessory organs (Figure 1-27)

Essential Organs

Testes (Gonads)

Produce sperm (male gamete)

Covered by tunica albuginea, located in scrotum

Produce testosterone

Vas Deferens

Is a tube

End of epididymis

Accessory Organs

- Ducts (carry sperm from testes to exterior), sex glands (produce solutions that mix with sperm), and external genitalia
- Seminal vesicles produce most seminal fluid
- Prostate gland produces some seminal fluid and activates sperm
- Bulbourethral gland (Cowper's glands) secretes a very small amount of seminal fluid
- External genitalia: penis and scrotum
  - Penis contains three columns of erectile tissue: two corpora cavernosa and one spongiosum
  - Scrotum encloses testes

COMBINING FORMS

1. andr/o male
2. balan/o glans penis

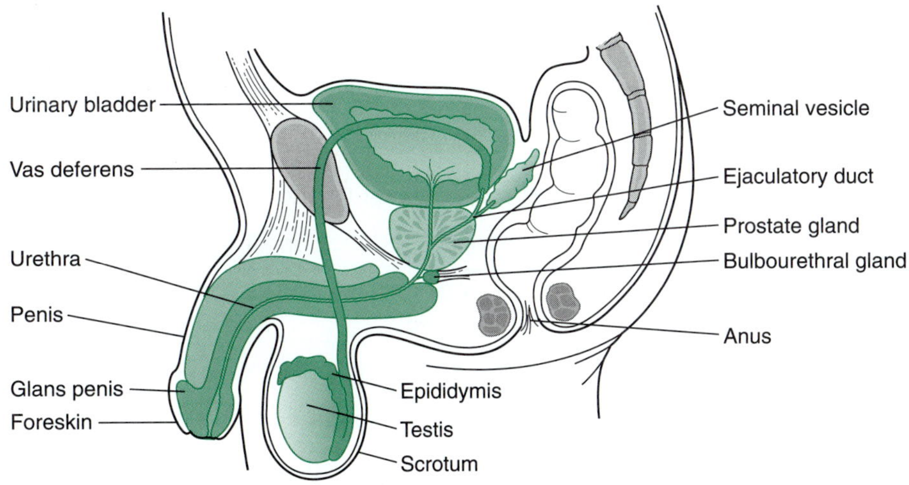

Figure 1-27 Male reproductive system.

Copyright © 2005, Elsevier Inc. All rights reserved.
CPT only © 2004. *Current Procedural Terminology, 2005, Professional Edition*, American Medical Association. All rights reserved.

3. epididym/o	epididymis
4. orch/i	testicle
5. orch/o	testicle
6. orchi/o	testicle
7. orchid/o	testicle
8. prostat/o	prostate gland
9. semin/i	semen
10. sperm/o	sperm
11. spermat/o	sperm
12. test/o	testicle
13. vas/o	vessel, vas deferens
14. vesicul/o	seminal vesicles

SUFFIXES

1. -one	hormone
2. -pexy	fixation

MEDICAL ABBREVIATIONS

1. BPH	benign prostatic hypertrophy
2. PSA	prostate-specific antigen
3. TURBT	transurethral resection of bladder tumor
4. TURP	transurethral resection of prostate

MEDICAL TERMS

Cavernosa	Connection between the cavity of the penis and a vein
Cavernosography	Radiographic recording of a cavity, e.g., the pulmonary cavity or the main part of the penis
Cavernosometry	Measurement of the pressure in a cavity, e.g., the penis
Chordee	Condition resulting in the penis being bent downward
Corpora cavernosa	The two cavities of the penis
Epididymectomy	Surgical removal of the epididymis
Epididymis	Tube located at the top of the testes that stores sperm
Epididymovasostomy	Creation of a new connection between the vas deferens and epididymis
Meatotomy	Surgical enlargement of the opening of the urinary meatus
Orchiectomy	Castration, removal of the testes
Orchiopexy	Surgical procedure to release undescended testis and fixate within the scrotum

Copyright © 2005, Elsevier Inc. All rights reserved.
CPT only © 2004. *Current Procedural Terminology, 2005, Professional Edition*, American Medical Association. All rights reserved.

Penoscrotal	Referring to the penis and scrotum
Plethysmography	Determining the changes in volume of an organ part or body
Priapism	Painful condition in which the penis is constantly erect
Prostatotomy	Incision into the prostate
Transurethral resection, prostate	Procedure performed through the urethra by means of a cystoscopy to remove part or all of the prostate
Tumescence	State of being swollen
Tunica vaginalis	Covering of testes
Varicocele	Swelling of a scrotal vein
Vas deferens	Tube that carries sperm from the epididymis to the urethra
Vasogram	Recording of the flow in the vas deferens
Vasotomy	Creation of an opening in the vas deferens
Vasovasorrhaphy	Suturing of the vas deferens
Vasovasostomy	Reversal of a vasectomy
Vesiculectomy	Excision of the seminal vesicle
Vesiculotomy	Incision into the seminal vesicle

Copyright © 2005, Elsevier Inc. All rights reserved.
CPT only © 2004. *Current Procedural Terminology, 2005, Professional Edition,* American Medical Association. All rights reserved.

MALE GENITAL SYSTEM QUIZ

1. This gland activates the sperm and produces some seminal fluid:
   a. seminal vesicle
   b. bulbourethral
   c. prostate gland
   d. scrotum

2. Carries the sperm from the testes to the exterior:
   a. duct
   b. sex gland
   c. tunica
   d. seminal

3. The penis contains these erectile tissues:
   a. one corpora cavernosa and two spongiosa
   b. two corpora cavernosa and two spongiosa
   c. one corpora cavernosa and one spongiosum
   d. two corpora cavernosa and one spongiosum

4. Also known as Cowper's gland:
   a. seminal vesicles
   b. bulbourethral
   c. prostate gland
   d. scrotum

5. Which of the following is NOT an accessory organ:
   a. gonads
   b. seminal vesicles
   c. prostate
   d. penis

6. Combining form meaning male:
   a. andr/o
   b. balan/o
   c. orchi/o
   d. test/o

7. Combining form meaning glans penis:
   a. balan/o
   b. vas/o
   c. vesicul/o
   d. orch/o

8. The testes are covered by the:
   a. seminal vesicles
   b. androgen
   c. chancre
   d. tunica albuginea

Copyright © 2005, Elsevier Inc. All rights reserved.
CPT only © 2004. *Current Procedural Terminology, 2005, Professional Edition*, American Medical Association. All rights reserved.

9. This abbreviation describes a surgical resection of the prostate that is accomplished by means of an endoscope inserted into the urethra:
   a. TURBT
   b. BPH
   c. UPJ
   d. TURP

10. This abbreviation describes a condition of the prostate in which there is an enlargement that is benign:
    a. TURBT
    b. BPH
    c. UPJ
    d. TURP

Copyright © 2005, Elsevier Inc. All rights reserved.
CPT only © 2004. *Current Procedural Terminology, 2005, Professional Edition*, American Medical Association. All rights reserved.

MALE GENITAL SYSTEM—PATHOPHYSIOLOGY

Male Genital System Disorders

Disorders of the scrotum, testes, and epididymis

Cryptorchidism

- Undescended testes
  - Unilateral or bilateral
  - Primarily result from obstruction
- Treatment
  - May descend spontaneously
  - Administration of hormone to stimulate testosterone production
  - Surgical intervention

Orchitis

- Inflammation of testes
- Most common cause is virus
  - Such as mumps orchitis
- May be associated with
  - Gonorrhea
  - Syphilis
  - Tuberculosis
- Symptoms
  - Mild to severe pain in testes
  - Mild to severe edema
  - Feeling of weight in testicular area
- Treatment
  - Depends upon presence of underlying condition

Epididymitis

Inflammation of epididymis

Inflammatory response to trauma or infection

Abscess may form

Types

- Sexually transmitted epididymitis
  - Gonorrhea
  - *T. pallidum*
  - *T. vaginalis*
- Nonspecific bacterial epididymitis
  - *E. coli*
  - Streptococci
  - Staphylococci
  - Associated with underlying urological disorder
- Symptoms
  - Scrotal pain
  - Swelling

Copyright © 2005, Elsevier Inc. All rights reserved.
CPT only © 2004. *Current Procedural Terminology, 2005, Professional Edition*, American Medical Association. All rights reserved.

- Erythema
- Perhaps hydrocele formation
- Treatment
  - Antibiotic
  - Bed rest
  - Ice packs
  - Scrotal support
  - Analgesics

Hydrocele (Figure 1-28)

Collection of fluid in membranes of tunica vaginalis

May be congenital or acquired

Congenital hydrocele may reabsorb due to a communication between the scrotal sac and peritoneal cavity and require no intervention

- Symptoms
  - Scrotal enlargement
  - Usually painless
    - Unless infection is present

Varicocele

Abnormal dilation of the plexus of veins in the spermatic cord leading to the scrotum

Decreases sperm production and motility

- Symptoms
  - Usually painless
  - In elderly, may signal renal tumor
- Treatment
  - Surgical intervention

Torsion of the testes (Figure 1-29)

Twisting of testes

Congenital abnormal development of the tunica vaginalis and spermatic cord

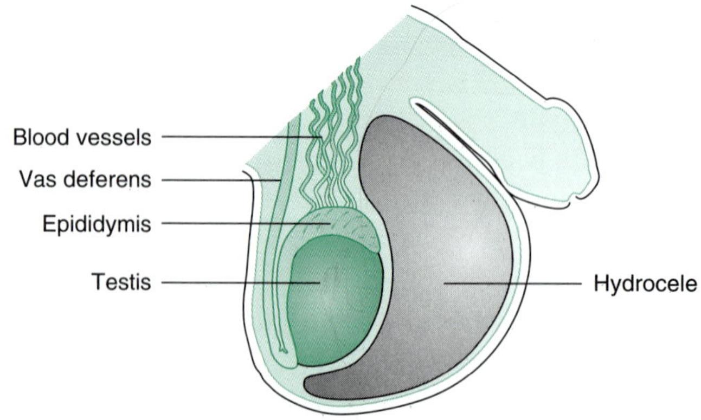

Figure 1-28 Hydrocele.

Copyright © 2005, Elsevier Inc. All rights reserved.
CPT only © 2004. *Current Procedural Terminology, 2005, Professional Edition*, American Medical Association. All rights reserved.

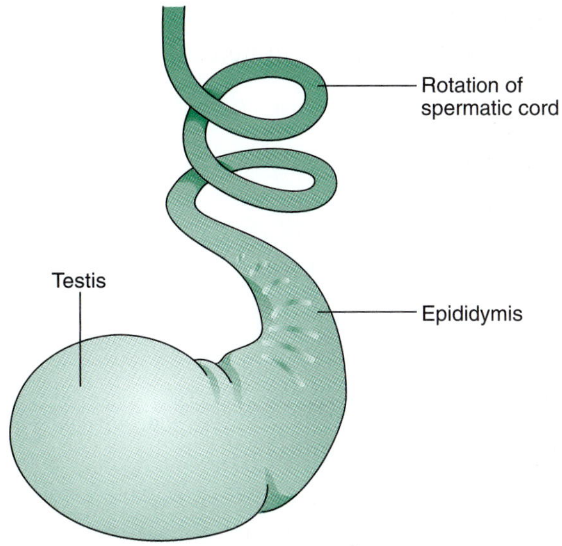

Figure 1-29 Torsion of testis.

Trauma may precipitate

- Symptoms
    - Sudden onset of severe pain
    - Nausea
    - Vomiting
    - Scrotal edema and tenderness
    - Fever
- Treatment
    - Immediate surgical intervention

Cancer of testes

Usually occurs in younger men

- Two main groups
    - Germ cell tumors (GCT)
    - Sex cord tumors

Cancer of scrotum

- Rare form of cancer
    - Squamous cell carcinoma
- Symptoms
    - Asymptomatic in early stages
    - Ulcerations in later stages
- Treatment
    - Wide local excision
    - Mohs' microscopic technique
        - Precise removal of tumor
        - Layers are removed until no further microscopic evidence of abnormal cells is seen

Copyright © 2005, Elsevier Inc. All rights reserved.
CPT only © 2004. *Current Procedural Terminology, 2005, Professional Edition*, American Medical Association. All rights reserved.

- Laser therapy
- Lymph nodes are examined for metastasis

Disorders of the urethra

Epispadias

Congenital anomaly

Urethral meatus is located on dorsal side of penis

Usually occurs in conjunction with other abnormalities

Treatment

- Surgical reconstruction

Hypospadias

- Most common abnormality of the penis
- Urethral opening on the ventral side of penis
- Results in curvature of penis
  - Due to chordee
- Treatment
  - Surgical reconstruction

Urethritis

Inflammation of urethra

Infectious urethritis can be gonococcal or nongonococcal

Nongonococcal organisms

- *C. trachomatis*
- *U. urealyticum*

- Symptoms
  - Discharge
  - Inflammation of meatus
  - Burning
  - Itching
  - Urgent and frequent urination
  - In nongonococcal, symptoms are less
- Treatment
  - Antibiotics based on organism

Disorders of the penis

Balanitis

Inflammation of the glans

- Causes
  - Syphilis
  - Trichomoniasis
  - Gonorrhea
  - *Candida albicans*
  - Tinea

Copyright © 2005, Elsevier Inc. All rights reserved.
CPT only © 2004. *Current Procedural Terminology, 2005, Professional Edition*, American Medical Association. All rights reserved.

    - Underlying disease
    - No circumcision
- Symptoms
    - Irritation
    - Tenderness
    - Discharge
    - Edema
    - Ulceration
    - Swelling of lymph nodes
- Treatment
    - Culture of discharge
    - Saline irrigation
    - Antibiotics

Phimosis and paraphimosis

Phimosis

Condition in which prepuce (foreskin) is constricted
    - Prepuce cannot be retracted over the glans penis

Can occur at any age

Associated with poor hygiene and chronic infection in uncircumcised males
- Symptoms
    - Erythema
    - Edema
    - Tenderness

Treatment
    - Surgical circumcision

Paraphimosis

Condition in which prepuce (foreskin) is constricted

Prepuce is retracted over glans penis and cannot be moved forward

Symptoms
    - Edema

Treatment
    - Surgical

Peyronie disease

Also known as bent nail syndrome

Fibrotic condition
    - Results in lateral curvature of penis during erection

Occurs most often in middle-aged men
- Cause is unknown but associated with
    - Diabetes
    - Keloid development
    - Dupuytren contracture (flexion deformity of toes and fingers)

Copyright © 2005, Elsevier Inc. All rights reserved.
CPT only © 2004. *Current Procedural Terminology, 2005, Professional Edition*, American Medical Association. All rights reserved.

- Treatment
  - Sometimes spontaneous remission
  - Pharmacologic oxygenation increasing therapies
  - Surgical resection of fibrous bands

Cancer of penis

Occurs most often in men over 60

- Increased risks
  - More common in uncircumcised men
  - Sexual partner with cervical carcinoma
  - Human papillomavirus
- Usually begins with small lesion beneath prepuce
- Intraepithelial neoplasia is also known as
  - Bowen's disease
  - Erythroplasia of Queyrat
  - Begins as noninvasive

Progresses to invasive if untreated

Metastasis to lymph nodes

- Treatment
  - Excision
  - Moh's micrographic technique
  - Radiation therapy
  - Laser therapy
  - Cryosurgery
  - Advanced tumors are treated with partial or total penectomy and chemotherapy

Disorders of the prostate gland

Benign prostatic hyperplasia (BPH)

Multiple fibroadenomatous nodules

  - Related to aging

- Growth compresses prostate
  - Prostate obstructs bladder neck and urethra
  - Decreases urine flow

It is thought that increased levels of estrogen/androgen cause BPH

- Symptoms
  - Increased frequency and urgency of urination
  - Nocturia
  - Incontinence
  - Hesitancy
  - Diminished force
  - Postvoiding dribble
- Screening
  - Prostate-specific antigen (PSA)
  - Digital rectal examination (DRE)

Copyright © 2005, Elsevier Inc. All rights reserved.
CPT only © 2004. *Current Procedural Terminology, 2005, Professional Edition,* American Medical Association. All rights reserved.

- Treatment
    - Partial prostatectomy
    - Transurethral resection of prostate (TURP)
    - Excision of nodules
    - Hormone therapy
    - Placement of urethral stents

Prostatitis

Inflammation of prostate

- Acute or chronic

- Causes

Bacterial

- *Escherichia coli*
- Enterococci
- Staphylococci
- Streptococci
- *Chlamydia trachomatis*
- *Ureaplasma urealyticum*
- *Neisseria gonorrhea*

Nonbacterial

- Spontaneous

- Symptoms

Acute prostatitis

- Fever and chills
- Lower back pain
- Perineal pain
- Dysuria
- Tenderness, suprapubic
- Urinary tract infection

Chronic prostatitis

- Same as acute only with no infection in urinary tract

- Treatment

Acute

- Antibiotic based on culture

Chronic

- No treatment available

Cancer of prostate

Indications are the cause is related to androgens

Predominately adenocarcinoma (95%)

No relationship between BPH and cancer of prostate

- Symptoms
    - Asymptomatic in early stages
    - Later symptoms include
        - Dysuria
        - Back pain

Copyright © 2005, Elsevier Inc. All rights reserved.
CPT only © 2004. *Current Procedural Terminology, 2005, Professional Edition*, American Medical Association. All rights reserved.

WHITMORE-JEWETT STAGES:

Stage A is clinically undetectable tumor confined to the gland and is an incidental finding at prostate surgery.
A1: well-differentiated with focal involvement
A2: moderately or poorly differentiated or involves multiple foci in the gland

Stage B is tumor confined to the prostate gland.
B0: nonpalpable, PSA-detected
B1: single nodule in one lobe of the prostate
B2: more extensive involvement of one lobe or involvement of both lobes

Stage C is a tumor clinically localized to the periprostatic area but extending through the prostatic capsule; seminal vesicles may be involved.
C1: clinical extracapsular extension
C2: extracapsular tumor producing bladder outlet or ureteral obstruction

Stage D is metastatic disease.
D0: clinically localized disease (prostate only) but persistently elevated enzymatic serum acid phosphatase
D1: regional lymph nodes only
D2: distant lymph nodes, metastases to bone or visceral organs
D3: D2 prostate cancer patients who relapse after adequate endocrine therapy

Figure 1-30 Whitmore-Jewett stages.

TNM STAGES:

Primary Tumor (T)

TX: Primary tumor cannot be assessed
T0: No evidence of primary tumor
T1: Clinically inapparent tumor not palpable or visible by imaging
- T1a: Tumor incidental histologic finding in 5% or less of tissue resected
- T1b: Tumor incidental histologic finding in more than 5% of tissue resected
- T1c: Tumor identified by needle biopsy (e.g., because of elevated PSA)

T2: Tumor confined within the prostate
- T2a: Tumor involves half a lobe or less
- T2b: Tumor involves more than half of a lobe, but not both lobes
- T2c: Tumor involves both lobes; extends through the prostatic capsule

T3a: Unilateral extracapsular extension
T3b: Bilateral extracapsular extension
T3c: Tumor invades the seminal vesicle(s)
T4: Tumor is fixed or invades adjacent structures other than the seminal vesicle(s)
- T4a: Tumor invades any of bladder neck, external sphincter, or rectum
- T4b: Tumor invades levator muscles and/or is fixed to the pelvic wall

Regional lymph nodes (N)

NX: Regional lymph nodes cannot be assessed
N0: No regional lymph node metastasis
N1: Metastasis in a single lymph node, 2 cm or less in greatest dimension
N2: Metastasis in a single lymph node, more than 2 cm but not more than 5 cm in greatest dimension; or multiple lymph node metastases, none more than 5 cm in greatest dimension
N3: Metastasis in a single lymph node more than 5 cm in greatest dimension

Distant metastases (M)

MX: Presence of distant metastasis cannot be assessed
M0: No distant metastasis
M1: Distant metastasis
- M1a: Nonregional lymph node(s)
- M1b: Bone(s)
- M1c: Other site(s)

Figure 1-31 TNM stages.

        - Hematuria
        - Frequent urination
        - Urinary retention
        - Increased incidence of uremia
- Stages
    - Two systems used to stage prostate cancer
        - Whitmore-Jewett stages as indicated in **Figure 1-30**
        - Tumor node metastasis (TNM) as indicated in **Figure 1-31**
- Treatment
    - Dependent upon stage

Copyright © 2005, Elsevier Inc. All rights reserved.
CPT only © 2004. *Current Procedural Terminology, 2005, Professional Edition,* American Medical Association. All rights reserved.

MALE GENITAL SYSTEM PATHOPHYSIOLOGY QUIZ

1. What is the condition in which the testes do not descend?
   a. cryptorchidism
   b. Bowen's disease
   c. torsion
   d. hypospadias

2. Orchitis is most often caused by a _______.
   a. bacteria
   b. virus
   c. parasite
   d. fungus

3. A condition that can be either congenital or acquired through trauma and that involves twisting of the testes is
   a. hydrocele
   b. hypospadias
   c. cryptorchidism
   d. torsion

4. Cancer of the _______ is divided into two main groups of germ cell tumors and sex cord tumors.
   a. testes
   b. penis
   c. scrotum
   d. prostate

5. This type of surgical technique involves excision of a lesion in layers until no further evidence of abnormality is seen.
   a. Bowen's
   b. Addison's
   c. Mohs'
   d. laser

6. Epispadias is a disorder of the urethra in which the urethral meatus is located on the _______ side of the penis.
   a. ventral
   b. dorsal
   c. lateral
   d. medial

7. Inflammation of the glans is _______.
   a. phimosis
   b. paraphimosis
   c. urethritis
   d. balanitis

8. This disease is also known as the bent nail syndrome.
   a. Bowen's
   b. Peyronie
   c. Addison's
   d. Whitmore-Jewett

Copyright © 2005, Elsevier Inc. All rights reserved.
CPT only © 2004. *Current Procedural Terminology, 2005, Professional Edition*, American Medical Association. All rights reserved.

9. The condition in which multiple fibroadenomatous nodules form and lead to decreased urine flow. The condition is thought to be related to increased levels of estrogen/androgen.
   a. BPH
   b. DRE
   c. GCT
   d. TNM

10. Cancer of the prostate is predominately this type of cancer.
   a. sex cord
   b. adenocarcinoma
   c. squamous cell
   d. seminoma

Copyright © 2005, Elsevier Inc. All rights reserved.
CPT only © 2004. *Current Procedural Terminology, 2005, Professional Edition,* American Medical Association. All rights reserved.

URINARY SYSTEM

- Removes waste materials
- Regulates fluid volume
- Maintains electrolytes, water, and acid balance
- Assists liver in detoxification

Organs (Figure 1-32)

Kidneys

Ureters

Urinary bladder

Urethra

Kidneys (Figure 1-33)

Electrolytes and fluid balance

Controls pH balance

Two organs located behind peritoneum (retroperitoneal space)

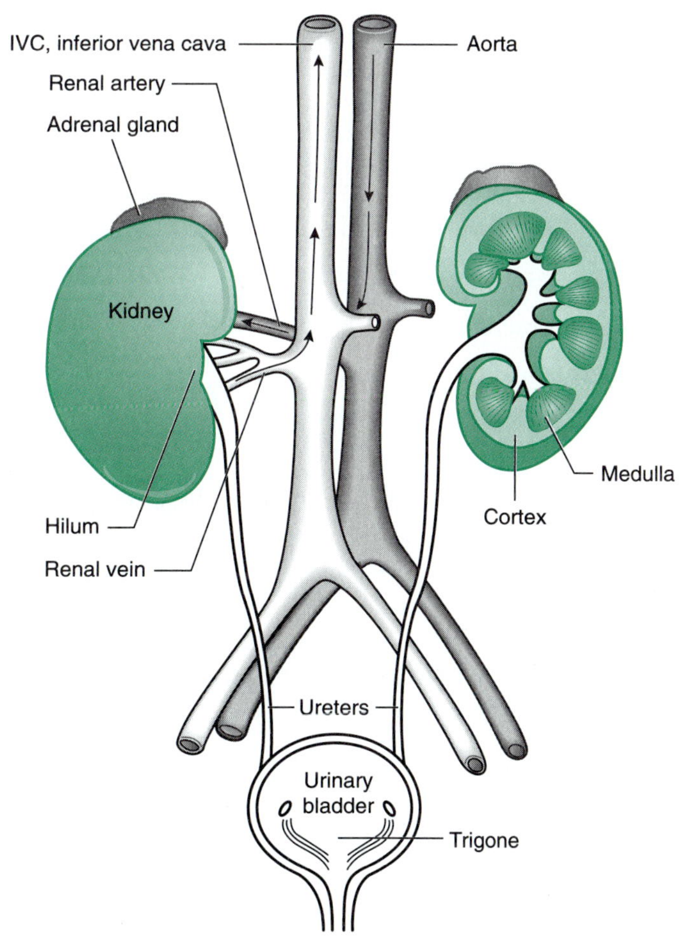

Figure 1-32 Urinary system.

Copyright © 2005, Elsevier Inc. All rights reserved.
CPT only © 2004. *Current Procedural Terminology, 2005, Professional Edition*, American Medical Association. All rights reserved.

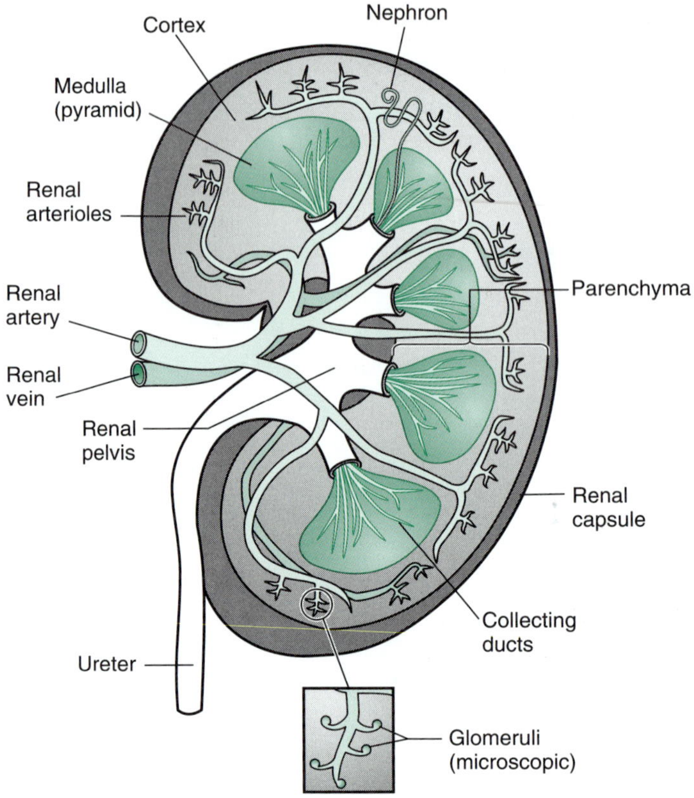

Figure 1-33 Kidney.

Cortex (outer layer)

Medulla (inner portion)

Pyramids (divisions of medulla)

Papilla (inner part of pyramids)

Pelvis (receptacle for urine within the kidney)

Calyces surround top of renal pelvis

Ureters

Narrow tubes connecting kidney and bladder

Urinary Bladder

Reservoir for urine

Shaped like an upside down pear with three surfaces

- Posterior (base)
- Anterior (neck)
- Superior (peritoneum)

Trigone

- Smooth area inside bladder
- Formed by openings of the ureters and urethra

Copyright © 2005, Elsevier Inc. All rights reserved.
CPT only © 2004. *Current Procedural Terminology, 2005, Professional Edition*, American Medical Association. All rights reserved.

Urethra

Canal from bladder to exterior of body

Urinary meatus, outside opening of the urethra

COMBINING FORMS

1. albumin/o	albumin
2. azot/o	urea
3. cyst/o	bladder
4. glomerul/o	glomerulus
5. glyc/o	sugar
6. glycos/o	sugar
7. hydr/o	water
8. lith/o	stone
9. meat/o	meatus
10. nephr/o	kidney
11. noct/i	night
12. olig/o	scant, few
13. pyel/o	renal pelvis
14. ren/o	kidney
15. son/o	sound
16. ur/o	urine
17. ureter/o	ureter
18. urethr/o	urethra
19. urin/o	urine
20. vesic/o	bladder

PREFIXES

1. dys-	painful
2. peri-	surrounding
3. poly-	many
4. retro-	behind

SUFFIXES

1. -eal	pertaining to
2. -lithiasis	condition of stones
3. -lysis	separation
4. -plasty	repair
5. -rrhaphy	suture
6. -tripsy	crush

Copyright © 2005, Elsevier Inc. All rights reserved.
CPT only © 2004. *Current Procedural Terminology, 2005, Professional Edition*, American Medical Association. All rights reserved.

MEDICAL ABBREVIATIONS

1. ARF	acute renal failure
2. BUN	blood urea nitrogen
3. ESRD	end-stage renal disease
4. HD	hemodialysis
5. IVP	intravenous pyelogram
6. KUB	kidney, ureter, bladder
7. pH	symbol for acid/base level
8. sp gr	specific gravity
9. UA	urinalysis
10. UPJ	ureteropelvic junction
11. UTI	urinary tract infection

MEDICAL TERMS

Bulbocavernosus	Muscle that constricts the vagina in a female and the urethra in a male
Bulbourethral	Gland with duct leading to the urethra
Calculus	Concretion of mineral salts, also called a stone
Calycoplasty	Surgical reconstruction of recess of renal pelvis
Calyx	Recess of renal pelvis
Cystolithectomy	Removal of a calculus (stone) from urinary bladder
Cystometrogram	CMG, measurement of the pressures and capacity of the urinary bladder
Cystoplasty	Surgical reconstruction of the bladder
Cystorrhaphy	Suture of the bladder
Cystoscopy	Use of a scope to view the bladder
Cystostomy	Surgical creation of an opening into the bladder
Cystotomy	Incision into the bladder
Cystourethroplasty	Surgical reconstruction of the bladder and urethra
Cystourethroscopy	Use of a scope to view the bladder and urethra
Dilation	Stretching or expansion
Dysuria	Painful urination
Endopyelotomy	Procedure involving the bladder and ureters, including the insertion of a stent into the renal pelvis
Extracorporeal	Occurring outside of the body
Fundoplasty	Repair of the bottom of the bladder
Hydrocele	Sac of fluid
Kock pouch	Surgical creation of a urinary bladder from a segment of the ileum

Copyright © 2005, Elsevier Inc. All rights reserved.
CPT only © 2004. *Current Procedural Terminology, 2005, Professional Edition*, American Medical Association. All rights reserved.

Nephrocutaneous fistula	A channel from the kidney to the skin
Nephrolithotomy	Removal of a kidney stone through an incision made into the kidney
Nephrorrhaphy	Suturing of the kidney
Nephrostomy	Creation of a channel into the renal pelvis of the kidney
Transureteroureterostomy	Surgical connection of one ureter to the other ureter
Transvesical ureterolithotomy	Removal of a ureter stone (calculus) through the bladder
Ureterectomy	Surgical removal of a ureter, either totally or partially
Ureterocutaneous fistula	Channel from ureter to exterior skin
Ureteroenterostomy	Creation of a connection between the intestine and the ureter
Ureterolithotomy	Removal of a stone from the ureter
Ureterolysis	Freeing of adhesions of the ureter
Ureteroneocystostomy	Surgical connection of the ureter to a new site on the bladder
Ureteropyelography	Ureter and renal pelvis radiography
Ureterotomy	Incision into the ureter
Urethrocystography	Radiography of the bladder and urethra
Urethromeatoplasty	Surgical repair of the urethra and meatus
Urethropexy	Fixation of the urethra by means of surgery
Urethroplasty	Surgical repair of the urethra
Urethrorrhaphy	Suturing of the urethra
Urethroscopy	Use of a scope to view the urethra
Vesicostomy	Surgical creation of a connection of the viscera of the bladder to the skin

Copyright © 2005, Elsevier Inc. All rights reserved.
CPT only © 2004. *Current Procedural Terminology, 2005, Professional Edition*, American Medical Association. All rights reserved.

URINARY SYSTEM QUIZ

1. The outer covering of the kidney:
   a. medulla
   b. pyramids
   c. cortex
   d. papilla

2. Which is not a division of the kidneys:
   a. pelvis
   b. pyramids
   c. cortex
   d. trigone

3. The inner portion of the kidneys:
   a. medulla
   b. pyramids
   c. cortex
   d. papilla

4. The smooth area inside the bladder:
   a. pyramids
   b. calyces
   c. trigone
   d. cystocele

5. The narrow tube connecting the kidney and bladder:
   a. urethra
   b. ureter
   c. meatus
   d. trigone

6. Which of the following is NOT a surface of the urinary bladder:
   a. posterior
   b. anterior
   c. superior
   d. inferior

7. Combining form that means stone:
   a. azot/o
   b. cyst/o
   c. lith/o
   d. olig/o

8. Term meaning painful urination:
   a. pyuria
   b. dysuria
   c. diuresis
   d. hyperemia

Copyright © 2005, Elsevier Inc. All rights reserved.
CPT only © 2004. *Current Procedural Terminology, 2005, Professional Edition*, American Medical Association. All rights reserved.

9. Combining form meaning scant:
   a. glyc/o
   b. hydr/o
   c. meat/o
   d. olig/o

10. Term that describes renal failure that is acute:
    a. ARF
    b. ESRD
    c. HD
    d. BPH

Copyright © 2005, Elsevier Inc. All rights reserved.
CPT only © 2004. *Current Procedural Terminology, 2005, Professional Edition*, American Medical Association. All rights reserved.

URINARY SYSTEM—PATHOPHYSIOLOGY

Renal Failure

Acute renal failure

Sudden onset of renal failure

Cause

- Trauma
- Infection
- Inflammation
- Toxicity

Symptoms

- Uremia
- Oliguria (decreased output) or anuria (no output)
- Hyperkalemia (high potassium in blood)
- Pulmonary edema

Types

- Prerenal
  - Associated with poor systemic perfusion
  - Decreased renal blood flow
    - Such as with congestive heart failure
- Intrarenal
  - Associated with renal parenchyma disease (functional tissue of kidney)
    - Such as acute interstitial nephritis
- Postrenal
  - Resulting from urine flow obstruction out of kidney

Treatment

- Underlying condition
- Dialysis
- Monitoring of fluid and electrolyte balance

Chronic renal failure

Gradual loss of function

- Progressively more severe renal insufficiency until end stage of:
  - End-stage renal disease
  - Irreversible kidney failure

Cause

- Long-term exposure to nephrotoxins
- Diabetes
- Hypertension

Copyright © 2005, Elsevier Inc. All rights reserved.
CPT only © 2004. *Current Procedural Terminology, 2005, Professional Edition*, American Medical Association. All rights reserved.

Symptoms

- No symptoms until well advanced
- Polyuria
- Nausea or anorexia
- Dehydration
- Neurologic manifestations

Stages of nephron loss

- Decreased reserve
  - 60% loss
- Renal insufficiency
  - 75% loss
- End-stage renal failure
  - 90% loss

Treatment

- No cure
- Dialysis
- Kidney transplant

Urinary Tract Infections (UTI)

Cystitis—bacterial

Cause

- Bacteria, usually *E. coli*

Symptoms

- Lower abdominal pain
- Dysuria
- Lower back pain
- Urinary frequency and urgency
- Cloudy, foul-smelling urine

Systemic signs

- Fever
- Malaise
- Nausea

Treatment

- Antibiotics
- Increased fluid intake

Copyright © 2005, Elsevier Inc. All rights reserved.
CPT only © 2004. *Current Procedural Terminology, 2005, Professional Edition*, American Medical Association. All rights reserved.

Cystitis—nonbacterial

Cause

- Unknown
- May later produce bacterial infection

Treatment

- No known treatment

Acute pyelonephritis (Figure 1-34)

Infection of the renal pelvis and medullary tissue

- May involve one or both kidneys

Cause

- *E. coli*
- *Proteus*
- *Pseudomonas*

Symptoms

- Fever
- Chills
- Groin or flank pain

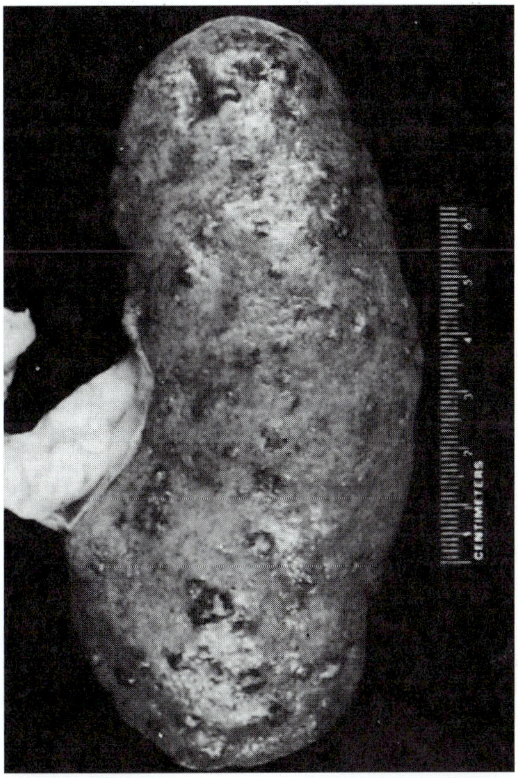

Figure 1-34 Acute pyelonephritis. Cortical surface is dotted with abscesses. (From Cotran R, Kumar V, Robbins S: *Robbins pathologic basis of disease,* Philadelphia, 1994, WB Saunders, p 969.)

Copyright © 2005, Elsevier Inc. All rights reserved.
CPT only © 2004. *Current Procedural Terminology, 2005, Professional Edition,* American Medical Association. All rights reserved.

- Dysuria
- Pyuria
- Nocturia

Treatment

- Antibiotics

Chronic pyelonephritis

Recurrent infection that causes scarring of kidney

Cause is difficult to determine

- Repeated infections
- Obstructive conditions

Symptoms

- Hypertension
- Dysuria
- Flank pain
- Increased frequency of urination

Glomerular Disorders

Function of the glomerulus is blood filtration

Nephrotic syndrome

Disease of the kidneys that includes damage to the membrane of the glomerulus

Accompanied by:

- Hypoalbuminemia
- Hypercholesterolemia
- Edema

Damage to the glomerulus results from

- Infection
- Immune response
    - Most predominant cause of dysfunction is exposure to toxins

May be a manifestation of an underlying condition, such as diabetes

Symptoms

- Edema
- Weight gain
- Pallor

Treatment

- Glucocorticoids, such as prednisone
    - Reduces inflammation
- Sodium reduction
- Careful monitoring for continued inflammation

Copyright © 2005, Elsevier Inc. All rights reserved.
CPT only © 2004. *Current Procedural Terminology, 2005, Professional Edition*, American Medical Association. All rights reserved.

Acute poststreptococcal glomerulonephritis (APSGN)

Cause

- Streptococcus infection
  - With certain types of group A beta-hemolytic streptococcus
- Creates an antigen-antibody complex
  - Infiltrates the glomerular capillaries
  - Results in inflammation in kidneys
  - Inflammation interferes with normal kidney function
  - Fluid and waste build-up
  - Can lead to acute renal failure and scarring

Usually occurs in children 3 to 7 years of age
  - Most often in boys

Symptoms

- Back and flank pain
- Cloudy, dark urine
- Oliguria (decreased output)
- Edema
- Elevated blood pressure
- Fatigue
- Malaise
- Headache
- Nausea
- Elevated blood pressure

Treatment

- Sodium reduction
- Antibiotics
- Careful monitoring for continued inflammation

Urinary Tract Obstructions

Interference with urine flow

Causes dilation of urinary system

Increased urinary tract infection

Obstruction can be
- Functional
- Anatomic
  - Also known as obstructive uropathy

Kidney stones

- Formed of mineral salts
- Develop anywhere in urinary tract
- Tend to form in presence of excess salt and decreased fluid intake
  - Most stones are formed of calcium salts
  - Staghorn calculus form in the renal pelvis

Copyright © 2005, Elsevier Inc. All rights reserved.
CPT only © 2004. *Current Procedural Terminology, 2005, Professional Edition*, American Medical Association. All rights reserved.

Symptoms

- Asymptomatic until obstruction occurs
- Obstruction results in renal colic
    - Extremely intense pain in flank
    - Nausea
    - Vomiting
    - Cold, clammy skin
    - Increased pulse rate

Treatment

- Stone usually passes spontaneously
- May use extracorporeal shock wave lithotripsy (ESWL) to break up stone
    - Laser lithotripsy may also be used
- Drugs may be used to dissolve the stone
- Preventative treatment to adjust pH level
    - Increased fluid intake

Bladder carcinoma

- Tumors originate in the transitional epithelial lining
- Tends to recur
- Often metastatic to the liver and bone

Symptoms

- Often asymptomatic in early stage
- Hematuria
- Dysuria
- Frequent urination
- Infections common

Increased risks

- Cigarette smoking
- Working with industrial chemicals
- Analgesics used in large amounts
- Recurrent bladder infections

Treatment

- Immuno-therapy (bacillus Calmette-Guérin vaccine, BCG)
- Excision
- Chemotherapy
- Radiation therapy

Hydronephrosis

Distention of kidney with urine

- Due to an obstruction
- Usually as a result of a kidney stone
- May also be due to scarring, tumor, edema from infection, or other obstruction

Copyright © 2005, Elsevier Inc. All rights reserved.
CPT only © 2004. *Current Procedural Terminology, 2005, Professional Edition*, American Medical Association. All rights reserved.

Symptoms

- Usually asymptomatic
- Mild flank pain
- Infection may develop
- May lead to chronic renal failure

Treatment

- Treat the underlying condition, such as removal of the stone or antibiotics for infection
- Dilation of the stricture

Vascular Disorders

Nephrosclerosis

Excessive hardening and thickening of vascular structure of kidney

- Reduces blood supply
  - Increases blood pressure
  - Results in atrophy and ischemia of structures
  - May lead to chronic renal failure

Symptoms

- Asymptomatic in early stages

Treatment

- Diuretics
- ACE inhibitors (angiotensin-converting enzyme)
- Beta blockers that block the release of resin
- Antihypertensive drugs
- Sodium intake reduction

Congenital Disorders

Polycystic kidney

- Numerous kidney cysts
- Genetic disease

Symptoms

- Asymptomatic until 40s
- Develops chronic renal failure
- Cysts may spread to other organs, such as liver

Treatment

- As for chronic renal failure

Copyright © 2005, Elsevier Inc. All rights reserved.
CPT only © 2004. *Current Procedural Terminology, 2005, Professional Edition*, American Medical Association. All rights reserved.

Wilms' tumor

- Usually unilateral kidney tumors
- Most common tumor in children

Usually advanced at time of diagnosis

- Metastasis to lungs at time of diagnosis is common

Symptoms

- Asymptomatic until abdominal mass becomes apparent at age 1 to 5

Treatment

- Excision
- Radiation therapy
- Chemotherapy
- Usually a combination of above

Copyright © 2005, Elsevier Inc. All rights reserved.
CPT only © 2004. *Current Procedural Terminology, 2005, Professional Edition*, American Medical Association. All rights reserved.

URINARY SYSTEM PATHOPHYSIOLOGY QUIZ

1. Which of the following is NOT a type of acute renal failure?
   a. prerenal
   b. intrarenal
   c. interrenal
   d. postrenal

2. The loss of nephron function in end-stage renal disease is
   a. 60%
   b. 70%
   c. 80%
   d. 90%

3. The cause of bacterial cystitis is usually
   a. proteus
   b. pseudomonas
   c. staphylococci
   d. *E. coli*

4. The primary treatment for acute pyelonephritis would be
   a. prednisone
   b. sodium reduction
   c. antibiotics
   d. BCG

5. APSGN stands for
   a. advanced poststaphylococcal glomerulonephritis
   b. acute poststreptococcal glomerulonephritis
   c. acute poststaphylococcal glomerulonephritis
   d. advanced poststreptococcal glomerulonephritis

6. Obstructive uropathy is also known as
   a. pyelonephritis
   b. renal failure
   c. urinary tract obstruction
   d. nephrotic syndrome

7. A treatment for kidney stone may be
   a. ESWL
   b. prednisone
   c. open surgical procedure
   d. diuretics

8. The treatment for hydronephrosis involves
   a. an open surgical procedure
   b. use of diuretics
   c. treatment of the underlying condition
   d. BCG

Copyright © 2005, Elsevier Inc. All rights reserved.
CPT only © 2004. *Current Procedural Terminology, 2005, Professional Edition*, American Medical Association. All rights reserved.

9. This is a congential condition in which numerous cysts form in the kidney.
   a. Wilms'
   b. polycystic kidney
   c. nephrosclerosis
   d. nephrotic syndrome

10. The treatment of Wilms' would NOT include which of the following:
    a. excision
    b. chemotherapy
    c. diuretic
    d. radiation therapy

Copyright © 2005, Elsevier Inc. All rights reserved.
CPT only © 2004. *Current Procedural Terminology, 2005, Professional Edition*, American Medical Association. All rights reserved.

DIGESTIVE SYSTEM

Function: digestion, absorption, and elimination

Includes gastrointestinal tract (alimentary canal) and accessory organs

Mouth (Figure 1-35)

Roof: hard palate, soft palate, uvula (projection at back of mouth)

Floor contains tongue (Figure 1-36), muscles, taste buds, and lingual frenulum, which anchors tongue to floor of mouth

Teeth

Thirty-two teeth (permanent)

Names of teeth: incisor, cuspid, bicuspid, and tricuspid

Tooth has crown (outer portion), neck (narrow part below gum line), root (end section), and pulp cavity (core)

Salivary Glands (Figure 1-37)

Surround the mouth and produce saliva

Parotid

Submandibular

Sublingual

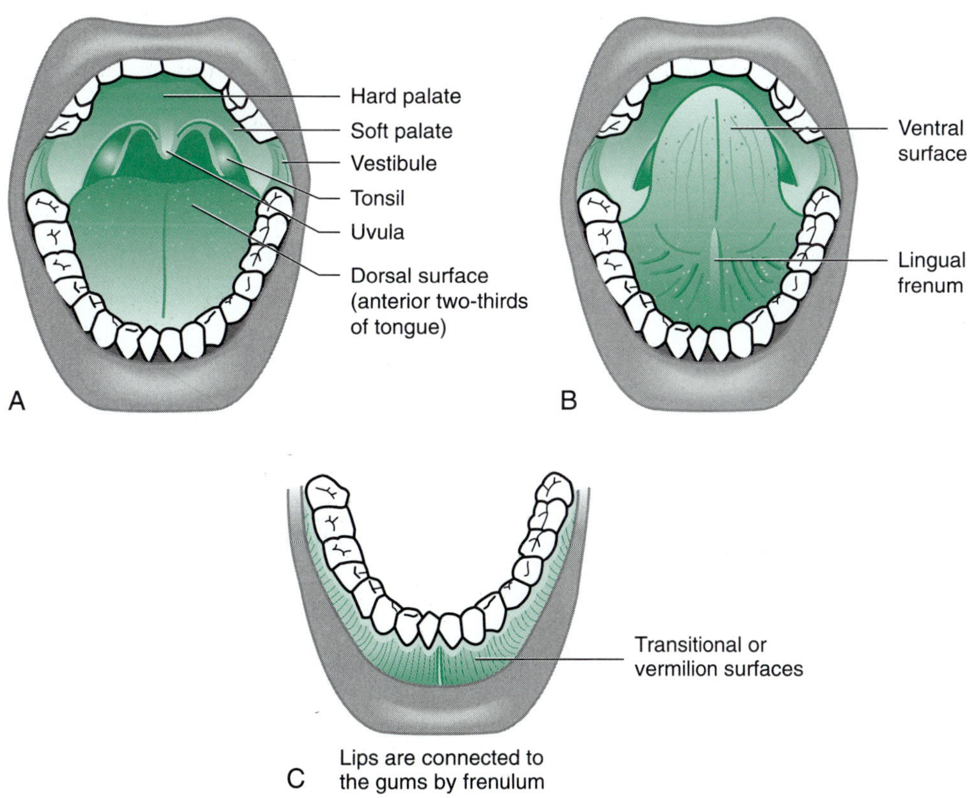

Figure 1-35 Anatomic structure of the mouth.

Copyright © 2005, Elsevier Inc. All rights reserved.
CPT only © 2004. *Current Procedural Terminology, 2005, Professional Edition*, American Medical Association. All rights reserved.

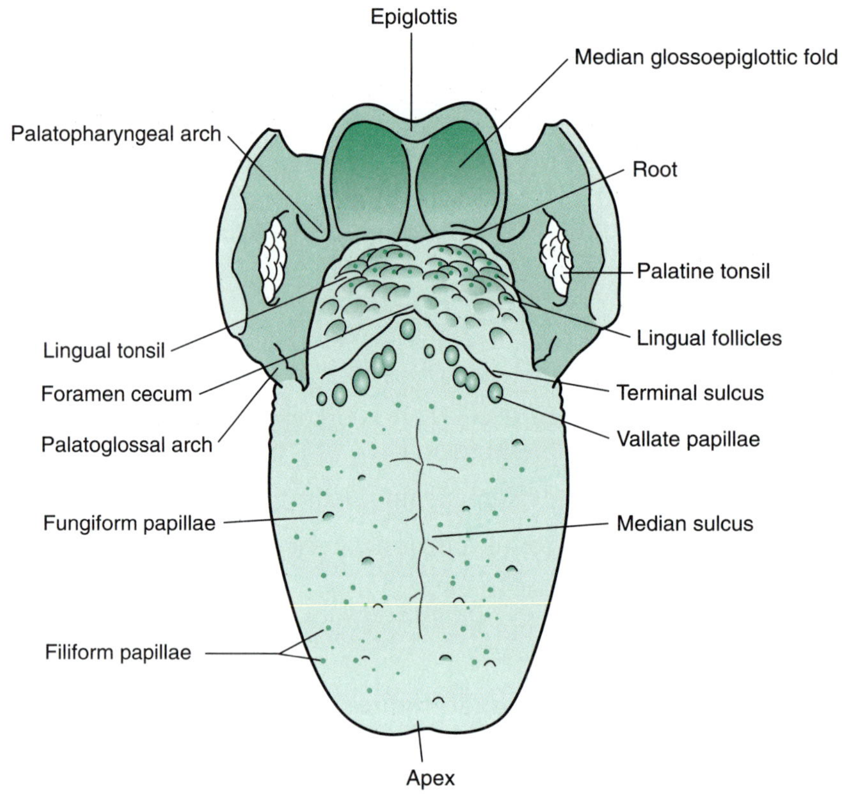

Figure 1-36 Dorsum of the tongue.

Pharynx or Throat (Figure 1-38)

Muscular tube through which air and food/water travel

Epiglottis covers larynx when swallowing

Esophagus

Muscular tube that carries food to stomach by means of peristalsis (rhythmic contractions)

Stomach

Sphincter (ring of muscles) at entry into stomach (gastroesophageal or cardiac)

Three parts of stomach: fundus (upper part), body (middle part), antrum/pylorus (lower part)

Lined with rugae (folds of mucosal membrane)

Pyloric sphincter opens to allow food to leave stomach and enter small intestine

Small Intestine

Duodenum

Jejunum

Ileum

Copyright © 2005, Elsevier Inc. All rights reserved.
CPT only © 2004. *Current Procedural Terminology, 2005, Professional Edition*, American Medical Association. All rights reserved.

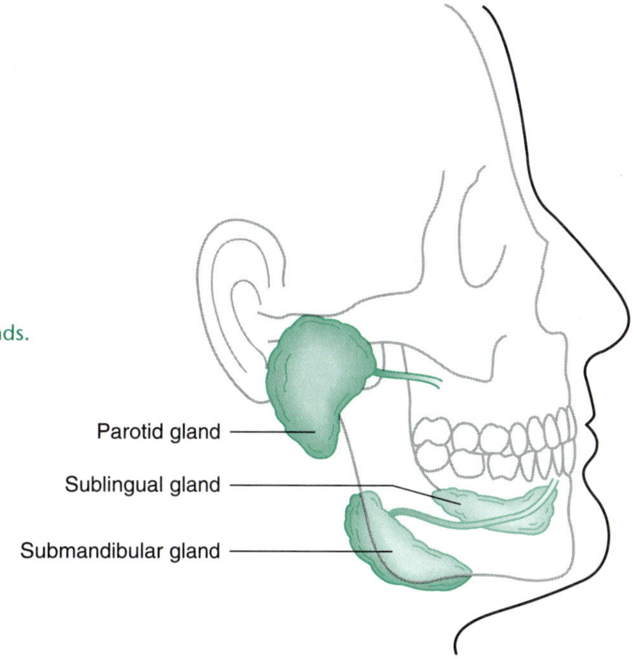

Figure 1-37 Major salivary glands.

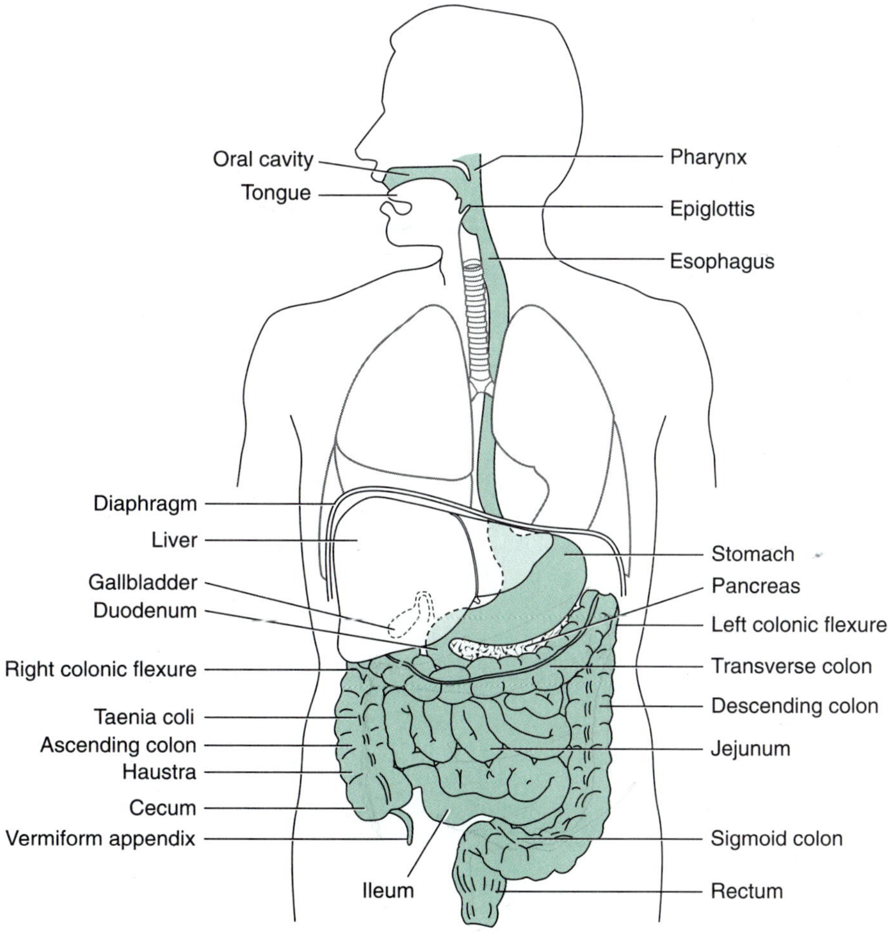

Figure 1-38 Digestive system.

Copyright © 2005, Elsevier Inc. All rights reserved.
CPT only © 2004. *Current Procedural Terminology, 2005, Professional Edition,* American Medical Association. All rights reserved.

Large Intestine

Extends from ileum to anus

Cecum, from which appendix extends, connects ileum and colon

Colon, divided into ascending, transverse, descending, and sigmoid

Sigmoid colon, connected to rectum that terminates at anus

Accessory Organs

Liver produces bile, sent to gallbladder via hepatic duct and cystic duct

Gallbladder stores bile, sent to duodenum via common bile duct

Pancreas produces enzymes sent through pancreatic duct to common bile duct then to duodenum

Islets of Langerhans produce insulin and glucagon

Peritoneum

Serous membrane lines abdominal cavity and maintains organs in correct anatomic place

COMBINING FORMS

1. abdomin/o — abdomen
2. an/o — anus
3. appendic/o — appendix
4. bil/i — bile
5. bilirubin/o — bile pigment
6. cec/o — cecum
7. celi/o — abdomen
8. chol/e — gall/bile
9. cholangio/o — bile duct
10. cholecyst/o — gallbladder
11. choledoch/o — common bile duct
12. col/o — colon
13. dent/i — tooth
14. diverticul/o — diverticulum
15. duoden/o — duodenum
16. enter/o — small intestine
17. esophag/o — esophagus
18. gastr/o — stomach
19. gingiv/o — gum

Copyright © 2005, Elsevier Inc. All rights reserved.
CPT only © 2004. *Current Procedural Terminology, 2005, Professional Edition*, American Medical Association. All rights reserved.

20. gloss/o tongue
21. hepat/o liver
22. herni/o hernia
23. ile/o ileum
24. jejun/o jejunum
25. lapar/o abdomen
26. lingu/o tongue
27. lip/o fat
28. lith/o stone
29. or/o mouth
30. palat/o palate
31. pancreat/o pancreas
32. peritone/o peritoneum
33. polyp/o polyp
34. proct/o rectum
35. pylor/o pylorus
36. rect/o rectum
37. sial/o saliva
38. sigmoid/o sigmoid colon
39. steat/o fat
40. stomat/o mouth
41. uvul/o uvula

SUFFIXES

1. -cele hernia
2. -chezia defecation
3. -phagia eating

MEDICAL ABBREVIATIONS

1. EGD esophagogastroduodenoscopy
2. EGJ esophagogastric junction
3. ERCP endoscopic retrograde cholangiopancreatography
4. GERD gastroesophageal reflux disease
5. GI gastrointestinal

Copyright © 2005, Elsevier Inc. All rights reserved.
CPT only © 2004. *Current Procedural Terminology, 2005, Professional Edition*, American Medical Association. All rights reserved.

6. HJR hepatojugular reflux
7. LLQ left lower quadrant
8. LUQ left upper quadrant
9. PEG percutaneous endoscopic gastrostomy
10. RLQ right lower quadrant
11. RUQ right upper quadrant

MEDICAL TERMS

Anastomosis	Surgical connection of two tubular structures, such as two pieces of the intestine
Biliary	Refers to gallbladder, bile, or bile duct
Cholangiography	Radiographic recording of the bile ducts
Cholecystectomy	Surgical removal of the gallbladder
Cholecystoenterostomy	Creation of a connection between the gallbladder and intestine
Colonoscopy	Fiberscopic examination of the entire colon that may include part of the terminal ileum
Colostomy	Artificial opening between the colon and the abdominal wall
Diverticulum	Protrusion in the wall of an organ
Dysphagia	Difficulty swallowing
Enterolysis	Releasing of adhesions of intestine
Eventration	Protrusion of the bowel through an opening in the abdomen
Evisceration	Pulling the viscera outside of the body through an incision
Exstrophy	Condition in which an organ is turned inside out
Fulguration	Use of electric current to destroy tissue
Gastrointestinal	Pertaining to the stomach and intestine
Gastroplasty	Operation on the stomach for repair or reconfiguration
Gastrostomy	Artificial opening between the stomach and the abdominal wall
Hernia	Organ or tissue protruding through the wall or cavity that usually contains it
Ileostomy	Artificial opening between the ileum and the abdominal wall
Imbrication	Overlapping
Incarcerated	Regarding hernias, a constricted, irreducible hernia that may cause obstruction of an intestine
Intussusception	Slipping of one part of the intestine into another part
Jejunostomy	Artificial opening between the jejunum and the abdominal wall
Laparoscopy	Exploration of the abdomen and pelvic cavities using a scope placed through a small incision in the abdominal wall
Lithotomy	Incision into an organ or a duct for the purpose of removing a stone

Copyright © 2005, Elsevier Inc. All rights reserved.
CPT only © 2004. *Current Procedural Terminology, 2005, Professional Edition*, American Medical Association. All rights reserved.

Lithotripsy	Crushing of a stone by sound wave or force
Paraesophageal hiatus hernia	Hernia that is near the esophagus
Perinephric cyst	Cyst in the tissue around the kidney
Perirenal	Around the kidney
Proctosigmoidoscopy	Fiberscopic examination of the sigmoid colon and rectum
Sialolithotomy	Surgical removal of a stone of the salivary gland or duct
Varices	Varicose veins
Volvulus	Twisted section of the intestine

Copyright © 2005, Elsevier Inc. All rights reserved.
CPT only © 2004. *Current Procedural Terminology, 2005, Professional Edition*, American Medical Association. All rights reserved.

DIGESTIVE SYSTEM QUIZ

1. NOT a part of the small intestine:
   a. ileum
   b. cecum
   c. duodenum
   d. jejunum

2. Term meaning a ring of muscles:
   a. pyloric
   b. parotid
   c. epiglottis
   d. sphincter

3. The throat is also known as the:
   a. larynx
   b. epiglottis
   c. esophagus
   d. pharynx

4. The three parts of the stomach:
   a. pyloric, rugae, fundus
   b. fundus, body, antrum
   c. antrum, pyloric, rugae
   d. ilium, fundus, pyloric

5. The projection at the back of the mouth:
   a. palate
   b. sublingual
   c. uvula
   d. parotid

6. Mucosal membrane that lines the stomach:
   a. cecum
   b. rugae
   c. frenulum
   d. fundus

7. The parts of the colon are:
   a. ascending, transverse, descending, sigmoid
   b. ascending, descending, sigmoid
   c. transverse, descending, sigmoid
   d. descending, sigmoid

8. Combining form meaning abdomen:
   a. an/o
   b. cec/o
   c. celi/o
   d. col/o

Copyright © 2005, Elsevier Inc. All rights reserved.
CPT only © 2004. *Current Procedural Terminology, 2005, Professional Edition*, American Medical Association. All rights reserved.

9. Term that means tying together of two ends of a tube:
   a. anastomosis
   b. amylase
   c. aphthous stomatitis
   d. atresia

10. Abbreviation that means a scope placed through the esophagus, into the stomach, and to the duodenum:
    a. ERCP
    b. EGD
    c. GERD
    d. PEG

Copyright © 2005, Elsevier Inc. All rights reserved.
CPT only © 2004. *Current Procedural Terminology, 2005, Professional Edition*, American Medical Association. All rights reserved.

DIGESTIVE SYSTEM—PATHOPHYSIOLOGY

Disorders of the Oral Cavity

Cleft lip and cleft palate (Figure 1-39)

- Congenital defect
- Cleft lip and palate is a condition in which the lip and palate do not properly join together

Causes feeding problems

- Infants cannot create sufficient suction for feeding
- Danger of aspirating food
- Results in speech defects

Treatment

- Surgical repair of defects

Ulceration

- Canker sore
    - Ulceration of the oral mucosa

Also known as

- Aphthous ulcer (aphtha = small ulcer)
- Aphthous stomatitis

Heals spontaneously

Infections

Candidiasis

Candida albicans is naturally found in mouth

Thrush (oral candidiasis) is overarching infection

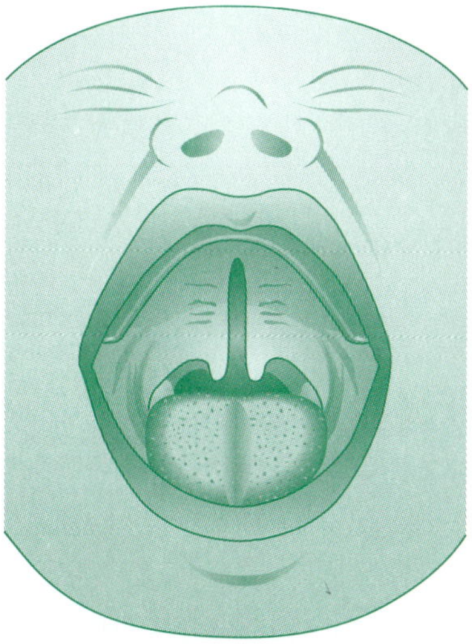

Figure 1-39 Cleft palate.

Copyright © 2005, Elsevier Inc. All rights reserved.
CPT only © 2004. *Current Procedural Terminology, 2005, Professional Edition*, American Medical Association. All rights reserved.

- Result of
  - Antibiotic regimen
  - Chemotherapy
  - Glucocorticoids
- Common in diabetics and AIDS patients

Treatment

- Nystatin (topical fungal agent)

Herpes simplex type 1

Herpetic stomatitis

- Viral cold sores and blisters
- Associated with herpes simplex virus type 1 (HSV-1)

Treatment

- No cure
- May be alleviated somewhat by antiviral medications

Cancer of the oral cavity

- Most common type is squamous cell carcinoma
  - Kaposi's sarcoma is type seen in AIDS patients
- Increased in smokers
- Lip cancer also increased in smokers
- Poor prognosis
- Usually asymptomatic until later stages
- Metastasis through lymph nodes

Esophageal Disorders

Scleroderma

- Also known as progressive systemic sclerosis
- Atrophy of the smooth muscles of the lower esophagus

Lower esophageal sphincter (LES) does not close properly

- Leads to esophageal reflux
- Strictures form

Symptom

- Predominantly dysphagia

Esophagitis

Inflammation of esophagus

Types

Acute

- Most common type is that caused by hiatal hernia
- Infectious esophagitis is common in patients with AIDS

Copyright © 2005, Elsevier Inc. All rights reserved.
CPT only © 2004. *Current Procedural Terminology, 2005, Professional Edition*, American Medical Association. All rights reserved.

- Ingestion of strong alkaline or acid substances
  - Such as those in household cleaners
- Inflammation leads to scarring

Chronic
- Most common type is that caused by LES reflux

Cancer of the esophagus

Most common type is leiomyoma (smooth muscle tumor)

Usually caused by continued irritation
- Smoking
- Alcohol
- Hiatal hernia
- Chronic esophagitis

Poor prognosis

Hiatal hernia

Diaphragm goes over the stomach
- Esophagus passes through the diaphragm at natural opening (hiatus)
- Part of the stomach protrudes (herniates) through the opening in the diaphragm into the thorax

Types (Figure 1-40)

- Sliding
  - Stomach and gastroesophageal junction protrudes through the hiatus
- Paraesophageal
  - Part of fundus protrudes

Symptoms

- Heartburn
- Reflux
- Belching
- Lying down causes discomfort
- Dysphagia
- Substernal pain after eating

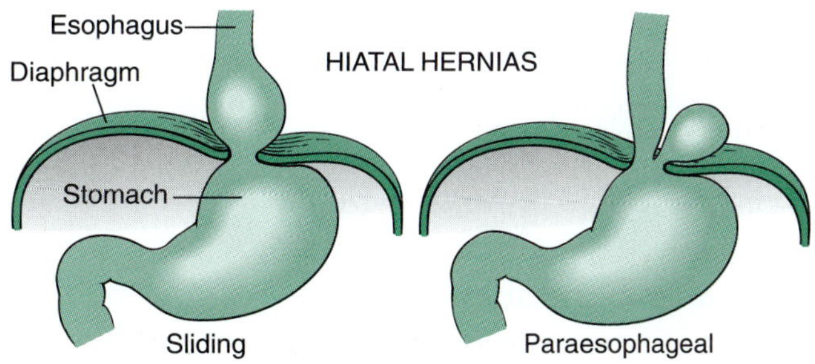

Figure 1-40 Sliding and paraesophageal hernias (hiatal hernias).

Copyright © 2005, Elsevier Inc. All rights reserved.
CPT only © 2004. *Current Procedural Terminology, 2005, Professional Edition*, American Medical Association. All rights reserved.

Gastroesophageal reflex disease (GERD)

Associated with hiatal hernias
- Reflux of gastric contents

Lower esophageal sphincter does not constrict properly

Treatment

- Reduce irritants, such as:
    - Smoking
    - Spicy foods
    - Alcohol
- Antacids
- Elevate the head of the bed
- Avoid tight clothing

Stomach and Duodenum Disorders

Gastritis

Inflammation of the stomach

Acute superficial gastritis

Mild, transient irritation

Causes

- Excessive alcohol
- Infection
- Food allergies
- Spicy foods
- Aspirin

Symptoms

- Nausea
- Vomiting
- Anorexia
- Bleeding in more severe cases
- Epigastric pain

Treatment

- Usually spontaneous remission in 2 to 3 days
- Removal of underlying irritation
- Antibiotics for infection

Chronic atrophic gastritis

Progressive atrophy of epithelium

Types

- Type A, atrophic or fundal
    - Involves the fundus of the stomach
    - Autoimmune disease
        - Decreases acid secretion
        - Results in high gastrin levels

Copyright © 2005, Elsevier Inc. All rights reserved.
CPT only © 2004. *Current Procedural Terminology, 2005, Professional Edition*, American Medical Association. All rights reserved.

- Type B, antral
  - Involves the antrum region of the stomach
  - Often associated with the elderly
    - May be associated with pernicious anemia
  - Low gastrin levels
  - Usually caused by infection
  - Irritated by alcohol, drugs, and tobacco

Peptic ulcers

Erosive area on the mucosa

- Extends below epithelium
- Chronic ulcers have scar tissue at the base of the erosive area

Ulcers can occur anyplace on the gastrointestinal tract but typically are found on the:

- Lower esophagus
- Stomach
- Proximal duodenum

Some causes

- Alcohol
- Aspirin
- Severe stress
- Bacterial infection caused by *Helicobacter pylori (H. pylori)*, 90% of the time
- Genetic factor

Symptoms

- Epigastric pain when stomach is empty
  - Relieved by food or antacid
- Burning

May include

- Vomiting red blood
- Nausea
- Weight loss
- Anorexia

Severe cases may include

- Obstruction
- Hemorrhage
- Perforation

Treatment

- Surgical intervention
- Antacids
- Dietary restrictions
- Rest
- Antibiotics

Copyright © 2005, Elsevier Inc. All rights reserved.
CPT only © 2004. *Current Procedural Terminology, 2005, Professional Edition*, American Medical Association. All rights reserved.

Gastric cancer

Most often occurs in men over 40

Cause is unknown

Predisposing factors

- Atrophic gastritis
- Pernicious anemia
- History of nonhealing gastric ulcer
- Blood type A
- Geographic factors
- Environmental factors
- Carcinogenic foods
    - Smoked meats
    - Nitrates
    - Pickled foods

Symptoms

- Usually asymptomatic in early stages

Treatment

- Excision
- Chemotherapy
- Radiation

Prognosis is poor

Pyloric stenosis

- Narrowing of the pyloric sphincter
- Signs appear soon after birth
    - Failure to thrive
    - Projectile vomiting

Treatment

- Surgery to relieve the stenosis (pyloromyotomy)

Intestinal Disorders

Small intestine

Malabsorption conditions

Celiac disease

- Most important malabsorption condition
- Villi atrophy in response to food containing gluten and loose ability to absorb
    - Gluten is a protein found in wheat, rye, oats, and barley

Symptoms
- Diarrhea
- Fatigue

Copyright © 2005, Elsevier Inc. All rights reserved.
CPT only © 2004. *Current Procedural Terminology, 2005, Professional Edition*, American Medical Association. All rights reserved.

- ◦ Weakness
- ◦ Steatorrhea (excess fat in feces)

Treatment

- ◦ Gluten-free diet
- ◦ Steroids when necessary

Lactase deficiency

Enzyme deficiency

- Secondary to gastrointestinal damage, such as:
  - ◦ Regional enteritis
  - ◦ Infection
- Genetic defect

Symptoms

- Intolerance to milk

Treatment

- Elimination of milk

Crohn's disease (regional enteritis)

Cause

- Unknown

Symptoms

- Vary greatly
- Diarrhea
- Gas
- Fever
- Abdominal pain
- Malaise
- Anorexia
- Weight loss

Treatment

- No specific treatment
- Antidiarrheal drugs
- Palliative medications based on symptoms
- Resection of the affected section of intestine

Appendicitis

Inflammation of vermiform appendix that projects from the cecum

Obstruction of lumen leads to infection

- Appendix becomes hypoxic (decreased oxygen levels)
- May cause gangrene
- May rupture, causing peritonitis

Symptoms

- Periumbilical (around umbilicus) pain, initially
- Right lower quadrant (RLQ) pain as inflammation progresses

Copyright © 2005, Elsevier Inc. All rights reserved.
CPT only © 2004. *Current Procedural Terminology, 2005, Professional Edition*, American Medical Association. All rights reserved.

- Nausea
- Vomiting
- Possible diarrhea

Treatment

- Management of any perforation or abscess

Peritonitis

Inflammation of the peritoneum (membrane that lines the abdominal cavity)

Usually a result of

- Spread of infection from abdominal organ
- Puncture wound to abdomen
- Rupture of gastrointestinal tract

Abscesses form, resulting in adhesions

  - May result in obstruction

Types

- Acute
- Chronic

Symptoms

- Abdominal pain
- Vomiting
- Rigid abdomen
- Fever
- Leukocytosis (increased white cells in blood)

Treatment

- Antibiotics
- Suction of stomach and intestines
- If possible, surgical removal of origin of infection, such as appendix
- Fluid replacement
- Bed rest

Obstruction

Any interference with passage of intestinal contents

May be:

- Acute
- Chronic
- Partial
- Total

Copyright © 2005, Elsevier Inc. All rights reserved.
CPT only © 2004. *Current Procedural Terminology, 2005, Professional Edition*, American Medical Association. All rights reserved.

Types

Nonmechanical

- Paralytic ileus
- Result of trauma or toxin

Mechanical

- Result of tumors, adhesions, hernias
- Simple mechanical obstruction
  - One point of obstruction
- Closed-loop obstruction
  - At least two points of obstruction

Symptoms

- Abdominal distention
- Pain
- Vomiting
- Total constipation

Treatment

- Surgical intervention
- Symptomatic treatment

Large intestine

Diverticulosis

Herniation of intestinal mucosa

- Forms sacs in the lining, called diverticula

Diverticulitis

Sacs fill and become inflamed

- Common in aged

Symptoms

- Diarrhea or constipation
- Gas
- Abdominal discomfort

Complications

- Perforation
- Bleeding
- Peritonitis
- Abscess
- Obstruction

Treatment

- Antimicrobials as necessary
- Stool softeners

Copyright © 2005, Elsevier Inc. All rights reserved.
CPT only © 2004. *Current Procedural Terminology, 2005, Professional Edition*, American Medical Association. All rights reserved.

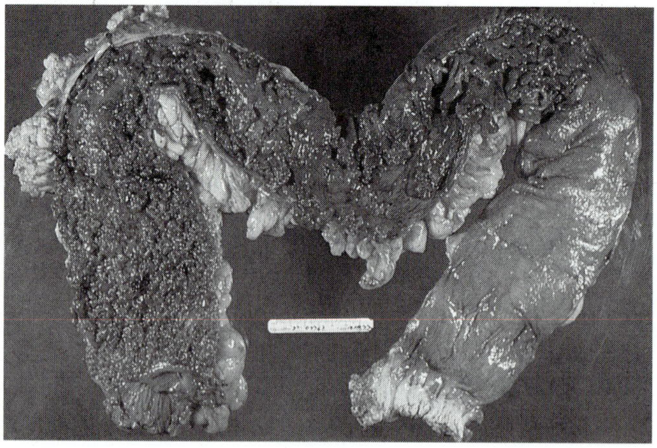

Figure 1-41 Ulcerative colitis. (From Damjanov I: *Pathology for the health-related professions,* ed. 2, Philadelphia, 2000, WB Saunders.)

- Dietary restrictions of solid foods
- Surgical intervention if necessary

Ulcerative colitis (Figure 1-41)

- Inflammation of rectum that progresses to colon
- May develop into toxic megacolon
    - Leads to obstruction and dilation of colon
- Increased risk of colorectal cancer

Symptoms

- Diarrhea
    - Blood and mucus may be present
- Cramping
- Fever
- Weight loss

Treatment

- Remove physical or emotional stressors
- Anti-inflammatory medications
- Antimotility agents
- Nutritional supplementation
- Surgical intervention, if necessary

Colorectal cancer

Usually develop from polyp

- In those 55

Increased risks

- Genetic factors
- 40 years of age and older

Copyright © 2005, Elsevier Inc. All rights reserved.
CPT only © 2004. *Current Procedural Terminology, 2005, Professional Edition*, American Medical Association. All rights reserved.

- Diets high in
  - Fat
  - Sugar
  - Red meat
- Low-fiber diets

Symptoms

- Asymptomatic until advanced
- Some may experience
  - Cramping
  - Ribbon stools
  - Feeling of incomplete evacuation
  - Fatigue
  - Weight loss
  - Change in bowel habits
  - Blood in the stool

Treatment

- Surgical excision
- Radiation
- Chemotherapy
- Combination of above

Disorders of Liver, Gallbladder, and Pancreas

Disorders of the liver

Jaundice (hyperbilirubinemia)

A symptom of biliary disease, not a disease itself
  - Results in yellow eyes and skin

Types

Prehepatic
- Excess destruction of red blood cells
- Result of hemolytic anemia or reaction to transfusion

Intrahepatic
- Impaired uptake of bilirubin and decreased blending of bilirubin by hepatic cells
- Result of liver disease, such as cirrhosis or hepatitis

Posthepatic
- Excess bile flows into blood
- Result of obstruction
  - Due to conditions such as inflammation of liver, tumors, cholelithiasis

Treatment

- Removal of the cause

Copyright © 2005, Elsevier Inc. All rights reserved.
CPT only © 2004. *Current Procedural Terminology, 2005, Professional Edition*, American Medical Association. All rights reserved.

Viral hepatitis

- Liver cells are damaged
- Results in inflammation and necrosis
- Damage can be mild or severe
- Scar tissue forms in liver
    - Leads to ischemia

Hepatitis A (HAV)

- Infectious hepatitis
- Transmission
    - Most commonly the oral-fecal route
    - Homosexual sexual transmission has occurred
- Does not have a chronic state
- Vaccine available for those who are traveling
- Gamma globulin may be administered to those just exposed

Hepatitis B (HBV)

- Serum hepatitis
- Carrier state is common
    - Asymptomatic but contagious
- Long incubation period
- Transmission
    - Intravenous drug users
    - Transfusion
    - Exposure to blood and bodily fluids
    - Sexual transmission
    - Mother-to-fetus transmission
    - Immune globulin is temporary prophylactic
- Vaccine is now routine for children

Hepatitis C (HCV)

- Transmission
    - Most commonly by transfusion
- Half of the cases develop into chronic hepatitis
- Increases the risk of hepatocellular cancer
- Carrier state may develop

Hepatitis D (HDV)

- Transmission
    - Blood
    - Intravenous drug users
- Hepatitis B is present for this type to develop

Copyright © 2005, Elsevier Inc. All rights reserved.
CPT only © 2004. *Current Procedural Terminology, 2005, Professional Edition*, American Medical Association. All rights reserved.

Hepatitis E (HEV)

- Transmission
    - Oral-fecal
- Does not develop into chronic or carrier

Symptoms of hepatitis

Stages

- Preicteric
    - Anorexia
    - Nausea
    - Fatigue
    - Malaise
- Icteric
    - Jaundice
    - Hepatomegaly (enlarged liver)
    - Biliary obstruction
    - Light-colored stools
    - Pruritus
- Posticteric (recovery)
    - Reduction of symptoms

Treatment

- None
- In early stages gamma globulins may be used
- Interferon may be used for cases of chronic hepatitis B and C

Nonviral hepatitis

- Hepatitis that results from hepatotoxins
- Symptoms
    - Similar to viral hepatitis
- Treatment
    - Removal of hepatotoxin

Cirrhosis

Profuse liver damage

- Extensive fibrosis
    - Results in inflammation

Progressive disorder

Leads to liver failure

Types

- Alcoholic liver
    - Known as Laënnec's cirrhosis or portal
    - Largest group

Copyright © 2005, Elsevier Inc. All rights reserved.
CPT only © 2004. *Current Procedural Terminology, 2005, Professional Edition*, American Medical Association. All rights reserved.

- Biliary
  - Associated with immune disorders
  - Obstructions occur and disrupt normal function
- Postnecrotic
  - Associated with chronic hepatitis and exposure to toxins

Symptoms

- Asymptomatic in early stages
- Nausea
- Vomiting
- Fatigue
- Weight loss
- Pruritus
- Jaundice
- Edema

Treatment

- Symptomatic
- Dietary restrictions
  - Reduced protein and sodium
  - Increased vitamins and carbohydrates
- Diuretics
- Antibiotics
- Liver transplant

Disorders of the gallbladder

Cholecystitis

Inflammation of gallbladder and cystic duct

Cholangitis

Inflammation of bile duct

Cholelithiasis

Formation of gallstones **(Figure 1-42)**

- Consists of cholesterol or bilirubin
- Occur most often in those with high levels of cholesterol or bile salts

Stones cause irritation and inflammation

- May lead to infection
- Obstruction
  - May result in pancreatitis
  - Rupture is possible

Symptoms

- Often asymptomatic
- Upper right quadrant (URQ) pain

Copyright © 2005, Elsevier Inc. All rights reserved.
CPT only © 2004. *Current Procedural Terminology, 2005, Professional Edition*, American Medical Association. All rights reserved.

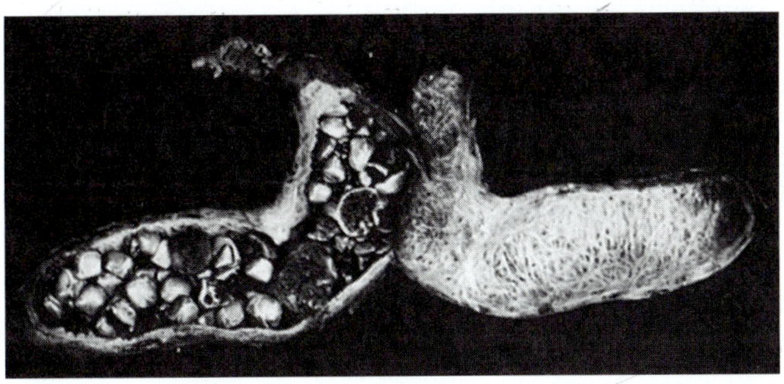

Figure 1-42 Resected gallbladder containing mixed gallstones. (From Kissane JM, editor: *Anderson's pathology*, ed 9, St. Louis, 1990, Mosby.)

- Pain in back and/or shoulder
- Epigastric discomfort
- Bloating
- Belching

Treatment

- Surgical intervention (cholecystectomy)
- Lithotripsy
- Medical management by use of drugs that break down stone

Disorders of the pancreas

Pancreatitis

- Inflammation of pancreas
- Acute and chronic forms

Symptoms

- Severe pain
- Fever
- Acute form is a medical emergency
- Neurogenic shock
- Septicemia
- General sepsis

Complications

- Adult respiratory syndrome (ARS)
- Renal failure

Treatment

- No oral intake
    - IV fluids given and carefully monitored
- Analgesics

Copyright © 2005, Elsevier Inc. All rights reserved.
CPT only © 2004. *Current Procedural Terminology, 2005, Professional Edition*, American Medical Association. All rights reserved.

Pancreatic cancer

Increased risk

- Cigarette smoking
- Diet high in fat and protein

Symptoms

- Weight loss
- Jaundice
- Anorexia
- Most types of pancreatic cancer are asymptomatic until well advanced

Treatment

- Palliative
- Pain management

Copyright © 2005, Elsevier Inc. All rights reserved.
CPT only © 2004. *Current Procedural Terminology, 2005, Professional Edition*, American Medical Association. All rights reserved.

DIGESTIVE SYSTEM PATHOPHYSIOLOGY QUIZ

1. This type of hyperbilirubinemia is hallmarked by excess bile flow into the blood.
   a. intrahepatic
   b. prehepatic
   c. posthepatic
   d. jaundice

2. This type of hepatitis is transmitted by the oral-fecal route.
   a. A
   b. B
   c. C
   d. D

3. Which of the following is the recovery stage of hepatitis?
   a. prehepatic
   b. posthepatic
   c. preicteric
   d. posticteric

4. This type of cirrhosis is also known as portal cirrhosis.
   a. biliary
   b. alcoholic liver
   c. postnecrotic
   d. traumatic

5. This condition is the inflammation of the bile ducts.
   a. cholangitis
   b. cholecystitis
   c. cholelithiasis
   d. cholangitis

6. Formation of gallstones most often occurs with high levels of the following:
   a. bile salts and toxins
   b. cholesterol and toxins
   c. cholesterol and bile salts
   d. toxins

7. The primary factor that increases the risk of pancreatic cancer is
   a. smoking
   b. alcohol
   c. intravenous drug use
   d. hepatitis

8. A potential complication of this condition is ARS.
   a. hyperbilirubinemia
   b. hepatitis
   c. pancreatitis
   d. pancreatic cancer

Copyright © 2005, Elsevier Inc. All rights reserved.
CPT only © 2004. *Current Procedural Terminology, 2005, Professional Edition*, American Medical Association. All rights reserved.

9. The primary treatment for jaundice is
   a. removal of cause
   b. antibiotics
   c. dialysis
   d. vaccine

10. This condition has as the largest group those that abuse alcohol.
    a. cirrhosis
    b. hepatitis
    c. pancreatitis
    d. pancreatic cancer

Copyright © 2005, Elsevier Inc. All rights reserved.
CPT only © 2004. *Current Procedural Terminology, 2005, Professional Edition*, American Medical Association. All rights reserved.

MEDIASTINUM AND DIAPHRAGM

Not an organ system

Mediastinum

That area between lungs that a median (partition) divides (Figure 1-43) into:

- superior
- anterior
- posterior
- middle

Diaphragm

A dome-shaped muscular partition that separates abdominal cavity from thoracic cavity

Assists in breathing

Expands to assist lungs in exhalation/relaxation of the diaphragm

Flattens out during inspiration/contraction of diaphragm

Diaphragmatic hernia: esophageal hernia

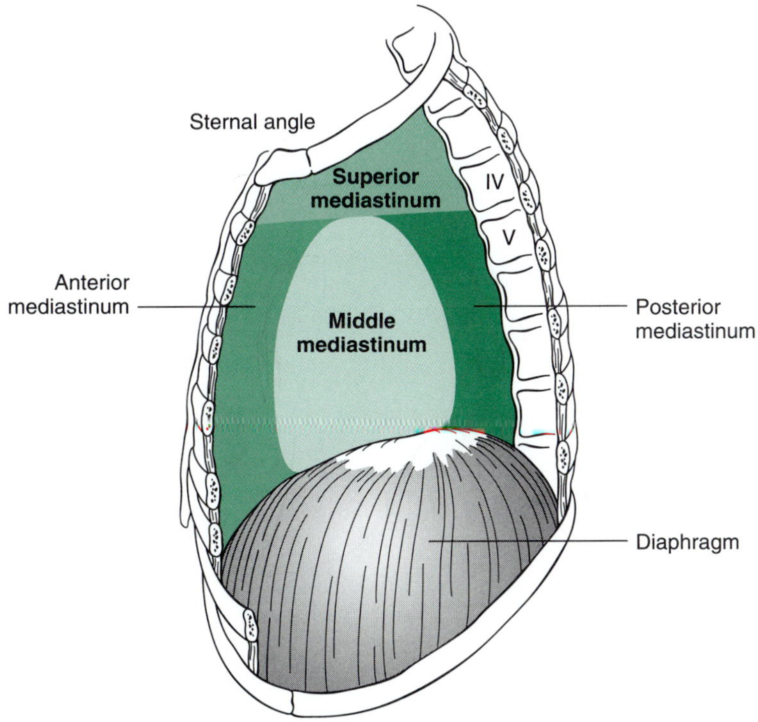

Figure 1-43 Mediastinum and diaphragm.

Copyright © 2005, Elsevier Inc. All rights reserved.
CPT only © 2004. *Current Procedural Terminology, 2005, Professional Edition*, American Medical Association. All rights reserved.

MEDIASTINUM AND DIAPHRAGM QUIZ

1. The mediastinum is not an organ system:
   a. true
   b. false

2. The mediastinum is divided into:
   a. superior, anterior, posterior
   b. superior, anterior, posterior, middle
   c. anterior, posterior, middle
   d. middle, anterior, superior

3. During inspiration, the diaphragm:
   a. expands
   b. moves upward
   c. collapses
   d. flattens out

4. The term means partition:
   a. middle
   b. medium
   c. median
   d. diaphragm

5. The diaphragm is said to be this shape:
   a. square
   b. flat
   c. dome
   d. round

6. This separates the abdominal cavity from the thoracic cavity:
   a. mediastinum
   b. diaphragm
   c. superior
   d. inferior

7. This is the area between the lungs:
   a. mediastinum
   b. diaphragm
   c. superior
   d. inferior

8. This is an esophageal hernia:
   a. mediastinal
   b. diaphragmatic
   c. paraesophageal
   d. hiatal

Copyright © 2005, Elsevier Inc. All rights reserved.
CPT only © 2004. *Current Procedural Terminology, 2005, Professional Edition,* American Medical Association. All rights reserved.

9. A diaphragmatic hernia is also known as:
   a. esophageal
   b. epiglottis
   c. partitional
   d. medial

10. The diaphragm assists in:
   a. percussion
   b. auscultation
   c. contraction
   d. breathing

Copyright © 2005, Elsevier Inc. All rights reserved.
CPT only © 2004. *Current Procedural Terminology, 2005, Professional Edition*, American Medical Association. All rights reserved.

HEMIC AND LYMPHATIC SYSTEM

Hemic refers to blood

Lymphatic system removes excess tissue fluid
- Located throughout body
- Composed of lymph, vessels, and organs

Lymph

Colorless fluid containing lymphocytes and monocytes

Originates in blood and after filtering, returns to blood

Transports fluids and proteins that have leaked from blood system back to veins

Absorbs and transports fats from villi of small intestine to blood system

Assists in immune function

Lymph Vessels

Similar to veins

Scattered throughout body

Lymph Organs

Lymph nodes, spleen, bone marrow, thymus, and tonsils

Lymph nodes, areas of concentrated tissue (Figure 1-44)

Spleen, located in upper left quadrant (ULQ) of abdomen

Composed of lymph tissue

Function is to filter blood; activates lymphocytes and B-cells to filter antigens

Stores blood

Thymus secretes thymosin causing T-cells to mature

Larger in infants and shrinks with age

Tonsils

Palatine tonsils

Pharyngeal tonsils/adenoids

Hematopoietic Organ

Bone marrow, contains tissue that produces RBCs, WBCs, and platelets

Produces stem cells

COMBINING FORMS

1. aden/o, adnen/o — gland
2. adenoid/o — adenoids
3. axill/o — armpit
4. cervic/o — neck/cervix

Copyright © 2005, Elsevier Inc. All rights reserved.
CPT only © 2004. *Current Procedural Terminology, 2005, Professional Edition*, American Medical Association. All rights reserved.

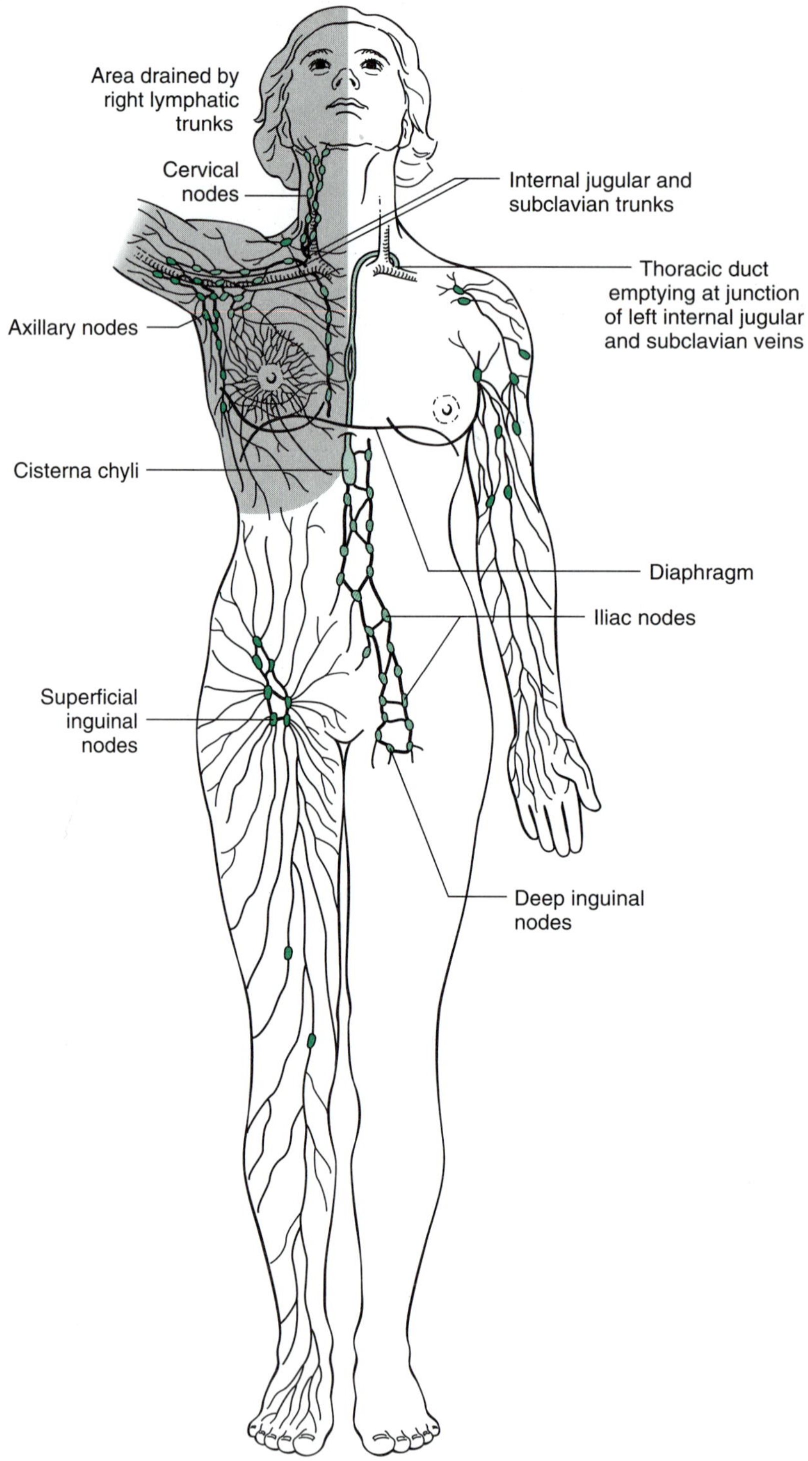

Figure 1-44 Lymphatic system.

5. immun/o immune
6. inguin/o groin
7. lymph/o lymph
8. lymphaden/o lymph gland
9. splen/o spleen

Copyright © 2005, Elsevier Inc. All rights reserved.
CPT only © 2004. *Current Procedural Terminology, 2005, Professional Edition*, American Medical Association. All rights reserved.

10. thym/o	thymus gland
11. tonsill/o	tonsil
12. tox/o	poison

PREFIXES

1. hyper-	excess
2. inter-	between
3. retro-	behind

SUFFIXES

1. -ectomy	removal
2. -edema	swelling
3. -itis	inflammation
4. -megaly	enlargement
5. -oid	resembling
6. -oma	tumor
7. -penia	deficient
8. -pexy	fixation
9. -phylaxis	protection
10. -poiesis	production

MEDICAL TERMS

Axillary nodes	Lymph nodes located in the armpit
Cloquet's node	Also called a gland; it is the highest of the deep groin lymph nodes
Inguinofemoral	Referring to the groin and thigh
Jugular nodes	Lymph nodes located next to the large vein in the neck
Lymph node	Station along the lymphatic system
Lymphadenectomy	Excision of a lymph node or nodes
Lymphadenitis	Inflammation of a lymph node
Lymphangiography	Radiographic recording of the lymphatic vessels and nodes
Lymphangiotomy	Incision into a lymphatic vessel
Parathyroid	Produces a hormone to mobilize calcium from the bones to the blood
Splenectomy	Excision of the spleen
Splenography	Radiographic recording of the spleen
Splenoportography	Radiographic procedure to allow visualization of the splenic and portal veins of the spleen
Stem cell	Immature blood cell
Thoracic duct	Collection and distribution point for lymph, and the largest lymph vessel located in the chest
Transplantation	Grafting of tissue from one source to another

Copyright © 2005, Elsevier Inc. All rights reserved.
CPT only © 2004. *Current Procedural Terminology, 2005, Professional Edition*, American Medical Association. All rights reserved.

HEMIC AND LYMPHATIC SYSTEM QUIZ

1. The spleen is located in this quadrant of the abdomen:
   a. URQ
   b. ULQ
   c. LLQ
   d. LRQ

2. Produces RBCs and platelets:
   a. thymus
   b. tonsils
   c. lymph node
   d. bone marrow

3. Which of the following is NOT a lymph organ:
   a. adrenal
   b. spleen
   c. thymus
   d. tonsil

4. Lymph transports fluids and ________ that have leaked from the blood system back to veins.
   a. stem cells
   b. lymphocytes
   c. B-cells
   d. proteins

5. This is largest in infants and shrinks with age:
   a. tonsils
   b. spleen
   c. thymus
   d. bone marrow

6. Combining form meaning gland:
   a. axill/o
   b. thym/o
   c. aden/o
   d. tox/o

7. Prefix meaning excess:
   a. hyper-
   b. hypo-
   c. inter-
   d. retro-

8. Suffix meaning enlargement:
   a. -edema
   b. -poiesis
   c. -penia
   d. -megaly

Copyright © 2005, Elsevier Inc. All rights reserved.
CPT only © 2004. *Current Procedural Terminology, 2005, Professional Edition*, American Medical Association. All rights reserved.

9. Lymph node located on neck:
   a. thoracic
   b. jugular
   c. Cloquet's
   d. axillary

10. These cells originate in the bone marrow:
    a. leucocytes
    b. erythrocytes
    c. monocytes
    d. stem cells

Copyright © 2005, Elsevier Inc. All rights reserved.
CPT only © 2004. *Current Procedural Terminology, 2005, Professional Edition,* American Medical Association. All rights reserved.

HEMIC AND LYMPHATIC SYSTEM—PATHOPHYSIOLOGY

Anemia

- Reduction in number of erythrocytes or decrease in quality of hemoglobin
  - Less oxygen is transported in the blood

Aplastic anemia

Diverse group of anemias

Characterized by bone marrow failure with reduced number of hematopoietic cells

Causes

- Genetic
- Toxin
- Radiation
- Immunologic
- Idiopathic (unknown)

Treatment

- Blood transfusion
- Bone marrow transplant

Iron deficiency anemia

Characterized by small erythrocytes and a reduced amount of hemoglobin

Caused by low or absent iron stores or serum iron concentrations

- Blood loss
- Decreased intake of iron
- Malabsorption of iron

Symptoms

- Pallor
- Headache
- Stomatitis
- Oral lesions
- Gastrointestinal complaints
- Retinal hemorrhages
- Thinning, brittle nails and hair

Treatment

- Iron supplement

Pernicious anemia

- Megaloblastic anemia
- Usually in older adults
- Caused by impaired intestinal absorption of vitamin B_{12}

Copyright © 2005, Elsevier Inc. All rights reserved.
CPT only © 2004. *Current Procedural Terminology, 2005, Professional Edition*, American Medical Association. All rights reserved.

Symptoms

- Pallor
- Weakness
- Neurologic manifestations
- Gastric discomfort

Treatment

- Injections of Vitamin B_{12}

Hemolytic anemia

May be acute or chronic

Shortened survival of mature erythrocytes

- Inability of bone marrow to compensate for decreased survival of erythrocytes

Treatment

- Treat the cause

Sickle cell anemia

- Occurs primarily in those of West African descent
- Abnormal sickle-shaped erythrocytes (sickle cell)

Symptoms

- Abdominal pain
- Ulceration of lower extremities
- Fatigue
- Dyspnea
- Increased heart rate

Treatment

- Symptomatic

Granulocytosis

- Increase in granulocytes
  - Neutrophils
  - Eosinophils
  - Basophils

Eosinophilia

Increase in number of eosinophils

Cause

- Allergic disorders
- Dermatologic disorders

Copyright © 2005, Elsevier Inc. All rights reserved.
CPT only © 2004. *Current Procedural Terminology, 2005, Professional Edition*, American Medical Association. All rights reserved.

- Parasitic invasion
- Drugs
- Malignancies

Monocytosis

Cause

- Infection
- Hematologic factors

Leukocytosis

Cause

- Acute viral infections, such as hepatitis
- Chronic infections, such as syphilis

Leukocytopenia

Cause

- Neoplasias
- Immune deficiencies
- Drugs
- Virus
- Radiation

Infectious mononucleosis

Acute infection of B cells

Epstein-Barr virus the most common cause

Symptoms

- Fatigue
- Lymph node enlargement
- Splenomegaly
- Hepatomegaly

Transmission

- Saliva
    - Known as kissing disease

Treatment

- Rest
- Treatment of symptoms

Copyright © 2005, Elsevier Inc. All rights reserved.
CPT only © 2004. *Current Procedural Terminology, 2005, Professional Edition,* American Medical Association. All rights reserved.

Leukemia

Malignant disorder of the blood and blood-forming organs

Leads to dysfunction of cells

- Primarily leads to proliferation of abnormal leukocytes

Acute leukemia

- Rapid onset
- Short survival time
- Most cases occur in children

Types

- Lymphocytic
- Myelogenous
- Monocytic

Symptoms

- Anemia
- Bleeding
- Fever
- Infection
- Anorexia

Treatment

- Chemotherapy
- Bone marrow transplant

Chronic leukemia

Types

- Myelogenous
- Lymphocytic

Cells are more differentiated

Gradual onset with milder symptoms

Survival time is longer than with acute leukemia

- Majority of cases are in adults

Symptoms

- Extreme fatigue
- Weight loss
- Splenomegaly
- Night sweats
- Fever
- Infections

Copyright © 2005, Elsevier Inc. All rights reserved.
CPT only © 2004. *Current Procedural Terminology, 2005, Professional Edition*, American Medical Association. All rights reserved.

Treatment

- Chemotherapy
- Bone marrow transplant

Lymphadenopathy

Lymphadenopathy

- Any abnormality of lymph node
- Enlargement of lymph node

Lymphangitis

- Inflammation of lymphatic vessel

Lymphadenitis

- Inflammation of lymph node
- Localized inflammation associated with inflamed lesion
- Generalized inflammation associated with disease
- Inflammation can occur as result of
    - Trauma
    - Infection
    - Drug reaction
    - Autoimmune disease
    - Immunologic disease

Malignant Lymphoma

Hodgkin disease

- Initial sign is a painless mass commonly located on the neck
- Giant Reed-Sternberg cells are present in the lymphatic tissue

Presentation

- Enlarged spleen (splenomegaly)
- Abdominal mass
- Mediastinal mass
- Localized node involvement
    - Orderly spreading of node involvement

Symptoms

- Night sweats
- Fever
- Weight loss
- Itching (pruritus)
- Anorexia

Copyright © 2005, Elsevier Inc. All rights reserved.
CPT only © 2004. *Current Procedural Terminology, 2005, Professional Edition*, American Medical Association. All rights reserved.

Treatment

- Radiation therapy
- Chemotherapy

Prognosis depends of the stage of the disease when diagnosed

Non-Hodgkin Lymphoma

No giant Reed-Sternberg cells present

Involves multiple nodes scattered throughout the body
  - Noncontiguous spread of node involvement

Usually begins as a painless enlargement of node

Symptoms

- Presents similar to Hodgkin disease

Treatment

- Chemotherapy
- Radiation

Prognosis depends on stage

Burkitt lymphoma

- Type of non-Hodgkin lymphoma
- Usually found in Africa
- Characterized by lesions in the jaw
- Epstein-Barr (herpes virus) has been found in Burkitt's lymphoma

Myeloma

Multiple myeloma

- B cell cancer
  - Also known as plasma cell myeloma
- Increased plasma cells replace bone marrow
- Multiple tumor sites cause bone destruction
- Result in weakened bone
- Cause is unknown

Treatment

- Chemotherapy
- Poor prognosis, with average life expectancy of 3 years

Copyright © 2005, Elsevier Inc. All rights reserved.
CPT only © 2004. *Current Procedural Terminology, 2005, Professional Edition,* American Medical Association. All rights reserved.

HEMIC AND LYMPHATIC SYSTEM PATHOPHYSIOLOGY QUIZ

1. This condition involves a reduced number of erythrocytes and decreased quality of hemoglobin.
   a. monocytosis
   b. eosinophilia
   c. anemia
   d. leukocytosis

2. This condition is hallmarked by a shortened survival of mature erythrocytes and inability of bone marrow to compensate for decreased survival.
   a. hemolytic anemia
   b. granulocytosis
   c. eosinophilia
   d. monocytosis

3. The most common type of this virus is Epstein-Barr.
   a. leukocytopenia
   b. infectious mononucleosis
   c. leukocytosis
   d. hemolytic anemia

4. Inflammation of the lymphatic vessels is
   a. lymphadenitis
   b. lymphoma
   c. lymphadenopathy
   d. lymphangitis

5. What giant cell is present in Hodgkin disease?
   a. B cell
   b. Reed-Sternberg
   c. T cell
   d. C cell

6. The average number of years of survival for multiple myeloma is
   a. 5
   b. 10
   c. 3
   d. 20

7. The most common type of sideroblastic anemia is
   a. acquired
   b. hereditary
   c. reversible
   d. nonreversible

8. These are large stem cells.
   a. megaloblasts
   b. leukocytes
   c. erythrocytes
   d. granulocytes

Copyright © 2005, Elsevier Inc. All rights reserved.
CPT only © 2004. *Current Procedural Terminology, 2005, Professional Edition*, American Medical Association. All rights reserved.

9. This is known as the kissing disease.
   a. monocytosis
   b. leukocytopenia
   c. infectious mononucleosis
   d. granulocytosis

10. This lymphoma is usually found in Africa.
   a. multiple
   b. Burkitt
   c. B cell
   d. T cell

Copyright © 2005, Elsevier Inc. All rights reserved.
CPT only © 2004. *Current Procedural Terminology, 2005, Professional Edition,* American Medical Association. All rights reserved.

ENDOCRINE SYSTEM

- Regulates body through hormones
- Affects growth, development, and metabolism

Nine Glands (Figure 1-45)

Pituitary (hypophysis): master gland

Located at base of brain in a depression in skull (sella turcica)

Anterior pituitary (adenohypophysis)

Adrenocorticotropic hormone (ACTH)—stimulates adrenal cortex

Follicle-stimulating hormone (FSH)—males, stimulates sperm production; females, stimulates secretion of estrogen and stimulates follicle development

Growth hormone (GH or somatotropin)—stimulates growth and fat metabolism, and maintains blood glucose levels

Luteinizing hormone (LH)—male, stimulates testosterone; females, stimulates secretion of progesterone and estrogen

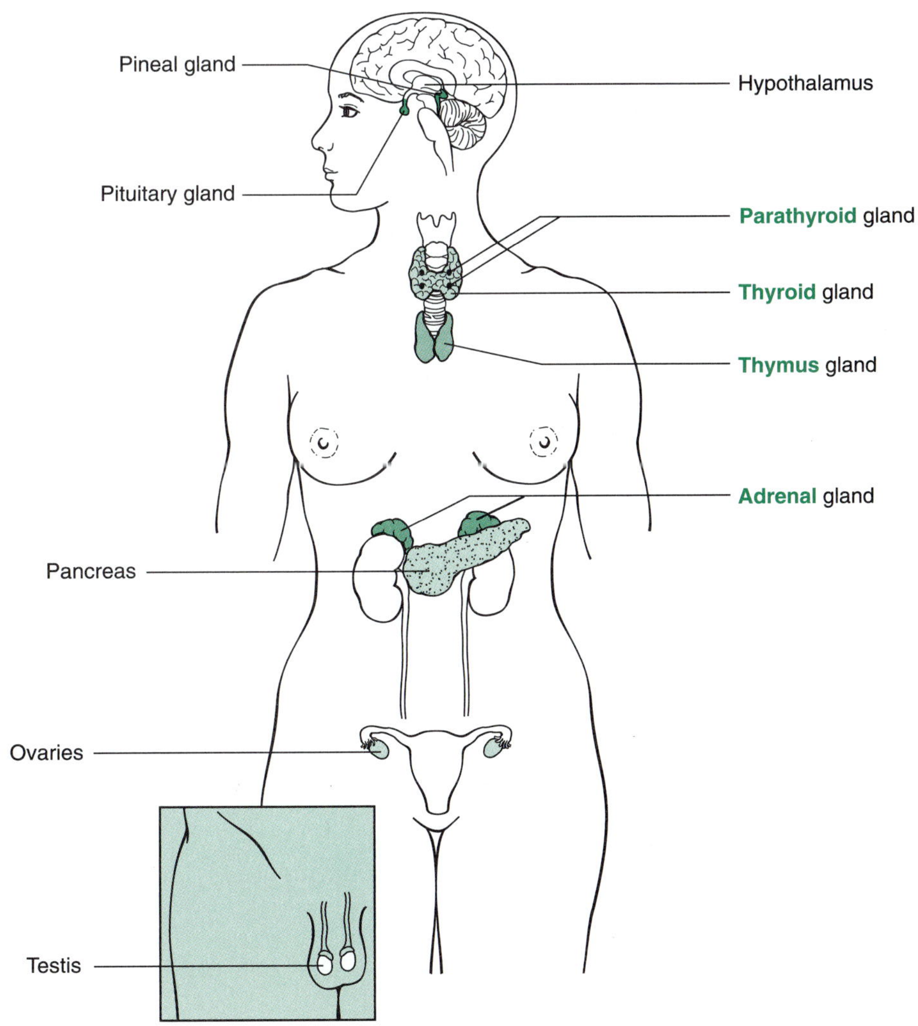

Figure 1-45 Endocrine system.

Copyright © 2005, Elsevier Inc. All rights reserved.
CPT only © 2004. *Current Procedural Terminology, 2005, Professional Edition*, American Medical Association. All rights reserved.

Melanocyte-stimulating hormone (MSH)—increases pigmentation

Prolactin (PRL)—stimulates milk production and breast development

Thyroid-stimulating hormone (TSH or thyrotropin)—stimulates thyroid gland

Posterior pituitary (neurohypophysis)—stores hormones

Antidiuretic hormone (ADH)—stimulates reabsorption of water by kidney tubules

Oxytocin—stimulates contractions during childbirth and release of milk

Thyroid

Two lobes overlying trachea (Adam's apple)

Secretes two hormones that increase metabolism—thyroxine (T_4) and triiodothyronine (T_3)

Secretes one hormone that decreases blood calcium—thyrocalcitonin

Parathyroid (4)

Located on posterior side of thyroid

Secretes PTH (parathyroid hormone)

Mobilizes calcium from bones

Adrenal (pair)

Located on top of each kidney

Adrenal cortex—outer region that secretes corticosteroids

Cortisol—increases blood glucose

Aldosterone—increases reabsorption of sodium (salt)

Androgen, estrogen, progestin—sexual characteristics

Adrenal medulla—inner region that secretes catecholamines (epinephrine and norepinephrine)

Pancreas

Located behind stomach

Contains specialized cells (islets of Langerhans) that produce hormones

Produces: insulin (decreases blood glucose), glucagon (converts glycogen to glucose), and somatostatin (regulates other cells of pancreas)

Thymus

Located behind sternum

Atrophies during adolescence

Produces thymosin—stimulates T-lymphocytes

Hypothalamus (part of brain)

Located below thalamus

Stimulates pituitary to release hormones

Copyright © 2005, Elsevier Inc. All rights reserved.
CPT only © 2004. *Current Procedural Terminology, 2005, Professional Edition*, American Medical Association. All rights reserved.

Pineal

Located behind hypothalamus

Secretes melatonin—affects brain and releases of hormones

Ovaries (pair, females)

Estrogen—female sex characteristics

Progesterone—maintains pregnancy

Placenta

Produces HCG (human chorionic gonadotropin) during pregnancy

Testes (pair, males)

Testosterone—male sex characteristics

COMBINING FORMS

1. aden/o, adnen/o	in relationship to a gland
2. adren/o	adrenal gland
3. adrenal/o	adrenal gland
4. andr/o	male
5. calc/o or calci/io	calcium
6. cortic/o	cortex
7. crin/o	secrete
8. dips/o	thirst
9. estr/o	female
10. gluc/o	sugar
11. glyc/o	sugar
12. gonad/o	ovaries and testes
13. home/o	same
14. hormon/o	hormone
15. kal/i	potassium
16. lact/o	milk
17. myx/o	mucus
18. natr/o	sodium
19. pancreat/o	pancreas
20. phys/o	growing
21. pituitar/o	pituitary gland
22. somat/o	body
23. ster/o or stere/o	solid, having three dimensions

Copyright © 2005, Elsevier Inc. All rights reserved.
CPT only © 2004. *Current Procedural Terminology, 2005, Professional Edition*, American Medical Association. All rights reserved.

24. thyroid/o	thyroid gland
25. toxic/o	poison

PREFIXES

1. eu-	good/normal
2. oxy-	sharp
3. pan-	all
4. tetra-	four
5. tri-	three
6. tropin-	act upon

SUFFIXES

1. -agon	assemble
2. -drome	run
3. -in	a substance
4. -ine	a substance
5. -tropin	act upon
6. -uria	urine

MEDICAL TERMS

Adrenals	Glands, located at the top of the kidneys, that produce steroid hormones
Contralateral	Opposite side
Hormone	Chemical substance produced by the body
Isthmus	Connection of two regions or structures
Isthmus, thyroid	Tissue connection between right and left thyroid lobes
Isthmusectomy	Surgical removal of the isthmus
Lobectomy	Removal of a lobe
Thymectomy	Surgical removal of the thymus
Thymus	Gland that produces hormones important to the immune response
Thyroglossal duct	Connection between the thyroid and the tongue
Thyroid	Part of the endocrine system that produces hormones that regulate metabolism
Thyroidectomy	Surgical removal of the thyroid

Copyright © 2005, Elsevier Inc. All rights reserved.
CPT only © 2004. *Current Procedural Terminology, 2005, Professional Edition*, American Medical Association. All rights reserved.

ENDOCRINE SYSTEM QUIZ

1. Which of the following is NOT affected by the endocrine system:
   a. growth
   b. development
   c. progesterone
   d. metabolism

2. Gland that overlies the Adam's apple:
   a. parathyroid
   b. adrenal
   c. pancreas
   d. thyroid

3. Gland that is located on the top of each kidney:
   a. parathyroid
   b. adrenal
   c. pancreas
   d. thyroid

4. The outer region of the adrenal gland that secretes corticosteroids:
   a. cortex
   b. medulla
   c. sternum
   d. medullary

5. Located on the thyroid:
   a. hypophysis
   b. thymus
   c. pineal
   d. parathyroid

6. Located at the base of the brain in a depression in the skull:
   a. pituitary
   b. thymus
   c. adrenal
   d. pineal

7. Stimulates contractions during childbirth:
   a. cortisol
   b. PTH
   c. ADH
   d. oxytocin

8. Produced only during pregnancy by the placenta:
   a. human chorionic gonadotropin
   b. melatonin
   c. thymosin
   d. adrenocorticotropic hormone

Copyright © 2005, Elsevier Inc. All rights reserved.
CPT only © 2004. *Current Procedural Terminology, 2005, Professional Edition,* American Medical Association. All rights reserved.

9. Combining form meaning secrete:
   a. dips/o
   b. crin/o
   c. gluc/o
   d. kal/i

10. Prefix meaning good:
    a. tri-
    b. tropin-
    c. pan-
    d. eu-

Copyright © 2005, Elsevier Inc. All rights reserved.
CPT only © 2004. *Current Procedural Terminology, 2005, Professional Edition*, American Medical Association. All rights reserved.

ENDOCRINE SYSTEM—PATHOPHYSIOLOGY

Diabetes Mellitus

Caused by a deficiency in insulin production or poor use of body cells

Types of diabetes mellitus

Type 1, IDDM (insulin-dependent diabetes mellitus), immune mediated

- Onset before age 30
- Acute onset
- Positive family history
- Require insulin

Type 2, NIDDM (non–insulin dependent diabetes mellitus)

- Adult onset, after age 30, but it is now occurring earlier
- Insidious onset
- Positive in immediate family
- Dietary management and/or oral hypoglycemics and/or insulin
- Most common type

Symptoms

- Polyuria
- Polydipsia
- Glycosuria
- Hyperglycemia

Acute complications

- Hypoglycemia
- Diabetic ketoacidosis

Chronic complications

- Diabetic neuropathy (Figure 1-46)
- Retinopathy
- Coronary artery disease
- Stroke
- Peripheral vascular disease
- Infection

Pituitary Disorders

- Tumors are the most common cause of pituitary disorders
- Tumors may secrete hormones, such as prolactin and ACTH

Anterior pituitary

Dwarfism

- Can be caused by deficiency of somatotrophin (GH) hormone

Copyright © 2005, Elsevier Inc. All rights reserved.
CPT only © 2004. *Current Procedural Terminology, 2005, Professional Edition*, American Medical Association. All rights reserved.

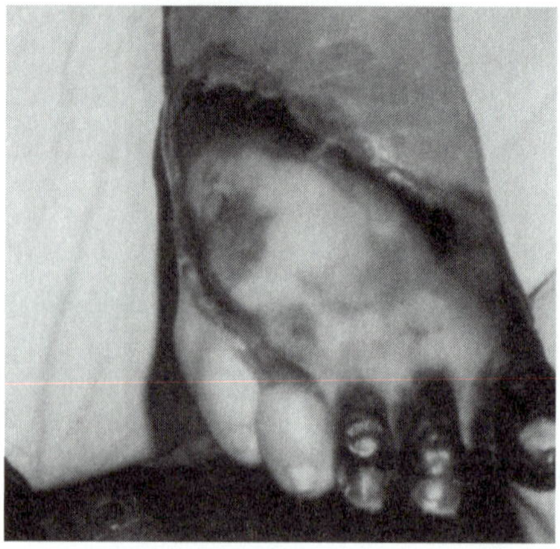

Figure 1-46 Diabetic patient with peripheral neuropathy. (From Levin ME: Pathogenesis and general management of foot lesions in the diabetic patient. In Bowker JH, Pfeifer MA, editors: *Levin and O'Neal's the diabetic foot,* ed 6, St Louis, 2001, Mosby.)

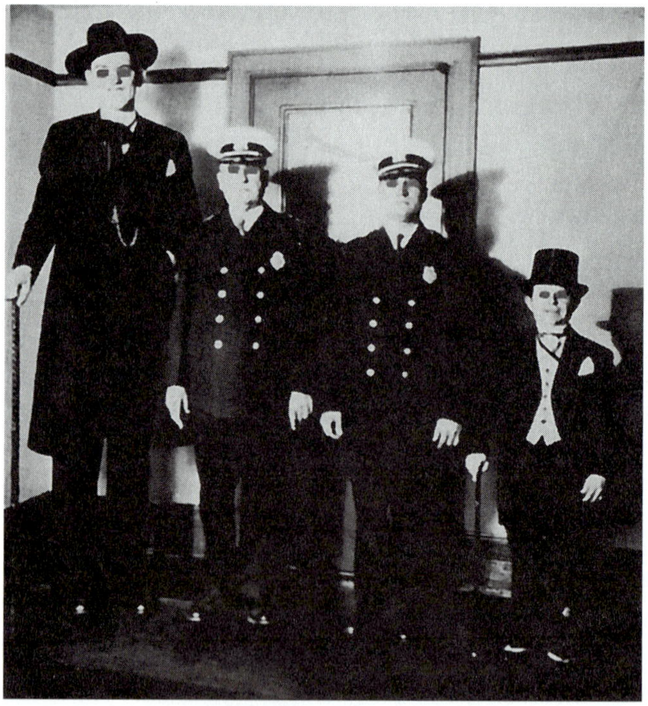

Figure 1-47 Giantism. A pituitary giant and dwarf contrasted with normal-size men. (From Thibodeau GA, Patton KT: *Anatomy & physiology,* ed 5, St Louis, 2003, Mosby.)

Gigantism (Figure 1-47)

- Can be caused by excess of somatotrophin (GH) hormone in childhood

Acromegaly

- Increased GH in adulthood
- Enlargement of facial bones, feet, and hands

Copyright © 2005, Elsevier Inc. All rights reserved.
CPT only © 2004. *Current Procedural Terminology, 2005, Professional Edition,* American Medical Association. All rights reserved.

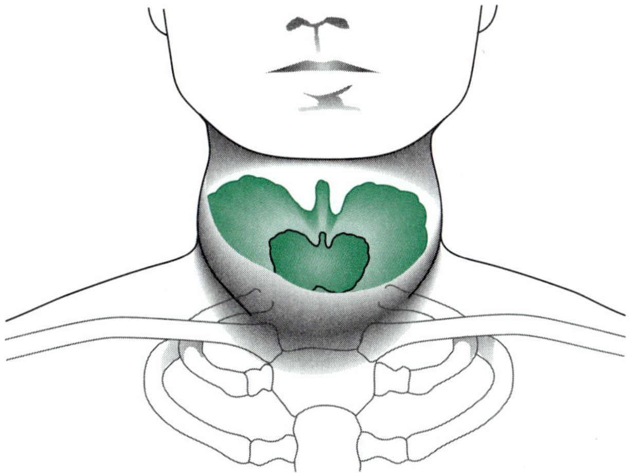

Figure 1-48 Goiter is an enlargement of the thyroid gland.

Diabetic insipidus

- Insufficient ADH
- Causes polyuria, polydipsia, and dehydration

Thyroid Disorders

Goiter (Figure 1-48)

Enlargement of thyroid gland

Cause

- Hypothyroid disorders
- Hyperthyroid disorders

Hyperthyroidism

Excessive thyroid hormone production

Characterized by

- Goiter
- Tachycardia
- Atrial fibrillation
- Pulse pressure
- Palpitations
- Fatigue
- Tremor
- Nervousness
- Weight loss
- Exophthalmos (protruding eyes)
    - Decreased blinking

Treatment

- Medication (antithyroid drugs)
- Radioactive iodine
- Surgical excision

Copyright © 2005, Elsevier Inc. All rights reserved.
CPT only © 2004. *Current Procedural Terminology, 2005, Professional Edition*, American Medical Association. All rights reserved.

Hypothyroidism

Decreased levels of thyroid hormone production

Types

- Cretinism
    - Congenital
    - Occurs in children
    - If not treated, it will cause a severe delay in physical mental development
- Myxedema
    - Severe form
    - Occurs in adults
    - Symptoms:
        - Cold intolerance
        - Weight gain
        - Mental sluggishness
        - Fatigue
- Hashimoto's thyroiditis
    - Autoimmune disorder

Treatment

- Medication (hormone replacement)

Parathyroid Disorders

Hyperparathyroidism

- Leads to hypercalcemia
    - Affects heart and bones

Symptoms

- Brittle bones
- Kidney stones
- Cardiac disturbances

Treatment

- Surgical excision

Hypoparathyroidism

Leads to hypocalcemia

Symptoms

- Nerve irritability
- Muscle cramps
- Tetany

Copyright © 2005, Elsevier Inc. All rights reserved.
CPT only © 2004. *Current Procedural Terminology, 2005, Professional Edition*, American Medical Association. All rights reserved.

Treatment

- Calcium and vitamin D

Adrenal Gland Disorders

Cushing syndrome

Excess levels of circulating cortisol (glucocorticoid)

Cause

- Hyperfunction of the adrenal cortex
- Excess levels of ACTH from the pituitary
- Long-term use of steroid medications

Symptoms

- Weight gain
    - Fat deposits on face and trunk
- Glucose intolerance
    - Diabetes may develop (20%)
- Muscle wasting
- Osteoporosis
- Change in mental status
- Delayed healing

Treatment

- Medication
- Radiation therapy
- Surgical intervention

Hyperaldosteronism

Excess aldosterone secreted by the adrenal cortex

Types

- Primary hyperaldosteronism (Conn's syndrome)
    - Caused by an abnormality of the adrenal cortex
        - Usually an adrenal adenoma
- Secondary hyperaldosteronism
    - Caused by other than adrenal secretion
- Symptoms
    - Hypertension
    - Hypokalemia
    - Neurologic disorders

Treatment

- Treat the underlying condition that caused hyperaldosteronism
    - Such as adrenal adenoma

Copyright © 2005, Elsevier Inc. All rights reserved.
CPT only © 2004. *Current Procedural Terminology, 2005, Professional Edition*, American Medical Association. All rights reserved.

Androgen and estrogen hypersecretion

Androgen, male characteristic hormone

- Virilization, development of male characteristics

Estrogen, female characteristic hormone

Cause

- Underlying condition
  - Adrenal tumor
  - Cushing syndrome

Treatment

- Surgical intervention for tumor
- Underlying condition

Addison disease

Deficiency of

- Glucocorticoids
- Adrenocorticoids
- Mineralocorticoids

Cause

- Tumors
- Autoimmune disorders
- Viral
- Tuberculosis
- Infection

Symptoms

- Decreased blood glucose levels
- Fatigue
- Lack of ability to handle stress
- Weight loss
- Infections
- Hypotension
- Decreased body hair
- Hyperpigmentation

Treatment

- Hormone replacement

Copyright © 2005, Elsevier Inc. All rights reserved.
CPT only © 2004. *Current Procedural Terminology, 2005, Professional Edition*, American Medical Association. All rights reserved.

ENDOCRINE SYSTEM PATHOPHYSIOLOGY QUIZ

1. This type of diabetes typically occurs before age 30:
   a. type 1
   b. type 2

2. The acronym that indicates that insulin is not required is
   a. IDDM
   b. NIDDM
   c. PIDDM
   d. NDDMI

3. The most common cause of pituitary disorders is
   a. hypersecretion
   b. hyposecretion
   c. tumor
   d. infection

4. In excess, this hormone can cause gigantism:
   a. somatotrophin
   b. thyroid
   c. mineralocorticoids
   d. adrenocortical

5. Goiter can be caused by which of the following:
   a. hypothyroidism
   b. parathyroidism
   c. hyperthyroidism
   d. both a and c

6. This type of hypothyroidism is an autoimmune disorder:
   a. myxedema
   b. Hashimoto's
   c. cretinism
   d. hypokalemia

7. Tetany can be caused by
   a. hypoparathyroidism
   b. hyperthyroidism
   c. hyperparathyroidism
   d. hyperaldosteronism

8. Conn's syndrome is also known as
   a. primary hypoparathyroidism
   b. primary hyperthyroidism
   c. primary hyperparathyroidism
   d. primary hyperaldosteronism

Copyright © 2005, Elsevier Inc. All rights reserved.
CPT only © 2004. *Current Procedural Terminology, 2005, Professional Edition,* American Medical Association. All rights reserved.

9. Development of male characteristics is known as
   a. virilization
   b. feminization
   c. hypertrophy
   d. hyperaldosteronism

10. The treatment for Addison disease is often
    a. chemotherapy
    b. radiation
    c. hormone replacement
    d. all of the above

Copyright © 2005, Elsevier Inc. All rights reserved.
CPT only © 2004. *Current Procedural Terminology, 2005, Professional Edition,* American Medical Association. All rights reserved.

NERVOUS SYSTEM

- Controlling, regulating, and communicating system
- Organization
  - Central nervous system (CNS), brain and spinal cord
  - Peripheral nervous system (PNS), cranial and spinal nerves

Cells of the Nervous System (Figure 1-49)

Neurons

Classified according to function:

Dendrites (receive signals)

Cell body (nucleus, within cell body)

Axon (carries signals from cell body)

Myelin sheath (insulation around axon)

Glia

Astrocytes

Microglia

Oligodendrocytes

Divisions (Figure 1-50)

Brain

Brainstem

Medulla oblongata

Pons

Midbrain

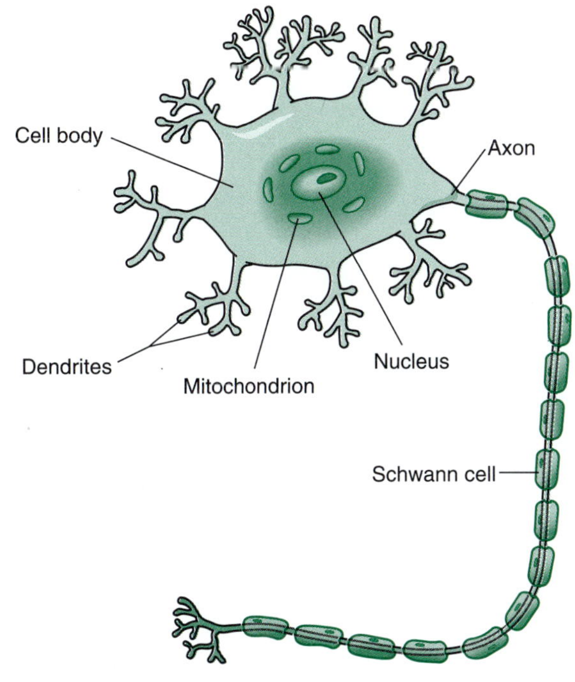

Figure 1-49 Myelinated axon.

Copyright © 2005, Elsevier Inc. All rights reserved.
CPT only © 2004. *Current Procedural Terminology, 2005, Professional Edition*, American Medical Association. All rights reserved.

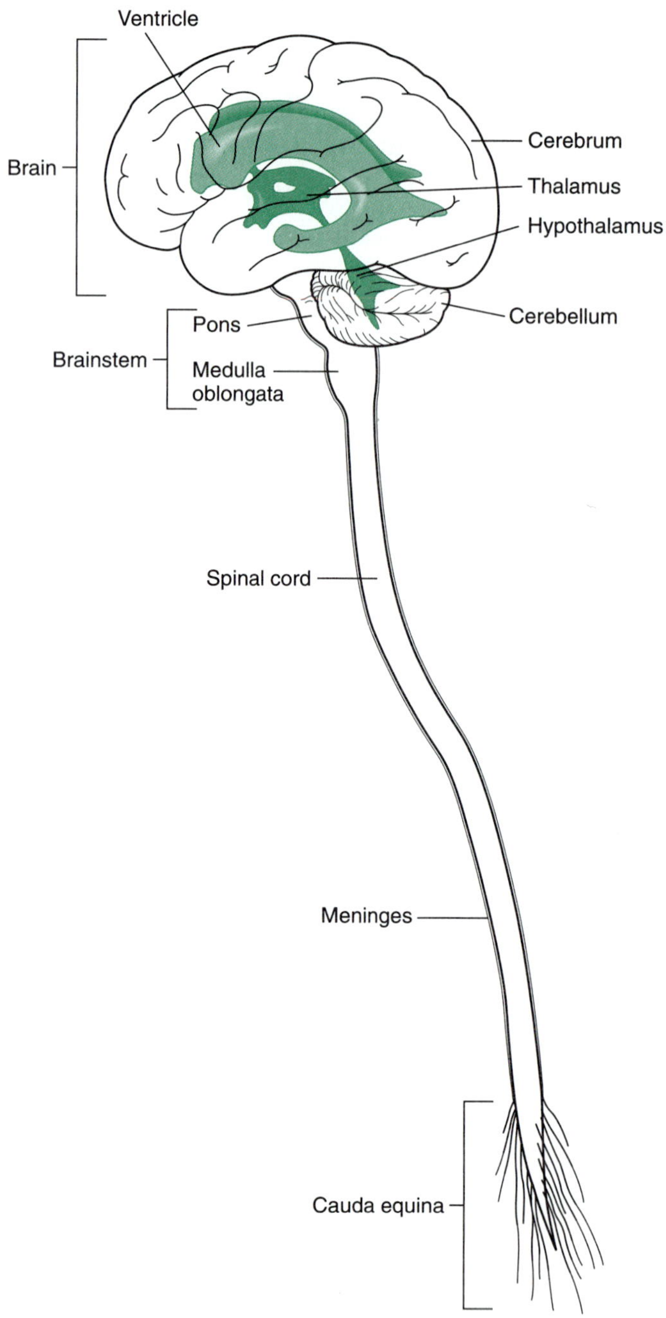

Figure 1-50 Brain and spinal cord.

Diencephalon

Hypothalamus controls autonomic nervous system

Thalamus relays impulses to cerebral cortex

Cerebellum

Controls muscle contractions

Balance

Copyright © 2005, Elsevier Inc. All rights reserved.
CPT only © 2004. *Current Procedural Terminology, 2005, Professional Edition,* American Medical Association. All rights reserved.

Cerebrum

Largest part of brain

Mental processes

Two hemispheres

Right controls left side of body

Left controls right side of body

Divided into five lobes

- Frontal
- Parietal
- Temporal
- Occipital
- Insula

Spinal Cord and Cranium

Spinal and cerebral meninges (coverings)

Spine and brain spaces containing cerebrospinal fluid (subarachnoid space)

Cavities within the brain containing cerebrospinal fluid (ventricles)

Peripheral Nervous System (PNS)

Cranial nerves, 12 pair

Spinal nerves, 31 pair

Autonomic Nervous System (ANS)

Two divisions

- Sympathetic system
- Parasympathetic system

COMBINING FORMS

1. cephal/o	head
2. cerebell/o	cerebellum
3. cerebr/o	cerebrum
4. crani/o	cranium
5. dur/o	dura mater
6. encephal/o	brain
7. gangli/o	ganglion
8. ganglion/o	ganglion
9. mening/o	meninges

Copyright © 2005, Elsevier Inc. All rights reserved.
CPT only © 2004. *Current Procedural Terminology, 2005, Professional Edition*, American Medical Association. All rights reserved.

10. meningi/o — meninges
11. ment/o — mind
12. mon/o — one
13. myel/o — bone marrow
14. neur/o — nerve
15. phas/o — speech
16. phren/o — mind
17. poli/o — gray matter
18. pont/o — pons
19. psych/o — mind
20. quadr/i — four
21. radic/o — nerve root
22. radicul/o — nerve root
23. rhiz/o — nerve root

PREFIXES

1. hemi- — half
2. per- — through
3. quadri- — four
4. tetra- — four

SUFFIXES

1. -algesia — pain sensation
2. -algia — pain
3. -cele — hernia
4. -esthesia — feeling
5. -iatry — medical treatment
6. -ictal — pertaining to
7. -paresis — incomplete paralysis
8. -plegia — paralysis

MEDICAL ABBREVIATIONS

1. ANS — autonomic nervous system
2. CNS — central nervous system
3. CSF — cerebrospinal fluid
4. CVA — stroke/cerebrovascular accident
5. EEG — electroencephalogram

Copyright © 2005, Elsevier Inc. All rights reserved.
CPT only © 2004. *Current Procedural Terminology, 2005, Professional Edition*, American Medical Association. All rights reserved.

6. LP lumbar puncture
7. PNS peripheral nervous system
8. TENS transcutaneous electrical nerve stimulation
9. TIA transient ischemic attack

MEDICAL TERMS

Burr	Drill used to create an entry into the cranium
Central nervous system	Brain and spinal cord
Craniectomy	Permanent, partial removal of skull
Craniotomy	Opening of the skull
Cranium	That part of the skeleton that encloses the brain
Diskectomy	Removal of a vertebral disk
Electroencephalography	Recording of the electric currents of the brain by means of electrodes attached to the scalp
Laminectomy	Surgical excision of the lamina
Peripheral nerves	12 pairs of cranial nerves, 31 pairs of spinal nerves, and autonomic nervous system; connects peripheral receptors to the brain and spinal cord
Shunt	An artificial passage
Skull	Entire skeletal framework of the head
Somatic nerve	Sensory or motor nerve
Stereotaxis	Method of identifying a specific area or point in the brain
Sympathetic nerve	Part of the peripheral nervous system that controls automatic body function and sympathetic nerves activated under stress
Trephination	Surgical removal of a disk of bone
Vertebrectomy	Removal of vertebra

Copyright © 2005, Elsevier Inc. All rights reserved.
CPT only © 2004. *Current Procedural Terminology, 2005, Professional Edition*, American Medical Association. All rights reserved.

NERVOUS SYSTEM QUIZ

1. Portion of the nervous system contains the cranial and spinal nerves:
   a. central
   b. peripheral
   c. autonomic
   d. parasympathetic

2. The part of the neuron that receives signals:
   a. dendrites
   b. cell body
   c. axon
   d. myelin sheath

3. NOT associated with glia:
   a. monocytes
   b. astrocytes
   c. microglia
   d. oligodendrocytes

4. Largest part of the brain:
   a. cerebellum
   b. cerebrum
   c. cortex
   d. pons

5. Divided into two hemispheres:
   a. cerebellum
   b. cerebrum
   c. cortex
   d. pons

6. The number of pairs of cranial nerves:
   a. 10
   b. 11
   c. 12
   d. 13

7. Controls the right side of the body:
   a. left cerebrum
   b. right cerebrum
   c. right cortex
   d. left cortex

8. Combining form that means brain:
   a. mening/o
   b. mon/o
   c. esthesi/o
   d. encephal/o

Copyright © 2005, Elsevier Inc. All rights reserved.
CPT only © 2004. *Current Procedural Terminology, 2005, Professional Edition*, American Medical Association. All rights reserved.

9. Prefix that means four:
   a. per-
   b. tetra-
   c. para-
   d. bi-

10. Combining form that means speech:
   a. phas/o
   b. rhiz/o
   c. poli/o
   d. myel/o

Copyright © 2005, Elsevier Inc. All rights reserved.
CPT only © 2004. *Current Procedural Terminology, 2005, Professional Edition,* American Medical Association. All rights reserved.

NERVOUS SYSTEM—PATHOPHYSIOLOGY

Dementias

Cognitive deficiencies

Causes

- Alzheimer's disease
- Vascular disease
- Head trauma
- Tumors
- Infection
- Toxins
- Substance abuse
- AIDS

Alzheimer's disease

Most common type of dementia

Progressive intellectual impairment

- Results in damage to neurons (neurofibrillary tangles)
- Fatal within 3 to 20 years

Causes

- Mostly unknown
- Perhaps genetic defect, autoimmune reaction, or virus

Symptoms

- Behavior change
- Memory loss
- Personality change
- Irritability
- Inability to complete activities of daily living

Treatment

- No cure
- Symptomatic treatment
- Support for the family

Vascular dementia

- Result of brain infarctions

Nutritional degenerative disease

Deficiency

- B vitamins
- Niacin
- Pantothenic acid

Associated with alcoholism

Copyright © 2005, Elsevier Inc. All rights reserved.
CPT only © 2004. *Current Procedural Terminology, 2005, Professional Edition*, American Medical Association. All rights reserved.

Amyotrophic lateral sclerosis (ALS)

- Motor neuron disease (MND)
- Also known as Lou Gehrig's disease
    - Baseball player who died of ALS
- Deterioration of neurons of the spinal cord and brain
- Results in atrophy of muscles and loss of fine motor skills
- Mental functioning remains normal
- Survival is 2 to 10 years after diagnosis
    - Death usually results from respiratory failure

Treatment

- Symptomatic only
- Emotional support
- No cure

Huntington's disease

- Inherited progressive atrophy of brain

Symptoms

- Restlessness
- Rapid, jerky movements in the arms and face
- Rigidity
- Intellectual impairment

Treatment

- No cure
- Symptomatic

Parkinson's disease

- Decreased secretion of dopamine
- Typically occurs after age 60

Symptoms

- Muscle rigidity and weakness
- Tremors
- Masklike facial appearance

Treatment

- Medications to reduce symptoms
- Dopamine replacement

Multiple sclerosis

- Common neurologic condition
    - Demyelination of the central nervous system

Copyright © 2005, Elsevier Inc. All rights reserved.
CPT only © 2004. *Current Procedural Terminology, 2005, Professional Edition*, American Medical Association. All rights reserved.

- Affects young adults
- Results in myelin destruction and gliosis of the white matter of the central nervous system
- Speculation that it is an autoimmune condition or the result of a virus

Symptoms

- Loss of feeling (paresthesias)
- Vision problems
- Bladder disorder
- Mood disorders
- Weakness of limbs

Treatment

- Symptomatic

Myasthenia gravis

- Means grave muscle weakness
- Speculation that it is an autoimmune condition

Symptoms

- Muscle weakness and fatigability
- May be localized or generalized

Often affects:
  - Swallowing
  - Breathing
  - Leading to crisis

Treatment

- Anticholinesterase drugs
  - Restores normal muscle strength and recoverability after fatigue

Poliomyelitis

- Contagious viral disease
- Affects motor neurons
- Causes paralysis and respiratory failure
- Prevent with vaccination

Postpolio syndrome (PPS)

Also known as postpoliomyelitis neuromuscular atrophy

Progressive muscle weakness
- Past history of paralytic polio

Symptoms

- Muscle weakness and fatigability
  - May include atrophy and muscle twitching

Copyright © 2005, Elsevier Inc. All rights reserved.
CPT only © 2004. *Current Procedural Terminology, 2005, Professional Edition*, American Medical Association. All rights reserved.

Treatment

- Symptomatic
- Maintenance of respiratory function

Guillain-Barré syndrome

Also known as:

- Idiopathic polyneuritis
- Acute inflammatory polyneuropathy
- Landry's ascending paralysis

Demyelination of peripheral nerves

Symptoms

- Primary ascending motor paralysis
- Variable sensory disturbances

Treatment

- Supportive

Congenital Neurologic Disorders

Hydrocephalus

- Excessive amounts of cerebrospinal fluid in the head
- Compresses brain
- Treatment is placement of a shunt

Spina bifida (Figure 1-51)

Defect in the vertebral column

- Myelomeningocele
  - Meninges and spinal cord protrude through the defect
- Meningocele
  - Meninges herniated through the defect
- Results in neurologic deficiencies

Treatment

- Surgical repair

Mental Disorders

Schizophrenia

- Variety of syndromes
- Results in changes in the brain
- Hereditary factors are considered a cause
  - Also, fetal brain damage is suspected
- Stress usually precipitates onset

Copyright © 2005, Elsevier Inc. All rights reserved.
CPT only © 2004. *Current Procedural Terminology, 2005, Professional Edition*, American Medical Association. All rights reserved.

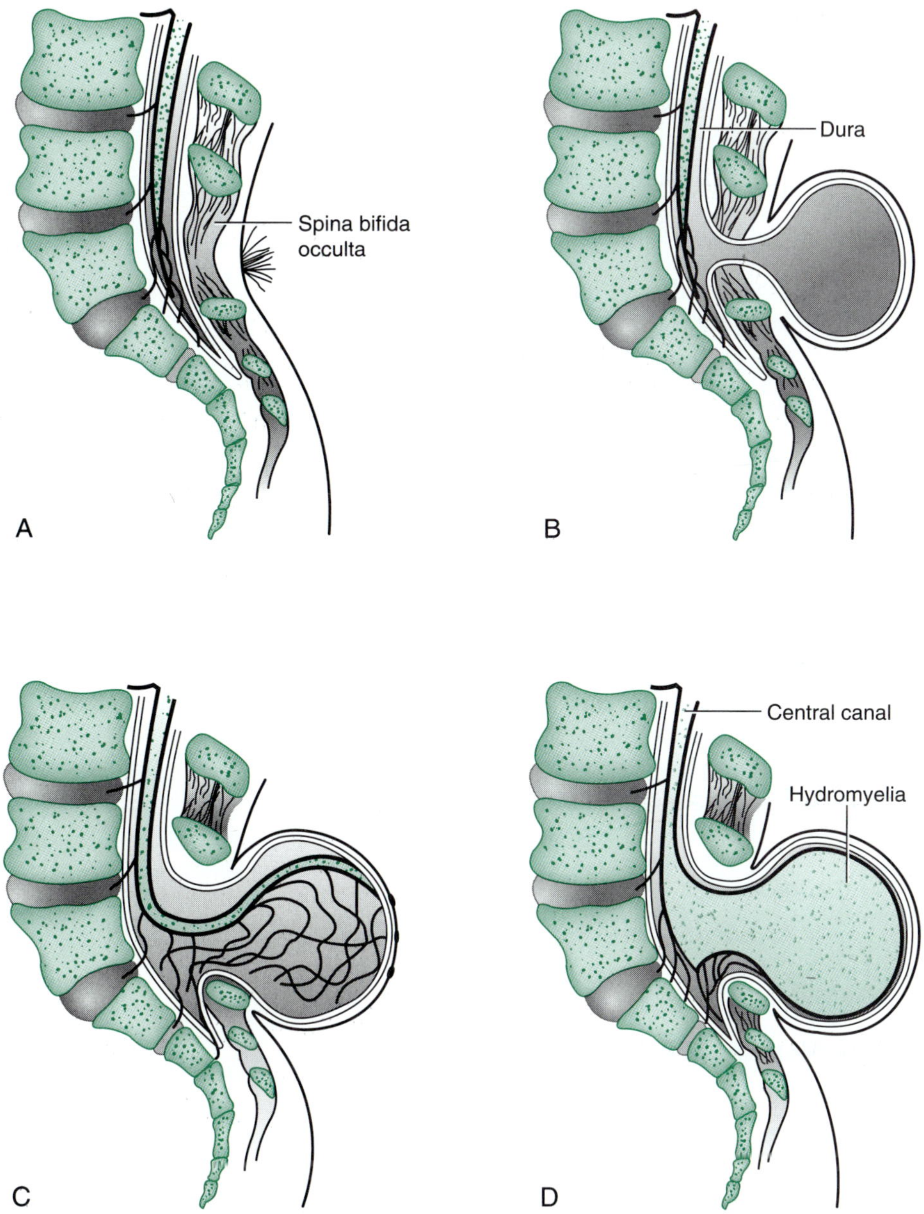

Figure 1-51 *A.* Spina bifida occulta. *B.* Meningocele. *C.* Myelomeningocele. *D.* Myelocystocele or hydromyelia.

Symptoms

- Delusions of persecution and/or grandeur
- Disorganized thought
- Repetitive behaviors
- Behavior issues
- Decreased speech
- Decreased ability to solve problems
- Loss of emotions
- Hallucinations

Types are based on characteristics

Copyright © 2005, Elsevier Inc. All rights reserved.
CPT only © 2004. *Current Procedural Terminology, 2005, Professional Edition,* American Medical Association. All rights reserved.

Treatment

- Antipsychotic drugs
- Drugs have very unpleasant side effects such as:
    - Excessive movement
    - Grimacing
    - Jerking
    - Tremors
    - Shuffling gait
    - Dry mouth
    - Blurred vision

Depression

- Common mood disorder
- Exact cause is unknown

Symptoms

- Sadness
- Hopelessness
- Lethargy
- Insomnia
- Anorexia

Treatment

- Antidepressant drugs
- Electroconvulsive therapy

Central Nervous System (CNS) Disorders

Vascular Disorder

Transient ischemic attack (TIA)

- Temporary reduction of blood flow to brain
- Often a warning sign of cerebrovascular accident

Symptoms

- Depend on location of ischemia
    - Usual recovery in 24 hours
- No loss of consciousness
- May display muscle weakness in legs/arms
- Paresthesia (numbness) of face
- Mental confusion may be present
- Repeated attacks common in the presence of atherosclerotic disease

Cerebrovascular accident (CVA) or stroke

- Infarction of brain due to lack of blood flow
- Necrosis of tissue with total occlusion of vessel

Copyright © 2005, Elsevier Inc. All rights reserved.
CPT only © 2004. *Current Procedural Terminology, 2005, Professional Edition*, American Medical Association. All rights reserved.

Causes

- Atherosclerotic disease
- Embolus
- Hemorrhage

Symptoms

- Depends on location of obstruction

Thrombus
- Gradual onset
- Often occurs at rest
- Intracranial pressure (ICP) minimal
- Localized damage

Embolus
- Sudden onset
- Occurs anytime
- ICP minimal
- Localized damage unless multiple emboli

Hemorrhage
- Sudden onset
- Occurs most often with activity
- ICP high
- Widespread damage
- May be fatal

Treatment

- Anticoagulant drugs if caused by thrombus or embolus
- Oxygen treatment
- Underlying condition treated, such as:
  - Hypertension
  - Atherosclerosis
  - Thrombus

Aneurysm

- Dilation of artery
  - May be localized or multiple
- Rupture possible, often on exertion
  - Fatal if rupture is massive

Symptoms

- May display visual effects, such as
  - Loss of visual fields
  - Photophobia
  - Diplopia
- Headache
- Confusion

Copyright © 2005, Elsevier Inc. All rights reserved.
CPT only © 2004. *Current Procedural Terminology, 2005, Professional Edition*, American Medical Association. All rights reserved.

- Slurred speech
- Weakness
- Stiff neck (nuchal rigidity)

Treatment

- Dependent on diagnosis prior to rupture
- Surgical intervention

Encephalitis

- Infection of parenchymal tissue of brain or spinal cord
  - Often viral
- Accompanying inflammation
- Usually results in some permanent damage

Symptoms

- Stiff neck
- Headaches
- Vomiting
- Fever
- May have seizure
- Lethargy

Some of the types of encephalitis

- Herpes simplex
- Lyme disease
- West Nile fever
- Western equine

Treatment

- Symptomatic
- Supportive

Reye's syndrome

Associated with viral infection

- Especially when aspirin has been administered

Changes occur in brain and liver

- Leads to intracranial pressure

Symptoms

- Headaches
- Vomiting
- Lethargy
- Seizures

Copyright © 2005, Elsevier Inc. All rights reserved.
CPT only © 2004. *Current Procedural Terminology, 2005, Professional Edition*, American Medical Association. All rights reserved.

Treatment

- Symptomatic treatment

Brain abscess

- Localized infection
- Necrosis of tissue
- Usually spread from infection elsewhere, such as ears or sinus

Symptoms

- Neurologic deficiencies
- Increased intracranial pressure

Treatment

- Antibiotics for bacterial infections
- Surgical drainage

Epilepsies

Chronic seizure disorder

Types

Partial

- State of altered focus but conscious

Generalized

Absence of seizures
- Brief loss of awareness
- Most common in children

Tonic-clonic
- Loss of consciousness
- Alternate contraction and relaxation
- Incontinence
- No memory of seizure

Causes

- Tumor
- Hemorrhage
- Trauma
- Edema
- Infection
- Excessive cerebrospinal fluid
- High fever
- Aura
    - Auditory or visual sign that precedes a seizure

Copyright © 2005, Elsevier Inc. All rights reserved.
CPT only © 2004. *Current Procedural Terminology, 2005, Professional Edition*, American Medical Association. All rights reserved.

Treatment

- Correct the cause
- Anticonvulsant drugs
- Neurosurgery

Trauma

Head injury

Concussion

- Mild blow to head
- Results in reversible interference with brain function
  - Recover in 24 hours with no residual damage

Contusion

- Bruising of the brain
- Force of the blow determines outcome

Hematomas

- Compresses surrounding structures
- Classified based on location

  Epidural
  - Develops between dura and skull

  Subdural
  - Develops between dura and arachnoid
    - Development within 24 hours is acute
    - Development within a week is subacute
  - ICP increases with enlargement of hematoma

  Subarachnoid
  - Develops between the pia and arachnoid
  - Blood mixes with cerebrospinal fluid
    - No localized hematoma forms

  Intracerebral
  - As a result of a contusion

  Symptoms
  - ICP symptoms
  - Others dependent on location and severity of injury

  Treatment
  - Identification of the location of hematoma
  - Medications to decrease edema
  - Antibiotics
  - Surgical intervention if necessary to decrease the ICP

Spinal cord injury

Result of trauma to vertebra, cord, ligaments, intravertebral disc

Copyright © 2005, Elsevier Inc. All rights reserved.
CPT only © 2004. *Current Procedural Terminology, 2005, Professional Edition*, American Medical Association. All rights reserved.

Vertebra injuries classified as

- Simple
- Compression
- Wedge (displaced angular section of bone)
  - Flexion injury in which hyperflexion compresses vertebra
- Dislocation
- Rotation

Symptoms

- Depends on location and severity
- Paralysis
- Loss of sensation
- Drop in blood pressure
- Loss of bladder and rectal control
- Decreased venous circulation

Treatment

- Identification of area of injury
- Immobilization
- Corticosteroids to decrease edema
- Bladder and rectal management
- Rehabilitation

Tumors of Brain and Spinal Cord

- Increases the ICP
- Life threatening
- Rarely metastasize outside of central nervous system
- Secondary brain tumors are common
- Metastasize from lung or breast

Gliomas common type

- Primary malignant tumor
- Types based on cell from which tumor arises and location of tumor

Glioblastoma

- Located in cerebral hemispheres
- Highly aggressive

Oligodendrocytoma

- Usually located in frontal lobes
- Oligodendroblastoma, more aggressive form

Copyright © 2005, Elsevier Inc. All rights reserved.
CPT only © 2004. *Current Procedural Terminology, 2005, Professional Edition*, American Medical Association. All rights reserved.

Ependymoma

- Located in ventricles
- Most often occurs in children
- Ependymoblastoma, more aggressive form

Astrocytoma

- Located anywhere in brain and spinal cord
- Invasive but slow growing

Pineal region

Germ cell tumors

- Usually in children
- Rare
- Variable growth rate

Several other pineal tumors

- Pineocytoma
- Teratoma
- Germinoma

Blood vessel

Angioma

- Usually located in posterior cerebral hemispheres
- Slow growing

Hemangioblastoma

- Located in cerebellum
- Slow growing

Medulloblastoma

- Aggressive tumor
- Located in posterior cerebellar vermis (fourth ventricle roof)

Meningioma

- Intradural tumor
- Slow growing

Pituitary tumor

- Related to aging
- Slow growing
    - Such as macroadenomas

Copyright © 2005, Elsevier Inc. All rights reserved.
CPT only © 2004. *Current Procedural Terminology, 2005, Professional Edition*, American Medical Association. All rights reserved.

Cranial nerve tumors

- Neurilemmomas
- Slow growing
- Metastatic

Spinal cord tumors

Manifestations include

- Seizure
- Visual disturbance
- Loss of balance

Intramedullary

- Originates in neural tissue

Extramedullary

- Originates outside the spinal cord

Metastatic tumors of spinal cord are usually

- Myeloma
- Lymphoma
- Carcinomas

Most common type of primary extramedullary tumor

- Meningiomas
- Neurofibromas

Copyright © 2005, Elsevier Inc. All rights reserved.
CPT only © 2004. *Current Procedural Terminology, 2005, Professional Edition*, American Medical Association. All rights reserved.

NERVOUS SYSTEM PATHOPHYSIOLOGY QUIZ

1. The most common dementia is
   a. Alzheimer's disease
   b. secondary
   c. nutritional degenerative disease
   d. Lou Gehrig's

2. MND stands for
   a. maximal neuron disorder
   b. migrating niacin disorder
   c. motor neuron disease
   d. motor neuropathic disorder

3. Dopamine replacement is useful in treating
   a. multiple sclerosis
   b. Parkinson's disease
   c. Huntington's disease
   d. CVA

4. The condition in which the primary symptoms are muscle weakness and fatigability:
   a. amyotrophic lateral sclerosis
   b. multiple sclerosis
   c. dyskinesis
   d. myasthenia gravis

5. Another name for idiopathic polyneuritis is
   a. Guillain-Barré syndrome
   b. multiple sclerosis
   c. amyotrophic lateral sclerosis
   d. postpolio syndrome

6. This condition is thought to be caused by genetic factors and possibly fetal brain damage.
   a. Parkinson's
   b. schizophrenia
   c. spina bifida
   d. Guillain-Barré syndrome

7. This condition is associated with viral infection, especially when aspirin has been administered.
   a. Reye's syndrome
   b. Guillain-Barré syndrome
   c. Lou Gehrig's
   d. Conn's syndrome

8. Concussion is a mild blow to the head in which recovery is expected within _______ hours.
   a. 12
   b. 24
   c. 48
   d. 1 week

Copyright © 2005, Elsevier Inc. All rights reserved.
CPT only © 2004. *Current Procedural Terminology, 2005, Professional Edition*, American Medical Association. All rights reserved.

9. ICP means
   a. intercranial pressure
   b. intracranial pressure
   c. interior cranial pressure
   d. intensive cranial pressure

10. In this type of hematoma, blood mixes with cerebrospinal fluid:
    a. epidural
    b. subdural
    c. subarachnoid
    d. intracerebral

Copyright © 2005, Elsevier Inc. All rights reserved.
CPT only © 2004. *Current Procedural Terminology, 2005, Professional Edition*, American Medical Association. All rights reserved.

SENSES

- Sight Eyes
- Hearing Ears
- Smell Nose
- Taste Tongue
- Touch Skin

Sight: Three Layers of the Eye (Figure 1-52)

Sclera (outer layer)

White of eye

Cornea, front transparent portion of sclera

Lies over iris

Choroid (middle layer)

Pigment layer

Ciliary muscle and iris on front portion of layer

Contracts

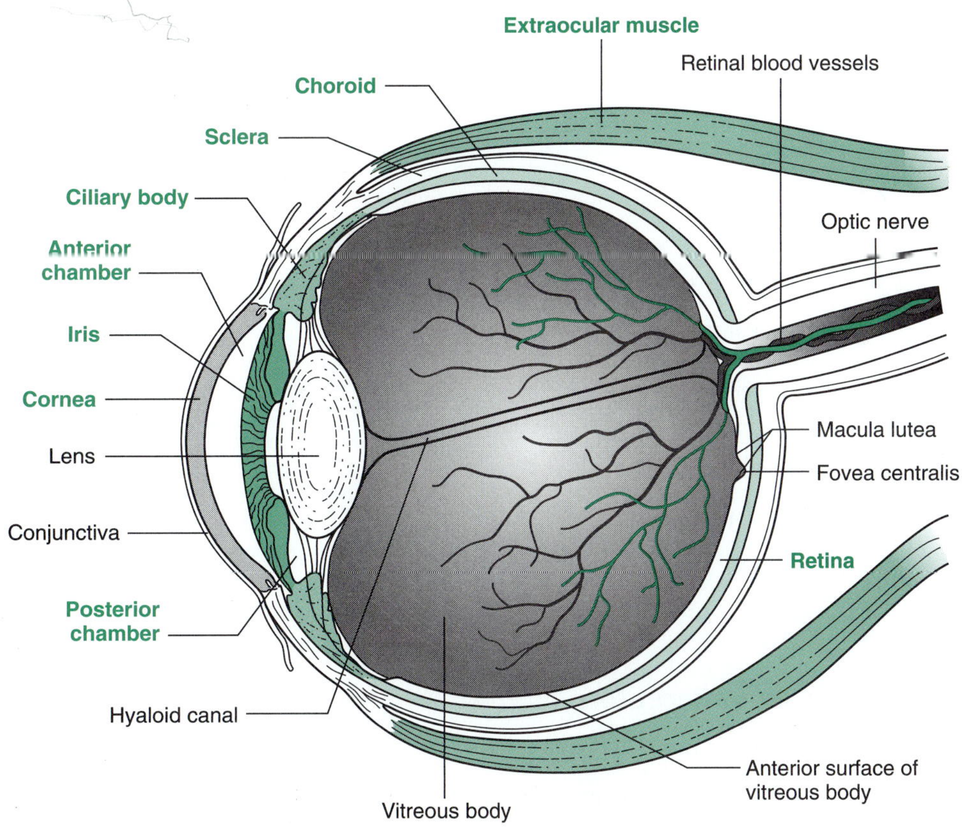

Figure 1-52 Eye and ocular adnexa.

Copyright © 2005, Elsevier Inc. All rights reserved.
CPT only © 2004. *Current Procedural Terminology, 2005, Professional Edition*, American Medical Association. All rights reserved.

Retina (inner layer)

Contains rods and cones

- Rods provide night vision
- Cones provide day and color vision

Conjunctiva

Covers front of sclera and lines eyelid

Lens

Behind pupils

Focuses light

Fluids

Aqueous humor (front of lens)

Vitreous humor (behind lens)

Hearing, Three Divisions of the Ear

External Ear

Auricle (pinna)

External auditory canal

Middle Ear

Ossicles

- Malleus
- Incus
- Stapes

Eustachian tube—leads to pharynx

Inner Ear

Vestibule

Semicircular canals/vestibular apparatus

Cochlea

Smell

Olfactory Sense Receptors

Located in nasal cavity

Closely related to sense of taste

Cranial nerve I

Copyright © 2005, Elsevier Inc. All rights reserved.
CPT only © 2004. *Current Procedural Terminology, 2005, Professional Edition*, American Medical Association. All rights reserved.

Taste

Gustatory sense

Taste buds located on tongue

Cranial nerves VII and IX

Touch

Mechanoreceptors

Widely distributed throughout body

Reacts to touch and pressure

- Meissner corpuscles (touch)
- Pacinian corpuscles (pressure)

Proprioceptors

Position and orientation

Thermoreceptors

Under skin

Sense temperature changes

Nociceptors

Pain sensors

In skin and internal organs

COMBINING FORMS

1. ambly/o	dim
2. aque/o	water
3. audi/o	hearing
4. blephar/o	eyelid
5. conjunctiv/o	conjunctiva
6. cor/o	pupil
7. corne/o	cornea
8. cycl/o	ciliary body
9. dacry/o	tear
10. essi/o, esthesi/o	sensation
11. ir/o	iris
12. irid/o	iris
13. kerat/o	cornea
14. lacrim/o	tear

Copyright © 2005, Elsevier Inc. All rights reserved.
CPT only © 2004. *Current Procedural Terminology, 2005, Professional Edition*, American Medical Association. All rights reserved.

15. myring/o ear drum
16. ocul/o eye
17. ophthalm/o eye
18. opt/o eye, vision
19. optic/o eye
20. ot/o ear
21. palpebr/o eyelid
22. papill/o optic nerve
23. phac/o eye lens
24. phak/o eye lens
25. pupill/o pupil
26. retin/o retina
27. scler/o sclera
28. staped/o stapes
29. tympan/o ear drum
30. uve/o uvea
31. vitre/o glassy

PREFIXES

1. audi- hearing
2. eso- inward
3. exo- outward

SUFFIXES

1. -opia vision
2. -tropia to turn

MEDICAL ABBREVIATIONS

1. AD right ear
2. AS left ear
3. AU both ears
4. H or E hemorrhage or exudate
5. IO intraocular
6. IOL intraocular lens
7. OD right eye
8. OS left eye
9. OU each eye
10. PERL pupils equal and reactive to light

Copyright © 2005, Elsevier Inc. All rights reserved.
CPT only © 2004. *Current Procedural Terminology, 2005, Professional Edition*, American Medical Association. All rights reserved.

11. PERRL pupils equal, round, and reactive to light
12. PERRLA pupils equal, round, and reactive to light and accommodation
13. REM rapid eye movement
14. TM tympanic membrane

MEDICAL TERMS

Anterior segment	Those parts of the eye in the front of and including the lens, orbit, extraocular muscles, and eyelid
Apicectomy	Excision of a portion of the temporal bone
Astigmatism	Condition in which the refractive surfaces of the eye are unequal
Aural atresia	Congenital absence of the external auditory canal
Cataract	Opaque covering on or in the lens
Cholesteatoma	Tumor that forms in middle ear
Conjunctiva	The lining of the eyelids and the covering of the sclera
Dacryostenosis	Narrowing of the lacrimal duct
Enucleation	Removal of an organ or organs from a body cavity
Episclera	Connective covering of sclera
Exenteration	Removal of an organ all in one piece
Exophthalmos	Protrusion of the eyeball
Exostosis	Bony growth
Fenestration	Creation of a new opening in the inner wall of the middle ear
Glaucoma	Eye diseases that are characterized by an increase of intraocular pressure
Hyperopia	Farsightedness, eyeball is too short from front to back
Keratomalacia	Softening of the cornea associated with a deficiency of vitamin A
Keratoplasty	Surgical repair of the cornea
Labyrinth	Inner connecting cavities, such as the internal ear
Labyrinthitis	Middle ear inflammation
Lacrimal	Related to tears
Mastoidectomy	Removal of the mastoid bone
Ménière's disease	Condition that causes dizziness, ringing in the ears, and deafness
Myopia	Nearsightedness, eyeball too long from front to back
Myringotomy	Incision into tympanic membrane
Ocular adnexa	Orbit, extraocular muscles, and eyelid
Ophthalmoscopy	Examination of the interior of the eye by means of a scope, also known as funduscopy
Otitis media	Noninfectious inflammation of the middle ear; serous otitis media produces liquid drainage (not purulent) and suppurative otitis media produces purulent (pus) matter

Copyright © 2005, Elsevier Inc. All rights reserved.
CPT only © 2004. *Current Procedural Terminology, 2005, Professional Edition*, American Medical Association. All rights reserved.

Otoscope	Instrument used to examine the ear
Papilledema	Swelling of the optic disk (papilla)
Posterior segment	Those parts of the eye behind the lens
Sclera	Outer covering of the eye
Strabismus	Extraocular muscle deviation resulting in unequal visual axes
Tarsorrhaphy	Suturing together of eyelids
Tinnitus	Ringing in the ears
Transmastoid	Creates an opening in mastoid for drainage antrostomy
Tympanolysis	Freeing of adhesions of the tympanic membrane
Tympanometry	Test of the inner ear using air pressure
Tympanostomy	Insertion of ventilation tube into tympanum
Uveal	Vascular tissue of the choroid, ciliary body, and iris
Vertigo	Dizziness

Copyright © 2005, Elsevier Inc. All rights reserved.
CPT only © 2004. *Current Procedural Terminology, 2005, Professional Edition*, American Medical Association. All rights reserved.

SENSES QUIZ

1. The middle layer of the eye:
   a. sclera
   b. retina
   c. episclera
   d. choroid

2. The covering of the front of sclera and lining of eyelid:
   a. aqueous humor
   b. ossicles
   c. vitreous
   d. conjunctiva

3. Which of the following is NOT a bone of the middle ear:
   a. cochlea
   b. stapes
   c. malleus
   d. incus

4. This cranial nerve controls the sense of smell:
   a. I
   b. II
   c. III
   d. IV

5. Which of the following is NOT part of the inner ear:
   a. pinna
   b. vestibule
   c. semicircular canals
   d. cochlea

6. These receptors react to touch:
   a. nociceptors
   b. mechanoreceptors
   c. proprioceptors
   d. thermoreceptors

7. These react to position and orientation:
   a. nociceptors
   b. mechanoreceptors
   c. proprioceptors
   d. thermoreceptors

8. Combining form meaning eyelid:
   a. aque/o
   b. blephar/o
   c. optic/o
   d. uve/o

Copyright © 2005, Elsevier Inc. All rights reserved.
CPT only © 2004. *Current Procedural Terminology, 2005, Professional Edition*, American Medical Association. All rights reserved.

9. Combining form meaning eye lens:
   a. cor/o
   b. irid/o
   c. ocul/o
   d. phak/o

10. Abbreviation meaning the pupils are round, reactive to light, equal, and reactive to accommodation:
    a. PERRLA
    b. PERRL
    c. PERL
    d. PURL

Copyright © 2005, Elsevier Inc. All rights reserved.
CPT only © 2004. *Current Procedural Terminology, 2005, Professional Edition*, American Medical Association. All rights reserved.

SENSES—PATHOPHYSIOLOGY

Eye

Visual disturbances

Astigmatism

- Irregular curvature of the refractive surfaces of the eye
- Can be congenital or acquired (as a result of disease or trauma)

Diplopia

- Double vision

Amblyopia

- Dimness of vision

Hyperopia

- Farsightedness
- Shortened eyeball
    - Can see objects in the distance, not close up

Presbyopia

- Age-related farsightedness

Myopia

- Nearsightedness
- Elongated eyeball
    - Can see objects up close, not in the distance

Nystagmus

- Rapid, involuntary eye movements

Movements can be:

- Vertical
- Horizontal
- Rotational
- Combination of above

- Due to underlying condition or adverse effect of drug
- Various types, such as:

Vestibular nystagmus

- Rhythmatic eye movements

Strabismus

- Cross-eyed
- Due to muscle weakness or neurologic defect
- Treatment
    - Eye exercises

Copyright © 2005, Elsevier Inc. All rights reserved.
CPT only © 2004. *Current Procedural Terminology, 2005, Professional Edition*, American Medical Association. All rights reserved.

  - Corrective lenses
  - Corrective surgery

Infections

Conjunctivitis (pink eye)

- Inflammation of the conjunctiva lining of the eyelid or covering of the sclera
- Due to
  - Infection
  - Allergy
  - Irritation
- Treatment
  - Varies with the cause
  - Antibiotic eye drops

Hordeolum (stye)

- Bacterial infection of eyelid hair follicle
  - Usually staphylococci
- Results in mass on eyelid
- Treatment
  - Antibiotics
  - Incision and drainage may be necessary

Keratitis

- Corneal inflammation
- Caused by herpes simplex virus
- Causes tearing and photophobia

Macular degeneration

- Destruction of the fovea centralis
  - Fovea centralis is the small pit in the center of the retina (fovea centralis retinae)
- Usually age related
- Results from exposure to ultraviolet rays or drugs
  - Also may have a genetic component
- Central vision is lost

Treatment

- Surgical intervention with laser
- Medications

Detached retina

- Retinal tear
  - Vitreous humor then leaks behind retina
  - Retina then pulls away from choroid
- Results in increasing blind spot in visual field

Copyright © 2005, Elsevier Inc. All rights reserved.
CPT only © 2004. *Current Procedural Terminology, 2005, Professional Edition*, American Medical Association. All rights reserved.

- Condition is painless
- Pressure continues to build if left unattended
- Final result is blindness

Treatment

Surgical intervention with laser to repair tear

Cataracts

Lens becomes opaque

Classified by morphology:

- Size
- Shape
- Location
- Also may be classified by etiology (cause) or time cataract occurs

Examples of classification:

- Congenital cataract
  - Bilateral opacity present at birth
  - Also known as developmental cataract
- Heat cataract
  - Also known as glassblowers' cataract
  - Caused by exposure to radiation
- Traumatic cataract
  - Result of injury to eye
- Senile cataract **(Figure 1–53)**
  - Age related
  - Usually forms on corneal area of lens

Symptoms

- Blurring of vision
- Halos around lights

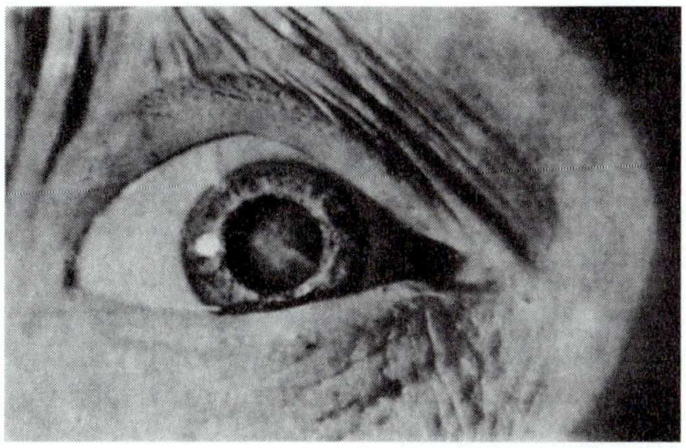

Figure 1-53 Mature cataract with gray fissures. (From Pau H: *Differential diagnosis of eye diseases*, Philadelphia, 1978, WB Saunders, p. 240.)

Copyright © 2005, Elsevier Inc. All rights reserved.
CPT only © 2004. *Current Procedural Terminology, 2005, Professional Edition*, American Medical Association. All rights reserved.

Treatment

- Removal of cataract with intraocular lens implantation

Glaucoma

Excess accumulation of intraocular aqueous humor

- Results in decreased blood flow and edema
- Damages the retinal cells and optic nerve

Narrow angle glaucoma

- Acute type of glaucoma

Chronic glaucoma

Also known as

- Wide angle glaucoma
- Open angle glaucoma

Asymptomatic

Treatment

- Medications that decrease output of aqueous humor and decreased intraocular pressure (IOP)
- Laser treatment to provide drainage

Ear

Infections

Otitis media

Infection or inflammation of middle ear cavity

Chronic infection produces adhesions

- Results in loss of hearing
- Often occurs in children in combination with URI (upper respiratory infection)
- Causes severe ear pain (otalgia)

Treatment

- Antibiotics
- Surgical intervention with placement of tubes to allow for drainage
  - Useful in patients with recurrent infection

Otitis externa

- Also known as swimmer's ear
- Infection of external auditory canal and pinna (exterior ear)
- Caused by bacteria or fungus
- Results in pain and discharge

Copyright © 2005, Elsevier Inc. All rights reserved.
CPT only © 2004. *Current Procedural Terminology, 2005, Professional Edition*, American Medical Association. All rights reserved.

Treatment

- Antibiotic
- Encouraged to keep ear dry

Hearing Loss

Conductive hearing loss

Due to a defect of the sound-conducting apparatus

- Accumulation of wax
- Scar tissue on the tympanic membrane

Also known as:

- Transmission hearing loss
- Conduction deafness

Sensorineural

Due to a lesion of the cochlea or central neural pathways

Also known as:

- Perceptive deafness

May be divided into

- Cochlear hearing loss
  - Due to a defect in the receptor or transducing mechanisms of cochlea
- Retrocochlear hearing loss
  - Due to defect located proximal to the cochlea (vestibulocochlear nerve or auditory area of brain)

Presbycusis is age-related sensorineural hearing loss

Ototoxic hearing loss

- Due to ingestion of toxic substance
- Also known as toxic deafness

Copyright © 2005, Elsevier Inc. All rights reserved.
CPT only © 2004. *Current Procedural Terminology, 2005, Professional Edition*, American Medical Association. All rights reserved.

SENSES PATHOPHYSIOLOGY QUIZ

1. This condition can be acquired or congenital and results in an irregular curvature of the refractive surfaces of the eye.
   a. diplopia
   b. hyperopia
   c. nystagmus
   d. astigmatism

2. In this condition the eyeball is shorter than normal and results in being able to see objects in the distance but not close up.
   a. diplopia
   b. hyperopia
   c. nystagmus
   d. astigmatism

3. Rapid, involuntary eye movement is the predominant symptom of this condition.
   a. diplopia
   b. hyperopia
   c. nystagmus
   d. astigmatism

4. Age-related farsightedness is
   a. presbyopia
   b. hyperopia
   c. diplopia
   d. myopia

5. Another name for a stye is
   a. keratitis
   b. hordeolum
   c. hyperopia
   d. strabismus

6. An inflammation of the cornea that is caused by herpes simplex virus is
   a. keratitis
   b. hordeolum
   c. hyperopia
   d. strabismus

7. In this condition there is destruction of the fovea centralis.
   a. macular degeneration
   b. detached retina
   c. glaucoma
   d. cataract

8. This is an infection that occurs in the middle ear cavity.
   a. otitis media
   b. otitis externa
   c. ototoxic
   d. retrocochlear

Copyright © 2005, Elsevier Inc. All rights reserved.
CPT only © 2004. *Current Procedural Terminology, 2005, Professional Edition*, American Medical Association. All rights reserved.

9. The hearing loss that can be due to a lesion on the cochlea is
   a. conductive
   b. sensorineural
   c. ototoxic
   d. transmission

10. This condition is also known as perceptive deafness.
    a. conductive
    b. sensorineural
    c. otitis media
    d. transmission

Copyright © 2005, Elsevier Inc. All rights reserved.
CPT only © 2004. *Current Procedural Terminology, 2005, Professional Edition*, American Medical Association. All rights reserved.

ANATOMY AND TERMINOLOGY QUIZ ANSWERS

INTEGUMENTARY SYSTEM QUIZ

1. c	6. c
2. d	7. d
3. a	8. b
4. b	9. c
5. d	10. c

MUSCULOSKELETAL SYSTEM QUIZ

1. b	6. d
2. c	7. b
3. a	8. d
4. c	9. a
5. a	10. c

RESPIRATORY SYSTEM QUIZ

1. b	6. c
2. d	7. c
3. c	8. b
4. a	9. d
5. a	10. d

CARDIOVASCULAR SYSTEM QUIZ

1. d	6. b
2. a	7. d
3. c	8. a
4. a	9. d
5. d	10. d

FEMALE GENITAL SYSTEM AND PREGNANCY QUIZ

1. d	6. a
2. a	7. b
3. a	8. b
4. b	9. c
5. c	10. d

MALE GENITAL SYSTEM QUIZ

1. c	6. a
2. a	7. a
3. d	8. d
4. b	9. d
5. a	10. b

Copyright © 2005, Elsevier Inc. All rights reserved.
CPT only © 2004. *Current Procedural Terminology, 2005, Professional Edition*, American Medical Association. All rights reserved.

URINARY SYSTEM QUIZ

1. c
2. d
3. a
4. c
5. b
6. d
7. c
8. b
9. d
10. a

DIGESTIVE SYSTEM QUIZ

1. b
2. d
3. d
4. b
5. c
6. b
7. a
8. c
9. a
10. b

MEDIASTINUM AND DIAPHRAGM QUIZ

1. a
2. b
3. d
4. c
5. c
6. b
7. a
8. b
9. a
10. d

HEMIC AND LYMPHATIC SYSTEM QUIZ

1. b
2. d
3. a
4. d
5. c
6. c
7. a
8. d
9. b
10. d

ENDOCRINE SYSTEM QUIZ

1. c
2. d
3. b
4. a
5. d
6. a
7. d
8. a
9. b
10. d

NERVOUS SYSTEM QUIZ

1. b
2. a
3. a
4. b
5. b
6. c
7. a
8. d
9. b
10. a

Copyright © 2005, Elsevier Inc. All rights reserved.
CPT only © 2004. *Current Procedural Terminology, 2005, Professional Edition*, American Medical Association. All rights reserved.

SENSES QUIZ

1. d
2. d
3. a
4. a
5. a
6. b
7. c
8. b
9. d
10. a

Copyright © 2005, Elsevier Inc. All rights reserved.
CPT only © 2004. *Current Procedural Terminology, 2005, Professional Edition*, American Medical Association. All rights reserved.

PATHOPHYSIOLOGY QUIZ ANSWERS

INTEGUMENTARY SYSTEM PATHOPHYSIOLOGY QUIZ

1. c
2. c
3. a
4. d
5. b
6. c
7. d
8. b
9. d
10. a

MUSCULOSKELETAL SYSTEM PATHOPHYSIOLOGY QUIZ

1. d
2. c
3. b
4. a
5. d
6. d
7. a
8. c
9. b
10. d

RESPIRATORY SYSTEM PATHOPHYSIOLOGY QUIZ

1. b
2. a
3. d
4. d
5. d
6. a
7. c
8. b
9. a
10. c

CARDIOVASCULAR PATHOPHYSIOLOGY QUIZ

1. b
2. a
3. d
4. c
5. d
6. a
7. c
8. c
9. a
10. d

FEMALE GENITAL SYSTEM AND PREGNANCY PATHOPHYSIOLOGY QUIZ

1. b
2. d
3. a
4. c
5. b
6. a
7. a
8. c
9. b
10. c

MALE GENITAL SYSTEM PATHOPHYSIOLOGY QUIZ

1. a
2. b
3. d
4. a
5. c
6. b
7. d
8. b
9. a
10. b

Copyright © 2005, Elsevier Inc. All rights reserved.
CPT only © 2004. *Current Procedural Terminology, 2005, Professional Edition*, American Medical Association. All rights reserved.

URINARY SYSTEM PATHOPHYSIOLOGY QUIZ

1. c
2. d
3. d
4. c
5. b
6. c
7. a
8. c
9. b
10. c

DIGESTIVE SYSTEM PATHOPHYSIOLOGY QUIZ

1. c
2. a
3. d
4. b
5. a
6. c
7. a
8. c
9. a
10. a

HEMIC AND LYMPHATIC SYSTEMS PATHOPHYSIOLOGY QUIZ

1. c
2. a
3. b
4. d
5. b
6. c
7. a
8. a
9. c
10. b

ENDOCRINE SYSTEM PATHOPHYSIOLOGY QUIZ

1. a
2. b
3. c
4. a
5. d
6. b
7. a
8. d
9. a
10. c

NERVOUS SYSTEM PATHOPHYSIOLOGY QUIZ

1. a
2. c
3. b
4. d
5. a
6. b
7. a
8. b
9. b
10. c

SENSES PATHOPHYSIOLOGY QUIZ

1. d
2. b
3. c
4. a
5. b
6. a
7. a
8. a
9. b
10. b

Copyright © 2005, Elsevier Inc. All rights reserved.
CPT only © 2004. *Current Procedural Terminology, 2005, Professional Edition,* American Medical Association. All rights reserved.

UNIT II

Reimbursement Issues

REIMBURSEMENT ISSUES

Your Responsibility

Ensure accurate coding based upon services provided and documented.

Obtain correct reimbursement for services rendered.

Upcoding (maximizing) or downcoding never appropriate.

Stay abreast of current and changing:

Reimbursement policies

Coding guidelines

Health Insurance Portability and Accountability Act (HIPAA) changes utilizing various resources such as:

- Centers for Medicare and Medicaid Policy Manuals
- National Correct Coding Guidelines

Health Information Management Professionals are bound by the AHIMA Code of Ethics and Standards of Ethical Coding (www.ahima.org).

> For the certification examination:
> You need a working knowledge of national reimbursement and regulatory guidelines.

Population Change = Reimbursement Change

Elderly fastest growing patient segment.

By 2030, there will be one elderly person for each person younger than 19 years.

Medicare primarily for elderly.

Medicare

Getting bigger all the time!

By 2008, Medicare spending will exceed $364 billion.

Health care will continue to expand to meet enormous future demands.

Job security for coders!

Those covered—beneficiaries

Originally established in 1965 for those 65 and older.

Added coverage for disabled and End Stage Renal Disease (ESRD) in 1972.

Basic Structure

Part A: Hospital and Institutional Care Coverage

> For the certification examination:
> You need to know what is covered and not covered under Part A and what can be reported outside the DRG payment.

Copyright © 2005, Elsevier Inc. All rights reserved.
CPT only © 2004. *Current Procedural Terminology, 2005, Professional Edition,* American Medical Association. All rights reserved.

Covered inpatient expenses include:

Room

- Semiprivate room rate
  Pays the same amount whether the patient has a:
    Private room that is or is not medically necessary
- Semiprivate room
- Ward accommodations
  Accommodations must meet program standards.

Patient pays the difference between private and semiprivate room when:

- Private room is not medically necessary
- Patient has requested the private room
  Provider must inform patient of the additional charge for private room

Patient does not pay the difference between private and semiprivate room when:

- Isolation is required to avoid jeopardizing the health or recovery of the patient or others.
  Examples:
    - Communicable diseases
    - Heart attacks
    - Cerebrovascular accidents
    - Psychotic episodes
    - Hospital has no semiprivate or ward accommodations available at the time of admission and
  Patient must require immediate hospitalization.

Patients may be assigned to ward accommodations if:

- All semiprivate accommodations are occupied.
- Facility has no semiprivate accommodations.
  Patient must be moved to semiprivate room when one is available.
    Accommodations meet program standards.

Nursing services and other related services

- Defined as use of hospital facilities and medical social services ordinarily furnished by the hospital for the care/treatment of inpatients

Drugs, biologicals, supplies, appliances, and equipment

- FDA-approved drugs and biologicals for use in the hospital
  Must usually be furnished by the hospital for the care/treatment of inpatients
- Supplies, appliances, and equipment
  Must be used for care/treatment solely during the inpatient hospital stay
  OR
  When unreasonable or impossible to limit the use to the inpatient period

Copyright © 2005, Elsevier Inc. All rights reserved.
CPT only © 2004. *Current Procedural Terminology, 2005, Professional Edition*, American Medical Association. All rights reserved.

Example:

- Items permanently installed in/attached to the patient's body while an inpatient, such as cardiac valves, cardiac pacemakers, and artificial limbs
- Items which are temporarily installed in/attached to the patient's body while an inpatient and are necessary to permit the patient's release from the hospital, such as tracheotomy or drainage tubes.

- Hospital must have purchased the item

  A cost was incurred by the hospital for the item

  - Excluded are items given to the hospital

  Example: free pharmaceutical samples

Certain other covered diagnostic or therapeutic services

- Diagnostic or therapeutic items/services ordinarily furnished inpatients by hospital

  This includes the supply by others under arrangements made by the hospital.

  Example:

  - Diagnostic or therapeutic services of an audiologist provided off the hospital premises but billed for by the hospital
  - Surgical dressings and splints, casts, and other devices used for the reduction of fractures and dislocations
- Prosthetic devices that are covered that replace all/part of an organ

  The function of a permanently inoperative or malfunctioning internal body organ

  Example

  - Braces, trusses, artificial replacements, such as legs, arms, and eyes
- Diagnostic/therapeutic inpatient services of a psychologist/physical therapist

  Must be a salaried member of the staff of a hospital
- Inpatient diagnostic services furnished by an independent, certified clinical lab under arrangements with the hospital

  Lab certified under CLIA

  CLIA = Clinical Laboratories Improvement Act
- Reasonable cost of medical/surgical services of medical/osteopathic interns or residents under an approved teaching program
- Transportation services

  Includes transport by ambulance

Additionally covered expenses when they meet certain criteria

- Inpatient rehabilitation
- Skilled nursing
- Some personal convenience items for long-term illness/disability
- Home health visit
- Hospice care

Noncovered inpatient-hospital expenses

- Nonmedically necessary services or supplies
- Private-duty nurse or other private-duty attendant
- Deluxe or nonmedically necessary private room
- Personal convenience items

  Those not routinely furnished to patients

Copyright © 2005, Elsevier Inc. All rights reserved.
CPT only © 2004. *Current Procedural Terminology, 2005, Professional Edition*, American Medical Association. All rights reserved.

- Nonphysician inpatient services
  - Have not been provided directly or arranged for by hospital staff

Coverage under Part A is compulsory

- Paid for by Social Security tax
- Eligibility is determined by the Social Security Administration (SSA).
- Reimbursement is for all covered and medically necessary services.
  - Once annual deductible is met
- ICD-9-CM codes are basis for Part A payment.
- Charges are submitted on UB92 form.
  - UB = Uniform Billing
  - Also known as CMS-1450

Part B: Supplemental

Provides coverage for nonhospital charges

- Physician services
- Outpatient hospital services
- Home health care
- Medically necessary supplies and equipment
- Those services and supplies not covered under Part A
- Payment for the hospital stay
- If the patient has exhausted all Part A benefit prior to admission

Beneficiaries purchase coverage with monthly premiums

Three coding systems used to report Part B services and supplies

- CPT
- HCPCS
- ICD-9-CM

Charges submitted on CMS-1500 (Figure 2-1)

Also known as Universal Health Care form

Part C: Medicare + Choice

Variety of health-care options are available.

Such as managed care

Added after Part A and B

Part D: Prescription Drug, Improvement, and Modernization Act of 2003

Prescription drug plan

Piloted through 2005

Open enrollment beginning January 1, 2006

Premium paid by beneficiary

Copyright © 2005, Elsevier Inc. All rights reserved.
CPT only © 2004. *Current Procedural Terminology, 2005, Professional Edition*, American Medical Association. All rights reserved.

PLEASE DO NOT STAPLE IN THIS AREA

PICA **HEALTH INSURANCE CLAIM FORM** PICA

CARRIER

1. MEDICARE (Medicare #) MEDICAID (Medicaid #) CHAMPUS (Sponsor's SSN) CHAMPVA (VA File #) GROUP HEALTH PLAN (SSN or ID) FECA BLK LUNG (SSN) OTHER (ID)

1a. INSURED'S I.D. NUMBER (FOR PROGRAM IN ITEM 1)

2. PATIENT'S NAME (Last Name, First Name, Middle Initial)

3. PATIENT'S BIRTH DATE MM DD YY SEX M F

4. INSURED'S NAME (Last Name, First Name, Middle Initial)

5. PATIENT'S ADDRESS (No., Street)

6. PATIENT RELATIONSHIP TO INSURED Self Spouse Child Other

7. INSURED'S ADDRESS (No., Street)

CITY STATE

8. PATIENT STATUS Single Married Other Employed Full-Time Student Part-Time Student

CITY STATE

ZIP CODE TELEPHONE (Include Area Code) ( )

ZIP CODE TELEPHONE (INCLUDE AREA CODE) ( )

9. OTHER INSURED'S NAME (Last Name, First Name, Middle Initial)

10. IS PATIENT'S CONDITION RELATED TO:

11. INSURED'S POLICY GROUP OR FECA NUMBER

a. OTHER INSURED'S POLICY OR GROUP NUMBER

a. EMPLOYMENT? (CURRENT OR PREVIOUS) YES NO

a. INSURED'S DATE OF BIRTH MM DD YY SEX M F

b. OTHER INSURED'S DATE OF BIRTH MM DD YY SEX M F

b. AUTO ACCIDENT? PLACE (State) YES NO

b. EMPLOYER'S NAME OR SCHOOL NAME

c. EMPLOYER'S NAME OR SCHOOL NAME

c. OTHER ACCIDENT? YES NO

c. INSURANCE PLAN NAME OR PROGRAM NAME

d. INSURANCE PLAN NAME OR PROGRAM NAME

10d. RESERVED FOR LOCAL USE

d. IS THERE ANOTHER HEALTH BENEFIT PLAN? YES NO *If yes*, return to and complete item 9 a-d.

READ BACK OF FORM BEFORE COMPLETING & SIGNING THIS FORM.

12. PATIENT'S OR AUTHORIZED PERSON'S SIGNATURE I authorize the release of any medical or other information necessary to process this claim. I also request payment of government benefits either to myself or to the party who accepts assignment below.

SIGNED DATE

13. INSURED'S OR AUTHORIZED PERSON'S SIGNATURE I authorize payment of medical benefits to the undersigned physician or supplier for services described below.

SIGNED

PATIENT AND INSURED INFORMATION

14. DATE OF CURRENT: MM DD YY ILLNESS (First symptom) OR INJURY (Accident) OR PREGNANCY(LMP)

15. IF PATIENT HAS HAD SAME OR SIMILAR ILLNESS. GIVE FIRST DATE MM DD YY

16. DATES PATIENT UNABLE TO WORK IN CURRENT OCCUPATION FROM MM DD YY TO MM DD YY

17. NAME OF REFERRING PHYSICIAN OR OTHER SOURCE

17a. I.D. NUMBER OF REFERRING PHYSICIAN

18. HOSPITALIZATION DATES RELATED TO CURRENT SERVICES FROM MM DD YY TO MM DD YY

19. RESERVED FOR LOCAL USE

20. OUTSIDE LAB? YES NO $ CHARGES

21. DIAGNOSIS OR NATURE OF ILLNESS OR INJURY. (RELATE ITEMS 1,2,3 OR 4 TO ITEM 24E BY LINE)

1. ___ . __ 3. ___ . __

2. ___ . __ 4. ___ . __

22. MEDICAID RESUBMISSION CODE ORIGINAL REF. NO.

23. PRIOR AUTHORIZATION NUMBER

24. A DATE(S) OF SERVICE From MM DD YY To MM DD YY	B Place of Service	C Type of Service	D PROCEDURES, SERVICES, OR SUPPLIES (Explain Unusual Circumstances) CPT/HCPCS MODIFIER	E DIAGNOSIS CODE	F $ CHARGES	G DAYS OR UNITS	H EPSDT Family Plan	I EMG	J COB	K RESERVED FOR LOCAL USE
1										
2										
3										
4										
5										
6										

25. FEDERAL TAX I.D. NUMBER SSN EIN

26. PATIENT'S ACCOUNT NO.

27. ACCEPT ASSIGNMENT? (For govt. claims, see back) YES NO

28. TOTAL CHARGE $

29. AMOUNT PAID $

30. BALANCE DUE $

31. SIGNATURE OF PHYSICIAN OR SUPPLIER INCLUDING DEGREES OR CREDENTIALS (I certify that the statements on the reverse apply to this bill and are made a part thereof.)

SIGNED DATE

32. NAME AND ADDRESS OF FACILITY WHERE SERVICES WERE RENDERED (If other than home or office)

33. PHYSICIAN'S, SUPPLIER'S BILLING NAME, ADDRESS, ZIP CODE & PHONE #

PIN# GRP#

PHYSICIAN OR SUPPLIER INFORMATION

(APPROVED BY AMA COUNCIL ON MEDICAL SERVICE 8/88) **PLEASE PRINT OR TYPE** APPROVED OMB-0938-0008 FORM CMS-1500 (12-90), FORM RRB-1500, APPROVED OMB-1215-0055 FORM OWCP-1500, APPROVED OMB-0720-0001 (CHAMPUS)

Figure 2-1 Example of CMS-1500 Health Insurance Claim Form. (Courtesy U.S. Department of Health and Human Services, Centers for Medicare and Medicaid Services.)

Copyright © 2005, Elsevier Inc. All rights reserved.
CPT only © 2004. *Current Procedural Terminology, 2005, Professional Edition,* American Medical Association. All rights reserved.

Officiating Office

Department of Health and Human Services (DHHS)

- Delegated to Centers for Medicare and Medicaid Services (CMS)
- CMS runs Medicare and Medicaid.
- CMS delegates daily operation to fiscal intermediaries (FI) and local carriers.
- FI and local carriers are usually insurance companies.

Funding for Medicare

Social security taxes

Equal match from government

CMS sends money to FI and local carriers.

FI and local carriers handle paperwork and pay claims.

Medicare Covers

Beneficiary responsibility

Part A (hospital)

An annual deductible which varies each year based upon:

- The previous year's deductible
- PPS (Prospective Payment System) payment rate

Varying co-insurance amount dependant upon length of stay

Days	Co-insurance Amount
61st through the 90th days	1/4 of inpatient hospital deductible for each day of hospital service
91st through the 150th days	1/2 of inpatient hospital deductible for each day of lifetime reserve*
21st through the 100th days	1/8 of inpatient hospital deductible for each day of skilled nursing facility care under extended care services

**Lifetime reserve is 60 days and may be used only once in a lifetime, benefit of Part A.*

Part B (physician)

Annual deductible of $110 (2005)

Begins each January 1

Medicare pays 80% of covered services.

Patient pays 20%.

Example: A participating physician provides service to a patient

- Service is a "Medicare covered service."
- Physician bills Medicare full cost of service of $500.
- Medicare's allowed amount for service is $400.
- Patient has not paid deductible for year.

Copyright © 2005, Elsevier Inc. All rights reserved.
CPT only © 2004. *Current Procedural Terminology, 2005, Professional Edition*, American Medical Association. All rights reserved.

Payments are as follows:

$400	Allowed amount
–$100	Patient deductible
$300	

80% × 300 = $240 Medicare pays

20% × 300 = $60 Patient pays

$300 payment to physician

Physician writes off $100 nonallowed charge.

Must not bill patient for nonallowed charge

Medicare responsibility

Part A (hospital)

Prospective Payment System (PPS) pays fixed amount for admission.

- Based on the condition
- Minus the annual deductible and co-insurance
- Deductible for 2005 is $912.

Services exempt from annual deductible and co-insurance

Paid at 100% of PPS or Fee Schedule amount

Example:

- Screening mammography
- Inpatient hospital radiology or pathology physician services

Physician must accept assignment

Exception:

1. The following furnished as a benefit of Part A and B home health:
   - Supplies
   - Drugs
   - DME (durable medical equipment)
   - Prosthetics
   - Orthotics
2. Clinical diagnostic laboratory tests
3. Certain surgical procedures performed in an ASC (ambulatory surgical center) or outpatient department of a hospital

Exemptions to the inpatient PPS (prospective payment system) are paid at 80% of allowed amount.

Patient pays deductible and 20% of these exceptions.

Copyright © 2005, Elsevier Inc. All rights reserved.
CPT only © 2004. *Current Procedural Terminology, 2005, Professional Edition,* American Medical Association. All rights reserved.

Medical necessity and frequency limitations

Defined in:

- LMRP (Local Medical Review Policies)
- NCD (National Coverage decisions) as:
  - Medical necessity
    - Medical need or reason for a service or procedure
  - Frequency limitations
    - Limits the amount or number of a specific service or procedure that are provided during a specified time period

PEER REVIEW ORGANIZATIONS (PRO)

Social Security Act was amended to establish PRO.

Also known as Quality Improvement Organizations (QIO)

Purpose: Ensure hospitals adhere to payment system.

Reviewed by Hospital Payment Monitoring Program (HPMP)

PRO Reviews

Admission

Discharge

Quality of care

DRG validation

Coverage

Procedure performed

The Review

Begins with nurse who screens records based on PRO guidelines

Out-of-compliance cases forwarded to physician reviewer

Violations can result in severe sanctions.

FEDERAL REGISTER

Government publishes changes in laws (Figure 2-2).

November and December issues contain outpatient facility proposed changes.

NATIONAL CORRECT CODING INITIATIVE (NCCI)

Developed by the Centers for Medicare and Medicaid Services to:

Promote national correct coding methods

Control improper coding that leads to inappropriate payment of Part B claims (physician)

Copyright © 2005, Elsevier Inc. All rights reserved.
CPT only © 2004. *Current Procedural Terminology, 2005, Professional Edition,* American Medical Association. All rights reserved.

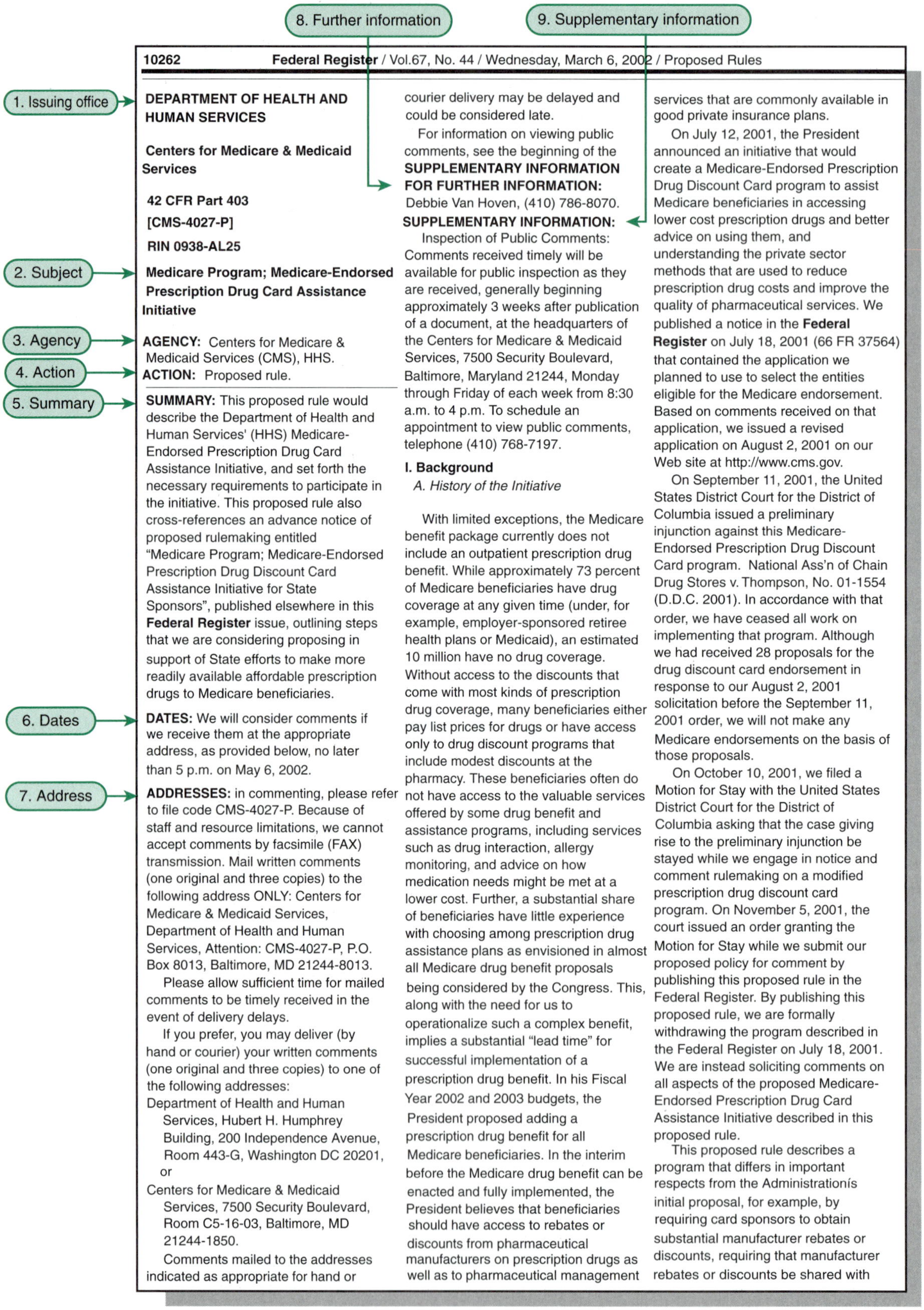

10262 **Federal Register** / Vol.67, No. 44 / Wednesday, March 6, 2002 / Proposed Rules

DEPARTMENT OF HEALTH AND HUMAN SERVICES

Centers for Medicare & Medicaid Services

42 CFR Part 403

[CMS-4027-P]

RIN 0938-AL25

Medicare Program; Medicare-Endorsed Prescription Drug Card Assistance Initiative

AGENCY: Centers for Medicare & Medicaid Services (CMS), HHS.

ACTION: Proposed rule.

SUMMARY: This proposed rule would describe the Department of Health and Human Services' (HHS) Medicare-Endorsed Prescription Drug Card Assistance Initiative, and set forth the necessary requirements to participate in the initiative. This proposed rule also cross-references an advance notice of proposed rulemaking entitled "Medicare Program; Medicare-Endorsed Prescription Drug Discount Card Assistance Initiative for State Sponsors", published elsewhere in this **Federal Register** issue, outlining steps that we are considering proposing in support of State efforts to make more readily available affordable prescription drugs to Medicare beneficiaries.

DATES: We will consider comments if we receive them at the appropriate address, as provided below, no later than 5 p.m. on May 6, 2002.

ADDRESSES: in commenting, please refer to file code CMS-4027-P. Because of staff and resource limitations, we cannot accept comments by facsimile (FAX) transmission. Mail written comments (one original and three copies) to the following address ONLY: Centers for Medicare & Medicaid Services, Department of Health and Human Services, Attention: CMS-4027-P, P.O. Box 8013, Baltimore, MD 21244-8013.

Please allow sufficient time for mailed comments to be timely received in the event of delivery delays.

If you prefer, you may deliver (by hand or courier) your written comments (one original and three copies) to one of the following addresses:

Department of Health and Human Services, Hubert H. Humphrey Building, 200 Independence Avenue, Room 443-G, Washington DC 20201, or

Centers for Medicare & Medicaid Services, 7500 Security Boulevard, Room C5-16-03, Baltimore, MD 21244-1850.

Comments mailed to the addresses indicated as appropriate for hand or courier delivery may be delayed and could be considered late.

For information on viewing public comments, see the beginning of the **SUPPLEMENTARY INFORMATION**

FOR FURTHER INFORMATION: Debbie Van Hoven, (410) 786-8070.

SUPPLEMENTARY INFORMATION: Inspection of Public Comments: Comments received timely will be available for public inspection as they are received, generally beginning approximately 3 weeks after publication of a document, at the headquarters of the Centers for Medicare & Medicaid Services, 7500 Security Boulevard, Baltimore, Maryland 21244, Monday through Friday of each week from 8:30 a.m. to 4 p.m. To schedule an appointment to view public comments, telephone (410) 768-7197.

I. Background

A. History of the Initiative

With limited exceptions, the Medicare benefit package currently does not include an outpatient prescription drug benefit. While approximately 73 percent of Medicare beneficiaries have drug coverage at any given time (under, for example, employer-sponsored retiree health plans or Medicaid), an estimated 10 million have no drug coverage. Without access to the discounts that come with most kinds of prescription drug coverage, many beneficiaries either pay list prices for drugs or have access only to drug discount programs that include modest discounts at the pharmacy. These beneficiaries often do not have access to the valuable services offered by some drug benefit and assistance programs, including services such as drug interaction, allergy monitoring, and advice on how medication needs might be met at a lower cost. Further, a substantial share of beneficiaries have little experience with choosing among prescription drug assistance plans as envisioned in almost all Medicare drug benefit proposals being considered by the Congress. This, along with the need for us to operationalize such a complex benefit, implies a substantial "lead time" for successful implementation of a prescription drug benefit. In his Fiscal Year 2002 and 2003 budgets, the President proposed adding a prescription drug benefit for all Medicare beneficiaries. In the interim before the Medicare drug benefit can be enacted and fully implemented, the President believes that beneficiaries should have access to rebates or discounts from pharmaceutical manufacturers on prescription drugs as well as to pharmaceutical management services that are commonly available in good private insurance plans.

On July 12, 2001, the President announced an initiative that would create a Medicare-Endorsed Prescription Drug Discount Card program to assist Medicare beneficiaries in accessing lower cost prescription drugs and better advice on using them, and understanding the private sector methods that are used to reduce prescription drug costs and improve the quality of pharmaceutical services. We published a notice in the **Federal Register** on July 18, 2001 (66 FR 37564) that contained the application we planned to use to select the entities eligible for the Medicare endorsement. Based on comments received on that application, we issued a revised application on August 2, 2001 on our Web site at http://www.cms.gov.

On September 11, 2001, the United States District Court for the District of Columbia issued a preliminary injunction against this Medicare-Endorsed Prescription Drug Discount Card program. National Ass'n of Chain Drug Stores v. Thompson, No. 01-1554 (D.D.C. 2001). In accordance with that order, we have ceased all work on implementing that program. Although we had received 28 proposals for the drug discount card endorsement in response to our August 2, 2001 solicitation before the September 11, 2001 order, we will not make any Medicare endorsements on the basis of those proposals.

On October 10, 2001, we filed a Motion for Stay with the United States District Court for the District of Columbia asking that the case giving rise to the preliminary injunction be stayed while we engage in notice and comment rulemaking on a modified prescription drug discount card program. On November 5, 2001, the court issued an order granting the Motion for Stay while we submit our proposed policy for comment by publishing this proposed rule in the Federal Register. By publishing this proposed rule, we are formally withdrawing the program described in the Federal Register on July 18, 2001. We are instead soliciting comments on all aspects of the proposed Medicare-Endorsed Prescription Drug Card Assistance Initiative described in this proposed rule.

This proposed rule describes a program that differs in important respects from the Administrationís initial proposal, for example, by requiring card sponsors to obtain substantial manufacturer rebates or discounts, requiring that manufacturer rebates or discounts be shared with

Figure 2-2 Example of page from the Federal Register. (From *Federal Register,* October 11, 2000, vol. 65 [197]: 60366.)

Copyright © 2005, Elsevier Inc. All rights reserved.
CPT only © 2004. *Current Procedural Terminology, 2005, Professional Edition,* American Medical Association. All rights reserved.

Unbundling

CMS defines as:

Billing multiple procedure codes for a group of procedures that are covered by a single comprehensive code

Examples

- Dividing one service into parts and coding for each part separately, such as:

  Reporting bilateral procedures unilaterally

  Example: Reporting 31231, bilateral or unilateral diagnostic nasal endoscopy, with the –50 (bilateral procedure), rather than correctly as 31231

- Downcoding in order to use an additional code

  Example: Downcoding one of two lacerations of same complexity and site to enable reporting of two separate repairs

- Separating the surgical approach from the major surgical service

  Example: Coding separately for a thoracic approach during an anterior spine procedure

RESOURCE-BASED RELATIVE VALUE SCALE (RBRVS)

Prior to implementation of RBRVS on January 1, 1992, payment to providers was based upon the customary, prevailing, and reasonable charge (CPR) for a service.

Based on the Following Three Components:

1. Physician work
2. Practice experience
3. Malpractice insurance premiums

CPR Paid the Lowest of:

- Customary charge

  Median of physician's charges for the service for a set period of time
- Prevailing charge

  Charge set at 90th percentile of customary charge for service
- Reasonable charge

  The lowest of the:
  - Physician's actual fee for the service
  - Customary charge or
  - Prevailing charge

Omnibus Budget Reconciliation Act of 1989

Enacted to replace the CPR payment method with:

Resource-based relative value scale fee schedule (RBRVS)

Copyright © 2005, Elsevier Inc. All rights reserved.
CPT only © 2004. *Current Procedural Terminology, 2005, Professional Edition*, American Medical Association. All rights reserved.

AMBULATORY PATIENT CLASSIFICATIONS (APC)

Omnibus Budget Reconciliation Act of 1986 (OBRA)

Prior to OBRA, Medicare hospital outpatient services paid on a cost-based system

Also known as a retrospective system

Act mandated:

- Replacement of cost-based system with a PPS (prospective payment system)
- Hospitals to report claims using CMS Healthcare Common Procedural Coding System (HCPCS)
- Certain data to be submitted to CMS about the specific outpatient services being provided
  - Data was used to develop Outpatient Prospective Payment System (OPPS)

Developed Ambulatory Patient Groups (APGs)

Grouped outpatient services

Differ from DRGs because an outpatient can be assigned multiple APGs

APCs for one encounter but an inpatient is assigned only one DRG

Final version of the classification system was Ambulatory Patient Classifications (APCs)

Implementation on August 1, 2000

APCs mandatory for:

- All Medicare hospital outpatient services
- Inpatient services covered under Part B
  - If beneficiary has exhausted Part A benefits
- Inpatient services not covered by Part A
- Partial hospitalization services
  - Furnished by community mental health centers

Used for reimbursement for hospital-based outpatient services

Such as:

- Outpatient surgery
- Outpatient clinics
- Emergency departments
- Outpatient ancillary services

Example: radiology and laboratory

APC Structure

Consists of over 500 groups of services

A HCPCS code can be placed in more than one APC within a group of "like" APCs (Figure 2-3)

Copyright © 2005, Elsevier Inc. All rights reserved.
CPT only © 2004. *Current Procedural Terminology, 2005, Professional Edition*, American Medical Association. All rights reserved.

APC	HCPCS	APC Description	HCPCS Description	SI	Rel. Wt.	Pay Rate	Natl. Coin.	Min. Coin.
0006		**Level I Incision & Drainage**		T	1.7487	$94.94	$24.12	$18.99
0006	10060		Drainage of skin abscess					
0006	10061		Drainage of skin abscess					
0006	10080		Drainage of pilonidal cyst					
0006	10120		Remove foreign body					
0006	17999		Skin tissue procedure					
0006	20000		Incision of abscess					
0006	20950		Fluid pressure, muscle					
0006	21725		Revision of neck muscle					
0006	23931		Drainage of arm bursa					
0006	26010		Drainage of finger abscess					
0006	69000		Drain external ear lesion					
0006	69020		Drain outer ear canal lesion					
0007		**Level II Incision & Drainage**		T	11.4943	$624.01		$124.80
0007	10081		Drainage of pilonidal cyst					
0007	10140		Drainage of hematoma/fluid					
0007	10180		Complex drainage, wound					
0007	26011		Drainage of finger abscess					
0007	51080		Drainage of bladder abscess					
0007	54015		Drain penis lesion					
0007	55100		Drainage of scrotum abscess					
0007	57022		I & D vaginal hematoma, pp					
0007	57023		I & D vaginal hematoma, non-ob					
0007	69005		Drain external ear lesion					

Figure 2-3 APC grouping of HCPCS codes.

Services in each APC are:

- Alike clinically
- In resource required to provide service

APC includes some items/services that contribute to cost of the service but

Medicare does not usually reimburse separately.

These incidentals are packaged into the APC payment.

Examples:

- Operating room
- Recovery room
- Anesthesia
- Supplies
- Observation services
- Certain drugs
- Blood
- Medical visits on the same day of service

Copyright © 2005, Elsevier Inc. All rights reserved.
CPT only © 2004. *Current Procedural Terminology, 2005, Professional Edition,* American Medical Association. All rights reserved.

Addendum D.—Payment status indicators for the hospital outpatient prospective payment system

Indicator	Service	Status
A	Services Paid under a Fee Schedule other than OPPS, e.g., Clinical Diagnostic Laboratory Services; Physical, Occupational and Speech Therapy; and Screening Mammography	Paid under a Payment System other than OPPS.
C	Inpatient Procedures	Not Paid under OPPS; Admit Patient; Bill as Inpatient.
D	Deleted Code	Not Paid under Medicare.
E	Non-Covered Items and Services; Codes not Payable in Hospital Outpatient Setting; Codes Not Recognized by OPPS but for Which an Alternate Code may be Applicable	Not Covered under Medicare, or not an Allowed Code when Performed in a Hospital Outpatient Setting.
F	Corneal Tissue Acquisition	Paid at Reasonable Cost.
G	Drug/Biological Pass-Through	Paid under OPPS; Separate APC Payment Includes Pass-Through Amount.
H	Device Category Pass-Through	Paid under OPPS; Separate Cost-Based Pass-Through Payment.
K	Non Pass-Through Drug/Biological, Radiopharmaceutical Agent, Certain Brachytherapy Sources	Paid under OPPS; Separate APC.
L	Influenza Vaccine; Pneumococcal Pneumonia Vaccine	Paid at Reasonable Cost; Not Subject to Deductible or Coinsurance.
N	Items and Services Packaged into APC Rate	Paid under OPPS; Payment is Packaged into Payment for Other Services.
P	Partial Hospitalization	Paid under OPPS; Per Diem APC.
S	Significant Procedure, Not Discounted when Multiple	Paid under OPPS; Separate APC.
T	Significant Procedure, Multiple Procedure Reduction Applies	Paid under OPPS; Separate APC.
V	Clinic or Emergency Department Visit	Paid under OPPS; Separate APC.
X	Ancillary Service	Paid under OPPS; Separate APC.

Figure 2-4 Payment Status Indicators for the Hospital Outpatient Prospective Payment System Addendum D. (From *Federal Register,* Vol. 69, Tuesday, May 18, 2004.)

Medicare does reimburse separately for some items and services that are not packaged, such as casting, splitting, and strapping services.

Further APC information available http://www.cms.hhs.gov/suppliers/asc/

APC Payment Status Indicators (SI) (Figure 2-4)

Passthrough codes

Services, procedures, and/or supplies not included in APC package

Paid in addition to APC payment

Copyright © 2005, Elsevier Inc. All rights reserved.
CPT only © 2004. *Current Procedural Terminology, 2005, Professional Edition,* American Medical Association. All rights reserved.

Cost outlier

May apply when cost for treatment and care is greatly increased in comparison to cost for other patients in the same DRG

Additional reimbursement for the outlier must be requested either:

- When claim is filed
- Within 60 days of receipt of intermediary's first determination

Payment rate and co-insurance

Co-insurance amount is 20% of the median charge for all services in the APC.

This means the payment rate and co-insurance will not change until the co-insurance amount becomes 20% of the individual APC payment.

Multiple significant surgical procedures performed on the same day that are not status indicator S procedures are discounted.

- Full payment made for the highest reimbursed procedure
- 50% reimbursed for each additional surgical procedure

APC Payment Status Indicators (SI)

One letter assigned to each HCPCS/CPT code

Indicates if service, procedure, or supply is reimbursable under the Hospital Outpatient Prospective Payment System (HOPPS)

Identifies need for separate APC for multiple procedures/supplies

Defines under which PPS charges are reimbursed

Example:

- HCPCS/CPT codes under SI "A" are not paid under HOPPS but are paid under a fee schedule or another payment method

Such as: 76092, mammogram screening (SI "A")

- Electrical bone stimulation, which is not paid under APC payment system
- Cannot exceed the inpatient deductible (2005 = $912)

Each APC is assigned a co-insurance amount and payment rate.

Adjusted by hospital's wage index (labor costs)

Figure 2-5 illustrates the payment rate and co-insurance amounts

CPT/ HCPCS	Status Indicator	Description	APC	Relative Weight	Payment Rate	National Unadjusted Copayment	Minimum Unadjusted Copayment
10060	T	Drainage of skin abscess	0006	1.7487	$94.94	$24.12	$18.99
10061	T	Drainage of skin abscess	0006	1.7487	$94.94	$24.12	$18.99
10080	T	Drainage of pilonidal cyst	0006	1.7487	$94.94	$24.12	$18.99
P9038	K	RBC irradiated	9505	1.8011	$97.78		$19.56
P9039	K	RBC deglycerolized	9504	3.9764	$215.87		$43.17
P9040	K	RBC leukoreduced irradiated	9504	3.9764	$215.87		$43.17

Figure 2-5 APC Payment Rate and Co-insurance Amount.

Copyright © 2005, Elsevier Inc. All rights reserved.
CPT only © 2004. *Current Procedural Terminology, 2005, Professional Edition,* American Medical Association. All rights reserved.

Examples:
- Drainage of skin abscess (10060) is paid at $94.94, co-insurance amount of 20% ($18.99).
- Red blood cell irradiation (P9038) is paid at $97.78, co-insurance amount of 20% ($19.56).

Can receive payment for multiple services provided on the same day

Multiple procedures provided on the same day are discounted

-CA Modifier

Used with status indicator "C" services provided on an emergency basis in the outpatient setting if:
- Patient expires before admission to the hospital
- Patient is transferred to hospital as inpatient

Due to an unexpected occurrence during a scheduled outpatient procedure necessitating an inpatient procedure

Modifier is assigned to inpatient-only procedure.

Payment is allowed for only one procedure.

All other services on same day are packaged into APC for -CA modified service.

Transitional passthrough payments

Payments made for certain innovative devices, drugs, and biologicals

Paid in addition to APC payment

Such as:
- Chemotherapeutic agents
  - Including supportive and adjunctive drugs used
- Immunosuppressive drugs
- Orphan drugs
- Some new drugs
- Radiopharmaceuticals
- Certain drugs given in the emergency room for heart attacks

Have co-insurance amounts that can be less than 20% of the Average Wholesale Price (AWP)

Payments for passthroughs made for at least 2 years but not more than 3 years

Reported devices and drugs with HCPCS C codes, a revenue code, and SI "H"

0272, 0275, 0276, 0278, 0279, 0280, 0289, or 0624 to bill implantable devices

When a passthrough transitional passthrough payment has expired:

C code removed from HCPCS

Payment is no longer made for item

C codes can be viewed and/or downloaded from the CMS Web site at http://www.cms.hhs.gov/manuals/pm_trans/A0096.pdf

Copyright © 2005, Elsevier Inc. All rights reserved.
CPT only © 2004. *Current Procedural Terminology, 2005, Professional Edition*, American Medical Association. All rights reserved.

(Note that there is an underline "_" between the pm and trans in the web address.)

Pass-through items can still be reported but will not be paid.

Most recent information concerning applications and requirements for APC payments for new technologies, additional device categories, and pass-through payments for drugs and biologicals is located on the CMS Web site at www.cms.hhs.gov/medlearn/refopps.htm.

Discounting

Multiple surgical procedures during the same operative procedure

- Status indicators "T" indicates multiple procedure payment reduction applied

Highest weighted procedure paid in full

- 50% for the other procedures

Terminated surgical procedures before the induction of anesthesia paid at 50%

- Indicated by use of modifier –73 added to surgical procedure code

Outlier adjustments

Some costs that exceed 2.5 times the payment rate are partially paid.

Inpatient-only procedures

CMS publishes a list of procedure that are "inpatient-only" procedures

- http://www.cms.hhs.gov/providers/hopps/2005p/AddendumE.pdf
- Example of Status Indicator "C" procedures:
  - 27258 Treat hip dislocation
  - 32900 Removal of rib(s)
  - 33535 CABG, arterial, three

CMS publishes a list of procedures approved for ASC procedures

- http://www.cms.hhs.gov/providers/pufdownload/default.asp#asc
- Example of approved ASC procedures:
  - 10121 Removal of foreign body
  - 19340 Immediate breast prosthesis
  - 23155 Removal of humerus lesion

Observation status

Paid only for the three clinical conditions

1. Congestive heart failure
2. Chest pain
3. Asthma

Copyright © 2005, Elsevier Inc. All rights reserved.
CPT only © 2004. *Current Procedural Terminology, 2005, Professional Edition,* American Medical Association. All rights reserved.

Hospital reports observation with:

- HCPCS codes

  G0263 (admission to observation)

  G0264 (initial nursing assessment in observation)
- Revenue code:

  0762

Outpatient Code Edit (OCE)

General functions of the OCE system

Edits claims data to identify errors and returns an edit flag(s)

Edits are based upon HCPCS and ICD-9-CM codes.

Assigns an APC number to each service covered under OPPS

PROSPECTIVE PAYMENT SYSTEM (PPS)

Established by the Social Security Amendments of 1983

For services provided in:

Skilled nursing facilities

Inpatient rehabilitation facilities

Long-term care hospital settings

Hospital/facility paid fixed amount for patient discharged in a treatment category or Diagnosis Related Groups (DRG)

DIAGNOSIS RELATED GROUPS (DRG)

System of Classifying Patients Into Groups by Relating the:

Hospital case mix

Types of patients

Types of illnesses

Volume treated

Cost incurred by the hospital to provide care

System Based On:

- Principal diagnosis
- Medical or surgical service
- Patient age
- Any complication or co-morbidity (preexisting conditions)

Excluded hospitals:

Psychiatric

Children's

Rehabilitation

Copyright © 2005, Elsevier Inc. All rights reserved.
CPT only © 2004. *Current Procedural Terminology, 2005, Professional Edition*, American Medical Association. All rights reserved.

Structure of DRGs

Divides all principal diagnoses into 25 major diagnostic categories (MDCs) (Figure 2-6)

16 MDCs correspond to major organ systems.

Example:

Respiratory

Gastrointestinal

Cardiology

9 MDCs correspond to an etiology (cause).

Example:

Lung cancer

Major Diagnostic Categories

1 - Diseases and Disorders of the Nervous System
2 - Diseases and Disorders of the Eye
3 - Diseases and Disorders of the Ear, Nose, Mouth and Throat
4 - Diseases and Disorders of the Respiratory System
5 - Diseases and Disorders of the Circulatory System
6 - Diseases and Disorders of the Digestive System
7 - Diseases and Disorders of the Hepatobiliary System and Pancreas
8 - Diseases and Disorders of the Musculoskeletal System and Connective Tissue
9 - Diseases and Disorders of the Skin, Subcutaneous Tissue and Breast
10 - Endocrine, Nutritional and Metabolic Diseases and Disorders
11 - Diseases and Disorders of the Kidney and Urinary Tract
12 - Diseases and Disorders of the Male Reproductive System
13 - Diseases and Disorders of the Female Reproductive System
14 - Pregnancy, Childbirth and the Puerperium
15 - Newborns and Other Neonates with Conditions Originating in the Perinatal Period
16 - Diseases and Disorders of the Blood and Blood Forming Organs and Immunological Disorders
17 - Myeloproliferative Diseases and Disorders, and Poorly Differentiated Neoplasms
18 - Infectious and Parasitic Diseases (Systemic or Unspecified Sites)
19 - Mental Diseases and Disorders
20 - Alcohol/Drug Use and Alcohol/Drug Induced Organic Mental Disorders
21 - Injuries, Poisonings and Toxic Effects of Drugs
22 - Burns
23 - Factors Influencing Health Status and Other Contacts with Health Services
24 - Multiple Significant Trauma
25 - Human Immunodeficiency Virus Infections

Figure 2-6 Major Diagnostic Categories of the Diagnosis-Related Groups. (From *Diagnosis Related Groups,* Version 14.0, Definitions Manual, 3M Health Information Systems.)

Copyright © 2005, Elsevier Inc. All rights reserved.
CPT only © 2004. *Current Procedural Terminology, 2005, Professional Edition,* American Medical Association. All rights reserved.

DRGs are then further defined by a particular set of patient attributes

By diagnosis:

Principal diagnosis — Defined in the Uniform Hospital Discharge Data Set (UHDDS) as "that condition established after study to be chiefly responsible for occasioning the admission of the patient to the hospital for care"

Secondary diagnosis — Conditions that co-exist at the time of admission, that develop subsequently to the admission, or that affect the treatment received and/or length of stay

By procedure:

Principal procedure — A procedure that is performed for definitive treatment rather than for diagnostic or exploratory purposes or that is necessary in order to take care of a complication

Significant procedure — Medicare defines a significant procedure as one that is:

- Surgical in nature
- Carries an anesthetic/procedural risk, and
- Requires specialized training.

By patient:

Age — At time of procedure

Sex — Male/Female

Discharge status — Condition and/or place to which the patient is being discharged, such as to home, skilled nursing facility, rehabilitation

Surgical classes in each MDC are defined in a hierarchical (least-to-most resource intense) order

Multiple procedures related to principal diagnosis during hospital stay are assigned to only the highest surgical class in the hierarchy.

Tree diagrams are flow charts (Figure 2-7)

Depicts the DRG structure for each MDC

Symbols indicate decisions made during DRG assignment.

DRG Grouper performs assignment.

- Computer program

Case Study

The principal diagnosis is congestive heart failure (428.0). Additional diagnoses are morbid obesity (278.01), diabetes (250.00), coronary atherosclerosis (414.00), psoriasis (69.1), depressive disorder (311), unspecified personality disorder (301.9), hypercholesterolemia (272.0), cardiomegaly (429.3), and initial episode of subendocardial infarction (410.71). The result of code 410.71 being listed as the tenth diagnosis is a reimbursement of $4,702. If 410.71 had been listed within the top nine diagnoses, the reimbursement would have been $7,055. Incorrect listing of the complication of subendocardial infarction resulted in a $2,353 loss to the hospital.

Copyright © 2005, Elsevier Inc. All rights reserved.
CPT only © 2004. *Current Procedural Terminology, 2005, Professional Edition*, American Medical Association. All rights reserved.

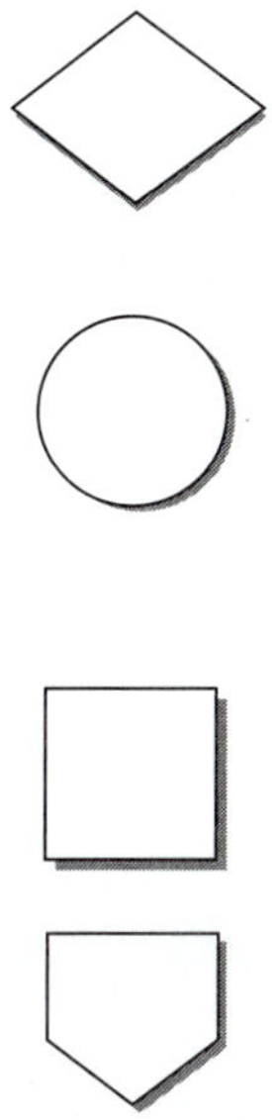

A diamond indicates that a decision is being made on a single variable as opposed to a search of several variables. This symbol is used when the decision variable in the DRG structure is principal diagnosis, discharge status, or age.

A circle indicates that a decision is being made by searching several variables. For example, a circle is used when all listed secondary diagnoses are searched to determine if a complication or comorbidity is present. A circle is also used when the decision in the DRG structure involves the presence of an operating room procedure or the presence of a particular diagnosis as either the principal diagnosis or as secondary diagnosis.

A square indicates that DRG assignment has been completed.

A pointer indicates that the tree diagram structure is continued on another page.

Figure 2-7 DRG symbols used in tree diagrams for each Major Diagnostic Category. (From *Diagnosis Related Groups,* Version 14.0, Definitions Manual, 3M Health Information Systems.)

DRG Classification

Begins with diagnosis and pre-MDC flow chart (**Figure 2-8**)

Pre-Major Diagnostic Categories (Pre-MDCs)

Pre-MDC DRGs are very resource intensive.

Services for these DRGs may be performed for diagnoses in many different MDCs.

Assigned independently of the MDC to indicate principal diagnosis.

For year 2004, there were 8 DRGs to which cases were directly assigned based on ICD-9-CM procedure codes.

Cases are assigned to these DRGs before they are assigned an MDC.

DRG 103	Heart Transplant
DRG 480	Liver Transplant
DRG 481	Bone Marrow Transplant
DRG 482	Tracheostomy for Face, Mouth, and Neck Diagnoses
DRG 483	Tracheostomy with Mechanical Ventilation 96+ hours or Principal Diagnosis of Except for Face, Mouth, and Neck Diagnoses
DRG 495	Lung Transplant
DRG 512	Simultaneous Pancreas/Kidney Transplant
DRG 513	Pancreas Transplant

If care involves a procedure/principal diagnosis contained within the pre-MDC flow chart, the patient is assigned to both:

- Pre-MDC
- MDC of the principal diagnosis

Copyright © 2005, Elsevier Inc. All rights reserved.
CPT only © 2004. *Current Procedural Terminology, 2005, Professional Edition*, American Medical Association. All rights reserved.

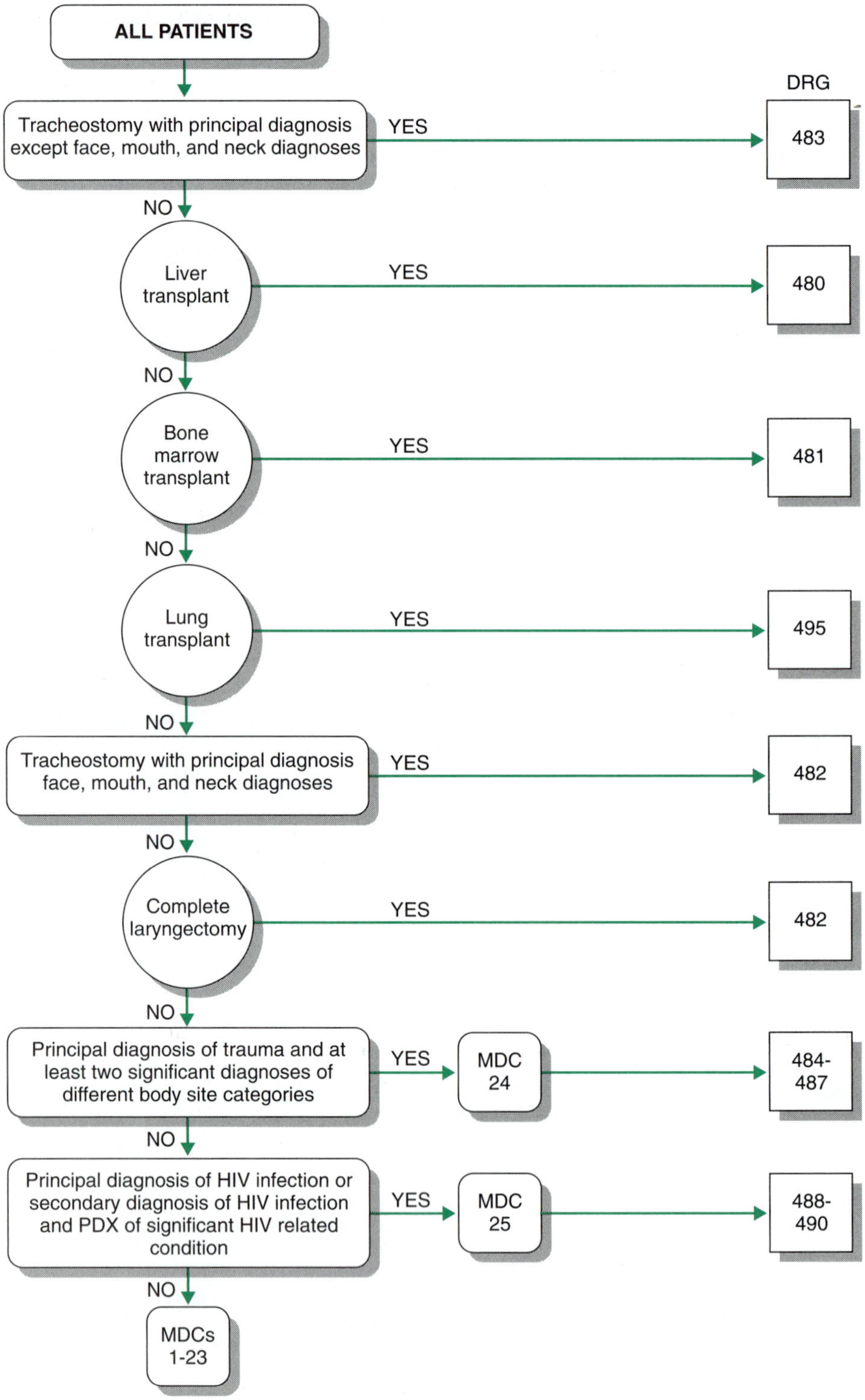

Figure 2-8 Pre-MDC flow chart, DRG Grouper Version 12.0. (From *Diagnosis Related Groups,* Version 14.0, Definitions Manual, 3M Health Information Systems.)

Copyright © 2005, Elsevier Inc. All rights reserved.
CPT only © 2004. *Current Procedural Terminology, 2005, Professional Edition,* American Medical Association. All rights reserved.

Example: HIV patient admitted for an appendectomy assigned to both MDC 25 and 6:

25 HIV

6 Diseases and disorders of the respiratory system

If admitting principal diagnosis/procedure is not one contained within the pre-MDCs flow chart, the remaining 23 MDCs are reviewed.

Use surgical procedure DRG if surgery was performed (Figure 2-9).

Surgical procedures pay more than nonsurgical MDCs.

Use principal diagnosis to select DRG if no surgery was performed.

DRG selection is based on:

- Patient's age
- Complications and co-morbidities (CC) (Figure 2-10)

Must be significant

Defined as condition that increases length of inpatient stay by at least 1 day in at least 75% of patients

Example:

Pneumonia is a CC; benign hypertension is not.

May be excluded if CC:

- Does not consistently increase cost to the hospital
- Is closely related to the principal diagnosis

Examples:

Leg edema is not considered a CC with congestive heart failure.

Dehydration is considered a CC with congestive heart failure.

Separate DRGs for:

- Burn patients
- Newborns transferred to another acute care facility
- Drug or alcoholism abuse patients leaving against medical advice
- Myocardial infarction patients and newborns who die

DRGs for patients whose medical records contain inconsistency or invalid information are classified to:

DRG 468	Extensive OR (operating room) Procedure Unrelated to the Principal Diagnosis
DRG 476	Prostatic OR Procedure Unrelated to the Principal Diagnosis
DRG 477	Non-Extensive OR Procedure Unrelated to the Principal Diagnosis
DRG 469	Principal Diagnosis Invalid as Discharge Diagnosis
DRG 470	Ungroupable (Medical record errors which affect DRG assignment)

- Hospital charges are reported on CMS 1450 (Figure 2-11).

Copyright © 2005, Elsevier Inc. All rights reserved.
CPT only © 2004. *Current Procedural Terminology, 2005, Professional Edition*, American Medical Association. All rights reserved.

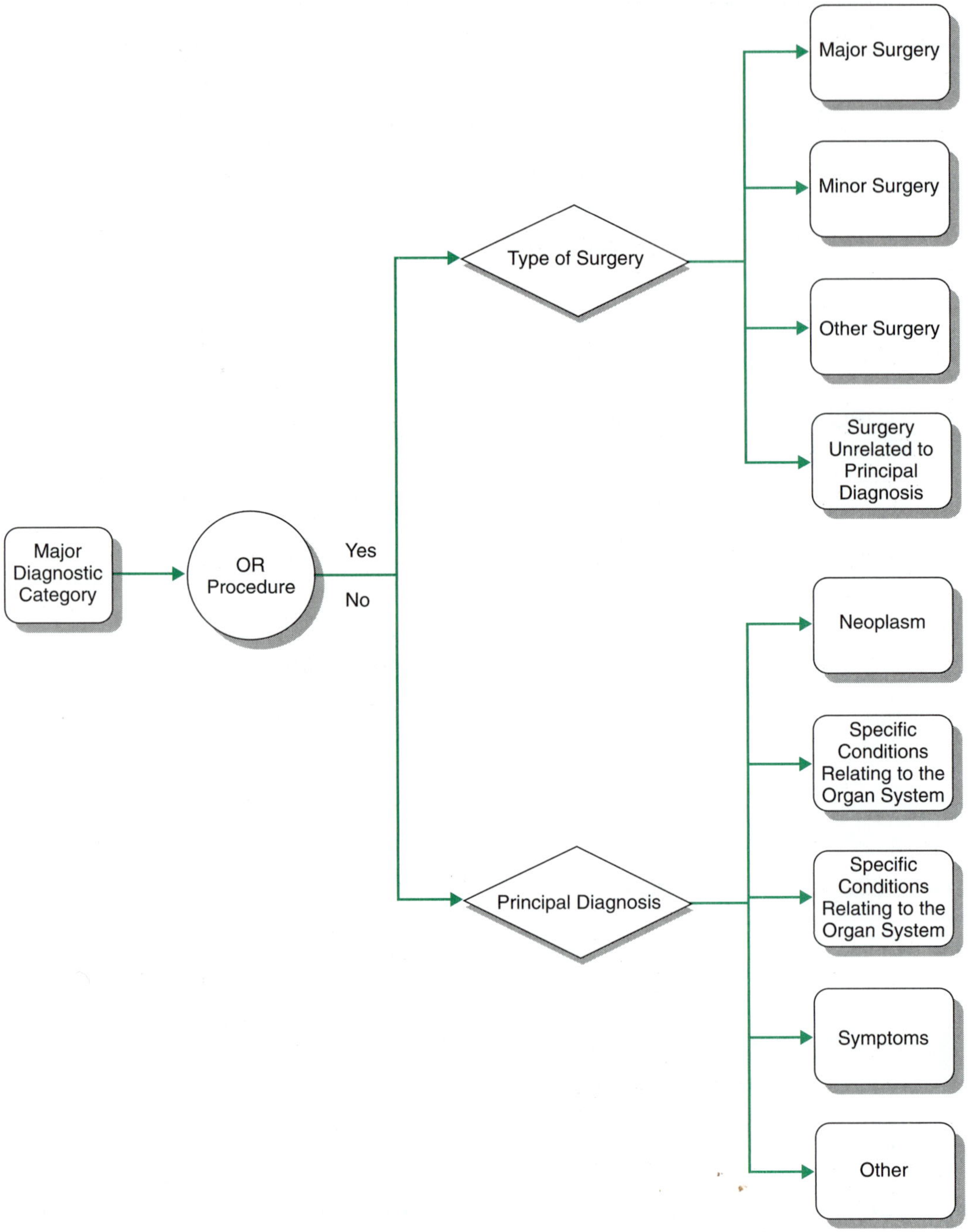

Figure 2-9 Typical DRG structure for a Major Diagnostic Category. The Medical and Surgical Classes are further divided according to the age of the patient or the presence of complications or co-morbidities. (From *Diagnosis Related Groups,* Version 14.0, Definitions Manual, 3M Health Information Systems.)

Copyright © 2005, Elsevier Inc. All rights reserved.
CPT only © 2004. *Current Procedural Terminology, 2005, Professional Edition,* American Medical Association. All rights reserved.

APPENDIX C - DIAGNOSES DEFINED AS COMPLICATIONS OR COMORBIDITIES

83901 Disloc 1st cerv vert-cl
80500-80518,80600-80619,
8068-8069,83900-83918,8470,
8488-8489,8798-8799,9290-9299,
95200-95209,9588,9598-9599

83902 Disloc 2nd cerv vert-cl
80500-80518,80600-80619,
8068-8069,83900-83918,8470,
8488-8489,8798-8799,9290-9299,
95200-95209,9588,9598-9599

83903 Disloc 3rd cerv vert-cl
80500-80518,80600-80619,
8068-8069,83900-83918,8470,
8488-8489,8798-8799,9290-9299,
95200-95209,9588,9598-9599

83904 Disloc 4th cerv vert-cl
80500-80518,80600-80619,
8068-8069,83900-83918,8470,
8488-8489,8798-8799,9290-9299,
95200-95209,9588,9598-9599

83905 Disloc 5th cerv vert-cl
80500-80518,80600-80619,
8068-8069,83900-83918,8470,
8488-8489,8798-8799,9290-9299,
95200-95209,9588,9598-9599

83906 Disloc 6th cerv vert-cl
80500-80518,80600-80619,
8068-8069,83900-83918,8470,
8488-8489,8798-8799,9290-9299,
95200-95209,9588,9598-9599

83907 Disloc 7th cerv vert-cl
80500-80518,80600-80619,
8068-8069,83900-83918,8470,
8488-8489,8798-8799,9290-9299,
95200-95209,9588,9598-9599

83908 Disloc mult cerv vert-cl
80500-80518,80600-80619,
8068-8069,83900-83918,8470,
8488-8489,8798-8799,9290-9299,
95200-95209,9588,9598-9599

83910 Disloc cerv vert NOS-opn
80500-80518,80600-80619,
8068-8069,83900-83918,8470,
8488-8489,8798-8799,9290-9299,
95200-95209,9588,9598-9599

83911 Disloc Ist cerv vert-opn
80500-80518,80600-80619,
8068-8069,83900-83918,8470,
8488-8489,8798-8799,9290-9299,
95200-95209,9588,9598-9599

83912 Disloc 2nd cerv vert-opn
80500-80518,80600-80619,
8068-8069,83900-83918,8470,
8488-8489,8798-8799,9290-9299,
95200-95209,9588,9598-9599

83913 Disloc 3rd cerv vert-opn
80500-80518,80600-80619,
8068-8069,83900-83918,8470,
8488-8489,8798-8799,9290-9299,
95200-95209,9588,9598-9599

83914 Disloc 4th cerv vert-opn
80500-80518,80600-80619,
8068-8069,83900-83918,8470,
8488-8489,8798-8799,9290-9299,
95200-95209,9588,9598-9599

83915 Disloc 5th cerv vert-opn
80500-80518,80600-80619,
8068-8069,83900-83918,8470,
8488-8489,8798-8799,9290-9299,
95200-95209,9588,9598-9599

83916 Disloc 6th cerv vert-opn
80500-80518,80600-80619,
8068-8069,83900-83918,8470,
8488-8489,8798-8799,9290-9299,
95200-95209,9588,9598-9599

83917 Disloc 7th cerv vert-opn
80500-80518,80600-80619,
8068-8069,83900-83918,8470,
8488-8489,8798-8799,9290-9299,
95200-95209,9588,9598-9599

83918 Disloc mlt cerv vert-opn
80500-80518,80600-80619,
8068-8069,83900-83918,8470,
8488-8489,8798-8799,9290-9299,
95200-95209,9588,9598-9599

8500 Concussion w/o coma
80000-80199,80300-80499,
8500-85219,85221-85419,
8738-8739,8798-8799,9050,
9251-9252,9290-9299,9588-9590,
9598-9599

8501 Concussion-brief coma
80000-80199,80300-80499,
8500-85219,85221-85419,
8738-8739,8798-8799,9050,
9251-9252,9290-9299,9588-9590,
9598-9599

8502 Concussion-moderate coma
80000-80199,80300-80499,
8500-85219,85221-85419,
8738-8739,8798-8799,9050,
9251-9252,9290-9299,9588-9590,
9598-9599

8503 Concussion-prolong coma
80000-80199,80300-80499,
8500-85219,85221-85419,
8738-8739,8798-8799,9050,
9251-9252,9290-9299,9588-9590,
9598-9599

8504 Concussion-deep coma
80000-80199,80300-80499,
8500-85219,85221-85419,
8738-8739,8798-8799,9050,
9251-9252,9290-9299,9588-9590,
9598-9599

8505 Concussion w coma NOS
80000-80199,80300-80499,
8500-85219,85221-85419,
8738-8739,8798-8799,9050,
9251-9252,9290-9299,9588-9590,
9598-9599

Figure 2-10 Appendix C, Diagnosis Defined as Complications or Comorbidities. (From *Diagnosis Related Groups,* Version 14.0, Definitions Manual, 3M Health Information Systems.)

Copyright © 2005, Elsevier Inc. All rights reserved.
CPT only © 2004. *Current Procedural Terminology, 2005, Professional Edition,* American Medical Association. All rights reserved.

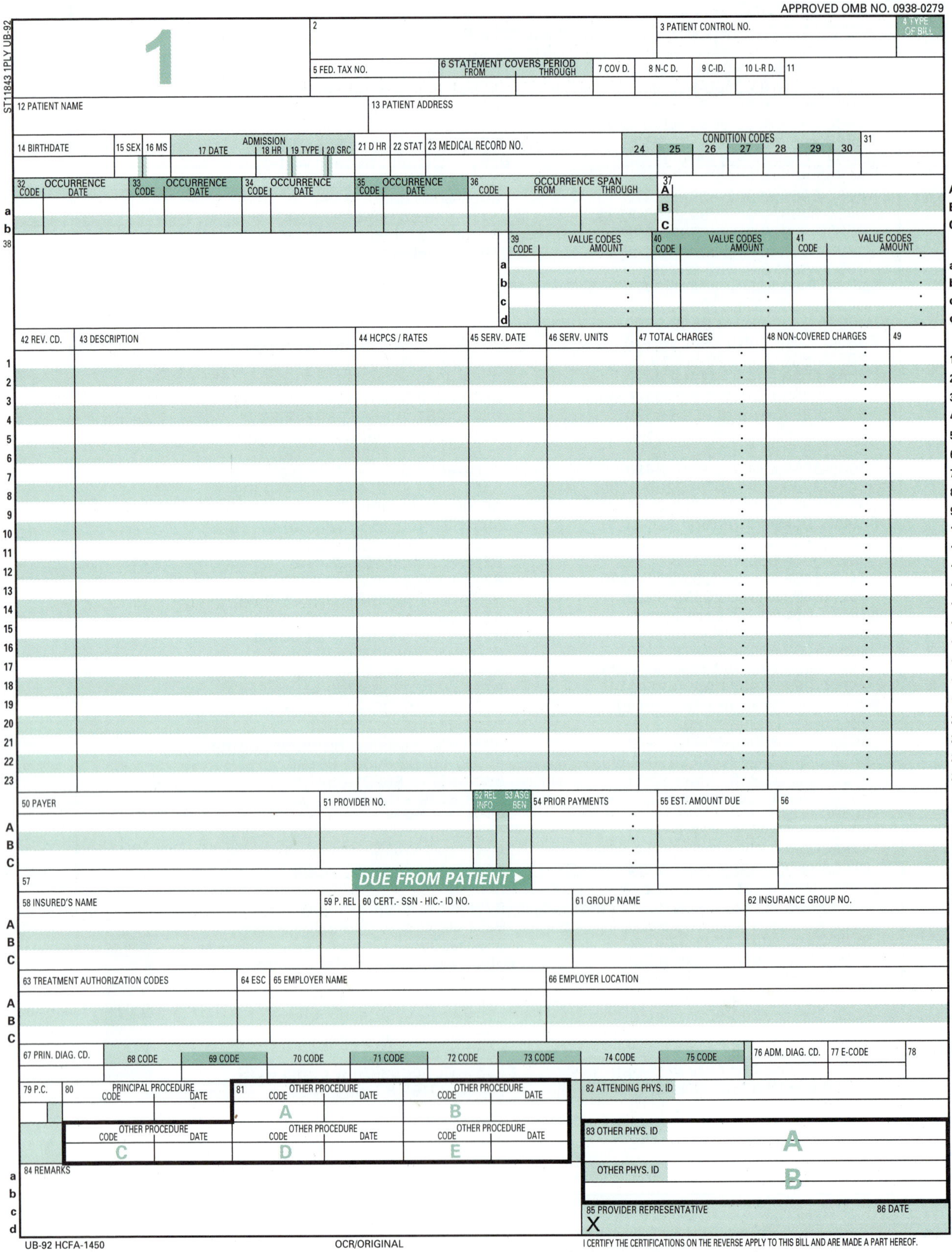

APPROVED OMB NO. 0938-0279

ST11843 1PLY UB-92

1 | 2 | 3 PATIENT CONTROL NO. | 4 TYPE OF BILL

5 FED. TAX NO. | 6 STATEMENT COVERS PERIOD FROM THROUGH | 7 COV D. | 8 N-C D. | 9 C-ID. | 10 L-R D. | 11

12 PATIENT NAME | 13 PATIENT ADDRESS

14 BIRTHDATE | 15 SEX | 16 MS | ADMISSION 17 DATE | 18 HR | 19 TYPE | 20 SRC | 21 D HR | 22 STAT | 23 MEDICAL RECORD NO. | CONDITION CODES 24 25 26 27 28 29 30 | 31

32 OCCURRENCE CODE DATE | 33 OCCURRENCE CODE DATE | 34 OCCURRENCE CODE DATE | 35 OCCURRENCE CODE DATE | 36 OCCURRENCE SPAN CODE FROM THROUGH | 37 A B C

38 | 39 VALUE CODES CODE AMOUNT | 40 VALUE CODES CODE AMOUNT | 41 VALUE CODES CODE AMOUNT (a b c d)

42 REV. CD. | 43 DESCRIPTION | 44 HCPCS / RATES | 45 SERV. DATE | 46 SERV. UNITS | 47 TOTAL CHARGES | 48 NON-COVERED CHARGES | 49 (lines 1–23)

50 PAYER | 51 PROVIDER NO. | 52 REL INFO | 53 ASG BEN | 54 PRIOR PAYMENTS | 55 EST. AMOUNT DUE | 56 (A B C)

57 | DUE FROM PATIENT ▶

58 INSURED'S NAME | 59 P. REL | 60 CERT.- SSN - HIC.- ID NO. | 61 GROUP NAME | 62 INSURANCE GROUP NO. (A B C)

63 TREATMENT AUTHORIZATION CODES | 64 ESC | 65 EMPLOYER NAME | 66 EMPLOYER LOCATION (A B C)

67 PRIN. DIAG. CD. | 68 CODE | 69 CODE | 70 CODE | 71 CODE | 72 CODE | 73 CODE | 74 CODE | 75 CODE | 76 ADM. DIAG. CD. | 77 E-CODE | 78

79 P.C. | 80 PRINCIPAL PROCEDURE CODE DATE | 81 OTHER PROCEDURE CODE DATE A | OTHER PROCEDURE CODE DATE B | 82 ATTENDING PHYS. ID

OTHER PROCEDURE CODE DATE C | OTHER PROCEDURE CODE DATE D | OTHER PROCEDURE CODE DATE E | 83 OTHER PHYS. ID A | OTHER PHYS. ID B

84 REMARKS (a b c d) | 85 PROVIDER REPRESENTATIVE X | 86 DATE

UB-92 HCFA-1450 | OCR/ORIGINAL | I CERTIFY THE CERTIFICATIONS ON THE REVERSE APPLY TO THIS BILL AND ARE MADE A PART HEREOF.

Figure 2-11 CMS—1450 / UB 92 Claim Form. (Courtesy U.S. Department of Health and Human Services, Centers for Medicare and Medicaid Services.)

Copyright © 2005, Elsevier Inc. All rights reserved.
CPT only © 2004. *Current Procedural Terminology, 2005, Professional Edition*, American Medical Association. All rights reserved.

Calculating DRG Payment

2005 DRG list of weights available at:

http://www.cms.hhs.gov/providers/hipps/ippspufs.asp

According to the list, DRG 84, Major Chest Trauma W/O CC is assigned the following weights and means:

Relative Weight	0.5539
Geometric mean LOS (GMLOS)	2.6
Arithmetic mean LOS (AMLOS)	3.2

A Medicare patient was admitted with a principal dx of closed fracture of three rigs (807.03). No surgical procedures were performed. The patient was discharged on day 3 with no complications or comorbidities indication in the documentation. The patient has not paid any of the Part A deductible for the year ($912). If the Hospital Specific Rate for DRG 84 was $2,000, calculation of the amount the hospital would receive from Medicare would be:

Relative Weight × Hospital Specific Rate – Medicare deductible = Amount Due from Medicare

0.5539 × $2,000 = $1,107.80 – $912 = $**195.80** amount due from Medicare

If the same patient developed pneumonia (486), which is a complication, the following would be the weights and means:

Relative Weight	0.9806
Geometric mean LOS	4.3
Arithmetic mean LOS	5.3

Calculation would be:

Relative Weight × Hospital Specific Rate – Medicare deductible = Amount Due from Medicare

0.9806 × $2,000 = $1,961.20 – $912 = $**1049.20** amount due from Medicare

CMS publishes a list of ICD-9-CM codes that are complications and co-morbidities.

Analyzing Case Mix

Refer to Figure 2-12, which illustrates seven hospital admissions with relative weights.

Relative Weight × Number of Cases = Total Value of Service

Example:

DRG 1: **3.3344** (Relative Weight) × **5** (number of cases) = **16.672** (Total Value of Services)

Total Value of Services / Number of cases = Case Mix Index (CMI)

Example:

115.1669 (Total Value of Services) / **78** (Total Number of Cases) = **1.48** (CMI)

Highest total reimbursement is DRG 10, Nervous system neoplasm W CC (28.1543)

Highest relative weight is DRG 1, Craniotomy age >17 W CC (3.3344)

Copyright © 2005, Elsevier Inc. All rights reserved.
CPT only © 2004. *Current Procedural Terminology, 2005, Professional Edition*, American Medical Association. All rights reserved.

DRG	MDC	Type	DRG Title	Relative Weight	Number of Cases	Total Value of Services
1	01	Surg	Craniotomy age >17 W CC	3.3344	5	16.672
2	01	Surg	Craniotomy age >17 W/O CC	1.9467	9	17.5203
3	01	Surg	Craniotomy age 0–17	1.9767	12	23.7204
9	01	Med	Spinal disorders and injury	1.2435	10	12.435
10	01	Med	Nervous system neoplasm W CC	1.2241	23	28.1543
11	01	Med	Nervous system neoplasm W/O CC	0.8771	19	16.6649
				10.6025	78	115.1669

Figure 2-12 Seven hospital admissions with relative weights.

Calculating DRG Payment In Transfers

Formula for payment for transferring hospital:

LOS (length of stay) + 1 day / GMLOS × Payment Amount

Formula for payment for hospital being transferred to:

Twice per day rate for Day 1 + per day rate for remaining days, up to total payment amount

> Patient is transferred from Hospital A to Hospital B after 2 days, where patient remains for the 10 days. Both hospitals are acute care PPS hospitals. The total payment for Hospital A would have been $10,000 and $15,000 for Hospital B. The geometric mean LOS (GMLOS) is 12.7 days.
>
> Transferring: 2 + 1 = 3 days/12.7 (GMLOS) = 2.2362204 × $10,000 (payment rate) = $2,362.20 Hospital A
>
> Transferred to: $15,000 / 12.7 = $1,181.10 per day rate; total days 10 + 1 (for first day) = 11 days × $1,181.10 (per day rate) = $12,992.10 Hospital B

Monitoring DRG Reimbursement

Accounts receivable (AR)

List of all cases not paid yet because codes are not available.

Bills have not yet been sent on these accounts.

Monitor AR amounts.

Remittance advice

Sent by Fiscal Intermediary (FI) listing amounts paid to hospital

Always verify correct amount was paid based on amount initially submitted.

Severity DRG (SDRG)

A revision of the DRG system to more accurately account for the severity of the patient

Developed but not implemented yet

Copyright © 2005, Elsevier Inc. All rights reserved.
CPT only © 2004. *Current Procedural Terminology, 2005, Professional Edition*, American Medical Association. All rights reserved.

All Payer DRG (APR-DRG)

DRGs were developed for Medicare patients.

- Reflects conditions of the older patient
- Does not reflect conditions of other populations
  Such as children

Resource Utilization Groups (RUGS)

Reimbursement system used in long-term skilled health-care settings

Long-term care hospitals (LTCH) are defined as those with average stays greater than 10 days

Based on ICD-9-CM codes

Utilizes information from the minimum data set (MDS):

- Rehabilitation services
- Special care needs
- Clinical requirements
- Activity of daily living
- Cognitive function
- Behavioral symptoms and resident's distressed mood

Assessment of patient must be on days 5, 14, 30, 60, and 90.

Defined by federal law

Home Health Prospective Payment System (HHPPS)

Reimbursement system used in home care agencies

Based on information in Outcome and Assessment Information Set (OASIS)

Payment based on the visit

Home Assessment Validation and Entry (HAVEN) is the CMS free data entry software utilized by most Home Health Agencies (HHA).

Inpatient Rehabilitation Facility (IRF) Prospective Payment System

Paid on a per-discharge basis

Utilizes information from an Inpatient Rehabilitation Facility Patient Assessment Instrument (IRF PAI)

Classifies patients into distinct groups based on clinical characteristics and expected resource needs

CMS 1450 CLAIM FORM

Also known as UB92

Submitted for reimbursement of facility-based services/supplies

Both electronic and paper format

Incomplete or incorrect completion may result in delays or denials of reimbursement.

More complicated than CMS-1500

Contains 86 Field Locators (FL)

FLs are numbered lines or blocks for the entry of data elements.

Copyright © 2005, Elsevier Inc. All rights reserved.
CPT only © 2004. *Current Procedural Terminology, 2005, Professional Edition*, American Medical Association. All rights reserved.

Following are the data entered into each FL:

FL 1 (Untitled) Provider Name, Address, and Telephone Number—**Required.**
FL 2 (Untitled) Not Required.
FL 3 Patient Control Number—**Required.**
FL 4 Type of Bill—Required.
—This three-digit alpha-numeric code ("frequency" code) gives three specific pieces of information.
—First digit identifies the type of facility (Figure 2-13).
—Second classifies the type of care (Figure 2-14).
—Third indicates the sequence of this bill in this particular episode of care (Figure 2-15).
FL 5 Federal Tax Number
FL 6 Statement Covers Period (From—Through)—**Required.**
—FI uses the "From" date to determine timely filing.
FL 7 Covered Days—**Required for inpatient.**
FL 8 Noncovered Days—**Required for inpatient.**
FL 9 Coinsurance Days—**Required for inpatient.**
FL 10 Lifetime Reserve Days—**Required.**
FL 11 (Untitled)—Not Required.
FL 12 Patient's Name—**Required.**
FL 13 Patient's Address—**Required.**
FL 14 Patient's Birth Date—**Required.**
—(MMDDCCYY) (CC is century, century, 2004. Cannot use just "04".)
FL 15 Patient's Sex—**Required.**
FL 16 Patient's Marital Status—Not Required.
FL 17 Admission Date—**Required For Inpatient and Home Health.**
FL 18 Admission Hour—Not Required.
FL 19 Type of Admission/Visit—**Required on inpatient bills only.**
FL 20 Source of Admission—**Required For Inpatient Hospital.**
FL 21 Discharge Hour—Not Required.
FL 22 Patient Status—**Required.**
FL 23 Medical Record Number—**Required.**
FLs 24, 25, 26, 27, 28, 29, 30 Condition Codes—**Required.**
—Provider enters the corresponding code to describe any conditions that apply to this billing period.
FL 31 Untitled—Not Required.
FL 32, 33, 34, and 35 Occurrence Codes and Dates—**Required.**
FL 36 Occurrence Span Code and Dates—**Required For Inpatient.**
FL 37 Internal Control Number (ICN)/Document Control Number (DCN)—**Required.**
FL 38 Untitled Except on Patient Copy of the Bill—Responsible Party Name and Address. Not Required.
FLs 39, 40, and 41 Value Codes and Amounts—**Required.**
FL 42 Revenue Code—**Required.**
FL 43 Revenue Description—Not Required.
FL 44 HCPCS/Rates—**Required**
—When using HCPCS to report outpatient services, the provider enters the HCPCS code describing the procedure here.
—On inpatient hospital bills the accommodation cost is shown here.
FL 45 Service Date—**Required.**
FL 46 Units of Service—**Required.**
FL 47 Total Charges—Not Applicable for Electronic Billers—**Required.**
—Provider sums the total charges for the billing period for each revenue code (in FL 42).

Copyright © 2005, Elsevier Inc. All rights reserved.
CPT only © 2004. *Current Procedural Terminology, 2005, Professional Edition*, American Medical Association. All rights reserved.

—The last revenue code entered in FL 42 is "0001," which represents the grand total of all charges billed.

—NOTE: Electronic billers do not submit revenue center code 0001.

FL 48 Noncovered Charges—**Required.**

FL 49 Untitled—Not Required.

FL 50A, B, and C Payer Identification—**Required.**

FL 51A, B, and C Provider Number—**Required.**

FLs 52A, B, and C Release of Information Certification Indicator—**Required.**

—NOTE: On the reverse side of CMS-1450 there is a certification that all necessary release statements are on file at the time the form is submitted.

FL 53A, B, and C Assignment of Benefits Certification Indicator—Not Required.

FLs 54A, B, and C Prior Payments—**Required.**

FL 55A, B, and C Estimated Amount Due From Patient—Not Required.

FL 56 Untitled—Not Required.

FL 57 Untitled—Not Required.

FLs 58A, B, and C Insured's Name—**Required.**

FL 59A, B, and C Patient's Relationship to Insured—**Required.**

FLs 60A, B, and C Certificate/Social Security Number/HI Claim/Identification Number (HICN)—**Required.**

FL 61A, B, and C Insurance Group Name—**Required.**

FL 62A, B, and C Insurance Group Number—**Required.**

FL 63 Treatment Authorization Code—**Required.**

FL 64 Employment Status Code—**Required.**

FL 65 Employer Name—**Required.**

FL 66 Employer Location—**Required.**

FL 67 Principal Diagnosis Code

Inpatient—Required

—The hospital enters the ICD-9-CM code for the principal diagnosis. The code must be the full ICD-9-CM diagnosis code, including all five digits where applicable.

—Where the proper code has fewer than five digits, the hospital may not fill with zeros.

Outpatient—Required

—The hospital reports the full ICD-9-CM code for the diagnosis shown to be chiefly responsible for the outpatient services.

FLs 68–75 Other Diagnosis Codes—Inpatient—**Required.**

FL 77 E-Code—Not Required.

FL 78 Untitled—Not Required.

FL 79 Procedure Coding Method Used—Not Required.

FL 80 Principal Procedure Code and Date—**Required for Inpatient Only.**

FL 81 Other Procedure Codes and Dates—**Required for Inpatient Only.**

FL 82 Attending/Requesting Physician ID—**Required**

Inpatient Part A

—Enter the provider's unique physician identification number as provided by Medicare and name of the attending physician.

Outpatient and Other Part B

—Enter the provider's unique physician identification number as provided by Medicare and name of the physician that requested the surgery, therapy, diagnostic tests, or other services.

FL 83 Other Physician ID

Inpatient Part A Hospital

—Required if a procedure is performed.

Copyright © 2005, Elsevier Inc. All rights reserved.
CPT only © 2004. *Current Procedural Terminology, 2005, Professional Edition,* American Medical Association. All rights reserved.

Outpatient Hospital

—Required where the HCPCS code reported is subject to the Ambulatory Surgical Center (ASC) payment limitation or where a reported HCPCS code is on the list of codes requiring Medicare approval

FL 84 Remarks—**Required**

—For reporting durable medical equipment such as orthotics or splints, the provider shows the rental rate, cost, and anticipated months of usage so that the provider's FI may determine whether to approve the rental or purchase of the equipment.

FL 85 Provider Representative Signature—**Required on Hardcopy.**

FL 86 Date—Not Required.

—This is the date of the provider representative's signature.

1st Digit-Type of Facility	
1	Hospital
4	Religious Non-Medical (Hospital)
5	Religious Non-Medical (Extended Care)
6	Intermediate Care
7	Clinic or Hospital Based Renal Dialysis Facility (requires special information in second digit below).
8	Special facility or hospital ASC surgery (requires special information in second digit below).
9	Reserved for National Assignment

Figure 2-13 First digit-type of service for UB92 bill type.

2nd Digit-Bill Classification (inpatient)	
1	Inpatient (Part A)
2	Hospital Based or Inpatient (Part B) (includes HHA visits under a Part B plan of treatment).
3	Outpatient (includes HHA visits under a Part A plan of treatment and use of HHA DME under a Part A plan of treatment)
4	Other - Part B - (includes HHA medical and other health services not under a plan of treatment, SNF diagnostic clinical laboratory services to nonpatients, and referenced diagnostic services).
7	Subacute Inpatient (Revenue Code 19X required)
8	Swing Bed (may be used to indicate billing for SNF level of care in a hospital with an approved swing bed agreement).
9	Reserved for National Assignment
2nd Digit Classification (clinic)	
1	*Rural Health Clinic (RHC)*
2	Hospital Based or Independent Renal Dialysis Facility
3	Free Standing
4	Other Rehabilitation Facility (ORF)
5	Comprehensive Outpatient Rehabilitation Facility (CORF)
6	Community Mental Health Center
7-8	Reserved for National Assignment
9	Other
2nd Digit Classification (Special Facilities)	
2	Hospice (Hospital Based)
3	Ambulatory Surgical Center Services to Hospital Outpatients
4	Free Standing Birthing Center
5	Critical Access Hospital
6	*Residential Facility (not used for Medicare)*
7-8	Reserved for National Assignment
9	Other

Figure 2-14 Second digit-bill classification for UB92 bill type.

Copyright © 2005, Elsevier Inc. All rights reserved.
CPT only © 2004. *Current Procedural Terminology, 2005, Professional Edition,* American Medical Association. All rights reserved.

3rd Digit-Frequency	Definition
1 Admit Through Discharge Claim	Use this code for bill encompassing an entire inpatient confinement or course of outpatient treatment for which you expect payment from the payer or which will update deductible for inpatient or Part B claims when Medicare is secondary to an EGHP.
2 Interim-First Claim	Use this code for the first of an expected series of bills for which utilization is chargeable or which will update inpatient deductible for the same confinement of course of treatment.
3 Interim-Continuing Claims (Not valid for PPS Bills)	Use this code when a bill for which utilization is chargeable for the same confinement or course of treatment had already been submitted and further billls are expected to be submitted later.
4 Interim-Last Claim (Not valid for PPS Bills)	Use this code for a bill for which utilization is chargeable, and which is the last of a series for this confinement or course of treatment. The "Through" date of this bill (FL 6) is the discharge for this treatment.
5 Late Charge Only	Use for outpatient claims only. Late charges are not accepted for Medicare inpatient or ASC claims.
7 Replacement of Prior Claim	Use to correct a previously submitted bill. Apply this code to the correct or "new" bill.
8 Void/Cancel of a Prior Claim	Use this code to indicate this bill is an exact duplicate of an incorrect bill previously submitted. A code "7" (Replacement of Prior Claim) is being submitted showing corrected information.

Figure 2-15 Third digit-frequency for UB92 bill type.

REVENUE CODES

Four digit classification system which:

- Identifies services or procedures
- Identifies location where services were rendered

Three Main Categories

1. Billing revenue codes

   Example:

   0137, replacement of a prior claim for a hospital outpatient charge

2. Accommodation revenue codes

   Example:

   0120, semiprivate room and board for obstetrical patient

3. Ancillary revenue codes

   Example:

   0314, laboratory pathological services for a biopsy

The digits and their placement further define elements of the revenue code (Figure 2-16).

Example:

Revenue code for laboratory pathological service is 031X.

The fourth digit (X) is assigned from one of five subcategory digits.

Subcategory identifies type of service/procedure within category.

Example:

Fourth digit (4) identifies biopsy services (0314).

Copyright © 2005, Elsevier Inc. All rights reserved.
CPT only © 2004. *Current Procedural Terminology, 2005, Professional Edition,* American Medical Association. All rights reserved.

				RVU Category
0	3	1	X	Laboratory Pathological
				Subcategory
			0	General Classification
			1	Cytology
			2	Histology
			4	Biopsy
			9	Other

Figure 2-16 Chart of Laboratory Pathological Revenue code category breakdown.

Medicare determines included and excluded services based on

- Revenue codes
- HCPCS codes (FL44)
- Principal and other diagnoses

  FL67 = PDx

  FLs 68–75 = Other Dx

Under the OPPS Medicare requires use of HCPCS codes by hospital outpatient departments when a code for that service is available

Example of services that require HCPCS codes:

0274	Prosthetic and orthotic devices
0331	Injected chemotherapy
0481	Cardiac catheterization laboratory
0623	Surgical dressing
0732	Telemetry
0901	Electroshock therapy

DATA QUALITY

Charge Description Master

Computer software used by hospitals

Includes all services, procedures, supplies, and drugs with a:

Corresponding description

Revenue code

CPT/HCPCS codes

Cost **(Figure 2-17)**

Copyright © 2005, Elsevier Inc. All rights reserved.
CPT only © 2004. *Current Procedural Terminology, 2005, Professional Edition,* American Medical Association. All rights reserved.

CPT/ HCPCS	Description	Active Date	Revenue Code	Charge
Q0171	Chlorpromazine Tablet 10 mg	11/02/2001	635	$2.23
Q0084	Chemotherapy Admin Infusion per visit	04/21/2003	261	$92.00
P9016	Red blood cells, leukocytes reduced, each unit	02/10/2003	380	$295.00
L3810	WHFO, addition to short and long opponens, thumb abduction © bar	05/14/2003	274	$403.23
Q0081	Infusion therapy, not chemotherapy drugs, per visit	08/02/2003	450	$153.00
J9370	Vincristine Sulfate, 1 mg	09/30/2003	636	$202.02

Figure 2-17 Example of basic "Charge Description Master."

Elements of a Charge Description Master

Procedure/service description

CPT/HCPCS codes to identify specific service

Revenue code

Charge for the specific procedure or service

Unique department coder number

Description number that is internally assigned to identify each procedure and service

Should be reviewed annually and updated as needed to assist in:

Reduction of claim denials

Accurate reimbursement

Compliance

Better data management and quality

Such as tracking of services and supplies

Review for:

Invalid/inaccurate codes

- Unclear/incorrect descriptions
- Omitted procedures or supplies
- Correct service/supply and revenue code linkage
- Appropriate fees

MEDICARE FRAUD AND ABUSE

Program established by Medicare

To decrease fraud and abuse

Beneficiary signatures on file

Service, charges submitted without need for patient signature

Presents opportunity for fraud

Copyright © 2005, Elsevier Inc. All rights reserved.
CPT only © 2004. *Current Procedural Terminology, 2005, Professional Edition*, American Medical Association. All rights reserved.

Fraud

Intentional deception to benefit

Example: Submitting for services not provided

Anyone who submits for Medicare services can be violator.

- Physicians
- Hospitals
- Laboratories
- Billing services
- YOU

Fraud Can Be

- Billing for services not provided
- Misrepresenting diagnosis, CPT, or HCPCS code(s)
- Kickbacks
- Unbundling services
- Falsifying medical necessity
- Consistent waiver of co-payment

Fraud Examples

> Patient presents with chest pain and is treated.
>
> Progress note indicates myocardial infarction (MI) is to be ruled out.
>
> Laboratory tests do not suggest or indicate MI.
>
> Coder assigns MI as PDx as the reason for encounter/admission.
>
> Chest pain pays less than MI.
>
> This is fraud!

Other examples of fraud:

- Upcoding is using a higher-level code for a lower-level service.
- Misrepresenting the diagnosis for a patient to justify the service or equipment furnished
- Unbundling or exploding charge

  Example: Reporting multichannel lab tests (many tests in one process) to appear as if the individual tests were performed
- Billing noncovered services

  Example: Routine foot care reported as more involved form of foot care that is paid under the Medicare program
- Applying for duplicate payment

  Example: Patient has Medicare and another insurance and both are billed without indicating that there is another third-party payer

OFFICE OF THE INSPECTOR GENERAL (OIG)

Each year develops work plan

Outlines Medicare monitoring program

FI monitors those areas identified in plan

Copyright © 2005, Elsevier Inc. All rights reserved.
CPT only © 2004. *Current Procedural Terminology, 2005, Professional Edition,* American Medical Association. All rights reserved.

Complaints of Fraud or Abuse

Submitted orally or in writing to FI or carrier

Allegations made by anyone against anyone

Allegations followed up by FI or carrier

Abuse

Generally involves
- Impropriety
- Lack of medical necessity for services reported

Review takes place after claim is submitted.

FI goes back and does historical review of claims.

Kickbacks

Bribe or rebate for referring patient for any service covered by Medicare

Any personal gain kickback

A felony
- 25,000 fine or
- 5 years in jail or
- Both

Protect Yourself

Use your common sense.

Submit only truthful and accurate claims.

If you are unsure about charges, check with physician or supervisor.

MANAGED HEALTH CARE

Network health-care providers and facilities that offer health-care services under one organization

Group hospitals, physicians, or other providers

90% of people with health-care coverage have organizational coverage (e.g., HMO)

Managed Care Organizations

Responsible for health-care services to an enrolled group or person

Coordinate various health-care services

Negotiate with facilities and providers

Capitation method common in managed care

Prepaid, fixed amount for each person in the plan

Regardless of resource use

Preferred Provider Organization (PPO)

Providers and facilities form network to offer health-care services as group.

Enrollees who seek health care outside PPO pay more.

Copyright © 2005, Elsevier Inc. All rights reserved.
CPT only © 2004. *Current Procedural Terminology, 2005, Professional Edition*, American Medical Association. All rights reserved.

Health Maintenance Organization (HMO)

Total package health care

Out-of-pocket expenses minimal

Assigned physician acts as gatekeeper to refer patient outside organization.

ABBREVIATIONS

AMLOS	Arithmetic Mean Length of Stay
APCs	Ambulatory Patient Classifications
APGs	Ambulatory Patient Groups
APR-DRG	All Payer DRG
AWP	Average Wholesale Price
CC	Complications and co-morbidities
CLIA	Clinical Laboratories Improvement Act
DCN	Document Control Number
DME	Durable Medical Equipment
DRG	Diagnosis Related Groups
EDI	Electronic Data Interchange
EIN	Employer Identification Number
EOB	Explanation of Benefits
ESRD	End Stage Renal Disease
FL	Field Locators
FUD	Follow-up Days
GMLOS	Geometric Mean Length of Stay
GPN	Group Provider Number
HAVEN	Home Assessment Validation and Entry
HCPCS	Healthcare Common Procedural Coding System
HHA	Home Health Agencies
HHPPS	Home Health Prospective Payment System
HICN	HI Claim/Identification Number
HIPAA	Health Insurance Portability and Accountability Act
HMO	Health Maintenance Organization
HOPPS	Hospital Outpatient Prospective Payment System
HPMP	Hospital Payment Monitoring Program
ICN	Internal Control Number
IRF	Inpatient Rehabilitation Facility
IRF PAI	Inpatient Rehabilitation Facility Patient Assessment Instrument
LMRP	Local Medical Review Policies
MDCs	Major Diagnostic Categories
NCCI	National Correct Coding Initiative
NCD	National Coverage Decisions
NPI	National Provider Identifier
OASIS	Outcome and Assessment Information Set
OBRA	Omnibus Budget Reconciliation Act of 1986
OCE	Outpatient Code Edit
OIG	Office of the Inspector General
OR	Operating Room
PDx	Principal Diagnosis
PIN	Provider Identification Number
PPO	Preferred Provider Organization
PPS	Prospective Payment System
PRO	Peer Review Organizations
QIO	Quality Improvement Organizations
RBRVS	Resource-Based Relative Value Scale
RUGs	Resource Utilization Groups
SDRG	Severity DRG
SI	Status Indicators
UCR	Usual, Customary, and Reasonable
UHDDS	Uniform Hospital Discharge Data Set

Copyright © 2005, Elsevier Inc. All rights reserved.
CPT only © 2004. *Current Procedural Terminology, 2005, Professional Edition,* American Medical Association. All rights reserved.

REIMBURSEMENT TERMINOLOGY

Advance Beneficiary Notice	ABN: notification in advance of services that Medicare may not pay for them, including the estimated cost to the patient
Ancillary Service	A service that is supportive of care of a patient, such as laboratory services
APC	A classification system used to group like services based upon clinical similarities and resources utilized
Assignment	A legal agreement that allows the provider to receive direct payment from a payer and the provider to accept payment as payment in full for covered services
Attending Physician	The physician legally responsible for oversight of an inpatient's care
Beneficiary	The person who benefits from insurance coverage; also known as subscriber, dependent, enrollee, member, or participant
Birthday Rule	When both parents have insurance coverage, the parent with the birthday earliest in the year is the primary coverage for a dependent
Certified Registered Nurse Anesthetist	CRNA: an individual with specialized training and certification in nursing and anesthesia
Charge Description Master	Record of services, procedures, supplies, and drugs with corresponding codes, descriptions, and charges billed
Co-insurance	Cost-sharing of covered services
Compliance Plan	Written strategy developed by medical facilities to ensure appropriate, consistent documentation within the medical record and ensure compliance with third-party payer guidelines
Concurrent Care	More than one physician providing care to a patient at the same time
Coordination of Benefits	COB: management of multiple third-party payments to ensure overpayment does not occur
Co-payment	Cost-sharing between beneficiary and payer
Correct Coding Initiative	CCI: developed by CMS to control improper unbundling of CPT codes leading to inappropriate payment
Deductible	That portion of covered services paid by the beneficiary before third-party payment begins
Denial	Statement from the payer that reimbursement is denied
Documentation	Detailed chronology of facts and observations regarding a patient's health
Diagnosis Related Groups	DRGs: A case mix classification system established by CMS consisting of classes of patients who are similar clinically and in consumption of hospital resources
Durable Medical Equipment	DME: medically related equipment that is not disposable, such as wheelchairs, crutches, and vaporizers
Electronic Data Interchange	EDI: computerized submission of health-care insurance information exchange
Employer Identification Number	EIN: an Internal Revenue Service (IRS)–issued identification number used on tax documents

Copyright © 2005, Elsevier Inc. All rights reserved.
CPT only © 2004. *Current Procedural Terminology, 2005, Professional Edition,* American Medical Association. All rights reserved.

Encounter Form	Medical document that contains information regarding a patient visit for health-care services
Explanation of Benefits	EOB: written, detailed listing of medical service payments by third-party payer to inform beneficiary and provider of payment
Fee Schedule	Established list of established payment for medical services
Follow-up Days	FUD, established by third-party payers and listing the number of days after a procedure for which a provider must provide normal uncomplicated related services to a patient for no fee (also known as global days, global package, or global period)
Group Provider Number	GPN: numeric designation for a group of providers that is used instead of the individual provider number
Hospital Payment Monitoring System	HPMS: an inpatient PPS audit system used by CMS to reduce improper payments
Invalid Claim	Claim that is missing necessary information and cannot be processed or paid
Inpatient	CMS defines an inpatient as a person who has been formally admitted to a hospital as inpatient with the expectation that he or she will remain at least overnight and occupy a bed even if it later develops that the patient can be discharged or transferred to another hospital and not actually use a hospital bed overnight.
Medical Record	Documentation about the health care of a patient
Noncovered Services	Any service not included by a third-party payer in the list of services for which payment is made
National Provider Identifier	NPI: 10-digit number assigned to provider and used for identification purposes when submitting services to third-party payers
Hospital Outpatient	An individual who is not an inpatient of a hospital but who is registered as an outpatient at the hospital
Prior Authorization	Also known as preauthorization, which is a requirement by payer to receive written permission prior to patient services if the service is to be considered for payment by the payer
Provider Identification Number	PIN, or UPIN, assigned by the third-party payer to providers to be used for identification purposes when submitting services to third-party payers
Rejection	A claim that does not pass edits and is returned to the provider as rejected
Reimbursement	Payment from a third-party payer for services rendered to a patient covered by the payer's health-care plan
State License Number	Identification number issued by a state to a physician who has been granted the right to practice in that state
Usual, Customary, and Reasonable	UCR: used by third-party payers to establish a payment rate for a service in an area with the usual (standard fee in area), customary (standard fee by the physician), and reasonable (as determined by payer) rate

Copyright © 2005, Elsevier Inc. All rights reserved.
CPT only © 2004. *Current Procedural Terminology, 2005, Professional Edition*, American Medical Association. All rights reserved.

REIMBURSEMENT QUIZ

1. Any person who is identified as receiving life or medical benefits:
   a. primary
   b. beneficiary
   c. participant
   d. recipient

2. The Social Security Amendments of 1983 established the _______, which pays a fixed amount intended to cover the cost of treating a typical patient for a particular DRG.
   a. OPPS
   b. HOPPS
   c. DRG
   d. PPS

3. The set of patient attributes that is used to define each DRG consist of
   a. Principal diagnosis, secondary diagnosis, insurance policy rules, principal procedure, and patient age
   b. Principal procedure, discharge status, patient age and sex, and principal diagnosis
   c. Principal and secondary diagnosis, principal procedure, patient age and sex, and discharge status
   d. Discharge status, principal and secondary diagnosis, principal procedure

4. A four-digit classification system that identifies and explains services or procedures and the location in which they were rendered is called a(n)
   a. ancillary code
   b. revenue code
   c. billing code
   d. accommodation code

5. CMS delegates the daily operation of the Medicare program to
   a. DHHS
   b. PRO
   c. RVU
   d. FI and carriers

6. The Omnibus Budget Reconciliation Act of 1986 required a PPS-based payment system to replace the one based on existing outpatient hospital cost. This system is what classification system?
   a. DRGs
   b. APCs
   c. CPT
   d. ICD-9-CM

7. This part of Medicare covers the inpatient hospital portion:
   a. Part A
   b. Part B
   c. Part C
   d. Part D

Copyright © 2005, Elsevier Inc. All rights reserved.
CPT only © 2004. *Current Procedural Terminology, 2005, Professional Edition*, American Medical Association. All rights reserved.

8. This issue of the Federal Register contains outpatient facility changes for CMS programs for the coming year:
   a. October/November
   b. November/December
   c. December/October
   d. November/August

9. Using the UB92 claim form in Figure 2-11, choose the fields in which the patient's name, address, and date of birth would be placed.
   a. 10, 5, and 14
   b. 12, 13, and 18
   c. 1, 2, and 3
   d. 12, 13, and 14

10. Entity responsible for development of the plan that outlines monitoring of the Medicare program:
    a. FI
    b. OIG
    c. DHSS
    d. HEW

Copyright © 2005, Elsevier Inc. All rights reserved.
CPT only © 2004. *Current Procedural Terminology, 2005, Professional Edition*, American Medical Association. All rights reserved.

REIMBURSEMENT QUIZ ANSWERS

1. b
2. d
3. b
4. b
5. d
6. b
7. a
8. b
9. d
10. b

Copyright © 2005, Elsevier Inc. All rights reserved.
CPT only © 2004. *Current Procedural Terminology, 2005, Professional Edition*, American Medical Association. All rights reserved.

UNIT III

Overview of CPT, ICD-9-CM, and HCPCS Coding

INTRODUCTION TO MEDICAL CODING

- Translate services/procedures/supplies/drugs into CPT/HCPCS/ICD-9-CM procedural codes.
- Translate diagnosis into ICD-9-CM codes.

Three Levels of Service Codes

1. Level I CPT
2. Level II HCPCS, National Codes
3. Level III Local Codes—phased out

Diagnosis Codes, ICD-9-CM

ICD-9-CM, Volumes 1 and 2, *International Classification of Diseases,* 9th ed., Clinical Modification

1. Classification system
2. Translates diagnosis (dx) into standarized codes
3. Diabetes becomes 250.XX

CPT

Developed by the American Medical Association (AMA) in 1966

Five-digit codes to report services provided to patients

Updated in November for use January 1

Incorrect Coding

Results in providers being paid inappropriately (either too much or too little)

Inpatient Services

Reported on insurance form

CMS-1450/ Universal Billing Form 92 (UB92) **(Figure 3-1)**

Outpatient Services

Reported on CMS-1500

CPT/HCPCS Level I Modifiers

Indicates anatomical site of procedure or service

Alters CPT or HCPCS code

Full list, CPT, Appendix A

Two separate lists

One for physicians to use

One for hospital outpatient facilities to use

Copyright © 2005, Elsevier Inc. All rights reserved.
CPT only © 2004. *Current Procedural Terminology, 2005, Professional Edition*, American Medical Association. All rights reserved.

APPROVED OMB NO. 0938-0279

ST11843 1PLY UB-92

1

2

3 PATIENT CONTROL NO. | 4 TYPE OF BILL

5 FED. TAX NO. | 6 STATEMENT COVERS PERIOD FROM THROUGH | 7 COV D. | 8 N-C D. | 9 C-ID. | 10 L-R D. | 11

12 PATIENT NAME | 13 PATIENT ADDRESS

14 BIRTHDATE | 15 SEX | 16 MS | ADMISSION 17 DATE | 18 HR | 19 TYPE | 20 SRC | 21 D HR | 22 STAT | 23 MEDICAL RECORD NO. | CONDITION CODES 24 25 26 27 28 29 30 | 31

32 OCCURRENCE CODE DATE | 33 OCCURRENCE CODE DATE | 34 OCCURRENCE CODE DATE | 35 OCCURRENCE CODE DATE | 36 OCCURRENCE SPAN CODE FROM THROUGH | 37 A B C

a b

38

39 VALUE CODES CODE AMOUNT | 40 VALUE CODES CODE AMOUNT | 41 VALUE CODES CODE AMOUNT

a b c d

	42 REV. CD.	43 DESCRIPTION	44 HCPCS / RATES	45 SERV. DATE	46 SERV. UNITS	47 TOTAL CHARGES	48 NON-COVERED CHARGES	49	
1									1
2									2
3									3
4									4
5									5
6									6
7									7
8									8
9									9
10									10
11									11
12									12
13									13
14									14
15									15
16									16
17									17
18									18
19									19
20									20
21									21
22									22
23									23

50 PAYER | 51 PROVIDER NO. | 52 REL INFO | 53 ASG BEN | 54 PRIOR PAYMENTS | 55 EST. AMOUNT DUE | 56

A B C

57 DUE FROM PATIENT ▸

58 INSURED'S NAME | 59 P. REL | 60 CERT.- SSN - HIC.- ID NO. | 61 GROUP NAME | 62 INSURANCE GROUP NO.

A B C

63 TREATMENT AUTHORIZATION CODES | 64 ESC | 65 EMPLOYER NAME | 66 EMPLOYER LOCATION

A B C

67 PRIN. DIAG. CD. | 68 CODE | 69 CODE | 70 CODE | 71 CODE | 72 CODE | 73 CODE | 74 CODE | 75 CODE | 76 ADM. DIAG. CD. | 77 E-CODE | 78

79 P.C. | 80 PRINCIPAL PROCEDURE CODE DATE | 81 OTHER PROCEDURE CODE DATE A | OTHER PROCEDURE CODE DATE B | 82 ATTENDING PHYS. ID

OTHER PROCEDURE CODE DATE C | OTHER PROCEDURE CODE DATE D | OTHER PROCEDURE CODE DATE E | 83 OTHER PHYS. ID A | OTHER PHYS. ID B

a b c d

84 REMARKS

a b c d

85 PROVIDER REPRESENTATIVE X | 86 DATE

UB-92 HCFA-1450 | OCR/ORIGINAL | I CERTIFY THE CERTIFICATIONS ON THE REVERSE APPLY TO THIS BILL AND ARE MADE A PART HEREOF.

Figure 3-1 CMS 1450 UB92 Health Insurance Claim Form. *(Courtesy U.S. Department of Health and Human Services, Centers for Medicare and Medicaid Services.)*

Copyright © 2005, Elsevier Inc. All rights reserved.
CPT only © 2004. *Current Procedural Terminology, 2005, Professional Edition*, American Medical Association. All rights reserved.

Modifier Functions

Altered (i.e., more or less)

Bilateral

Multiple

Only portions of service (i.e., professional service only)

More than one surgeon

ASC Modifiers

-25 SIGNIFICANT, SEPARATELY IDENTIFIABLE E/M SERVICE, SAME PHYSICIAN/AND DAY OF PROCEDURE/SERVICE

- Documentation must support service
  Example: Patient seen for sinus congestion, physician performs H&P, prescribes decongestant, notes lesion on back, and removes it.
- Code: Procedure+E/M-25

-27 MULTIPLE OUTPATIENT HOSPITAL E/M ENCOUNTERS ON THE SAME DAY

- Separate and distinct E/M encounters
- Performed in multiple outpatient hospital settings
- Used only with E/M services

-50 BILATERAL PROCEDURE

- Body is bilateral.
  Example: Procedure on hands
- *Caution:* Some codes describe bilateral procedures.

Typically not used on integumentary codes

-52 REDUCED SERVICES

- Service reduced from those in code description
- Physician directed reduction
- Documentation substantiates reduction.
- Procedure discontinued after IV sedation administered
- Not for patient unable to pay

-58 STAGED/RELATED BY SAME PHYSICIAN DURING POSTOPERATIVE PERIOD

- Subsequent procedure planned at time of first surgery
  - During post-op of previous surgery in series
    Example: Multiple skin grafts completed in several sessions
  - Do not use when code describes a session.
    Example: 67208: lesion destruction of retina, one or more sessions
- Therapeutic procedure performed during the global period of a diagnostic procedure
  Example: Surgical biopsy of breast followed by subsequent mastectomy

Copyright © 2005, Elsevier Inc. All rights reserved.
CPT only © 2004. *Current Procedural Terminology, 2005, Professional Edition*, American Medical Association. All rights reserved.

-73 DISCONTINUED OUTPATIENT HOSPITAL/AMBULATORY SURGERY CENTER PROCEDURE PRIOR TO THE ADMINISTRATION OF ANESTHESIA

- Procedure stopped due to patient's condition
- After surgical preparation and sedation
- Prior to administration of anesthesia

-74 DISCONTINUED OUTPATIENT HOSPITAL/AMBULATORY SURGERY CENTER PROCEDURE AFTER ADMINISTRATION OF ANESTHESIA

- Procedure stopped due to patient's condition
- After administration of anesthesia
- May be after procedure begins

  Example: Intubation started or incision was made

-76 REPEAT PROCEDURE/SERVICE BY SAME PHYSICIAN

- *Note:* "Same Physician"
- Used to indicate necessary service

  Example: X-rays before and after fracture repair

-77 REPEAT PROCEDURE/SERVICE BY ANOTHER PHYSICIAN

- *Note:* "Another Physician"
- Performed by one physician, repeated by another physician
- Submitted with written report to establish medical necessity

-78 RETURN TO OPERATING ROOM FOR A RELATED PROCEDURE DURING POSTOPERATIVE PERIOD

- For complication of first procedure

  Example: Patient has outpatient procedure in morning, returned to operating room in afternoon with severe hemorrhage
- Indicates charge is not typographical error

-79 UNRELATED PROCEDURE OR SERVICE BY SAME PHYSICIAN DURING POSTOPERATIVE PERIOD

Example: Several days after discharge for procedure, patient returns for unrelated office service.

- Diagnosis code would also be different.

-99 MULTIPLE MODIFIERS

- Used when service needs more than one modifier but payer only allows for one modifier with each code

HCPC Level II Modifiers

Anatomical modifiers

-LT Left side

-RT Right side

-E1 Upper left, eyelid

Copyright © 2005, Elsevier Inc. All rights reserved.
CPT only © 2004. *Current Procedural Terminology, 2005, Professional Edition,* American Medical Association. All rights reserved.

-E2	Lower left, eyelid
-E3	Upper right, eyelid
-E4	Lower left, eyelid
-FA	Left hand, thumb
-F1	Left hand, second digit
-F2	Left hand, third digit
-F3	Left hand, fourth digit
-F4	Left hand, fifth digit
-F5	Right hand, thumb
-F6	Right hand, second digit
-F7	Right hand, third digit
-F8	Right hand, fourth digit
-F9	Right hand, fifth digit
-TA	Left foot, great toe
-T1	Left foot, second digit
-T2	Left foot, third digit
-T3	Left foot, fourth digit
-T4	Left foot, fifth digit
-T5	Right foot, great toe
-T6	Right foot, second digit
-T7	Right foot, third digit
-T8	Right foot, fourth digit
-T9	Right foot, fifth digit
-LC	Left circumflex, coronary artery
-LD	Left anterior descending coronary artery
-RC	Right coronary artery

Anatomical modifiers are not used with skin procedures.

Example: Removal of skin tags, any area

Exception is with codes that indicate feet, hands, fingers, legs, arms, and eyelids.

The Index

Used to locate service/procedure terms and codes

Speeds up code location

Like a dictionary

- First entries and last entries on top of page
- Code display in index:
  Single code: 38115

Copyright © 2005, Elsevier Inc. All rights reserved.
CPT only © 2004. *Current Procedural Terminology, 2005, Professional Edition*, American Medical Association. All rights reserved.

Multiple codes: 26645, 26650
Range of codes: 22305–22325

Location Methods

Service/procedure: Repair, excision

Anatomical site: Medial nerve, elbow

Condition or disease: Cleft lip, clot

Synonym: Toe and interphalangeal joint

Eponym: Jones Procedure, Heller Operation

Abbreviation: ECG, PEEP (Positive end-expiratory pressure)

"See" in Index

Cross-reference terms: "Look here for code"

Index: Stem, Brain: *See* Brainstem

Appendices of CPT

1. Appendix A: Modifiers and Modifiers for ASC
2. Appendix B: Additions, Deletions, Revisions
3. Appendix C: Clinical Examples, E/M Codes
4. Appendix D: Add-On Codes
5. Appendix E: -51 Exempt Codes
6. Appendix F: Modifier -63 (Appendix F-I new in 2005)
7. Appendix G: Conscious Sedation
8. Appendix H: Genetic Testing Modifiers
9. Appendix I: Category II Modifiers

EVALUATION AND MANAGEMENT (E/M) SECTION (99201-99499)

Outpatient

One who has not been admitted to a health-care facility

Example: Patient receives services at clinic or same-day surgery center.

Inpatient

One who has been formally admitted to a health-care facility

Physician dictates:

Admission orders

H&P

Requests consultations

Copyright © 2005, Elsevier Inc. All rights reserved.
CPT only © 2004. *Current Procedural Terminology, 2005, Professional Edition,* American Medical Association. All rights reserved.

Emergency Department (ED) Services (99281-99288)

No distinction between new and established patients

To qualify as ED (ER), facility must be open 24 hours a day.

5 ED codes do not lend themselves to reporting ED services.

These codes measure only physician services during an encounter, not all interventions provided during encounter **(Figure 3-2).**

Services provided in addition to the interventions are reported separately.

Such as sutures, debridement, etc.; these are reported in addition the ED CPT code.

Critical Care and ED Codes (99291-99296)

ED services often require additional codes from Critical Care Services.

Example: Multiple organ failure

Level 1—99281	Level 2—99282	Level 3—99283
1. Initial (triage) assessment 2. Suture removal 3. Wound recheck 4. Note for work or school 5. Simple discharge information	Interventions from previous level plus any of the following: 1. OTC med administration 2. Tetanus booster 3. Bedside diagnostic tests (stool hemoccult, glucometer) 4. Visual acuity 5. Orthostatic vital signs 6. Simple trauma not requiring x-ray 7. Simple discharge information	Interventions from previous level plus any of the following: 1. Heparin/saline lock 2. Crystalloid IV therapy 3. X-ray, one area 4. RX med administration 5. Fluorescein stain 6. Quick cath 7. Foley cath 8. Receipt of ambulance patient 9. Mental health emergencies (mild) not requiring parenteral medications or admission 10. Moderate complexity discharge instructions
Level 4—99284	**Level 5—99285**	**Critical care 99291, 99292**
Interventions from previous level plus any of the following: 1. X-ray, multiple areas 2. Special imaging studies (CT, MRI, ultrasound) 3. Cardiac monitoring 4. Multiple reassessments of patient 5. Parenteral [1]medications (including insulin) 6. Nebulizer treatment (1 or 2) 7. NG placement 8. Pelvic exam 9. Mental health emergencies (moderate). May require parenteral medications but not admission [1]*not through the alimentary canal but rather by injection through some other route, such as subcutaneous, intramuscular, intraorbital, intracapsular, intraspinal, intrasternal, or intravenous*	Interventions from previous level plus any of the following: 1. Monitor/stabilize patient during in hospital transport and/or testing (CT, MRI, ultrasound) 2. Vasoactive medication 3. Administration (dopamine, dobutamine, multiple) nebulizer treatments (3 or more) 4. Conscious sedation 5. Lumbar puncture 6. Thoracentesis 7. Sexual assault exam 8. Admission to hospital 9. Mental health emergency (severe) psychotic and/or agitated/combative 10. Requires admission 11. Fracture/dislocation reduction 12. Suicide precautions 13. Gastric lavage 14. Complex discharge instructions	Interventions from any previous level plus any of the following: 1. Multiple parenteral medications 2. Continuous monitoring 3. Major trauma care 4. Chest tube insertion 5. CPR 6. Defibrillation/cardioversion 7. Delivery of baby 8. Control of major hemorrhage 9. Administration of blood or blood products

Figure 3-2 ED acuity sheet.

Copyright © 2005, Elsevier Inc. All rights reserved.
CPT only © 2004. *Current Procedural Terminology, 2005, Professional Edition,* American Medical Association. All rights reserved.

Critical Care Services are provided to patients in life-threatening (critically ill or injured) situations.

99281-99285 collapse into Level 1, 2, or 3 under APC system

- Hospital determines what level the codes are in
  - For example,
    - 99281 = Level 1
    - 99282 & 99283 = Level 2
    - 99284 & 99285 = Level 3
    - OR
    - 99281 & 99282 = Level 1
    - 99283 & 99284 = Level 2
    - 99285 = Level 3

Levels are reimbursed at different rates by CMS

- For example, for 2004 ED levels reimbursed:
  - Level 1 ED $74.70
  - Level 2 ED $130.77
  - Level 3 ED $226.30

Both Critical Care codes (99291 & 99292) are included in Level 4, Critical Care and reimbursed in 2004 at $491.01 (not a time based payment)

APC Levels of Service

Facilities report emergency department (ED) services for non-OPPS patients using CPT codes.

There are five ED CPT codes (99281–99285) **(Figure 3-2)**.

Under OPPS, these five codes collapse into 3 to 5 levels.

Three levels are 610, 611, and 612.

Number of levels is dependent upon facility protocol.

Example:

610 Low Level Emergency Visits (would be equal to 99281 and 99282)

611 Mid Level Emergency Visits (would be equal to 99283 and 99284)

612 High Level Emergency Visits (would be equal to 99285)

Another facility may define the levels as follows:

610 Low Level Emergency Visits (would be equal to 99281)

611 Mid Level Emergency Visits (would be equal to 99282 and 99283)

612 High Level Emergency Visits (would be equal to 99284 and 99285)

Each level includes a baseline level of service.

Baseline services are:

- Registration
- Initial Nursing Assessment
- Periodic Vital Signs
- Discharge Instructions
- Exam Room set up/clean up
- Limited intervention using

Copyright © 2005, Elsevier Inc. All rights reserved.
CPT only © 2004. *Current Procedural Terminology, 2005, Professional Edition*, American Medical Association. All rights reserved.

Minimal resources

10 Minutes or less staff contact

Examples:

Administration of oral medications

Initiation of oxygen therapy

Obtaining lab specimens

Levels ascend based upon

Increase in staff time

Additional interventions

Examples:

- Extended initial nursing assessment or discharge
- Starting an IV
- Insertions of tubes (catheters, Foleys, or nasogastric)

Each hospital creates its own set of internal guidelines to determine in which level each Critical Care and ED CPT code is included.

CMS directs only that the system is reasonable and relates to resource intensity.

Does not direct which CPT codes go in each APC level

Critical care codes collapse into 1 APC

620 Critical Care

Uses of Anesthesia

Relieve pain

Manage unconscious patients, life functions, and resuscitation

Analgesia

Relief of pain

Some Methods of Anesthesia

Endotracheal: Through mouth

Local: Application to area (injection or topical)

Epidural: Between vertebral spaces

Regional: Field or nerve

MAC: Monitored anesthesia care

Patient-Controlled Analgesia (PCA)

Patient administers drug.

Used to relieve chronic pain

Conscious Sedation

To be used when surgeon administers sedation himself/herself

Decreased level of consciousness

Copyright © 2005, Elsevier Inc. All rights reserved.
CPT only © 2004. *Current Procedural Terminology, 2005, Professional Edition*, American Medical Association. All rights reserved.

Report with 99141 or 99142 (Medicine), unless procedure code is marked with a bulls-eye.

Presence of trained observer, such as a nurse, is required.

If administered by a physician other than the one performing the procedure, use Anesthesia section code.

SURGERY SECTION (10021-69990)

Largest CPT section

Each year CMS publishes a list of CPT surgery codes that are paid only as an inpatient procedure.

For example, 33300-33335, repair of wounds of the heart and great vessels, are inpatient procedures.

Whereas 33282-33284, implantation or removal of cardiac event recorders, are paid as outpatient procedures

Inpatient procedures reported with Volume 3 procedure codes

Outpatient procedures reported with CPT surgery codes

Section Format

Divided by subspecialty (e.g., integumentary, cardiovascular)

Notes and Guidelines

Throughout section

Information varied and extensive

"Must reading"

Subsection notes apply to entire subsection.

Subheading notes apply to entire subheading.

Category notes apply to entire category.

Parenthetical information **(Figure 3-3)**

Unlisted Procedure Codes

Used only when more specific code not found

Written report accompanies submission.

Each unlisted code service paid on case-by-case basis

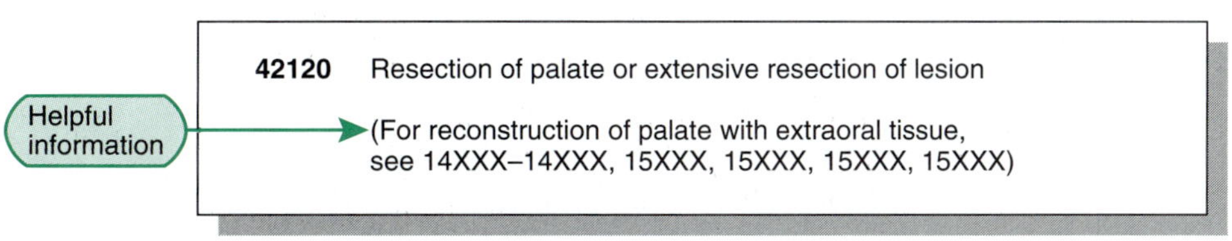

Figure 3-3 Parenthetical information in the CPT manual

Copyright © 2005, Elsevier Inc. All rights reserved.
CPT only © 2004. *Current Procedural Terminology, 2005, Professional Edition*, American Medical Association. All rights reserved.

Separate Procedures

"(Separate procedure)" follows code description.

Usually minor surgical procedure

Incidental to more major procedure

Breast biopsy

Biopsy before radical mastectomy would not be coded

Separate procedures reported when:

- Only procedure performed
- With another procedure
  - On different site
  - Unrelated to major procedure

GENERAL SUBSECTION (10021-10022)

Fine needle aspirations with or without (w/wo) imaging guidance

- Excludes bone marrow aspirations (38220)

INTEGUMENTARY SYSTEM SUBSECTION (10040-19499)

Often used in all specialties of medicine

Used not just by surgeons or dermatologists but by a wide range of physicians

Subheadings of Integumentary Subsection

1. Skin, Subcutaneous, and Accessory Structures
2. Nails
3. Repair (Closure)
4. Destruction
5. Breast

Skin, Subcutaneous, and Accessory Structures (10040-11646)

Incision & Drainage (10040-10180)

- I&D of abscess, carbuncle, boil, cyst, infection, hematoma, pilonidal cyst
  - Lancing (cutting of skin)
  - Aspiration (removal with needle)
- Gauze or tube may be inserted for continued drainage.

Excision—Debridement (11000-11044)

Dead tissue cut away and washed away with saline

11000-11001 eczematous or infected skin

11010-11012 foreign material with fracture or dislocation

11040-11044 skin, subcutaneous muscle, bone

Copyright © 2005, Elsevier Inc. All rights reserved.
CPT only © 2004. *Current Procedural Terminology, 2005, Professional Edition*, American Medical Association. All rights reserved.

Paring or Cutting (11055-11057)

- Removal by scraping or peeling (e.g., removal of corn or callus)
- Codes indicate number: 1, 2–4, 4+.

Biopsy (11100-11101)

- Skin, subcutaneous tissue, or mucous membrane biopsy
- Not all of lesion removed

All of lesion removed = excision

Codes indicate number: 1 or each additional

Tissue that is removed during excision, shave, etc. and submitted to pathology is NOT reported separately as a biopsy.

Rather, it is included in the code for the excision.

Skin Tag Removal (11200-11201)

- Benign lesions
- Removed with scissors, blade, chemicals, electrosurgery, etc.
- Codes indicate number: up to 15 and each additional 10 lesions.

Shaving of Lesions (11300-11313)

- Removed by transverse incision or sliced horizontally
- Based on:
  - Size (e.g., 1.1–2 cm)
  - Location (e.g., arm, hand, nose)
- Does not require suture closure

Benign/Malignant Lesions (11400-11646)

- Codes divided: Benign or malignant
- Physician assesses lesion as benign or malignant.
- Codes include local anesthesia and simple closure.
- Report each excised lesion separately.
- Lesion size
  - Taken from physician's notes
  - Do not take size from pathology report—storage solution shrinks tissue
  - Includes greatest diameter plus margins
  - Margins (healthy tissue) are also taken for comparison with unhealthy tissue.
  - *Example:* 1 cm lesion with 2 cm margin left and right of lesion
    - 1 + 2 + 2 = 5 cm
  - Re-excisions following initial excision of malignant lesion
    - Coded as excision of malignant lesion
- All excised tissue pathologically examined
- Destroyed lesions have no pathology samples.
  - *Example:* Laser or chemical

Copyright © 2005, Elsevier Inc. All rights reserved.
CPT only © 2004. *Current Procedural Terminology, 2005, Professional Edition*, American Medical Association. All rights reserved.

- Lesion closure
  - Simple or subcutaneous closure included in removal
  - Reported separately

Layered or intermediate, 12031–12057 (Repair—Intermediate)

Complex, 13100–13153 (Repair—Complex)

  - Local anesthesia included

Nails (11719-11765)

Both toes and fingers

Types of services:

- Trimming, debridement, removal, biopsy, repair

Introduction (11900-11983)

Types of services. Lesion injections, tattooing, tissue expansion, contraceptive insertion/removal, hormone implantation services, and insertion/removal of nonbiodegradable drug-delivery implant

Repair (12001-13160)

Repair Factors in Wound Repair

- As types of wounds vary, types of wound repair also vary.
- Length, complexity (simple, intermediate, complex), and site

  Length measured in centimeters

  Measured prior to closure

Types of Wound Repair

Simple: Superficial, epidermis, dermis, or subcutaneous tissue

One-layer closure

Dermabond closure

Medicare use G0168

Intermediate: Layered closure of deeper layers of subcutaneous tissue and superficial fascia with skin closure

Simple closure can be coded as intermediate if extensive debridement is required.

Complex: Greater than layered

Example: Scar revision, complicated debridement, extensive undermining, stents, extensive retention sutures

Included in Wound Repair Codes

1. Simple ligation of vessels
2. Simple exploration of wound
3. Normal debridement

Additional codes for debridement can be used when:

Gross contamination requires prolonged cleaning.

Copyright © 2005, Elsevier Inc. All rights reserved.
CPT only © 2004. *Current Procedural Terminology, 2005, Professional Edition*, American Medical Association. All rights reserved.

Appreciable amounts of devitalized/contaminated tissue are removed to expose healthy tissue.

Debridement is provided without immediate primary closure.

Grouping of Wound Repair

- Add together lengths by:
  1. Complexity
     Simple, intermediate, complex
  2. Location
     e.g., face, ears, eyelids, nose, lips

Do Not Group Wound Repairs That Are

- Different complexities
  Example: Simple repair and complex repair
- Different locations
  Example: Simple repairs of scalp (12001) and nose (12011)

Adjacent Tissue Transfer, Flaps, and Grafts (14000-15776)

Information Needed to Code Graft

1. Type of graft—adjacent, free, flap, etc.
2. Donor site (from)
3. Recipient site (to)
4. Any repair to donor site
5. Size

Adjacent Tissue Transfer/Rearrangement (14000-14300)

Includes excision and/or repair (e.g., Z-plasty, W-plasty, V-plasty, rotation flap, advancement flap)

Measure site of defect from excision plus size of defect from flap design for total size

Free Skin Graft

15000-15001 preparation of recipient site codes

15050-15261 graft codes

Split graft: Epidermis and some dermis **(Figure 3-4)**

Full-thickness: Epidermis and all dermis

Grafts (15342-15401)

- Bilaminate skin substitute
  Artificial skin
- Allograft: Donor graft
- Xenograft: Nonhuman donor

Copyright © 2005, Elsevier Inc. All rights reserved.
CPT only © 2004. *Current Procedural Terminology, 2005, Professional Edition*, American Medical Association. All rights reserved.

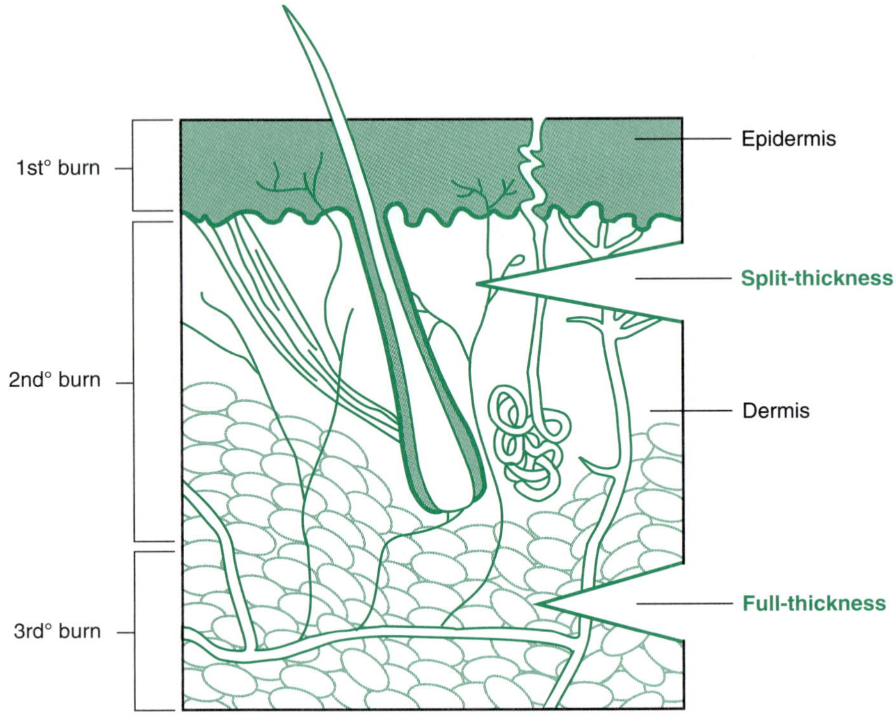

Figure 3-4 Split-thickness and full-thickness skin grafts.

Flap (15570-15776)

- Some skin left attached to blood supply
  Keeps flap viable
- Donor site may be far from recipient site.
- Flaps may be in stages.
- Formation of flap (15570-15576)
  Based on location: trunk, scalp, nose, etc.
- Transfer of flap (15650): Previously placed flap released from donor site
  Also known as walking or walk up of flap
- Muscle, Myocutaneous, or Fasciocutaneous Flaps (15732-15738)
  - Repairs made with
    - Muscle
    - Muscle and skin
    - Fascia and skin
  - Flaps rotated from donor to recipient site
  - Includes closure donor site
  - Codes divided on location, i.e.:
    - Trunk
    - Extremity

Pressure Ulcers (15920-15999)

- Excision and various closures
  Primary, skin flap, muscle, etc.

Copyright © 2005, Elsevier Inc. All rights reserved.
CPT only © 2004. *Current Procedural Terminology, 2005, Professional Edition*, American Medical Association. All rights reserved.

- Many codes "with ostectomy"
  Bone removal
- Locations
  1. Coccygeal (end of spine)
  2. Sacral (between hips)
  3. Ischial (lower hip)
  4. Trochanteric (outer hip)
- Site prep only 15936, 15946, or 15956
  Defect repair or donor site reported separately

Burns (16000-16036)

- Codes for small, medium, and large
- Most calculate percentage of body burn using Rule of Nines for adults (Figure 3-5)
  $<4\frac{1}{2}$ small
  $4\frac{1}{2}$ to 9 medium
  >9 large
- Lund-Browder for children (**Figure 3-6**)
  - Proportions of children differ from those of adults.
  - Heads are larger

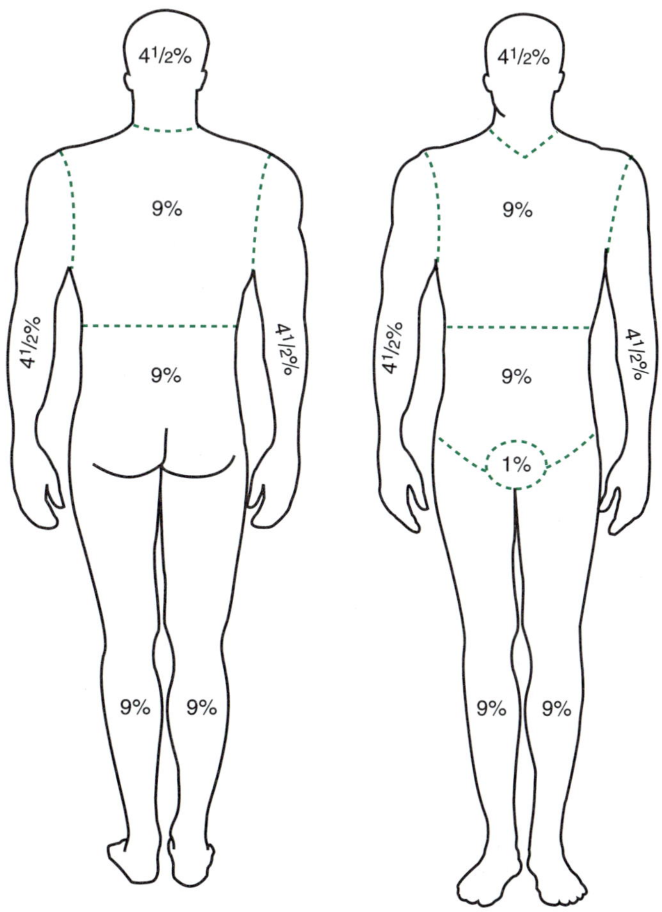

Figure 3-5 The Rule of Nines is used to calculate burn area on an adult.

Copyright © 2005, Elsevier Inc. All rights reserved.
CPT only © 2004. *Current Procedural Terminology, 2005, Professional Edition*, American Medical Association. All rights reserved.

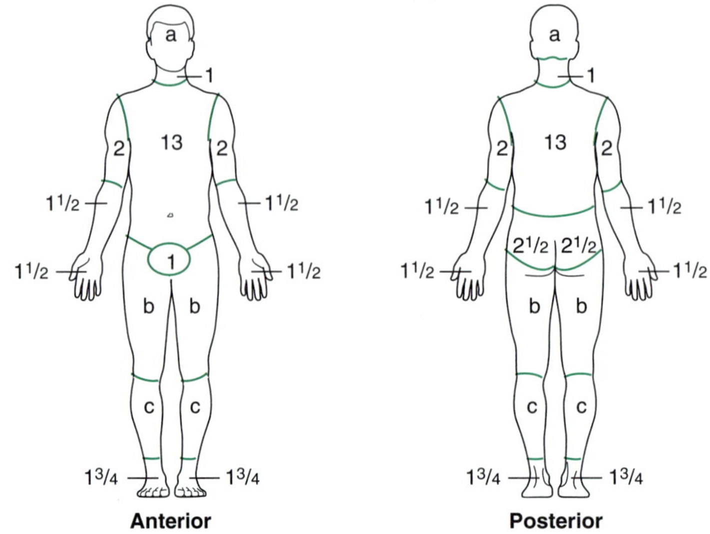

Relative percentage of body surface areas (% BSA) affected by growth

	0 yr	1 yr	5 yr	10 yr	15 yr
a – 1/2 of head	9 1/2	8 1/2	6 1/2	5 1/2	4 1/2
b – 1/2 of 1 thigh	2 3/4	3 1/4	4	4 1/4	4 1/2
c – 1/2 of lower leg	2 1/2	2 1/2	2 3/4	3	3 1/4

Figure 3-6 Lund-Browder chart for estimating the extent of burns on children.

- Often require multiple debridement and redressing
- Based on:
  1. Initial or subsequent service
  2. Size
  3. With or without anesthesia
- Report % of burn and depth (Refer to Figure 3-4 for depth)
- Escharotomies are performed only on an inpatient basis (16035-16036)

Destruction (17000-17286)

Ablation (destruction) of tissue

- Laser, electrosurgery, cryosurgery, chemosurgery, etc.

Benign/premalignant or malignant tissue

- Based on location and size

Mohs' Microscope (17304-17310)

- Surgeon acts as pathologist and surgeon.
- Removes one layer of lesion at time
- Until no malignant cells remain
- Based on stages stated in report

Copyright © 2005, Elsevier Inc. All rights reserved.
CPT only © 2004. *Current Procedural Terminology, 2005, Professional Edition,* American Medical Association. All rights reserved.

Other Procedures (17340-17999)

Treatment of acne
- Cryotherapy
- Chemical exfoliation

Electrolysis

Unlisted procedures

Breast Procedures (19000-19499)

Divided based on procedure, e.g.:

Aspiration

Incision

Excision

Repair

Reconstruction

Use excision-of-lesion codes if entire lesion is removed during incisional biopsy

Use additional codes for placement of radiological markers.

Mastectomies based on extent of procedure

Wide excision

Removal of neoplasm, capsule, and surrounding margins

Radical

Wide excision and anatomical structure surrounding neoplasm

Example: Muscle or fascia

Performed on an inpatient basis (19200–19920)

Code removal of lymph node separately unless included in code description

MUSCULOSKELETAL SYSTEM SUBSECTION (20000-29999)

- Subsection divided: Anatomical site, then service (e.g., excision)
- Used extensively by orthopedic surgeons
  Many codes commonly used by variety of physicians
- Extensive notes
- Most common:
  Fracture and dislocation treatments
  "General" subheading
  Arthroscopic procedures
  Casting and strapping

Fracture Treatment

Type of treatment depends on type and severity of fracture.

Open: Surgically opened to view or remotely opened to place nail across fracture site

Copyright © 2005, Elsevier Inc. All rights reserved.
CPT only © 2004. *Current Procedural Terminology, 2005, Professional Edition*, American Medical Association. All rights reserved.

Closed: Not surgically opened

Percutaneous: Insertion of devices through skin or a remote site

Traction

- Application of force to align bone
- Force applied by internal device (e.g., wire, pin) inserted into bone (skeletal fixation)
- Application of force by means of adhesion to skin (skin traction)

Manipulation

Use of force to return bone back to normal alignment

Codes often divided based on whether manipulation was or was not used

Dislocation

Bone displaced from normal joint position

Treatment: Return bone to normal joint location

Subheading—"General"

Begins "Incision" (20000-20005)

Depth makes difference between choice of Integumentary or Musculoskeletal incision codes

Musculoskeletal code used when underlying bone or muscle is involved

Wound Exploration (20100-20103)

Traumatic penetrating wounds

Divided on wound location

Includes:

- Surgical Exploration
- Enlargement
- Debridement
- Removal of foreign body (bodies)
- Ligation
- Repair of tissue and muscle

Use additional code for repair of major structures or blood vessels

Not used for integumentary repairs

Unless the repair requires extension, enlargement, or exploration

Excision (20150-20251)

Biopsies for bone and muscle

Divided by:

- Type of biopsy (bone/muscle)
- Depth
- Some by method

Copyright © 2005, Elsevier Inc. All rights reserved.
CPT only © 2004. *Current Procedural Terminology, 2005, Professional Edition*, American Medical Association. All rights reserved.

Can be percutaneous or excisional

Does not include tumor excision, which is coded separately

Biopsy with excision, only code excision

Introduction and Removal (20500-20694)

Codes for:

1. Injections
2. Aspirations
3. Insertions
4. Applications
5. Removals
6. Adjustments

Therapeutic sinus tract injection procedures:

- Not nasal sinus
- Abscess or cyst with passage (sinus tract) to skin
- Antibiotic injected with use of radiographic guidance

Removal of foreign bodies lodged in muscle or tendon sheath

Integumentary removal codes for removal from skin

Injection into:

- Tendon sheath
- Tendon origin
- Ligament
- Ganglion cyst
- Trigger points

Arthrocentesis injection "and/or" aspiration of a joint

- Both aspiration and injection reported with one code
- Do not unbundle and report with two codes.

Replantation (20802-20838)

Used to report reattachment of amputated limb

Code by body area

Performed only on an inpatient basis

Grafts (20900-20938)

Used to report harvesting through separate incision of:

1. Bone
2. Cartilage
3. Fascia lata
4. Tissue

Copyright © 2005, Elsevier Inc. All rights reserved.
CPT only © 2004. *Current Procedural Terminology, 2005, Professional Edition*, American Medical Association. All rights reserved.

Fascia lata grafts: from lower thigh where fascia is thickest

Some codes include obtaining grafting material (then, not coded separately).

Other Procedures (20950-20999)

Monitoring muscle fluid pressure (interstitial)

- Pressure increases when blood supply decreases due to increased accumulation of fluids.

Bone grafts identified by site taken from (donor site)

Free osseocutaneous flaps: bone grafts

- Taken along with skin and tissue overlying bone

Electrical stimulation

- Used to speed bone healing
- Placement of stimulators externally or internally
- Ultrasound also used externally

External Fixation (20690-20692)

Application of device that holds bone in place

Code fracture treatment and external fixation

- Unless treatment and fixation both included in fracture care code description

Arthrodesis

Fixation of joint

Often performed with other procedure, such as fracture repair

Subsequent Subheadings

After General subheading, divided by anatomical location

- Anatomical subheadings divided by type procedure

Example: Subheading "Head" divided by procedure:

1. Incision
2. Excision
3. Introduction or Removal
4. Repair, Revision, and/or Reconstruction
5. Other Procedures
6. Fracture and/or Dislocation

Spinal Instrumentation and Fixation

Spine (Ventral Column), 22100–22855 divided by repair location:

1. Cervical (C1–C7)

   C1 = Atlas

   C2 = Axis

Copyright © 2005, Elsevier Inc. All rights reserved.
CPT only © 2004. *Current Procedural Terminology, 2005, Professional Edition*, American Medical Association. All rights reserved.

2. Lumbar (L1–L5)
3. Thoracic (T1–T12)

Percutaneous vertebroplasty:

Use of polymethylmethacrylate injected into the vertebral space

Polymethylmethacrylate is a type of bone cement/glue like silicone but not silicone.

Adheres bone fragments together

Fills vertebral body defects

Types of Spinal Instrumentation

Segmental: Devices at each end of repair area plus at least one other attachment

Nonsegmental: Devices at each end of defect only

Spinal instrumentation procedures are performed only on an inpatient basis.

Casting and Strapping (29000-29799)

Replacement procedure or initial placement to stabilize when provided without additional restorative treatment

Example: Application of wrist splint or cast for wrist sprain

Initial fracture treatment includes placement and removal of first cast.
- Subsequent cast applications coded separately

Application not coded when part of surgical procedure

Example: Repair of radial fracture includes application of cast or splint.

Ace bandage applications not billed separately

Removal bundled into surgical procedure

Supplies reported separately

Subheading Endoscopy/Arthroscopy (29800-29999)

Surgical arthroscopy always includes diagnostic arthroscopy.

Codes divided on joint
- Subdivided on procedure
- Be aware of subterms and bundled procedures within code descriptions.

NOTE: Parenthetical information following codes indicates codes to use if procedure was an open procedure.

RESPIRATORY SYSTEM SUBSECTION (30000-32999)

- Anatomical site arrangement:
  Nose
  Larynx
- Further subdivided by procedure:
  Incision
  Excision

Copyright © 2005, Elsevier Inc. All rights reserved.
CPT only © 2004. *Current Procedural Terminology, 2005, Professional Edition*, American Medical Association. All rights reserved.

Endoscopy

Endoscopy in all subheadings except Nose

Each preceded by "Notes"

Endoscopy Rule One

- Code full extent.

  Example: Procedure begins at mouth and ends at bronchial tube.

Bronchial tube = full extent

Endoscopy Rule Two

- Code correct approach.

  Example: For removal:

  Interior lung lesion via endoscopy inserted through mouth

  Exterior lung lesion via laparoscope inserted through skin
- Incorrect approach = incorrect code = incorrect reimbursement

Endoscopy Rule Three

- Diagnostic always included in surgical

  Example:
  - Diagnostic bronchial endoscopy begins
  - Identifies foreign body
  - Removed foreign body (surgical endoscopy)

Nose (30000-30999)

Used extensively by otorhinolaryngologists (ear, nose, and throat specialists, ENT)

Also used by wide variety of physicians

When approach to nose:

- External approach, use Integumentary System
- Internal approaches, use Respiratory System

Incision (30000-30020)

- Insertion and removal of drain or gauze bundled into incision codes
- Supplies reported separately

Excision (30100-30160)

- Contains intranasal biopsy codes
- Polyp excision, by complexity

Excision includes any method of destruction, even laser.

Copyright © 2005, Elsevier Inc. All rights reserved.
CPT only © 2004. *Current Procedural Terminology, 2005, Professional Edition*, American Medical Association. All rights reserved.

Introduction (30200-30220)

- Common procedures

  Example: Injections to shrink nasal tissue or displacement therapy (saline flushes) to remove mucus

Displacement therapy performed through nose

Removal of Foreign Body (30300-30320)

- Divided by whether the removal occurred at office or in hospital (requires general anesthesia)

Repair (30400-30630)

Many plastic procedures, e.g.:

- Rhinoplasty (reshaping nose internal and/or external)
- Septoplasty (rearrangement of nasal septum)

Destruction (30801-30802)

Use of cauterization or ablation (removing by cutting)

Used for removal of excess nasal mucosa or to reduce turbinate inflammation

Based on intramural or superficial extent of destruction

Intramural: Deeper mucosa

Superficial: Outer layer of mucosa

Other Procedures (30901-30999)

- Control of nasal hemorrhage
  - Packing
  - Ligation
  - Cauterization
- Anterior packing for less severe bleeding
- Posterior packing for more severe bleeding

Accessory Sinuses, Incision (31000-31090)

Codes for lavage (washing) of sinuses

- Cannula (hollow tube) placed into sinus
- Saline solution flushed through

Endoscopic procedures may involve multiple codes when multiple locations are accessed.

Example: 31020, sinusotomy, maxillary can be coded with 31050 sinusotomy, sphenoid and 31070 sinusotomy frontal.

Repair of fractures occurring during procedure may be coded separately if not included in code description

Copyright © 2005, Elsevier Inc. All rights reserved.
CPT only © 2004. *Current Procedural Terminology, 2005, Professional Edition*, American Medical Association. All rights reserved.

Larynx (31000-31599)

Excision (31300-31402)

- Laryngotomy: open surgical procedure to expose larynx

  For removal procedure (e.g., tumor)
- May be confused with Trachea/Bronchi codes for tracheostomy used to establish air flow

Introduction (31500-31502)

- Endotracheal intubation, establishment of airway
- Based on planned (ventilation support) or emergency procedure

Endoscopy (31515-31656)

- Bronchoscopy tube may be inserted into nose or mouth.
- Rigid endoscopy performed under general anesthesia
- Flexible endoscopy performed under local or conscious sedation

Laryngoscopic Procedures (31505-31579)

- Uses terms *indirect* and *direct*

  Indirect: Tongue depressor with mirror used to view larynx

  Direct: Endoscope passed into larynx, physician directly views vocal cords

Repair (31580-31590)

- Several plastic procedures and fracture repairs
- Laryngoplasty procedures based on purpose
- Fracture codes based on whether manipulation used

Trachea and Bronchi (31600-31899)

Incision (31600-31614)

- Most codes: Tracheostomy divided by:

  Planned (ventilation support)

  Emergency
- Divided by type:

  Transtracheal or cricothyroid (position of incision)

Introduction (31700-31730)

- Catheterization
- Instillation
- Injection
- Aspiration
- Trachea tube placement
- Some include inhaled gas as contrast material

Copyright © 2005, Elsevier Inc. All rights reserved.
CPT only © 2004. *Current Procedural Terminology, 2005, Professional Edition*, American Medical Association. All rights reserved.

Repair (31750-31830)

- Plastic repairs of tracheoplasty and bronchoplasty

Lungs and Pleura (32000-32999)

Incision (32000-32225)

Thoracentesis: Needle inserted into pleural space for aspiration (withdrawal) of fluid or air

Thoracotomy: Surgical opening of chest to expose to view; used for:

1. Biopsy
2. Cyst
3. Foreign body removal
4. Cardiac massage, etc.

Excision (32310-32540)

- Biopsy codes in both Excision and Incision categories
  Excision biopsy with percutaneous needle
  Incision biopsy with chest open
- Also services of pleurectomy, pneumocentesis, and lung removal
  Segmentectomy: 1 segment
  Lobectomy: 1 lobe
  Bilobectomy: 2 lobes
  Total Pneumonectomy: 1 lung

CARDIOVASCULAR (CV) SYSTEM (33010-37799)

CV coding may require codes for

Surgery: Open and percutaneous

Cardiology Coding Terminology

Invasive: Enters body by method of

Incisional

Example: Opening chest for removal (e.g., tumor on heart)

Percutaneously

Placement of catheter into artery or vein by means of

Wire threaded through needle and catheter slid over wire

Cut down—small nick made and catheter inserted

Example: Catheter inserted into femoral or brachial artery

Common Catheters are:

Broviac

Copyright © 2005, Elsevier Inc. All rights reserved.
CPT only © 2004. *Current Procedural Terminology, 2005, Professional Edition*, American Medical Association. All rights reserved.

Hickman

HydroCath

Arrow multi-lumen

Groshong

Dual-lumen type

Triple-lumen type

Both Medicine and Surgery sections contain invasive procedures.

Noninvasive: Procedures that do not break skin

Example: Electrocardiogram

Electrophysiology (EPS): Study of electrical system of heart

Example: Study of irregular heartbeat (arrhythmia)

Nuclear Cardiology: Diagnostic and treatment specialty; uses radioactive substances for cardiac conditions

Example: MRI

Cardiovascular in Surgery Section

Codes for Procedures

Heart/Pericardium (33010-33999)

- Pacemakers, valve disorders

Arteries/Veins (34001-37799)

- Many of same types of procedures but noncoronary procedures

Heart/Pericardium (33010-33999)

Both percutaneous and open surgical

Extensive notes throughout

Frequent changes with medical advances

Examples of categories in Heart/Pericardium subheading:

- Pericardium
- Cardiac Tumor
- Pacemaker or Pacing Cardioverter-Defibrillator

Example of services:

- Pericardiocentesis: Percutaneous withdrawal of fluid from pericardial space
- Cardiac Tumor: Open surgical procedure for removal of tumor on heart

Pacemakers and Cardioverter-Defibrillators (33200-33249)

- Devices that assist heart in electrical function
- Divided by location of placement, approach, and type of service
- Patient record indicates revision or replacement.
- Codes include all services provided within 14 days related to repair, revision, or replacement.

Copyright © 2005, Elsevier Inc. All rights reserved.
CPT only © 2004. *Current Procedural Terminology, 2005, Professional Edition,* American Medical Association. All rights reserved.

Placed

Atrium

Ventricle

Both

Biventricular, both ventricles and atrium (uses 3 leads)

Approach

Epicardial: Open procedure to place on heart

Transvenous: Through vein to place in heart

Type of Service

Initial placement or replacement of all or part of device

Number of leads placed is important in code selection.

Electrophysiologic Operative Procedures (33250-33261)

- Surgeon repairs defect causing abnormal rhythm.
- Chest opened to full view
  Cardiopulmonary (CP) bypass usually used
- Codes based on reason for procedure and if CP bypass used

  Performed only on an inpatient basis

Patient-Activated Event Recorder (33282-33284)

- Also known as cardiac event recorder or loop recorder
- Internal surgical implantation required
- Divided based on device being implanted or removed

Cardiac Valves (33400-33496)

- Divided by valve:
  1. Aortic
  2. Mitral
  3. Tricuspid
  4. Pulmonary
- Subdivided according to whether cardiopulmonary bypass was used
- Code descriptions are all similar, requiring careful reading.
- Performed only on an inpatient basis

Coronary Artery Bypass (CAB)

- CAB performed for severely clogged coronary arteries (atherosclerosis)
- Performed only on an inpatient basis

Copyright © 2005, Elsevier Inc. All rights reserved.
CPT only © 2004. *Current Procedural Terminology, 2005, Professional Edition*, American Medical Association. All rights reserved.

Arteries and Veins Subheading (34001-37799)

Only for noncoronary vessels

- Divided based on whether artery or vein involved
  Example: Different codes for embolectomy, depending on whether artery or vein involved

Catheters placed into vessels for monitoring, removal, repair

Using nonselective or selective catheter placement

Nonselective: Direct placement without further manipulation

Selective: Place and then manipulate into further order(s).

Selective placement includes nonselective placement.

Catheter Placement Example

Nonselective: 36000 Introduction of needle into vein

Selective: 36012 Placement of catheter into second order venous system

Vascular Families Are Like a Tree

- Main branch—first order
- Second-order branch
- Third-order branch
- Brachiocephalic Vascular Family **(Figure 3-7)**

Report farthest extent of catheter placement in a vascular family

Embolectomy and Thrombectomy (34001-34490)

Embolus: Dislodged thrombus

Thrombus: Mass of material in vessel located in place of formation

May be removed by dissection or balloon

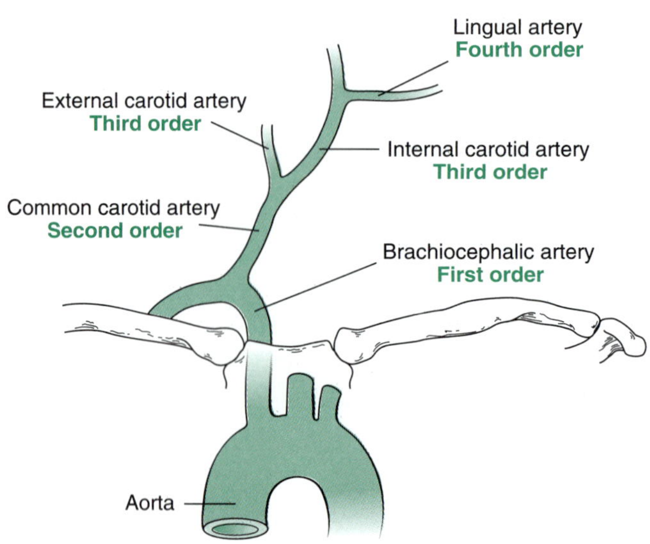

Figure 3-7 Brachiocephalic vascular family with first-, second-, third-, and fourth-order vessels.

Copyright © 2005, Elsevier Inc. All rights reserved.
CPT only © 2004. *Current Procedural Terminology, 2005, Professional Edition*, American Medical Association. All rights reserved.

Balloon Removal: Threaded into vessel, inflated under mass, pulled out with mass

Codes are divided by site of incision and artery/vein

Venous Reconstruction—CV Repairs (34501-34530)

Types of Repair:

Valve

Vein

Aneurysm

Aneurysm

- Aneurysm: Weakened arterial wall causing a bulge or ballooning
- Repair by removal or bypass
- Endovascular repair (34800-34832) from inside vessel
- Direct (35001-35162) from outside vessel

Endovascular Repair of Abdominal Aortic Aneurysm (34800-34834)

- Performed only on an inpatient basis

Repair Arteriovenous Fistula (35180-35190)

Abnormal passage

Divided based on fistula type:

- Congenital
- Acquired/Traumatic
- By site

Repair methods

- Autogenous graft—fistula created artery to vein
- Nonauto fistula—biocompatible tube connecting artery to vein

Angioplasty and Atherectomy

Divided by whether open or percutaneous and by vessel

Transluminal: By way of vessel

Transluminal Angioplasty: Catheter passed into vessel and stretched

Placement of eluding or noneluding stents is coded in addition to catheter placement.

Transluminal Atherectomy: Guide wire threaded into vessel and clots destroyed

Noncoronary Bypass Grafts (35500–35671)

- Divided by:
  1. Vein
  2. In Situ Vein (veins repaired in their original place)
  3. Other Than Vein

Copyright © 2005, Elsevier Inc. All rights reserved.
CPT only © 2004. *Current Procedural Terminology, 2005, Professional Edition*, American Medical Association. All rights reserved.

- Code by type of graft and vessels being used to bypass

  Example: 35506, Bypass graft, with vein; carotid-subclavian

  Graft attached to carotid and to subclavian, bypassing defect of subclavian

Procurement of saphenous vein graft is included and not reported separately.

Harvesting of upper extremity vein or femoropopliteal vein is reported separately.

Vascular Injection Procedures (36000-36015)

- Divided into:
  1. Intravenous
  2. Intraarterial—Intraaortic
  3. Venous
- Used for many procedures, including:

  Local anesthesia

  Introduction of needle

  Catheter

  Injection of contrast material

  Preoperative and postoperative care

  Example: Injection of opaque substance for venography (radiography of vein)

  Bypass grafts are performed only on an inpatient basis.

  Harvesting of veins for bypass grafts can be performed on outpatient basis.

Central Venous Access Procedures

- Peripheral = long term, used for medication/chemotherapy administration
- Central = short term, used for monitoring
- Five categories
  1. Insertion
  2. Repair
  3. Partial replacement
  4. Complete replacement
  5. Removal

Insertion (36555-36571)

Insertion of newly established venous access

Tunneled under skin (i.e., Hickman, Broviac, Groshong)

Nontunneled (i.e., Hohn catheter, triple lumen, PICC)

Central (i.e., subclavian, intrajugular, femoral, inferior vena cava)

Peripheral (anything else)

Codes divided by tunneled/nontunneled, central/peripheral, and age

Copyright © 2005, Elsevier Inc. All rights reserved.
CPT only © 2004. *Current Procedural Terminology, 2005, Professional Edition*, American Medical Association. All rights reserved.

Repair (36575, 36576)

Repair of malfunction without replacement

Repair of central venous access device

No differentiation between age of patient or central/peripheral insertion

Replacement

Partial (36578) is replacement of catheter only.

Complete (36580-36585) is replacement through same venous access site.

Differentiated by tunneled/nontunneled, central/peripheral, and with or without subcutaneous port or pump

Removal (36589, 36590)

To be used for tunneled catheter

Removal of nontunneled catheter is not reported separately

Guidance for Vascular Access

75998, fluoroscopic guidance for central venous access device placement, replacement, or removal

Reported in addition to primary procedure

76937, ultrasound guidance for vascular access

Reported in addition to primary procedure

HEMIC AND LYMPHATIC SYSTEMS SUBSECTION (38100-38999)

Divisions

1. Spleen
2. General
3. Lymph Nodes and Lymphatic Channels

Spleen Subheading (38100-38200)

Spleen easily ruptured, causes massive hemorrhage

May require splenectomy

Splenectomy: total or partial/open or laparoscopic

Often done as part of more major procedure

Bundled into major procedure

General (38204-38242)

Codes divided on:

Presentation

Preparation

Copyright © 2005, Elsevier Inc. All rights reserved.
CPT only © 2004. *Current Procedural Terminology, 2005, Professional Edition*, American Medical Association. All rights reserved.

Purification

Aspiration

Biopsy

Harvesting

Transplantation

Stem Cells

Immature blood cells originating in bone marrow

Used in treatment of leukemia

Types of stem cells

Allogenic: Close relative

Autologous: Patient's own

Lymph Nodes and Lymphatic Channels Subheading (38300-38999)

Two types of lymphadenectomies:

Limited: Lymph nodes only

Radical: Lymph nodes, submandibular gland, and surrounding tissue

Often bundled into more major procedure (e.g., prostatectomy)

Do not unbundle and report lymphadenectomy separately.

MEDIASTINUM (39000-39499)

- Incision codes for foreign body removal or biopsy
- Excision codes for removal of cyst or tumor
- All procedures, except for 39400 (mediastinoscopy), are performed on an inpatient basis

DIAPHRAGM (39501-39599)

Only category: Repair

Most codes hernia or laceration repairs

DIGESTIVE SYSTEM (40490-49999)

Divided by anatomical site from mouth to anus + organs that aid digestive process

Example: Liver and gallbladder

Many bundled procedures

Endoscopy

- Diagnostic endoscopy is always bundled into a surgical endoscopy
- Code to furthest extent of procedure.

Copyright © 2005, Elsevier Inc. All rights reserved.
CPT only © 2004. *Current Procedural Terminology, 2005, Professional Edition,* American Medical Association. All rights reserved.

Endoscopy Terminology

Notes define specific terminology.

Code descriptions are specific regarding

Technique and depth of scope

Esophagoscopy: esophagus only

Esophagogastroscopy: esophagus to past diaphragm

Esophagogastroduodenoscopy: esophagus to beyond pyloric channel

Read notes preceding 45300-45387:

Proctosigmoidoscopy: Rectum and sigmoid colon (6–25 cm)

Sigmoidoscopy: Entire rectum, sigmoid colon, and may include part of descending colon (26–60 cm)

Colonoscopy: Entire colon, rectum to cecum, and may include terminal ileum (greater than 60 cm)

Laparoscopy and Endoscopy

Some subheadings have both laparoscopy (outside) and endoscopy (inside) procedures.

Example: Subheading Esophagus

- Endoscopy views inside
- Laparoscopy inserted through umbilicus, views from outside

Hemorrhoidectomy and Fistulectomy Codes (46221-46320)

Divided by

Complexity

Simple: No plastic procedure involved

Complex: Includes plastic procedure and fissurectomy

Anatomy

Subcutaneous: No muscle involvement

Submuscular: Splinter muscle

Complex fistulectomy involves excision/incision of multiple fistulas.

Hernia Codes (49491-49611)

Divided by:

1. Type of hernia

   Example: Inguinal, femoral, incisional, ventral

2. Initial or subsequent repair
3. Age of patient

Copyright © 2005, Elsevier Inc. All rights reserved.
CPT only © 2004. *Current Procedural Terminology, 2005, Professional Edition,* American Medical Association. All rights reserved.

4. Clinical presentation:

   Strangulated: Blood supply cut off

   Incarcerated: Cannot be returned to cavity (not reducible)

   Additional code is used for implantation of mesh or prosthesis.

URINARY SYSTEM (50010-53899)

Anatomical division:

- Kidney
- Ureters
- Bladder
- Urethra

Further divided by procedure:

- Incision
- Excision
- Introduction
- Repair
- Laparoscopy
- Endoscopy

Kidney Subheading (50010-50590)

Endoscopy codes are used for procedures done through a previously established stoma or incision.

Introduction Category (50390-50398)

- Catheters for drainage and injections for radiography
- Aspirations
- Insertion of guide wires
- Tube changes
- Usually reported with radiology component

Ureter Subheading (50600-50980)

Divided on type of procedure:

Incision

Excision

Introduction

Repair

Laparoscopy codes describe surgical procedures.

Bladder Subheading (51000-52700)

Includes codes for

Incision

Excision

Copyright © 2005, Elsevier Inc. All rights reserved.
CPT only © 2004. *Current Procedural Terminology, 2005, Professional Edition,* American Medical Association. All rights reserved.

Introduction

Urodynamics

Repair

Laparoscopy

Endoscopy

Cystoscopy

Urethroscopy

Cystourethroscopy

Transurethral surgery

Many bundled codes

Example: Urethral dilation is included with insertion of cystoscope.

Read all descriptions carefully.

Urodynamics (51725-51798)

- Procedures relate to motion and flow of urine.
- Used to diagnose urine flow obstructions
- Bundled: All usual, necessary instruments, equipment, supplies, and technical assistance

MALE GENITAL SYSTEM (54000-55899)

1. Penis (most codes)
2. Testes
3. Epididymis
4. Tunica Vaginalis
5. Scrotum
6. Vas Deferens
7. Spermatic Cord
8. Seminal Vesicles
9. Prostate

Biopsy Codes

Located all in anatomical subheading to which the codes refer

Example: Biopsy codes in subheadings:

- Epididymis (Excision)
  Example: 54800, needle biopsy of epididymis
- Testis (Excision)
  Example: 54500, needle biopsy of testis

Penis (54000-54450)

Incision codes (54000-54015) differ from Integumentary System codes.

- Penis incision codes for deeper structures

Copyright © 2005, Elsevier Inc. All rights reserved.
CPT only © 2004. *Current Procedural Terminology, 2005, Professional Edition*, American Medical Association. All rights reserved.

Destruction (54050-54065)

- Codes divided on:
  Extent: simple or extensive
  Method of destruction (e.g., chemical, cryosurgery)
- Extensive destruction can be by any method.

Excision (54100-54164)

- Commonly used codes for biopsy and circumcision

Introduction (54200-54250)

- Many procedures for corpora cavernosum (spongy body of penis)
  - Injection procedures for Peyronie disease (toughening of corpora cavernosum)
  - Treatments for erectile dysfunction

Repair (54300-54450)

- Many plastic repairs
- Some repair staged
  Stage indicated in code description

INTERSEX SURGERY (55970-55980)

There are only two codes within subsection.

1. Male to female
2. Female to male

Complicated procedures completed over extended period of time

Performed by physicians with extensive specialized training

FEMALE GENITAL SYSTEM (56405-58999)

Anatomical division: From vulva to ovaries

- Many bundled services

Vulva, Perineum, & Introitus (56405-56821)

Skene's gland coded with Urinary System, Incision or Excision codes

- Group of small mucous glands, lower end of urethra
  - Paraurethral duct

Incision (56405-56441)

I & D of abscess: Vulva, perineal area or Bartholin's gland

Marsupialization:

- Cyst incised
- Drained
- Edges sutured to sides to keep cyst open

Copyright © 2005, Elsevier Inc. All rights reserved.
CPT only © 2004. *Current Procedural Terminology, 2005, Professional Edition*, American Medical Association. All rights reserved.

Destruction (56501-56515)

- Lesions destroyed by variety of methods
    - Destruction = eradication, not excision. Excision is removal
- Divided by whether destruction is simple or extensive
  Complexity based on physician's judgment
  Stated in record
- Destruction has no pathology report.

Excision (56605-56740)

Biopsy includes:

1. Local anesthetic
2. Biopsy
3. Simple closure
4. Code based on number of lesions biopsied

Vulvectomy: Surgical Removal of Portion of Vulva (56620-56640)

Based on extent and size of area removed

Extent:

1. Simple: Skin and superficial subcutaneous tissues
2. Radical: Skin and deep subcutaneous tissues

Size:

1. Partial: <80% vulvar area
2. Complete: >80% vulvar area

Extent and size, indicated in operative report

Repair (56800-56810)

- Many plastic repairs
- Read notes following category.
  If repair procedure involves wound of genitalia, use Integumentary System code.

Endoscopy (56820-56821)

- By means of a colposcopy
  With or without biopsy

Vagina (57000-57425)

Codes divided based on service (e.g., incision, excision)

Introduction (57150-57180)

- Includes vaginal irrigation, insertion of devices, diaphragm, cervical caps
- Report the inserted device separately—99070 or HCPCS, such as A4261 (cervical cap)

Copyright © 2005, Elsevier Inc. All rights reserved.
CPT only © 2004. *Current Procedural Terminology, 2005, Professional Edition,* American Medical Association. All rights reserved.

Repair (57200-57335)

- For nonobstetric repairs:

  For obstetric repairs, use Maternity Care & Delivery codes.

Manipulation (57400-57415)

Dilation: Speculum inserted into vagina and enlarged using dilator

Endoscopy (57420, 57425)

- Colposcopy codes based on purpose (e.g., biopsy, diagnostic)

Cervix Uteri (57452-57820)

Cervix uteri, narrow lower end of uterus

Services include excision, manipulation, repair.

Excision (57500-57556)

Conization codes

Conization: Removal of cone of tissue from cervix

LEEP (loop electrocautery excision procedure) technology can be used for conizations.

Corpus Uteri (58100-58579)

Many complex procedures

- Often very similar wording in code descriptions
- Requires careful reading

Excision (58100-58294)

- Dilation & curettage (D & C, 58120) of uterus
  After dilation, curette scrapes uterus.
  Coded according to circumstances: obstetrical or nonobstetrical
- Do not report postpartum hemorrhage service with 58120.
  Use 59160—Maternity & Delivery code.
- Many hysterectomy codes
  Based on approach (vaginal, abdominal) and extent (uterus, fallopian tubes, etc.)
- Often secondary procedures performed with hysterectomy
- Do not code secondary, related minor procedures separately.
- Only 58110 (endometrial biopsy), 58120 (dilation and curettage), and 58145 (myomectomy, vaginal approach) are performed on an outpatient basis.

Introduction (58300-58353)

- Common procedures (e.g., insertion of an IUD)
- Report supply of device separately.
- Specialized services (e.g., artificial insemination procedures)

Copyright © 2005, Elsevier Inc. All rights reserved.
CPT only © 2004. *Current Procedural Terminology, 2005, Professional Edition*, American Medical Association. All rights reserved.

- Used to report physician component of service
- Component coding:
  Necessary with catheter procedures for hysterosonography
  Notes following codes indicate radiology guidance component codes.

Oviduct/Ovary (58600-58770)

Oviduct: Fallopian Tube

Incision category contains tubal ligations.

- When it occurs during the same hospitalization as delivery, ligation is coded separately.

Laparoscopy (58660-58679)

- Through abdominal wall
- Based on purpose of procedure (e.g., lysis, lesion removal)
- *Caution:* If only diagnostic laparoscopy:
  Do not use Female Genital System codes.
  Use 49320, Digestive System.
- Many codes can be reported separately with appropriate modifiers.
  Example: 58660 Laparoscopy, surgical; with lysis of adhesions can be coded with any of the indented codes that follow 58660 (58661, 58662, 85670)

Ovary (58800-58960)

Two categories only: Incision and Excision

Incision: Primarily for drainage of cysts and abscesses

- Divided on surgical approach

Excision: Biopsy, wedge resection, and oophorectomy

In Vitro Fertilization (58970-58999)

Specialized codes usually used by physicians trained in fertilization procedures

- Codes divided by type of procedure and method used

MATERNITY CARE & DELIVERY SUBSECTION (59000-59899)

Divided by service:

- Antepartum
- Delivery
- Postpartum
- Abortion

Gestation

Fetal gestation: Approximately 266 days (40 weeks)

EDD: Estimated Date of Delivery

- 280 days from last menstrual period (LMP)

Copyright © 2005, Elsevier Inc. All rights reserved.
CPT only © 2004. *Current Procedural Terminology, 2005, Professional Edition*, American Medical Association. All rights reserved.

Trimesters

First, LMP to Week 12

Second, Weeks 13–27

Third, Week 28–EDD

Excision (59100-59160)

Postpartum curettage: Removes remaining pieces of placenta or clotted blood (59160)

Nonobstetric curettage: 58120 (Corpus Uteri, Excision)

Introduction (59200)

Insertion of cervical dilator: Used to prepare cervix for an abortive procedure or delivery (for abortive procedures, see 59855)

Cervical ripening agents may be introduced to prepare cervix.

- Is a "separate procedure" and not reported when part of more major procedure

Repair (59300–59350)

Only for repairs during pregnancy

Episiotomy or vaginal repair by other than attending

Suture repair (cerclage) of cervix or uterus (hysterorrhaphy)

Episiotomies and use of forceps

Included in delivery

Not reported separately

Abortion Services (59812-59857)

Spontaneous: Happens naturally

Incomplete: Requires medical intervention

Missed: Fetus dies naturally during first half of pregnancy

Septic: Missed abortion with infection

Medical intervention:

- Dilation & curettage or evacuation (suction removal)
- Intraamniotic injections (saline or urea)
- Vaginal suppositories (prostaglandin)

ENDOCRINE SYSTEM SUBSECTION (60000-60699)

Nine glands in endocrine system, only four included in subsection:

1. Thyroid
2. Parathyroid
3. Thymus
4. Adrenal

Copyright © 2005, Elsevier Inc. All rights reserved.
CPT only © 2004. *Current Procedural Terminology, 2005, Professional Edition*, American Medical Association. All rights reserved.

Pituitary & Pineal: See Nervous System subsection

Pancreas: Digestive System

Ovaries and Testes: Respective genital systems

Divided into two subheadings:

Thyroid Gland

Parathyroid, Thymus, Adrenal Glands, & Carotid Body

Carotid Body:

Refers to area adjacent to carotid artery

Can be site of tumors

Thyroid Gland, Excision Category (60001-60281)

Code descriptions often refer to:

- **Partial or subtotal:** Something less than total
- **Total:** All

Thyroid 1 gland with 2 lobes

NERVOUS SYSTEM SUBSECTION (61000-64999)

Divided anatomically:

- Skull, Meninges, and Brain
- Spine and Spinal Cord
- Extracranial Nerves, Peripheral Nerves, and Autonomic Nervous System

Skull, Meninges, and Brain Subheading (61000-62258)

Categories:

- Injection, Drainage, or Aspiration
- Twist Drills, Burr Hole(s), or Trephine

Conditions that require openings into brain to:

1. Relieve pressure
2. Insert monitoring devices
3. Place tubing
4. Inject contrast material

Craniotomy or Craniotomy Category

- Removal of portion of skull, usually as operative site
- Codes divided by site and condition for which procedure is performed
- Performed only on an inpatient basis

Copyright © 2005, Elsevier Inc. All rights reserved.
CPT only © 2004. *Current Procedural Terminology, 2005, Professional Edition*, American Medical Association. All rights reserved.

Surgery at Skull Base Category

Skull base: Area at base of cranium

- Lesion removal from this area very complex

Extensive category notes

Surgery at Skull Base Terminology

- Approach procedure used to gain exposure of lesion
- Definitive procedure is what is done to lesion
- Repair/reconstruction procedure reported separately only if extensive repair

Surgery of Skull Base (61580-61616)

- Approach procedure and definitive procedure coded separately
  Example: Removal of an intradural lesion using middle cranial fossa approach
  - 61590 approach procedure, middle cranial fossa and
  - 61608 definitive procedure of intradural resection of lesion
- Most of these procedures are performed only on an inpatient basis.

Cerebrospinal Fluid (CSF) Shunt Category (62180-62258)

- Used to drain fluid
- Codes describe placement of:
  1. Devices
  2. Repair
  3. Replacement
  4. Removal of shunting devices
- Most performed only on an inpatient basis

Spine and Spinal Cord Subheading (62263-63746)

Codes divided on condition and approach

Often used are:

- Unilateral or bilateral procedures (–50)
- Radiologic supervision and fluoroscopic guidance are coded separately.

Includes codes for

- Spinal Anesthetic injections 62310–62319
- Intrathecal catheter placement/implantation 62350–62355

Introduction/Injection of Anesthetic Agent, Diagnostic or Therapeutic Category (64400-64530)

- Includes codes for
  - Nerve blocks 64400-64450
  - Facet joint injections 64470-64476
  - Epidural Injections 64479-64484

Copyright © 2005, Elsevier Inc. All rights reserved.
CPT only © 2004. *Current Procedural Terminology, 2005, Professional Edition,* American Medical Association. All rights reserved.

- Used to provide pain relief
- As compared to an epidural catheter placement used for anesthetic purposes

EYE AND OCULAR ADNEXA SUBSECTION (65091-68899)

Terminology extremely important

- Code descriptions often vary only slightly

Codes divided anatomically, e.g.:

- Eyeball
- Conjunctiva
- Anterior segment
- Posterior segment
- Ocular adnexa

Some codes specifically for patients previously operated on

Much bundling:

Example: Subheading Posterior Segment, Prophylaxis category notes indicate:

- "The following descriptors intended to include (67141–67145) sessions in defined treatment period."

Removal Cataract Category (66830-66990)

Cataract excision types

Intracapsular extraction

Extracapsular extraction

Pars plana

Phacofragmentation technique

Phacoemulsification technique

The following are included in cataract removal and are not reported separately:

Lateral canthotomy

Iridectomy

Iridotomy

Anterior capsulotomy

Posterior capsulotomy

Use of viscoelastic agents

Enzymatic zonulysis

Pharmacologic agents

Subconjunctival injections

AUDITORY SYSTEM SUBSECTION (69000-69990)

Codes divided on:

1. External Ear
2. Middle Ear
3. Internal Ear

Copyright © 2005, Elsevier Inc. All rights reserved.
CPT only © 2004. *Current Procedural Terminology, 2005, Professional Edition*, American Medical Association. All rights reserved.

Further divisions on procedure:

1. Incision
2. Excision
3. Removal
4. Repair

Operating Microscope (+69990)

Employed with procedures using microsurgical techniques

Code in addition to primary procedure performed.

Do not report separately when primary procedure description includes microsurgical techniques.

Example: 15758, Free fascial flap with microvascular anastomosis

Note that following 15758 is the statement:

"(Do not report code 69990 in addition to code 15758)" indicating to the coder not to report the use of operating microscope separately.

HCPCS CODING

Developed by Centers for Medicare & Medicaid Services, CMS
- Formerly HCFA

HCPCS developed in 1983
CPT did not contain all codes necessary for Medicare services reporting.

One of Two Levels of Codes

1. Level I, CPT
2. Level II, HCPCS, also known as national codes

Phased out Level III, Local Codes

Developed by Medicare carriers for use at local level

Varied by locale

Discontinued October 2002
- Some codes incorporated into HCPCS

Level II, National Codes

Codes for wide variety providers
- Physicians
- Dentists
- Orthodontists

Codes for wide variety services
- Specific drugs
- Durable medical equipment (DME)
- Ambulance services

Copyright © 2005, Elsevier Inc. All rights reserved.
CPT only © 2004. *Current Procedural Terminology, 2005, Professional Edition*, American Medical Association. All rights reserved.

Format

Begins with letter, followed by four digits

Example: E0608, apnea monitor

Each letter represents group codes.

Example: "J" codes used to report drugs

Temporary Codes

Certain letters indicate temporary codes.

Example: K0006, heavy-duty wheelchair
- ◦ K codes are temporary codes.

HCPCS Index

Directs coder to specific codes

Do not code directly from index.

Reference main portion of text before assigning code.

Alphabetical order

Ambulance Modifiers

Origin and destination used in combination:
- First letter origin
- Second letter destination

Example:
- -R = Residence
- -H = Hospital
- -RH origin (first letter) residence and destination (second letter) hospital

PET Modifiers

Positron Emission Tomography: Noninvasive Imaging Procedure

Assesses metabolic organ activity

PET scan modifiers were deleted in 2004.

Table of Drugs

Listed by generic name, not brand name

Often used when reporting immunizations or injections

ICD-9-CM

On the CCS examination, you will be assigning ICD-9-CM codes to both inpatient and outpatient (ASC) services using Volume 1-3.

Copyright © 2005, Elsevier Inc. All rights reserved.
CPT only © 2004. *Current Procedural Terminology, 2005, Professional Edition*, American Medical Association. All rights reserved.

Introduction

Morbidity (illness)

Mortality (death)

CM = clinical modification

Provides continuity of data

WHO's ICD-9 used globally

1977: U.S. develops ICD-9 version
- Has more code subsets
- Data collapse back to ICD-9 for uniformity of data.

Medicare

- Medicare Catastrophic Act of 1988
  Required use of ICD-9-CM codes for outpatient claims
- Act abolished but codes still used

Uses of ICD-9-CM

- Facilitate payment of health services
- Evaluate patients' use of health services
- Fiscal entities track health-care costs.
- Research
  Health-care quality
  Future needs
  Newer cancer center built if patient use warrants
- Predict health-care trends
- Plan for future health-care needs

ICD-9-CM on Insurance Forms

- Diagnoses establish medical necessity.
- Services and diagnoses must correlate.
- CMS-1450 (UB92) field location placement
  67 Principal Diagnosis
  68–75 Additional or secondary diagnoses
  76–77 Admitting Diagnosis and External cause
  80–81 ICD-9-CM procedural codes **(Figure 3-8)**

Ethics
Documentation must support diagnosis and service/procedure
Example:
Services provided
Diagnosis justifies services.
If in doubt, check it out; don't make assumptions.
Your Job: Translate documentation into ICD-9-CM codes.

Copyright © 2005, Elsevier Inc. All rights reserved.
CPT only © 2004. *Current Procedural Terminology, 2005, Professional Edition*, American Medical Association. All rights reserved.

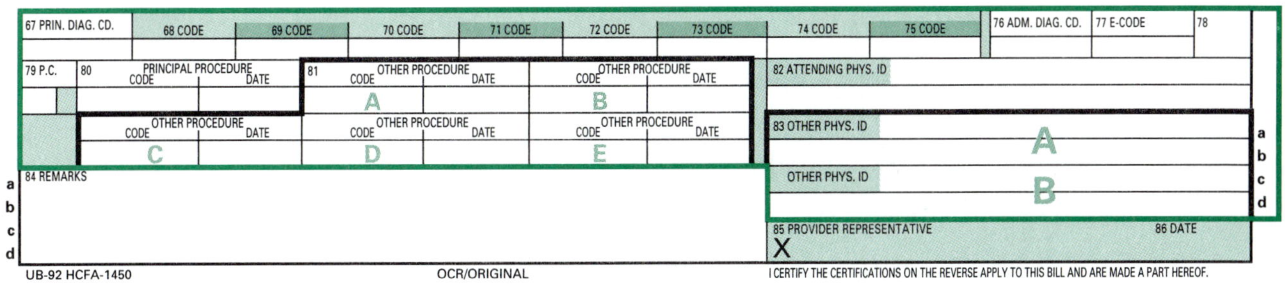
67 PRIN. DIAG. CD. | 68 CODE | 69 CODE | 70 CODE | 71 CODE | 72 CODE | 73 CODE | 74 CODE | 75 CODE | 76 ADM. DIAG. CD. | 77 E-CODE | 78
79 P.C. | 80 PRINCIPAL PROCEDURE CODE DATE | 81 OTHER PROCEDURE CODE DATE A | OTHER PROCEDURE CODE DATE B | 82 ATTENDING PHYS. ID
OTHER PROCEDURE CODE DATE C | OTHER PROCEDURE CODE DATE D | OTHER PROCEDURE CODE DATE E | 83 OTHER PHYS. ID A
84 REMARKS a b c d | OTHER PHYS. ID B a b c d
85 PROVIDER REPRESENTATIVE X | 86 DATE
UB-92 HCFA-1450 OCR/ORIGINAL I CERTIFY THE CERTIFICATIONS ON THE REVERSE APPLY TO THIS BILL AND ARE MADE A PART HEREOF.

Figure 3-8 Blocks 67–81 of CMS 1450 UB92. *(Courtesy U.S. Department of Health and Human Services, Centers for Medicare and Medicaid Services.)*

Format of ICD-9-CM

Volume 1: Diseases, Tabular List

Volume 2: Diseases, Alphabetic Index

Volume 3: Procedures, Tabular and Alphabetic Index

Volume 1, Diseases, Tabular List

- Contains code numbers
- 001.0-999.9 diagnosis codes describe condition.
- V & E codes = supplemental information

Volume 2, Diseases, Alphabetic Index

- Appears first in book
- Refers coder to code numbers in Volume 1
- Never code directly from Index!

Volume 3, Procedures, Tabular List and Alphabetic Index

- Index and Tabular List used for procedures and therapies
- Inpatient settings
- Procedures and therapies

ICD-9-CM Conventions

Symbols, abbreviations, punctuation, and notations

NEC: Not elsewhere classifiable

- No more specific code exists

NOS: Not otherwise specified

- Unspecified in documentation

[ ] BRACKETS

Enclose synonyms, alternative wording, or explanatory phrases

Helpful, additional information

Can affect code

Found only in Tabular List (001.0-999.9)

Copyright © 2005, Elsevier Inc. All rights reserved.
CPT only © 2004. *Current Procedural Terminology, 2005, Professional Edition*, American Medical Association. All rights reserved.

( ) PARENTHESES

Contain nonessential modifiers

- Take them or leave them

Found in Tabular List and Index

Do not affect code

COLON & BRACE

: **Colon:** Tabular List, completes statement with one or more modifiers

} **Brace:** Tabular List, modifying statements to left of brace

LOZENGE, SECTION MARK, & BOLD TYPE

[ ] **Lozenge:** Can indicate codes unique to ICD-9-CM

§ **Section:** Can be footnote indicator

Bold type: Codes and code titles in Tabular List, Volume 1

ITALICIZED TYPE

All excludes notes

Codes NOT used as principal diagnosis

SLANTED BRACKETS *[ ]*

Enclose manifestations of underlying condition

Code underlying condition first

INCLUDES, EXCLUDES, USE ADDITIONAL CODE

Includes notes: In chapter, section, or category

Excludes notes: Conditions are coded elsewhere.

Use additional code: Assignment of other code(s) is necessary.

AND/WITH

And: Means and/or

With: One condition with (in addition to) another condition

CODE, IF APPLICABLE, ANY CAUSAL CONDITION FIRST:

May be principal diagnosis if no causal condition applicable or known

Example: 707.10, Ulcer of lower limb, except decubitus; states:

- Chronic venous hypertension with ulcer (459.31)

If ulcer caused by chronic venous hypertension:

First: 459.31 chronic venous hypertension

Second: 707.10 ulcer of lower limb

Copyright © 2005, Elsevier Inc. All rights reserved.
CPT only © 2004. *Current Procedural Terminology, 2005, Professional Edition*, American Medical Association. All rights reserved.

Volume 2, Alphabetic Index

Nonessential modifiers: have no effect on code selection

Enclosed in parentheses

Clarify diagnosis

Example: Ileus (adynamic) (bowel) . . .

Terms

Main terms (bold typeface)

- Subterms
- Indented two spaces to right
- Not bold

Cross References

- Directs you: *See, see* also
- "*see*" directs you to specific term.
  Example: Panotitis—"*see*" Otitis media
- "*see* also" directs you to another term for more information.
  Example: Perivaginitis (*see* also Vesiculitis)
- "*see* category" Volume 1, Tabular List, specific information about use of code.
  Esxample: Mesencephalitis (*see* also Encephalitis) 323.9; late effect—*see* category 326

Notes

- Define terms
- Give further coding instructions
  Example: Index: "Melanoma"
  NOTE: "Except where otherwise indicated . . ."
- Mandatory fifth digits also appear as notes (one reason never to code from Index).

Eponyms

- Disease or syndromes named for person
  Example: Arnold-Chiari (see also Spina bifida)

Etiology and Manifestation of Disease

Etiology = cause of disease

Manifestation = symptom

Combination codes = etiology and manifestation in one code

Neoplasm

- In Volume 2, Index, locate Neoplasm Table under "Ns"

Copyright © 2005, Elsevier Inc. All rights reserved.
CPT only © 2004. *Current Procedural Terminology, 2005, Professional Edition,* American Medical Association. All rights reserved.

Sections

Section 1, Index to Diseases

Section 2, Table of Drugs and Chemicals

Section 3, Index to External Causes of Injuries and Poisonings (E Codes)

Section 1, Index to Diseases

- Largest part of Volume 2—Index
- First step in coding, locate main term in Index
- Subterms indented two spaces to right
- May have more than one subterm

Section 2, Table of Drugs and Chemicals

- Drug name placed alphabetically on left under heading "Substance" **(Figure 3-9)**
- First column: "Poisoning" code for substance involved
- E codes identify how poisoning occurred.

Headings

Accident: Unintentional

Therapeutic: Correct dosage, correctly administered with adverse effects **(This is the only E code reported on the CCS examination)**

Suicide attempt: Self-inflicted

Assault: Intentionally inflicted by another person

Undetermined: Unknown cause

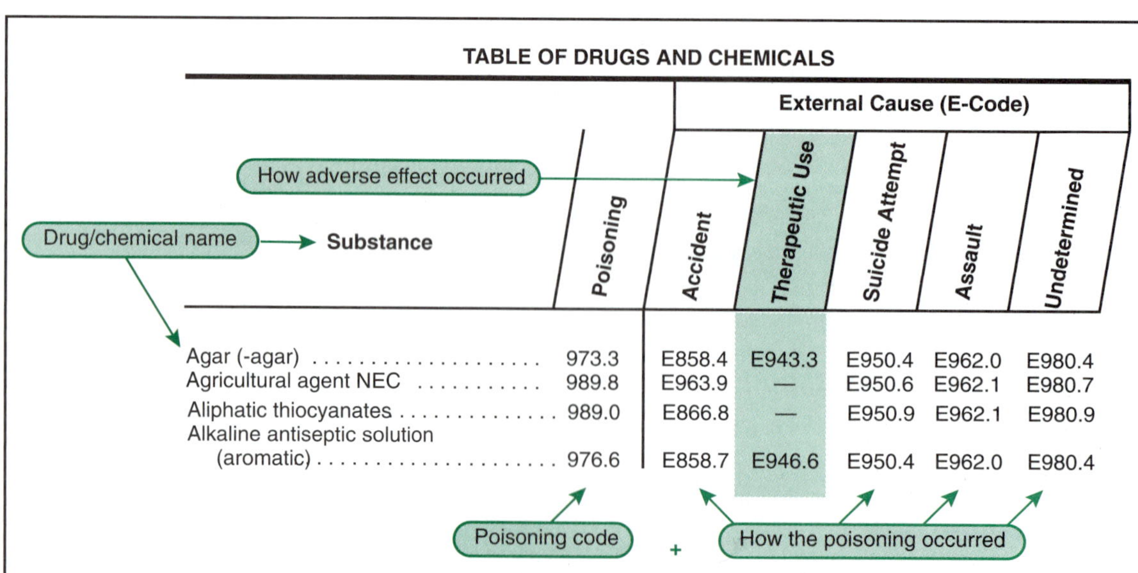

Figure 3-9 Section 2, Table of Drugs and Chemicals. *(From International Classification of Diseases, 9th Revision. U.S. Department of Health and Human Services, Public Health Service, Center for Medicare and Medicaid Services.)*

Copyright © 2005, Elsevier Inc. All rights reserved.
CPT only © 2004. *Current Procedural Terminology, 2005, Professional Edition,* American Medical Association. All rights reserved.

Section 3, E Codes

- Alphabetic Index to External Causes of Injuries and Poisonings
- Provides additional information
- Never principal (inpatient) or primary (outpatient) diagnosis
- Separate Index to External Causes
  Alphabetical, main terms in bold
  Subterms indented two spaces to right under main term

A word of caution about the alphabetic index

- Some words in Index do not appear in Tabular—saves space.
- Exact word may not be in code Tabular description.
  - But found in Alphabetic Index
  - That is why you must locate term in Index and then locate Tabular.

Volume 1, Tabular List

Two Major Divisions:

1. Classification of Diseases and Injuries (codes 001.0–999.9)
2. Supplementary Classification (V codes and E codes)

Classification of Diseases and Injuries

- Main portion of ICD-9-CM
- Codes from 001.0–999.9
- Most chapters are body systems.

  Example:

  Digestive System
  Respiratory System

Divisions of Classification of Diseases and Injuries

Chapters: 1 through 17

Section: A group of related conditions

Category: Represents single disease/condition

Subcategory: More specific

Subclassification: Most specific

Remember
Assign to highest level of specificity, based on documentation.
If four-digit code exists, do not report three-digit code.
If five-digit code exists, do not report four-digit code.

Copyright © 2005, Elsevier Inc. All rights reserved.
CPT only © 2004. *Current Procedural Terminology, 2005, Professional Edition,* American Medical Association. All rights reserved.

USING ICD-9-CM

Guidelines developed by Cooperating Parties

- AHA
- AHIMA
- CMS
- NCHS

General Guidelines

Appendix A of this text contains Official Guidelines for Coding and Reporting.

Inpatient coders use Sections I–III.

Outpatient coders primarily use Section I and IV; however

Diagnostic Coding and Reporting Guidelines do NOT cover all situations.

- Outpatient coders also use many Section II and III guidelines.

Guidelines for following labels

"(I)" indicates inpatient setting guidelines.

"(O)" indicates outpatient setting guidelines.

"(I/O)" guidelines apply to both inpatient and outpatient setting.

Steps to Diagnosis Coding (I/O)

Identify MAIN term(s) in diagnosis.

Locate MAIN term(s) in Index.

Review subterms.

Follow cross-reference instructions (e.g., *see, see also*).

Verify code(s) in Tabular.

Remember (I/O)

Read Tabular notes.

Code to highest specificity.

NEVER CODE FROM INDEX!

Guideline Section I, B, 3, Level of Specificity in Coding (I/O)

Assign diagnosis to highest level of specificity.

Do NOT use three-digit code if there is fourth.

Do NOT use four-digit code if there is fifth.

Section I, A, 2, Other (NEC) and Unspecified (NOS) (I/O)

NEC = Not elsewhere classifiable

More specific code does NOT exist.

Copyright © 2005, Elsevier Inc. All rights reserved.
CPT only © 2004. *Current Procedural Terminology, 2005, Professional Edition,* American Medical Association. All rights reserved.

NOS = Not otherwise specified (means "unspecified")

Available information NOT specific enough

Use ONLY if more specific code NOT available.

Section I, 10B and 103, Acute and Chronic Conditions (I/O)

Exists alone or together

May be separate or combo codes

If two codes, code acute first

Example: Acute and chronic pancreatitis

When two separate codes exist, code:

Acute cystitis 595.0

Chronic cystitis 595.2

Combination code: Both acute and chronic condition

Diarrhea (acute) (chronic) 787.91

Acute and subacute bacterial endocarditis 421.0

Otitis acute and subacute 382.9

Section I, 11A, Combination Code (I/O)

Always use combination code if one exists.

Example: Encephalomyelitis (diagnosis) due to rubella (manifestation), 056.01

Section I, B, 9, Multiple Diagnoses Coding (I/O)

Etiology (cause)

Manifestation (symptom)

Slanted brackets [ ]

Example: Retinopathy, diabetic 250.5 [362.01]

Must check Tabular notes to assign correct fifth digit for diabetes

Tabular: 362.0, Diabetic retinopathy, instructs to "Code first diabetes 250.5"

Section II, H, Uncertain Conditions (I)

If diagnosis at time of discharge states:

probable,

suspected,

likely,

questionable,

possible,

rule out

Code condition as if condition existed until proven otherwise.

Example: "Cough and fever, probably pneumonia" (I/O)

Copyright © 2005, Elsevier Inc. All rights reserved.
CPT only © 2004. *Current Procedural Terminology, 2005, Professional Edition*, American Medical Association. All rights reserved.

Inpatient: Code pneumonia; do NOT code cough and fever.

Outpatient: Code cough and fever; do NOT code pneumonia.

Section I, B, Impending or Threatened Condition (I)

Code any condition described at time of discharge as impending or threatened.

Did occur: Code as confirmed

Did NOT occur: Code as impending or threatened (MAIN terms)

Selection of Principal Diagnosis (I)

Condition established after study (tests)

Responsible for patient admission

Selection of Primary Diagnosis (O)

Condition for encounter

Documented

Responsible for services provided

Also list co-existing conditions.

Diagnosis and Services (I/O)

Diagnosis and procedure MUST correlate.

Medical necessity established

No correlation = no reimbursement

Section II, A, Symptoms, Signs, and Ill-Defined Conditions (I)

Inpatient coders do NOT use when definitive diagnosis has been established

Can be the provisional diagnosis if no more specific diagnosis available

Section I, C17, Codes in Brackets (I/O)

Never sequence as principal diagnosis.

Always sequence in order listed.

Index lists: Diabetes, gangrene 250.7 *[785.4]*

785.4 = gangrene

Tabular: 785.4 indicates "Code first any associated underlying condition: diabetes (250.7X). . . . "

Code first diabetes, then gangrene

250.7X = diabetes (X = fifth digit)

785.4 = gangrene

Copyright © 2005, Elsevier Inc. All rights reserved.
CPT only © 2004. *Current Procedural Terminology, 2005, Professional Edition*, American Medical Association. All rights reserved.

Section II, B, Two or More Interrelated Conditions (I/O)

When two or more interrelated conditions exist and either could be principal diagnosis, either sequenced first

Example: Patient with mitral valve stenosis and coronary artery disease (two interrelated conditions)

Either can be principal diagnosis and sequenced first.

Resource intensiveness affects choice.

Section II, C, Two or More Equal Diagnoses (I/O)

Either can be sequenced first

Example: Diagnosis of viral gastroenteritis and dehydration

Section II, D, Comparative or Contrasting Conditions (I)

"Either/or" diagnoses coded as confirmed

If determination can NOT be made, either can be sequenced first.

Pneumonia or lung cancer

Lung cancer or pneumonia

Section II, E, Symptom(s) Followed by Contrasting/Comparative Diagnosis (I)

Symptom code sequenced first

Then other diagnoses

Section I, C18, Observation and Eval. for Suspected Conditions Not Found (I/O)

V71.0–V71.9

Assigned as principal diagnosis for:

1. Admissions for evaluation
2. Following an accident that would ordinarily result in health problem, BUT there is none

Example: Car accident, driver hits head, no apparent injury, admit to R/O head trauma

Section II, F, Original Treatment Plan Not Carried Out (I)

Principal diagnosis becomes

Condition that after study was reason for admission

Treatment does NOT have to be carried out for condition.

Example: Patient admitted for elective surgery, develops pneumonia, surgery canceled

Code reason for surgery first.

Code "Surgical or other procedure NOT carried out because of contraindication" (V64.1).

Also code pneumonia.

Copyright © 2005, Elsevier Inc. All rights reserved.
CPT only © 2004. *Current Procedural Terminology, 2005, Professional Edition*, American Medical Association. All rights reserved.

V Codes

Located after 999.9 in Tabular

Two digits before decimal (e.g., V10.1)

Index for V codes Alphabetic Index to Diseases

Main terms: Contraception, counseling, dialysis, status, examination

Uses of V Codes (I/O)

Not sick BUT receives health care (e.g., vaccination)

Services for known disease/injury (e.g., chemotherapy)

A circumstance/problem that influences patient's health BUT NOT current illness/injury

Example: Organ transplant status

Example: Birth status and outcome of delivery (newborn)

Special Note About "History of" (I/O)

Index to Disease, MAIN term "History"

Entries between "family" and "visual loss V19.0" = "family history of"

Entries before "family" and after "visual loss V19.0" = "personal history of"

Section I, 12, Late Effects (I/O)

Late effect residual of (remaining from) previous illness/injury

e.g., Burn that leaves scar

Residual coded first (scar)

Cause (burn) coded second

ICD-9-CM, Chapter 1 (I/O)

Infectious and Parasitic Diseases

Divided based on etiology (cause of disease)

Many combination codes

Multiple Codes (I/O)

Sequencing must be considered.

UTI due to *Escherichia coli*

599.0 (UTI) etiology

041.4 (*E. coli*) organism

Section I, C1, Human Immunodeficiency Virus (I/O)

Code HIV or HIV-related illness ONLY if stated as confirmed in diagnostic statement

042 HIV or HIV-related illness

Copyright © 2005, Elsevier Inc. All rights reserved.
CPT only © 2004. *Current Procedural Terminology, 2005, Professional Edition,* American Medical Association. All rights reserved.

V08 Asymptomatic HIV or HIV-related illness

795.71 Nonspecific HIV and infants with inconclusive HIV tests

Section I, C1, Previously Diagnosed HIV-Related Illness (I/O)

Code prior diagnosis HIV-related disease 042 (HIV)

NEVER assign these patients to:

1. V08 (asymptomatic) or
2. 795.71 (nonspecific serologic evidence of HIV)

Section I, C1, HIV Sequencing (I)

If admitted for HIV-related illness (e.g., pneumonia)

Code 042 (HIV)

Followed by current illness (pneumonia)

If admitted for other than HIV-related illness

Code reason for admittance

Then 042 (HIV)

Section I, C1, HIV Sequencing (O)

Sequence first reason most responsible for encounter

Followed by secondary diagnosis that affects encounter or patient care

Section I, C18, A, HIV and Pregnancy (I/O)

This is an exception to HIV sequencing.

During pregnancy, childbirth, or puerperium, code:

647.8X (Other specified infections and parasitic diseases),

Followed by 042 (HIV)

Asymptomatic HIV during pregnancy, childbirth, or puerperium

647.8X (Other specified infections and parasitic diseases) and

V08 (Asymptomatic HIV infection status)

Section I, C1, Inconclusive Laboratory Test for HIV (I/O)

795.71 (Inconclusive serologic test for HIV)

Section I, C1, HIV Screening (I/O)

Code V73.89 (Screening for other specified viral disease)

Patient in high-risk group for HIV

V69.8 (Other problems related to lifestyle)

Patients returning for HIV screening results = V65.44 (HIV counseling)

Copyright © 2005, Elsevier Inc. All rights reserved.
CPT only © 2004. *Current Procedural Terminology, 2005, Professional Edition*, American Medical Association. All rights reserved.

Caution (I/O)

Incorrectly applying these HIV coding rules can cause patient hardship.

Insurance claims for patients with HIV usually need patient's written agreement to disclosure.

Septicemia and Septic Shock (I)

1. Code septicemia.
2. Use additional code for systemic inflammatory response syndrome if sepsis develops.
3. If applicable, code organ dysfunction codes.
4. Septic shock second

Sepsis and septic shock associated with OB codes:

Also use code 630–633, Ectopic and Molar Pregnancy

ICD-9-CM, Chapter 2, Neoplasms (I/O)

Two steps for coding neoplasms:

1. Index: Locate histologic type of neoplasm (e.g., sarcoma, melanoma).

   Review all instructions.
2. Locate code identified (usually in Neoplasm Table in Index) by body site.

Coded as primary site unless specified as secondary site (metastasis)

Bone	Meninges	Brain
Peritoneum	Diaphragm	Pleura
Heart	Retroperitoneum	Liver
Lymph nodes	Spinal cord	Mediastinum

Unknown status of neoplasm is always reported with 199.1.

Types of neoplasm are associated with morphology behavior codes (M-codes).

Section I, C2, Neoplasms

Treatment directed at malignancy: Neoplasm is principal diagnosis.

Except for chemotherapy or radiotherapy:

1. Therapy (treatment) listed first
2. Neoplasm listed second

Chemotherapy: V58.1

Radiotherapy: V58.0

Section I, C2, Neoplasms (I/O)

Surgical removal of neoplasm and subsequent chemotherapy or radiotherapy

Code malignancy as principal diagnosis.

Copyright © 2005, Elsevier Inc. All rights reserved.
CPT only © 2004. *Current Procedural Terminology, 2005, Professional Edition*, American Medical Association. All

Surgery to determine extent of malignancy

Code malignancy as principal diagnosis.

Section I, C2, Neoplasms (I/O)

V10, "Personal history of malignant neoplasm" if:

1. Neoplasm was previously destroyed
2. No longer being treated

If patient receives treatment for secondary neoplasm (metastasis):

Secondary neoplasm is principal diagnosis.

Even though primary is known

Section I, C2, Neoplasms (I)

Admission for symptoms of primary or secondary neoplasm

Malignancy principal diagnosis

Do NOT code symptoms or signs.

Section I, C2, Neoplasm (I/O)

Patient treated for anemia or dehydration due to neoplasm or therapy

Code:

1. Anemia or dehydration
2. Neoplasm
3. E-code for antineoplasm drug adverse effect

Patient admitted to repair complication of surgery for an intestinal malignancy

Complication principal diagnosis

Complication reason for encounter

Malignancy secondary diagnosis

V Codes and Neoplasms (I/O)

Patient receiving chemotherapy or radiotherapy post-op removal of neoplasm

Code:

1. Therapy
2. Active neoplasm

Do NOT report H/O (history of) neoplasm.

ICD-9-CM, Chapter 3 (I/O)

Endocrine, Nutritional, and Metabolic Diseases and Immunity Disorders

Copyright © 2005, Elsevier Inc. All rights reserved.
CPT only © 2004. *Current Procedural Terminology, 2005, Professional Edition*, American Medical Association. All rights reserved.

Disorders of Other Endocrine Glands (I/O)

Diabetes Mellitus 250 coded frequently

Often requires two codes

Example:

Diabetic iritis 250.5X for diabetes (etiology)

[364.42] for iritis (manifestation)

Fifth digit indicates type of diabetes.

0 = Type II or unspecified controlled

1 = Type I (juvenile) controlled

2 = Type II or unspecified uncontrolled

3 = Type I (juvenile) uncontrolled

Adult or juvenile

Type II (noninsulin-dependent)

Type I (insulin-dependent)

Other Metabolic and Immunity Disorders Section (I/O)

Disorders such as gout and dehydration

Disorders often have many names.

242.0X Toxic diffuse goiter also known as:

- Basedow's disease
- Graves' disease
- Primary thyroid hyperplasia

ICD-9-CM: Chapter 4 (I/O)

Diseases of Blood and Blood-Forming Organs

Short chapter with 10 sections

Includes anemia, blood disorders, coagulation defects

Often used code: anemia

Many different types of anemia:

- Hereditary hemolytic
- Iron deficiency
- Acquired hemolytic

Acute and/or chronic condition

Must be documented by a physician

Multiple coding often necessary

Identify underlying disease condition.

Copyright © 2005, Elsevier Inc. All rights reserved.
CPT only © 2004. *Current Procedural Terminology, 2005, Professional Edition*, American Medical Association. All rights reserved.

ICD-9-CM, Chapter 5, Mental Disorders (I/O)

Includes codes for

- Personality disorders
- Stress disorders
- Neuroses
- Psychoses
- Sexual dysfunction, etc.

Fifth digit = status of episode

Example: 304, Drug dependence has following fifth digits:

0: Unspecified (episode)

1: Continuous

2: Episodic

3: In remission

ICD-9-CM, Chapter 6 (I/O)

Diseases of Nervous System and Sense Organs

Central Nervous System

Peripheral Nervous System

Disorders of Eye

Diseases of Ear

ICD-9-CM, Chapter 7—Diseases of Circulatory System (I/O)

Three types of hypertension:

1. Malignant accelerated, severe, poor prognosis
2. Benign continuous, mild controllable
3. Unspecified NOT indicated as either malignant or benign

Section I, C7, Hypertension, Essential, or NOS (I/O)

Assign hypertension (arterial, essential, primary, systemic, NOS) to 401.

Fourth digit to indicate type

Section I, C7, Hypertension with Heart Disease (I/O)

402 Category

Certain heart conditions when stated "due to hypertension" or implied ("hypertensive")

Add fourth digit for type.

Use additional code to specify type of heart failure.

Copyright © 2005, Elsevier Inc. All rights reserved.
CPT only © 2004. *Current Procedural Terminology, 2005, Professional Edition*, American Medical Association. All rights reserved.

Section I, C7, Hypertensive Renal Disease with Chronic Renal Failure (I/O)

Cause-and-effect relationship assumed in chronic renal failure with hypertension

Category 403, Hypertensive renal disease, used when following present:

- Chronic renal failure (585)
- Renal failure, unspecified (586)
- Renal sclerosis, unspecified (587)

Section I, C7, Hypertensive Heart and Renal Disease (I/O)

Assign 404 when both hypertensive renal disease and hypertensive heart disease are stated.

Assume cause-and-effect relationship.

Assign fifth digit for mention of renal and/or congestive heart failure.

- Use additional code to specify type of heart failure.

Section I, C7, Hypertensive Cerebrovascular Disease (I/O)

Code:

- Cerebrovascular disease (430–438)
- Type of hypertension (401–405)

Section I, C7, Hypertensive Retinopathy (I/O)

Code:

- Hypertensive retinopathy
- Type of hypertension (401–405)

Section I, C7, Hypertension, Secondary (I/O)

Hypertension caused by an underlying condition

Code:

1. Underlying condition
2. Type of hypertension (401–405)

Section I, C7, Hypertension, Transient (I/O)

Transient hypertension: Temporary elevation of BP

DO NOT assign 401–405 Hypertensive Disease

- Hypertension diagnosis NOT established
  - Use:
    - 796.2, Elevated blood pressure
    - 642.3X, Transient hypertension of pregnancy

Copyright © 2005, Elsevier Inc. All rights reserved.
CPT only © 2004. *Current Procedural Terminology, 2005, Professional Edition*, American Medical Association. All rights reserved.

Section I, C7, Hypertension, Controlled (I/O)

Hypertension controlled by therapy

Assign code from 401–405

Section I, C7, Hypertension, Uncontrolled (I/O)

Untreated hypertension

Uncontrolled hypertension

Documentation must state malignant hypertension for use of 404 code.

Assign code from 401–405.

Section I, C7, Elevated Blood Pressure (I/O)

Elevated blood pressure coded 796.2

Elevated BP reading without hypertension is diagnosis.

Hypertension NOT stated, NOT coded to 401

Chapter 8, Diseases of Respiratory System (I/O)

Watch for "Use additional code to identify infectious organism."

Some codes indicate specific organism and do not need an additional code.

Respiratory Failure Sequencing

If the respiratory failure is due to an acute condition (such as MI) or acute exacerbation of a chronic condition (such as COPD), sequence the acute condition first

Example: MI (acute condition) and respiratory failure

Sequence MI first and respiratory failure second.

If the respiratory failure (acute condition) is due to a chronic nonrespiratory condition (such as myasthenia gravis), sequence the respiratory failure first.

Example: Acute respiratory failure (acute) and myasthenia gravis (chronic)

Sequence acute respiratory failure first and myasthenia gravis second.

Acute Respiratory Infection Section (I/O)

Frequently used codes, such as:

- Common cold
- Sore throat
- Acute tonsillitis
- Bronchitis
- Atelectasis

Not coded separately with a respiratory condition

Copyright © 2005, Elsevier Inc. All rights reserved.
CPT only © 2004. *Current Procedural Terminology, 2005, Professional Edition*, American Medical Association. All rights reserved.

Chapter 9 (I/O)

Diseases of Digestive System

Mouth to anus and accessory organs such as:

Extensive subcategories,

574 Cholelithiasis (10 subcategories)

Each has fifth digit subclassification.

Chapter 10 (I/O)

Diseases of Genitourinary System

Commonly used codes

- Urinary tract infection (599.0)
- Inflammation of prostate (601)
- Disorders of menstruation (625–627)

Chapter 11, Complications of Pregnancy, Childbirth, and Puerperium (I/O)

Extensive multiple coding with many fifth digit assignments and notes

Admission for pregnancy, complication

Obstetric complication = primary diagnosis

Codes 640–676.9 share same fifth digit subclassification

Denotes current episode of care

0 Unspecified as to episode of care or not applicable

1 Delivered, with or without mention of antepartum condition

2 Delivered, with mention of postpartum complication

3 Antepartum condition or complication

4 Postpartum condition or complication

Section I, C11, General Rules (I/O)

Not all encounters are pregnancy related.

Example: Pregnant woman, broken ankle; report:

1. Broken ankle
2. V22.2 Pregnant state incidental

Section I, C11, Complications of Pregnancy, Childbirth, and Puerperium (I/O)

Chapter 11 codes

Used on mother's medical record

Not on newborn medical record

Mother's record

Outcome of delivery code (V27.0-V27-9) when delivered

Copyright © 2005, Elsevier Inc. All rights reserved.
CPT only © 2004. *Current Procedural Terminology, 2005, Professional Edition*, American Medical Association. All rights reserved.

Section I, C11: Selection of Principal Diagnosis—Obstetric (I)

No delivery: Principal diagnosis = principal complication

If more than one complication, sequence any first

Section I, C11, Selection of Primary Diagnosis (O)

Routine prenatal visits no complications:

V22.0, Supervision, normal first pregnancy or

V22.1, Supervision, other normal pregnancy

Prenatal outpatient visits for high-risk pregnancies:

V23, Supervision of high-risk pregnancy

Section I, C11, Fifth Digit (I/O)

All categories EXCEPT 650 (Normal delivery)

Watch for

- Onset of delivery before 37 weeks gestation (644.2X)
- Post-term pregnancy 40–42 weeks gestation (645.1)
- Prolonged pregnancy beyond 42 weeks gestation (645.2)

Requires fifth digit for:

- Antepartum
- Postpartum

If delivery has occurred

Section I, C11, Fifth Digit (I/O)

Appropriate fifth digit listed under each code

640.0, Threatened abortion,

0: Unspecified episode

1: Delivered with or without complication

3: Antepartum condition or complication

Section I, C11, Normal Delivery, 650 (I)

Normal delivery includes

- Vaginal delivery
- Minimal or no assistance
- With or without episiotomy
- No fetal manipulation or instrumentation
- Full-term, single, liveborn infant

No complications, principal diagnosis = 650

With complications = NOT 650

Copyright © 2005, Elsevier Inc. All rights reserved.
CPT only © 2004. *Current Procedural Terminology, 2005, Professional Edition*, American Medical Association. All rights reserved.

V27.0 (Single liveborn)

Only outcome for 650 (Normal Delivery)

Section I, C11, Delivery Procedure Codes (I)

If delivered prior to admission

- In ambulance
- At home
- In ED

DO NOT CODE delivery

Code any postpartum repairs

Section I, C11, Postpartum Period (I/O)

After delivery and continues for 6 weeks

Section I, C11, Abortions (I/O)

No identifiable fetus

500 grams or less

Less than 22 weeks gestation

Codes 634–637 require fifth digits:

0: Unspecified

1: Incomplete (POC, product of conception) NOT expelled

May retain part or all of placenta or fetus

2: Complete, all (POC) expelled prior to care

Section I, C11, Abortions with Liveborn Fetus (I/O)

Attempted abortion results in liveborn fetus:

644.21 (Early onset of delivery) appropriately

Use V27 (Outcome of delivery)

Attempted abortion code also assigned

Chapter 12, Diseases of Skin and Subcutaneous Tissue (I/O)

SKIN

Epidermis

Dermis

Subcutaneous tissue

Infectious skin/subcutaneous tissue

Scar tissue

Copyright © 2005, Elsevier Inc. All rights reserved.
CPT only © 2004. *Current Procedural Terminology, 2005, Professional Edition*, American Medical Association. All rights reserved.

ACCESSORY ORGANS

Sweat glands

Sebaceous glands

Nails

Hair and hair follicles

Other

Multiple codes often necessary

Example: Cellulitis due to Staph, report:

1. Cellulitis 682
2. Staph 041

Chapter 13, Diseases of Musculoskeletal System and Connective Tissue (I/O)

Bone

Bursa

Cartilage

Fascia

Ligaments

Muscle

Synovia

Tendons

Chapter 13 Sections (I/O)

Arthopathies (joint disease) and Related Disorders

Dorsopathies (curvature of spine)

Rheumatism, Excluding back

Osteopathies, Chondropathies, and Acquired Musculoskeletal Deformities

Extensive notes and fifth digits

Chapters 14 and 15 (I/O)

Congenital Anomalies (abnormality at birth)

Conditions Originating in Perinatal Period

Perinatal period through 28th day following birth

Codes can be used after 28th day if it is documented that condition originated during perinatal period.

Section I, C15, Use of Codes V29 (I/O)

V29 Observation and evaluation of newborn

Suspected of having an abnormal condition

Infant 28 days or less

Copyright © 2005, Elsevier Inc. All rights reserved.
CPT only © 2004. *Current Procedural Terminology, 2005, Professional Edition*, American Medical Association. All rights reserved.

Section I, C15, Use of Codes V30–V39 (I)

V30–V39 liveborn infant(s)

Example:

V30, Single liveborn

V31, Liveborn twins

Inpatient: Principal diagnosis

NOTE: V30 used ONLY once, hospital where baby delivered (transfer cases)

Section I, C15, Coding Additional Diagnosis (I)

Code conditions that require:

- Treatment
- Further investigation
- Additional resource

Prolonged length of stay (LOS)

Implications for future care

Insignificant conditions, signs, symptoms

Resolve with no treatment

Need no code

EVEN IF documented

Section I, C15, Prematurity and Fetal Growth Retardation (I)

Codes from categories

764 (Slow fetal growth and fetal malnutrition) and

765 (Disorders relating to short gestation and unspecified low birthweight)

Not assigned solely on birthweight or gestational age

Use physician's assessment of maturity

Use additional code for weeks of gestation (765.20–765.29)

Chapter 16, Symptoms, Signs, and Ill-Defined Conditions (I/O)

Do NOT code a sign or symptom:

Definitive diagnosis made (symptoms are part of disease)

Used only if no specific diagnosis made

Chapter 17, Injury and Poisoning, Section Examples (I/O)

Fractures

Dislocations

Sprains and Strains

Copyright © 2005, Elsevier Inc. All rights reserved.
CPT only © 2004. *Current Procedural Terminology, 2005, Professional Edition*, American Medical Association. All rights reserved.

Intracranial Injury

With or without loss of consciousness

Internal Injury

Open or closed

Crushing Injury

Foreign Body

Burns

Late Effects

Code manifestation or reason for treatment first

Poisoning

E codes (I/O)

The only E codes assigned on the CCS examination are those for adverse effects of correct medication correctly given and correctly taken.

Section I, C19, Table of Drugs and Chemicals (I/O)

Alphabetic listing with codes

Do NOT code directly from Table.

Always reference Tabular.

Section I, C19, Late Effects of External Cause (I/O)

Should be used with late effect of a previous injury/poisoning

Should NOT be used with related current of injury code

Section I, C17, Sequence and Different Degree (I/O)

Do NOT code a sign/symptom if definitive diagnosis has been made.

Symptoms are part of disease.

Use only if no specific diagnosis is made.

Section I, C17, Burns Classified (I/O)

According to extent of body surface involved

Burn site NOT specified

Additional data required

Section I, C17, Category 948 (I/O)

Fourth digits = % body surface involved

Fifth digits = % body surface involved in third-degree burns

Rule of Nines applies.

Copyright © 2005, Elsevier Inc. All rights reserved.
CPT only © 2004. *Current Procedural Terminology, 2005, Professional Edition*, American Medical Association. All rights reserved.

Section I, C17, Debridement of Wounds, Infection, or Burn (I)

Excisional debridement (86.22)

- Cut away
- Performed by physician or other health-care provider

Nonexcisional procedure (86.28)

- Shaved or scraped
- Performed by physician or
- Nonphysician

Section I, C17, Coding for Multiple Injuries (I/O)

Separate code for each injury

Most serious injury first

Section I, C17, Vessel and Nerve Damage (I/O)

Code primary injury first.

Use additional code if nerve damage is minor.

Primary injury = nerve damage

Code nerve damage first.

Section I, C17, Multiple Fractures (I/O)

Same coding principles as with multiple injuries

Code multiple fractures, by site.

Sequenced by severity

Fractures (I/O)

Not indicated as closed or open = closed

Same bone fractured AND dislocated

Code fracture ONLY (highest level of injury)

Section IV, Diagnostic Coding and Reporting Guidelines for Outpatient Services (O)

Hospital-based outpatient services = OPPS

Part of Official Coding and Reporting Guidelines, Section IV

Guidelines A (O)

Use term first-listed diagnosis in lieu of principal diagnosis.

Guideline B (O)

Use codes 001.0 through V82.9 to code diagnosis, symptoms, conditions, problems, complaints, or other reason(s) for visit.

Copyright © 2005, Elsevier Inc. All rights reserved.
CPT only © 2004. *Current Procedural Terminology, 2005, Professional Edition*, American Medical Association. All rights reserved.

Guideline C (O)

Documentation should describe patient's condition using terminology that includes specific diagnoses as well as symptoms, problems, or reasons for encounter.

Guideline D (O)

Selection of codes 001.0 through 999.9 (Chapters 1–17) will frequently be used to describe reason for encounter.

Guideline E (O)

Codes that describe symptoms and signs, as opposed to diagnoses, are acceptable for reporting purposes when an established diagnosis has NOT been confirmed by physician.

Guideline F (O)

V codes deal with encounters for circumstances other than disease or injury.

- *Example:* Well-baby checkup

Guideline G (O)

Codes have either three, four, or five digits.

Fourth and/or fifth digit codes provide greater specificity.

Three-digit code is used ONLY if there is NO fourth or fifth digit.

Where fourth and/or fifth digits are provided, they must be assigned.

Diagnoses NOT coded to full digits available are invalid.

Guideline H (O)

List first code for diagnosis, condition, problem, or other reason for encounter/visit shown in medical record to be chiefly responsible for services provided.

List additional codes that describe any significant co-existing conditions or conditions also being treated.

Guideline I (O)

Do NOT code diagnoses documented as probable, suspected, questionable, ruled out, or working diagnoses.

Rather, code condition(s) to highest degree of certainty for that encounter/visit, such as symptoms, signs, abnormal test results, or other reason for visit.

Guideline J (O)

Chronic diseases treated on an ongoing basis may be coded and reported as many times as patient receives treatment and care for condition(s).

Guideline K (O)

Code all documented conditions that co-exist at time of visit and that require or affect patient care, treatment, or management.

Copyright © 2005, Elsevier Inc. All rights reserved.
CPT only © 2004. *Current Procedural Terminology, 2005, Professional Edition,* American Medical Association. All rights reserved.

Do NOT code conditions previously treated or no longer existing.

"History of" codes (V10- V19) may be used as secondary codes if:

Affects current care or treatment

Guidelines L and M (O)

For patients receiving diagnostic or therapeutic services ONLY

Sequence first

- Diagnosis
- Condition
- Problem
- Other reason shown in medical record to be chiefly responsible for encounter

Codes for other diagnoses (e.g., chronic conditions)

May be sequenced as secondary diagnoses

Exception:

Patients receiving chemotherapy, radiation therapy, or rehabilitation

V code first diagnosis, problem for which service being performed second.

Medical necessity principles apply

Multiple tests require supporting diagnosis for each test.

Guideline N (O)

For patients receiving preoperative evaluations ONLY

- Code from category V72.8 (Other specified examinations).
- Assign secondary code for reason for surgery.
- Code also any findings related to preoperative evaluation.

Guideline O (O)

Code diagnosis that required surgery.

Pre- and post-op diagnosis different

Code the post-op diagnosis

Guideline P (O)

Code routine prenatal visits with no complications:

V22.0, (Supervision of normal first pregnancy)

V22.1, (Supervision of other normal pregnancy)

DO NOT use these codes with pregnancy complication codes.

Copyright © 2005, Elsevier Inc. All rights reserved.
CPT only © 2004. *Current Procedural Terminology, 2005, Professional Edition*, American Medical Association. All rights reserved.

Volume 3, Procedures

90% of codes refer to surgical procedures.

10% refer to diagnostic and therapeutic procedures.

- Volume 3 codes are used by hospitals to report facility services provided to inpatients.
- Procedures done in physician's office or outpatient ASC are coded using CPT codes.
- Surgeon uses CPT to report services to inpatients.

Volume 3, Table of Contents

- Operations on body systems
- Miscellaneous Diagnostic and Therapeutic Procedures
- Most nonsurgical codes

Volume 3, Tabular List

- Conventions in Volume 3 are the same as those in Volumes 1 and 2.
- "Code also . . ." appears in Volume 3 and Volume 2.
- Additional information about coding various components or special adjunctive services of procedure

Volume 3, Alphabetic Index

Index often contains terms that do not appear in Volume 3, Tabular List.

Example: In Index, Volume 3, the entry Gastrostomy, subterm Janeway, directs you to 43.19.

Janeway not mentioned in Tabular List in the description of 43.19

Index terms in bold

Subterms not in bold

Alphabetical arrangement

Ignores single spaces and hyphens

Example: Opening and open reduction

"Opening" appears before "open reduction" because space between two words is ignored.

Often necessary and permissible to code individual components of a procedure

Example: During a procedure, a portion of intestine was removed and reconstruction of urinary bladder was done.

Both reconstruction (57.87) and resection (45.51) coded

Cross-reference features included in Volume 3 are

- *see*
- *see also*
- *see category*

Copyright © 2005, Elsevier Inc. All rights reserved.
CPT only © 2004. *Current Procedural Terminology, 2005, Professional Edition,* American Medical Association. All rights reserved.

Many operations named for surgeon who developed procedure (eponyms)

These procedures located under person's name or name of operation

Example: Watson-Jones is located under main term "Watson-Jones" and also as a subterm under "Operation."

Never code directly from Index

Volume 3, Tabular List

- Format same as Volume 1, Tabular List of Diseases, except Volume 3 codes have two digits before decimal
- Category, subcategory, and subclassification

Bundling

Included in all surgical procedures

Opening and closing of surgical site

Approach except where approach differs from code description

Example: Microscopic approach used instead of described approach

Do not unbundle and code these separately.

If closure takes place during separate surgical procedure, closure can be coded separately.

Copyright © 2005, Elsevier Inc. All rights reserved.
CPT only © 2004. *Current Procedural Terminology, 2005, Professional Edition*, American Medical Association. All rights reserved.

UNIT **IV**

Coding Challenge

EXAMINATIONS

You have three opportunities to practice taking an examination:

- Practice Examination (before study)
- Practice Examination (after study)
- Final Examination (at the end of your complete program of study)

You should have a current edition of the following texts for Part 2, but you may not use any text for Part 1 of the examinations:

- ICD-9-CM (International Classification of Diseases, 9th Edition, Clinical Modification)
- HCPCS (Health Care Common Procedural Coding System)
- CPT (Current Procedural Terminology)
- Medical Dictionary

No other reference material is allowed for the Practice Examination or Final Examination.

- For the Practice Examination, you will need a computer that can use a CD-ROM.
- For the Final Examination, you will not need a computer; rather, you will need paper, pencils, erasers, and the four coding references listed above (ICD-9-CM, HCPCS, CPT, Medical Dictionary).
- You should strive for an 80% to 90% on the second Practice Examination and 70% as a minimum on the Final Examination.

PRACTICE EXAMINATIONS

The Practice Examination contains 81 questions and is located on the **CD-ROM.** Take this examination before you begin your studies and then immediately on completion of your study. The software on the CD will automatically grade your first attempt at the examination and will store the results for comparison with your second effort. Ideally, you should complete the examination in one sitting (6 hours, or 360 minutes); if time does not allow, spread the examination times over several periods.

There are no time extensions in the real certification examination setting, and learning how to judge the amount of time you have to spend on each question is an important part of this learning experience to prepare you for the real certification experience.

There are rationales for each question in the Practice Examination, but do not read the rationales after the first Practice Examination; rather, wait until after you have taken the examination again before reviewing the rationales. The purpose of the Practice Examination is only to assess your beginning level of knowledge and skill—your starting place.

After your studies, take the same Practice Examination again. The software will display the results of the second examination and will compare these scores with the scores from the first examination to illustrate the improvements you have achieved. Keep track of your time; again you have 6 hours (360 minutes) to complete the examination.

Study the questions for which you did not choose the correct response. Did you misread the question, did you not know the material well enough to answer correctly, or did you run out of time? Knowing why you missed a question is an important step to improve your skill level.

FINAL EXAMINATION

If you scored well on both sections of the Practice Examination (at or above the minimum scores), you are ready to move on to the Final Examination, which, like the real certification, is a paper-and-pencil examination.

Copyright © 2005, Elsevier Inc. All rights reserved.
CPT only © 2004. *Current Procedural Terminology, 2005, Professional Edition*, American Medical Association. All rights reserved.

The time for the Final Examination is 6 hours (360 minutes). Located directly before the final examination text, there are answer sheets on which to place your answers. Remove the answer sheets from the text, and use a No. 2 pencil to enter your answer for each of the 81 questions.

If you change an answer, erase the previous entry completely. When you have finished the examination, review the score sheet to ensure that there are no stray pencil marks. Stray marks or incomplete erasures may be misread by the scan machine, registering an incorrect answer.

The grading for the Final Examination is as follows:

A. Part 1 contains **60** questions.
   a. Each correct answer is worth **2** points.
   b. Strive for a minimum score of **74,** or **37** correct answers, to consider the section successful.
B. Part 2 contains **21** coding cases.
   a. Each correct answer is worth **4** points.
   b. Strive for a minimum score of **172**, or **43** correct answers, to consider the section successful.

When calculating your score for Part 2, count the number of:

A. **correct** CPT, HCPC, or ICD-9-CM codes and modifiers, and **credit 4** points for each
B. **incorrect** or **unnecessary** CPT, HCPC or ICD-9-CM codes or modifiers, and **deduct 4** points for each

The scoring for the CCS examination includes deduction of points for unnecessary codes reported for conditions that the patient may have but for which the physician rendered no treatment or management. Consider, for example, an operative report on which it was documented that the surgeon performed a mastectomy for a patient with diabetes. The surgeon mentioned on the report that the patient had diabetes but provided no treatment or management for the condition. It would be unnecessary to report the diagnosis of diabetes; if you did report the diabetes, you would have to deduct 4 points from your score for reporting an unnecessary diagnosis code. Conversely, if the surgeon requested a test in order to manage or render treatment for the diabetes (i.e., glucose level), it would be correct to report the diabetes; if you didn't report the diagnosis code for the diabetes, you would have to deduct 4 points from your score for not reporting a necessary code.

Let's look at how this is calculated by reviewing the examination results of a student who received the following scores on her examination:

Part 1, 43 questions correct: $43 \times 2 = 86$ (The minimum is 74)

Part 2, 52 correct codes and/or modifiers:	$52 \times 4 = +208$
4 incorrect codes and/or modifiers:	$4 \times 4 = -16$
8 unnecessary codes and/or modifiers:	$8 \times 4 = -32$
	TOTAL: 160

This student carefully reviewed the incorrect and unnecessary codes and modifiers to determine her areas of weakness and then developed a plan to study those areas that had presented her with difficulties. One of these weaknesses was that she was overcoding the cases in Part 2.

After you have taken the examination and checked your answers in the Answers to Final section in this text, calculate your scores for Part 1 and Part 2 as indicated in the paragraph above. These two scores represent your Final Examination score. If you did not attain the minimum on each section, you should develop a plan to improve those particular areas where the examination indicates you had difficulties. After your additional study, you can take the Final Examination again for practice.

Copyright © 2005, Elsevier Inc. All rights reserved.
CPT only © 2004. *Current Procedural Terminology, 2005, Professional Edition*, American Medical Association. All rights reserved.

Although there are spaces for six procedure/service codes and four possible diagnosis codes, each case may not require this many codes to be correct or complete. However, no case will never require more than these numbers.

Do not assign E codes or M codes.

The Final Examination has more difficult questions and cases than the Practice Examination so as to ensure that you have had adequate practice with the more complex coding cases.

COMPUTERIZED CERTIFICATION EXAMINATIONS (CCS AND CCS-P) BEGIN IN 2005 FOR AHIMA

A testing service has been contracted by AHIMA to administer the CCS and CCS-P examinations in a computer-based format. The paper/pencil certification examination will no longer be available as both certification examinations will be administered exclusively in the computer-based format. The applications for the CCS and CCS-P submitted after January 1, 2005 will be for the computer-based format, and computer-based testing will be offered starting May 2005.

The new computer-based tests will be 4 hours long and contain:

- The CCS contains **60 multiple choice questions** to be completed in 1 hour in addition to **6 inpatient cases** (ICD-9-CM Volumes 1, 2, and 3) and **7 outpatient cases** (ICD-9-CM Volumes 1, 2, and CPT) to be completed in 3 hours.
- The CCS-P contains **60 multiple choice questions** to be completed in 1 hour in addition to **16 outpatient cases** (ICD-9-CM Volumes 1, 2, CPT, and HCPCS) to be completed in 3 hours.

Historically the tests were administered only twice a year, but with this new computer-based approach, there will be more opportunities throughout the year to take the tests. Application to take the examination is made in the same way to AHIMA. Visit the AHIMA web site (www.ahima.org/certification) for the latest information on this new computer-based testing.

The number of questions in this text reflects the configuration of the test prior to the January 2005 change. The competencies for the test remain the same, only the number of questions/cases and the length of time to complete the CCS and CCS-P examination have changed. So, your preparation for the test will need to be the same.

On a personal note, it is always difficult to take a test! But remember, this is just practice. It is your opportunity to test yourself against an examination and then to have an opportunity to develop a plan to work on the areas where you are having difficulties. You can always only do your best, so give this your very best and it will serve as a stepping stone to the success that you desire.

> *Don't let go of your dreams. If you have determination and belief in your dreams, you will succeed in spite of your desire to let go.*
>
> *Catherine Pulsifer*

Copyright © 2005, Elsevier Inc. All rights reserved.
CPT only © 2004. *Current Procedural Terminology, 2005, Professional Edition*, American Medical Association. All rights reserved.

Answer Sheet for Section 1

SECTION 1

1.	A	B	C	D	31.	A	B	C	D
2.	A	B	C	D	32.	A	B	C	D
3.	A	B	C	D	33.	A	B	C	D
4.	A	B	C	D	34.	A	B	C	D
5.	A	B	C	D	35.	A	B	C	D
6.	A	B	C	D	36.	A	B	C	D
7.	A	B	C	D	37.	A	B	C	D
8.	A	B	C	D	38.	A	B	C	D
9.	A	B	C	D	39.	A	B	C	D
10.	A	B	C	D	40.	A	B	C	D
11.	A	B	C	D	41.	A	B	C	D
12.	A	B	C	D	42.	A	B	C	D
13.	A	B	C	D	43.	A	B	C	D
14.	A	B	C	D	44.	A	B	C	D
15.	A	B	C	D	45.	A	B	C	D
16.	A	B	C	D	46.	A	B	C	D
17.	A	B	C	D	47.	A	B	C	D
18.	A	B	C	D	48.	A	B	C	D
19.	A	B	C	D	49.	A	B	C	D
20.	A	B	C	D	50.	A	B	C	D
21.	A	B	C	D	51.	A	B	C	D
22.	A	B	C	D	52.	A	B	C	D
23.	A	B	C	D	53.	A	B	C	D
24.	A	B	C	D	54.	A	B	C	D
25.	A	B	C	D	55.	A	B	C	D
26.	A	B	C	D	56.	A	B	C	D
27.	A	B	C	D	57.	A	B	C	D
28.	A	B	C	D	58.	A	B	C	D
29.	A	B	C	D	59.	A	B	C	D
30.	A	B	C	D	60.	A	B	C	D

Copyright © 2005, Elsevier Inc. All rights reserved.
CPT only © 2004. *Current Procedural Terminology, 2005, Professional Edition*, American Medical Association. All rights reserved.

Answer Sheet for Section 2

SECTION 2

Part A

1. Case 1
Diagnoses ICD-9-CM CODES: DX1 DX2 DX3 DX4
Procedures CPT CODES: PR1 PR2 PR3 PR4 PR5 PR6

2. Case 2
Diagnoses ICD-9-CM CODES: DX1 DX2 DX3 DX4
Procedures CPT CODES: PR1 PR2 PR3 PR4 PR5 PR6

3. Case 3
Diagnoses ICD-9-CM CODES: DX1 DX2 DX3 DX4
Procedures CPT CODES: PR1 PR2 PR3 PR4 PR5 PR6

4. Case 4
Diagnoses ICD-9-CM CODES: DX1 DX2 DX3 DX4
Procedures CPT CODES: PR1 PR2 PR3 PR4 PR5 PR6

5. Case 5
Diagnoses ICD-9-CM CODES: DX1 DX2 DX3 DX4
Procedures CPT CODES: PR1 PR2 PR3 PR4 PR5 PR6

6. Case 6
Diagnoses ICD-9-CM CODES: DX1 DX2 DX3 DX4
Procedures CPT CODES: PR1 PR2 PR3 PR4 PR5 PR6

7. Case 7
Diagnoses ICD-9-CM CODES: DX1 DX2 DX3 DX4
Procedures CPT CODES: PR1 PR2 PR3 PR4 PR5 PR6

8. Case 8
Diagnoses ICD-9-CM CODES: DX1 DX2 DX3 DX4
Procedures CPT CODES: PR1 PR2 PR3 PR4 PR5 PR6

9. Case 9
Diagnoses ICD-9-CM CODES: DX1 DX2 DX3 DX4
Procedures CPT CODES: PR1 PR2 PR3 PR4 PR5 PR6

10. Case 10
Diagnoses ICD-9-CM CODES: DX1 DX2 DX3 DX4
Procedures CPT CODES: PR1 PR2 PR3 PR4 PR5 PR6

11. Case 11
Diagnoses ICD-9-CM CODES: DX1 DX2 DX3 DX4
Procedures CPT CODES: PR1 PR2 PR3 PR4 PR5 PR6

Part B

12. Case 12
Diagnoses ICD-9-CM CODES: DX1 DX2 DX3 DX4 DX5 DX6 DX7 DX8 DX9 DX10
Procedures ICD-9-CM CODES: PR1 PR2 PR3 PR4 PR5 PR6

13. Case 13
Diagnoses ICD-9-CM CODES: DX1 DX2 DX3 DX4 DX5 DX6 DX7 DX8 DX9 DX10
Procedures ICD-9-CM CODES: PR1 PR2 PR3 PR4 PR5 PR6

14. Case 14
Diagnoses ICD-9-CM CODES: DX1 DX2 DX3 DX4 DX5 DX6 DX7 DX8 DX9 DX10
Procedures ICD-9-CM CODES: PR1 PR2 PR3 PR4 PR5 PR6

15. Case 15
Diagnoses ICD-9-CM CODES: DX1 DX2 DX3 DX4 DX5 DX6 DX7 DX8 DX9 DX10
Procedures ICD-9-CM CODES: PR1 PR2 PR3 PR4 PR5 PR6

16. Case 16
Diagnoses ICD-9-CM CODES: DX1 DX2 DX3 DX4 DX5 DX6 DX7 DX8 DX9 DX10
Procedures ICD-9-CM CODES: PR1 PR2 PR3 PR4 PR5 PR6

17. Case 17
Diagnoses ICD-9-CM CODES: DX1 DX2 DX3 DX4 DX5 DX6 DX7 DX8 DX9 DX10
Procedures ICD-9-CM CODES: PR1 PR2 PR3 PR4 PR5 PR6

18. Case 18
Diagnoses ICD-9-CM CODES: DX1 DX2 DX3 DX4 DX5 DX6 DX7 DX8 DX9 DX10
Procedures ICD-9-CM CODES: PR1 PR2 PR3 PR4 PR5 PR6

19. Case 19
Diagnoses ICD-9-CM CODES: DX1 DX2 DX3 DX4 DX5 DX6 DX7 DX8 DX9 DX10
Procedures ICD-9-CM CODES: PR1 PR2 PR3 PR4 PR5 PR6

20. Case 20
Diagnoses ICD-9-CM CODES: DX1 DX2 DX3 DX4 DX5 DX6 DX7 DX8 DX9 DX10
Procedures ICD-9-CM CODES: PR1 PR2 PR3 PR4 PR5 PR6

21. Case 21
Diagnoses ICD-9-CM CODES: DX1 DX2 DX3 DX4 DX5 DX6 DX7 DX8 DX9 DX10
Procedures ICD-9-CM CODES: PR1 PR2 PR3 PR4 PR5 PR6

Copyright © 2005, Elsevier Inc. All rights reserved.
CPT only © 2004. *Current Procedural Terminology, 2005, Professional Edition*, American Medical Association. All rights reserved.

FINAL EXAMINATION

The following emergency department acuity sheet will be used throughout Part 1 when reporting ED services. Remove this acuity sheet from the text for easier reference.

ACUITY SHEET

Level 1—99281	Level 2—99282	Level 3—99283
1. Initial (triage) assessment 2. Suture removal 3. Wound recheck 4. Note for work or school 5. Simple discharge information	Interventions from previous level plus any of the following: 1. OTC med administration 2. Tetanus booster 3. Bedside diagnostic tests (stool hemoccult, glucometer) 4. Visual acuity 5. Orthostatic vital signs 6. Simple trauma not requiring x-ray 7. Simple discharge information	Interventions from previous level plus any of the following: 1. Heparin/saline lock 2. Crystalloid IV therapy 3. X-ray, one area 4. RX med administration 5. Fluorescein stain 6. Quick cath 7. Foley cath 8. Receipt of ambulance patient 9. Mental health emergencies (mild) not requiring parenteral medications or admission 10. Moderate complexity discharge instructions
Level 4—99284	**Level 5—99285**	**Critical care 99291, 99292**
Interventions from previous level plus any of the following: 1. X-ray, multiple areas 2. Special imaging studies (CT, MRI, ultrasound) 3. Cardiac monitoring 4. Multiple reassessments of patient 5. Parenteral [1]medications (including insulin) 6. Nebulizer treatment (1 or 2) 7. NG placement 8. Pelvic exam 9. Mental health emergencies (moderate). May require parenteral medications but not admission [1]*not through the alimentary canal but rather by injection through some other route, such as subcutaneous, intramuscular, intraorbital, intracapsular, intraspinal, intrasternal, or intravenous*	Interventions from previous level plus any of the following: 1. Monitor/stabilize patient during in hospital transport and/or testing (CT, MRI, ultrasound) 2. Vasoactive medication 3. Administration (dopamine, dobutamine, multiple) nebulizer treatments (3 or more) 4. Conscious sedation 5. Lumbar puncture 6. Thoracentesis 7. Sexual assault exam 8. Admission to hospital 9. Mental health emergency (severe) psychotic and/or agitated/combative 10. Requires admission 11. Fracture/dislocation reduction 12. Suicide precautions 13. Gastric lavage 14. Complex discharge instructions	Interventions from any previous level plus any of the following: 1. Multiple parenteral medications 2. Continuous monitoring 3. Major trauma care 4. Chest tube insertion 5. CPR 6. Defibrillation/cardioversion 7. Delivery of baby 8. Control of major hemorrhage 9. Administration of blood or blood products

Copyright © 2005, Elsevier Inc. All rights reserved.
CPT only © 2004. *Current Procedural Terminology, 2005, Professional Edition,* American Medical Association. All rights reserved.

PART 1

1. A 2-year-old child was brought to the outpatient radiology department at the hospital by his father for an ultrasound of child's heart. At the age of 10 months, he was diagnosed with a heart murmur due to ventricular septal defect. At age 11 months, the child developed congestive heart failure, and at that time the physician prescribed diuretics and digitalis.

745.4	Bulbus cordis anomalies and anomalies of cardiac septal closure, ventricular septal deviation
785.2	Symptoms involving cardiovascular system, undiagnosed cardiac murmurs
747.29	Other congenital anomalies of circulatory system, other anomalies of aorta, other congenital
779.8	Other specified conditions originating in the perinatal period, other specified conditions originating in the perinatal period

A. 745.4
B. 745.4, 785.2
C. 747.29, 745.4
D. 745.4, 779.29

2. A patient is admitted to the hospital for bacterial endocarditis due to AIDS:

042	Human Immunodeficiency virus (HIV) disease
421.0	Acute and subacute bacterial endocarditis
421.1	Acute and subacute infective endocarditis in diseases classified elsewhere
421.9	Acute endocarditis, unspecified

A. 421.0, 042
B. 042, 421.9
C. 421.1, 042
D. 042, 421.0

3. The system that edits outpatient claims data to identify errors and returns a series of edit flags is known as:
A. APC
B. CCI
C. OCE
D. PPS

Copyright © 2005, Elsevier Inc. All rights reserved.
CPT only © 2004. *Current Procedural Terminology, 2005, Professional Edition*, American Medical Association. All rights reserved.

4. Female patient is admitted to the hospital for bilateral radical mastectomy. Final diagnosis is carcinoma of upper-outer quadrant of the breast.

85.42	Bilateral simple mastectomy
85.45	Unilateral radical mastectomy
85.46	Bilateral radical mastectomy
174.4	Malignant neoplasm of the female breast upper-outer quadrant
174.5	Malignant neoplasm of the female breast lower-outer quadrant
198.81	Secondary malignant neoplasm of the breast

A. 85.46, 174.4
B. 85.42, 174.5
C. 85.45, 174.4
D. 85.46, 198.81

5. A 26-year-old patient is seen in the ED with wrist pain received when he fell from a dirt bike. The patient is in apparent pain, and the wrist has begun to swell. He is unable to flex the wrist. The patient reports that he did strike his head on a log as a result of the fall. He denies any loss of consciousness. The ED physician ordered skull and wrist x-rays. The x-rays show no fracture of the skull but a small fracture of the wrist. The ED staff splinted the wrist. The physician prescribes acetaminophen with codeine, PO 325 mg q4h. The patient was discharged to home.

733.12	Pathologic fracture of distal radius and ulna, write NOS
814.00	Fracture of carpal bones, closed, unspecified, write NOS

A. Level 1, 733.12
B. Level 2, 814.00
C. Level 4, 814.00
D. Level 4, 733.12

6. Patient fell, struck his head, and was brought to the ED. He denies any loss of consciousness. He has significant bruising on the left side of his body and complains of pain under his left arm. A series of x-rays were ordered in addition to an MRI. Examination and review of the MRI and x-rays reveal a closed fracture of the skull, with extradural hemorrhage, and fracture of two ribs. Review of the medical record reveals hypertension. Patient is admitted to inpatient observation. Report the ED service, but not the radiology service:

803.21	Skull fracture, closed with subarachnoid, subdural, and extradural hemorrhage
807.02	Fracture, closed, two ribs
852.41	Extradural hemorrhage following injury without mention of open intracranial wound, no loss of consciousness
853.01	Other and unspecified intracranial hemorrhage following injury, without mention of open intracranial wound, no loss of consciousness

A. Level 4, 807.02, 803.21
B. Level 4, 803.21, 807.02
C. Level 3, 853.01, 852.41, 807.02
D. either A or B

Copyright © 2005, Elsevier Inc. All rights reserved.
CPT only © 2004. *Current Procedural Terminology, 2005, Professional Edition,* American Medical Association. All rights reserved.

7. A patient is admitted to the hospital with carcinoma of the prostate. The surgeon performed a bilateral pelvic lymphadenectomy with frozen section, radical retropubic prostatectomy, and plastic repair of the bladder neck using an open approach. The procedure was performed with spinal anesthetic. The pathology report later indicated T4a adenocarcinoma of the prostate.

40.29	Simple excision of other lymphatic structure, includes simple lymphadenectomy
57.85	Cystourethroplasty and plastic repair of bladder neck
60.69	Other prostatectomy, by any approach
60.5	Radical prostatectomy, by any approach
185	Malignant neoplasm of prostate

A. 60.69, 40.29, 57.85, 185
B. 60.5, 57.85, 185
C. 60.5, 57.85, 40.29, 185
D. 60.69, 57.85, 185

8. A 28-week pregnant woman is seen in the ED for a fracture of the right ankle, which is not affecting the pregnancy. Patient also complains of constant radiating pain down the left leg, which, after examination, is determined to be related to the pregnancy. The correct coding sequence is:
A. pregnancy related code, ankle fracture, leg pain
B. ankle fracture, pregnancy related code, leg pain
C. ankle fracture, leg pain, pregnancy related code
D. leg pain, ankle fracture, pregnancy related code

9. Patient is admitted to the hospital for congestive heart failure, hypertensive heart disease, and hypertensive renal disease. The coder assigns:
A. congestive heart failure and hypertensive renal disease
B. combination code for hypertensive heart and renal disease
C. hypertensive heart disease, hypertensive renal disease
D. combination code for hypertensive heart and renal disease and congestive heart failure

Copyright © 2005, Elsevier Inc. All rights reserved.
CPT only © 2004. *Current Procedural Terminology, 2005, Professional Edition,* American Medical Association. All rights reserved.

10. A 10-year-old boy presents to the ED for injuries caused by falling off his bike. All wounds were superficial. He has a 2-cm wound to his nose and a 1-cm wound to his cheek. He also has a 2.5-cm wound to his elbow. All injuries were simple repair by means of suture. Acetaminophen was administered, 325 mg. The patient's mother was advised to give the child acetaminophen if needed for pain. Directions for care of the wounds were given with follow-up with the child's pediatrician in 10 days. What would the code(s) be to report the wound repair?

12001	Simple repair of superficial wounds of scalp, neck, axillae, external genitalia, trunk and\or extremities (including hands and feet); 2.5 cm or less
12002	Simple repair of superficial wounds of scalp, neck, axillae, external genitalia, trunk and\or extremities (including hands and feet); 2.6 cm to 7.5 cm
12011	Simple repair of superficial wounds of face, ears, eyelids, nose, lips and\or mucous membranes; 2.5 cm or less
12013	Simple repair of superficial wounds of face, ears, eyelids, nose, lips and\or mucous membranes; 2.6 cm to 5.0 cm

A. Level 2, 12002
B. Level 2, 12013, 12001
C. Level 1, 12013, 12002
D. Level 1, 12011, 12002

11. Patient presents to the ASC for incisional biopsy of both breasts.

19102	Biopsy of breast; percutaneous, needle core, using imaging guidance
19101	Biopsy of breast; open incisional
19125	Excision of breast lesion identified by preoperative placement of radiological marker, open, single lesion
-50	Bilateral procedure
-LT	Left
-RT	Right

A. 19102-50
B. 19101-RT, 19101-LT
C. 19101-50
D. 19125-RT, 19125-LT

12. A patient with ovarian cancer is admitted to the hospital to receive chemotherapy. The patient develops uncontrolled nausea and vomiting. The principal diagnosis is:
A. uncontrolled nausea
B. ovarian cancer
C. chemotherapy
D. vomiting

Copyright © 2005, Elsevier Inc. All rights reserved.
CPT only © 2004. *Current Procedural Terminology, 2005, Professional Edition*, American Medical Association. All rights reserved.

13. Marsha presents to the ASC after having an abnormal shoulder x-ray in the clinic yesterday. The physician does a diagnostic arthroscopy and performs a limited debridement of the shoulder joint.

29805	Arthroscopy, shoulder, diagnostic, with or without synovial biopsy (separate procedure)
29822	Arthroscopy, shoulder, surgical; debridement, limited
29823	;debridement, extensive

A. 29805
B. 29823
C. 29822, 29805
D. 29822

14. Cole comes into the ED today with his mother after falling from the top bunk bed where he and his brother were wrestling. He is having pain in his left lower leg and is unable to bear weight on it. He also complains of a headache and nausea. Cole was taken to the x-ray department for views of the ankle and skull. After the physician talks with the radiologist regarding the diagnosis of ankle fracture and probable concussion, a walking short leg cast is applied from just below his knee to his toes. The patient is admitted to observation. What is the principal diagnosis reported by the hospital for the admission?
A. ankle fracture
B. concussion
C. headache
D. headache and nausea

15. A 17-year-old male is admitted to the hospital for a tonsillectomy and possible adenoidectomy due to chronic tonsillitis. On inspection, the adenoids were found not to be inflamed; a tonsillectomy was performed:

474.00	Chronic tonsillitis
474.02	Chronic tonsillitis and adenoiditis
474.10	Hypertrophy of tonsils with adenoids
28.2	Tonsillectomy without adenoidectomy
28.3	Tonsillectomy with adenoidectomy

A. 28.2, 474.00
B. 28.2, 474.02
C. 28.3, 474.10
D. 28.3, 474.00

Copyright © 2005, Elsevier Inc. All rights reserved.
CPT only © 2004. *Current Procedural Terminology, 2005, Professional Edition*, American Medical Association. All rights reserved.

16. A 62-year-old female presents to ASC for a sigmoidoscopy. The physician inserts a flexible scope into the patient's rectum and determines the rectum is clear of any polyps. The scope is advanced to the sigmoid colon, and three polyps are found. Using the snare technique, the polyps are removed. The remainder of the colon is free of polyps. The scope is withdrawn.

153.3	Malignant neoplasm of sigmoid colon
153.9	Malignant neoplasm of colon, unspecified
211.3	Benign neoplasm of colon
44110	Excision of one or more lesions of small or large intestine not requiring anastomosis, exteriorization, or fistulization; single enterotomy
44111	Excision of one or more lesions of small or large intestine not requiring anastomosis, exteriorization, or fistulization; multiple enterotomies
45383	Colonoscopy, flexible, proximal to splenic flexure; with ablation of tumor(s), polyp(s), or other lesion(s) not amenable to removal by hot biopsy forceps, bipolar cautery or snare technique
45338	Sigmoidoscopy, flexible; with removal of tumor(s), polyp(s), or other lesion(s) by snare technique

A. 45383, 211.3
B. 44110, 153.9
C. 45338, 211.3
D. 44111, 153.3

17. Margie, a 62-year-old female, presents to the ED with complaints of chest pain and shortness of breath. She has been experiencing these symptoms for the last 2 hours. The ED physician requests a portable two-view chest x-ray, various laboratory studies, and an ultrasound. It is decided to admit the patient to the hospital. The cardiologist will assume care for this patient. Report the ED services.

786	Symptoms involving respiratory system and other chest symptoms
786.05	Shortness of breath
786.50	Chest pain, unspecified

A. Level 4, 786.50, 786
B. Level 4, 786.50, 786.05
C. Level 5, 786, 786.05
D. Level 5, 786.50, 786.05

Copyright © 2005, Elsevier Inc. All rights reserved.
CPT only © 2004. *Current Procedural Terminology, 2005, Professional Edition*, American Medical Association. All rights reserved.

18. The physician lists the final diagnosis as cough and high fever for this inpatient. Physician documentation states possible acute bronchitis versus pneumonia. The following diagnoses codes are assigned:

466.0	Acute bronchitis
486	Pneumonia, organism unspecified
780.6	Fever
786.2	Cough

A. 466.0, 780.6
B. 780.6, 786.2, 486, 466.0
C. 486, 466.0
D. 786.2, 780.6

19. This 70-year-old male is taken to the ED with severe chest pain. While the ED physician is attempting to stabilize the patient, the patient's pressures drop and he goes into cardiac arrest. Cardiopulmonary resuscitation is performed on the patient, and his pressure returns to normal. The ED physician and staff spent 90 minutes providing services to this patient. He is transferred to the intensive care unit in critical condition.

92950	Cardiopulmonary resuscitation (e.g., in cardiac arrest)
92960	Cardioversion, elective, electrical conversion of arrhythmia; external
92970	Cardioassist-method of circulatory assist; internal
99291	Critical care, 30–74 minutes
99292	each additional 30 minutes
786.50	Chest pain
427.5	Cardiac arrest

A. 92950, 427.5
B. 92970, 427.5, 786.50
C. 99291, 92950, 427.5
D. 99291, 99292, 92950, 427.5, 786.50

20. This modifier indicates that an outpatient procedure was converted to an inpatient status due to an unexpected occurrence during a scheduled outpatient procedure:
A. -58
B. -73
C. -CA
D. -74

Copyright © 2005, Elsevier Inc. All rights reserved.
CPT only © 2004. *Current Procedural Terminology, 2005, Professional Edition,* American Medical Association. All rights reserved.

21. A 51-year-old male patient had surgery to remove two separate carbuncles of the left axilla. Pathology report indicated staphylococcal infection. Report the diagnoses.

680.3	Carbuncle and Furuncle Upper arm and forearm, Axilla, Shoulder
041.10	Staphylococcus, unspecified
041.19	Other staphylococcus
041.09	Other streptococcus

A. 680.3, 041.10
B. 680.3, 041.09
C. 680.3, 041.19
D. 041.09, 680.3

22. Richard, a 34-year-old male, was transferred to the ASC from the ED. He had fallen from a 4-foot scaffolding and hit his lower leg on the bottom rung of the support, fracturing his tibial shaft. The fracture sites were secured by means of percutaneous fixation.

27750	Closed treatment of tibial shaft fracture (with or without fibular fracture); without manipulation
27752	;with manipulation, with or without skeletal traction
27756	Percutaneous skeletal fixation of tibial shaft fracture (with or without fibular fracture) (e.g., pins or screws)
823.20	Shaft, closed tibia alone
823.30	Shaft, open tibia alone

A. 27750, 823.30
B. 27756, 823.30
C. 27752, 823.20
D. 27756, 823.20

23. Procedure performed is an endoscopic ethmoidectomy total with an endoscopic maxillary antrostomy with removal of maxillary tissue due to chronic sinusitis. Surgery was performed at ASC, located within the hospital. Code the procedure(s) and diagnosis.

31200	Ethmoidectomy; intranasal, anterior
31225	Maxillectomy; without orbital exenteration
31254	Nasal/sinus endoscopy, surgical; with ethmoidectomy, partial (anterior)
31255	Nasal/sinus endoscopy, surgical; with ethmoidectomy, total (anterior and posterior)
31256	Nasal/sinus endoscopy, surgical, with maxillary antrostomy;
31267	Nasal/sinus endoscopy, surgical, with maxillary antrostomy; with removal of tissue from maxillary sinus
461.9	Acute sinusitis, unspecified
473.9	Unspecified sinusitis (chronic)
-51	Multiple procedure

A. 31254, 31256-51, 473.9
B. 31255, 31267-51, 461.9
C. 31255, 31267-51, 473.9
D. 31200, 31225-51, 473.9

Copyright © 2005, Elsevier Inc. All rights reserved.
CPT only © 2004. *Current Procedural Terminology, 2005, Professional Edition*, American Medical Association. All rights reserved.

24. A 65-year-old gentleman is an inpatient who underwent left total hip arthroplasty and developed urinary retention. He has had several trials of voiding with both alpha blockade and bethanechol. The patient was given a spinal anesthetic, prepped, and draped in the lithotomy position. A 28 French resectoscope was passed under direct vision. Again, the prostate showed irregular ingrowth and obstruction. The bladder shows mild to moderate trabeculation. The prostate was thoroughly resected, chips evacuated from the bladder, and hemostasis achieved. A 22 French three-way catheter was inserted into the bladder and placed at continuous bladder irrigation. There was a large piece of tissue acting as a ball valve. A transurethral resection of the prostate was performed. The medical record indicates recurrent prostatic hyperplasia.

57.32	Other cystoscopy, transurethral cystoscopy
57.33	Closed (transurethral) biopsy of bladder
60.21	Transurethral (ultrasound) guided laser induced prostatectomy, TULIP
60.29	Other transurethral prostatectomy, TURP
601.8	Other specified inflammatory diseases of the prostate
600.91	Hyperplasia of prostate with urinary obstruction

A. 60.29, 57.32, 600.91
B. 60.21, 57.33, 600.91
C. 57.32, 60.29, 601.8
D. 60.29, 600.91

25. Susan was admitted to the hospital for dysfunctional uterine bleeding. She was taken to the operating room, where the bladder was straight catheterized. A weighted speculum was placed in the vagina. The anterior lip of the cervix was grasped with a single tooth tenaculum. Kevorkian curet was then used to obtain endocervical curetting. The uterus was then sounded to a depth of 6 cm. The cervical os was then serially dilated to allow passage of the hysteroscope. The hysteroscope was then passed, and uterine contents were examined, documented, and photographed. No evidence or polyps of fibroids were found. A fractional dilation and curettage was accomplished when a sharp curet was used to thoroughly sample endometrial cavity, with return of a moderate amount of tissue. The tenaculum was removed from the cervix, and the tenaculum site was oversewn with 3-0 chromic figure-of-eight sutures.

68.16	Closed biopsy of the uterus
69.09	Dilation and curettage of the uterus, other dilation and curettage
626.2	Disorders of menstruation and other abnormal bleeding from female genital tract, excessive or frequent menstruation
626.8	Disorders of menstruation and other abnormal bleeding from female genital tract, other, dysfunctional or functional uterine hemorrhage NOS

A. 68.16, 626.8
B. 68.16, 69.09, 626.8
C. 69.09, 626.8
D. 69.09, 626.2

Copyright © 2005, Elsevier Inc. All rights reserved.
CPT only © 2004. *Current Procedural Terminology, 2005, Professional Edition,* American Medical Association. All rights reserved.

26. A 16-year-old female with history of chronic renal failure due to cytomegalovirus infection and a failed kidney transplant was admitted to the hospital for her second transplant. The patient has an established AV fistula and received hemodialysis during the hospital stay prior to the transplant procedure. The failed kidney was removed and replaced with a donor organ. Postoperatively the donor organ was fully functional. The hospital course was without further complication, and the patient was subsequently discharged.

078.5	Cytomegalovirus disease
996.81	Complications of transplanted organ, kidney
586	Renal failure, unspecified
585	Chronic renal failure
55.53	Complete nephrectomy, removal of transplanted or rejected kidney
55.69	Transplant of kidney, other kidney transplant
39.95	Hemodialysis

A. 585, 996.81, 078.5, 55.53, 55.69, 39.95
B. 996.81, 078.5, 55.53, 55.69
C. 586, 996.81, 078.5, 55.53, 55.69, 39.95
D. 996.81, 078.5, 585, 55.53, 55.69, 39.95

27. A 21-year-old male patient is brought to the ED by ambulance. He is unresponsive, with tachycardia and tachypnea. He fell from scaffolding at work, approximately 40 feet. He has sustained multiple skull fractures and severe head trauma and has been unconscious about 20 minutes now. The ED physician placed an endotracheal tube for intubation and inserted a temporary central venous catheter (non-tunneled and centrally inserted). The ED physician had to hand bag the patient for 10 minutes until the neurologist arrived in the ED to assume care of this critically injured patient. The ED physician spent a total of 80 minutes caring for this patient.

99291	Critical care E/M, first 30–74 minutes
99292	each additional 30 minutes
31500	Intubation, endotracheal, emergency procedure
36556	Insertion of non-tunneled centrally inserted central venous catheter, over 5
36558	Insertion of tunneled centrally inserted central venous catheter, without subcutaneous port or pump, over 5
803.46	Other and unqualified skull fractures, closed with intracranial injury of other and unspecified nature, with loss of consciousness of unspecified duration
803.42	Other and unqualified skull fractures, closed with intracranial injury of other and unspecified nature, with brief [less than one hour] loss of consciousness

A. Level 5, 31500, 36556, 803.46
B. 99291, 31500, 36556, 803.46
C. 99291, 99292 × 2, 803.42
D. Level 5, 99291, 99292, 803.42

Copyright © 2005, Elsevier Inc. All rights reserved.
CPT only © 2004. *Current Procedural Terminology, 2005, Professional Edition*, American Medical Association. All rights reserved.

28. A patient is seen in the ASC for multiple colon polyps and diverticulosis. A flexible colonoscopy is inserted. A polyp was removed from the colon with a snare. A lesion was also noted on the cecum and was biopsied with a hot biopsy forceps. Another lesion was noted in the anal canal and biopsied. Areas of diverticulosis were noted and inspected. The pathology report later indicated that the lesion in the cecum was a benign polyp, the anal canal polyp a benign adenomatous polyp, and the polyp in the colon was benign.

45380	Colonoscopy, flexible, proximal to splenic flexure; with biopsy, single or multiple
45384	Colonoscopy, flexible, proximal to splenic flexure; with removal of tumor(s), polyp(s), or other lesions(s) by, hot biopsy forceps or bipolar cautery
45385	Colonoscopy, flexible, proximal to splenic flexure; with removal of tumor(s), polyp(s), or other lesions(s) by, snare technique
211.3	Benign neoplasm of other parts of digestive system, colon, including cecum and large intestine NOS
211.4	Benign neoplasm of other parts of digestive system, rectum and anal canal
211.9	Benign neoplasm of other parts of digestive system, other unspecified site
562.10	Diverticulosis of colon without mention of hemorrhage
-59	Distinct procedural service
-51	Multiple procedures

A. 45385, 211.3, 211.4, 562.10
B. 45380-59, 211.3, 211.4, 562.10
C. 45385, 45380-59, 211.3, 211.4, 562.10
D. 45385, 45384-51, 45380-51, 211.3, 211.9, 562.10

29. The patient presents to the ASC for removal of a 2.5-cm basal cell carcinoma from his chin and a 1.5-cm basal cell carcinoma of the nose. The surgeon excises the areas of carcinoma and repairs the areas with split-thickness skin grafts.

11643	Excision, malignant lesion including margins, face, ears, eyelids, nose, lips; excised diameter, 2.1-3.0 cm
15120	Split graft, face, scalp, eyelids, mouth, neck, ears, orbits, genitalia, hands, feet and/or multiple digits; first 100 sq cm or less, or one percent of body area of infants and children
173.3	Other malignant neoplasm of skin, skin of other and unspecified parts of the face, including cheek, chin, eyebrow, forehead, nose, temple
216.3	Benign neoplasm of skin, skin of other and unspecified parts of face, including cheek, eyebrow, nose, temple

A. 15120, 11643, 173.3
B. 15120, 11643 × 2, 173.3
C. 15120, 11643 × 2, 216.3
D. 15120, 11643, 216.3

Copyright © 2005, Elsevier Inc. All rights reserved.
CPT only © 2004. *Current Procedural Terminology, 2005, Professional Edition,* American Medical Association. All rights reserved.

30. A 6-year-old is brought to the ASC for removal of an impacted PE tube and placement of a new PE tube. General anesthesia was administered, and a 3.5-mm speculum was inserted into the right ear. The speculum was removed and inserted in the left ear. The impacted PE tube was then removed. There was some granulation tissue around this site. A new site was created posteriorly within some tympanosclerotic plaque. A new PE tube was inserted.

69405	Eustachian tube catheterization, transtympanic
69424	Ventilating tube removal requiring general anesthesia
69436	Tympanostomy (requiring insertion of ventilation tube), general anesthesia
388.8	Other disorders of the ear
996.59	Mechanical complication of other specified prosthetic device, implant, and graft; due to other implant and internal device not elsewhere classifiable
-LT	Left

A. 69424 × 2, 996.59
B. 69405-LT, 996.59
C. 69424, 388.8
D. 69424-LT, 69436-LT, 996.59

31. This outpatient was brought to the ASC for a section of the flexor retinaculum for carpal tunnel syndrome of the left hand. Under Bier block anesthesia and under tourniquet, the patient's left hand was prepped and draped in the usual manner. An incision was made in a curvilinear fashion over the flexor crease. The border of the flexor retinaculum was localized. It was cut along the ulnar side in its entirety up to the mid-palm area. The wound was then sutured in one layer with 4-0 nylon interrupted mattress sutures. A dressing was applied. The patient was then discharged to the recovery room. He has meds at home that he will be able to take for pain.

64716	Neuroplasty and/or transposition; cranial nerve (specify)
64772	Decompression; unspecified nerve(s) (specify)
64726	Decompression; unspecified nerve(s) (specify), plantar digital nerve
354.0	Mononeuritis of upper limb and mononeuritis multiplex, carpal tunnel syndrome
354.5	Mononeuritis multiplex, combination of a single condition classifiable to 354 or 355
-LT	Left
-RT	Right

A. 64772, 354.5
B. 64726-RT, 354.0
C. 64716-LT, 354.5
D. 64772-LT, 354.0

Copyright © 2005, Elsevier Inc. All rights reserved.
CPT only © 2004. *Current Procedural Terminology, 2005, Professional Edition,* American Medical Association. All rights reserved.

32. The patient presents to the ASC with a herniated disk. The surgeon performs a hemilaminectomy at L4-5 and L5-S1. The lower back area was opened; after decompression of the nerve roots, the interspace at L4-5 disk was excised. Next, the interspace at L5-S1 disk was excised.

63030	Laminotomy (hemilaminectomy), with decompression of nerve root(s), including partial facetectomy, foraminotomy and/or excision of herniated intervertebral disk, one interspace; lumbar
63035	Laminotomy (hemilaminectomy), with decompression of nerve root(s), including partial facetectomy, foraminotomy and/or excision of herniated intervertebral disk; each additional interspace, cervical or lumbar (list separately in addition to code for primary procedure)
63040	Laminotomy (hemilaminectomy), with decompression of nerve root(s), including partial facetectomy, foraminotomy and/or excision of herniated intervertebral disc, reexploration, single interspace; cervical
63045	Laminectomy, facetectomy and foraminotomy (unilateral or bilateral with decompression of spinal cord, cauda equina and/or nerve root(s), e.g., spinal or lateral recess stenosis), single vertebral segment; cervical
63043	each additional cervical interspace (list separately in addition to code for primary condition)
63048	each additional segment, cervical, thoracici, or lumbar (list separately in addition to code for primary condition)
722.10	Intervertebral disc disorders, displacement of thoracic or lumbar intervertebral disc without myelopathy, lumbar intervertebral disc without myelopathy
722.2	Displacement of intervertebral disc, site unspecified, without myelopathy
839.00	Other, multiple, and ill-defined dislocations; cervical vertebra, closed; cervical vertebra, unspecified

A. 63045, 63048, 722.2
B. 63040, 63043, 839.00
C. 63030, 63035, 722.10
D. 63040, 63043, 722.10

33. The patient was admitted for a malignant tumor of the thyroid. The surgeon performs a total thyroidectomy. The patient was prepped and draped. The neck area was opened. With careful radical dissection of the neck completed, one could visualize the size of the tumor. The decision was made to do a total thyroidectomy. The pathology report later indicated that the tumor was malignant.

06.2	Operations on thyroid and parathyroid glands, unilateral thyroid lobectomy
06.31	Operations on thyroid and parathyroid glands, other partial thyroidectomy, excision of lesion of thyroid gland
06.4	Operations on thyroid and parathyroid glands, complete thyroidectomy
06.52	Operations on thyroid and parathyroid glands, substernal thyroidectomy, complete substernal thyroidectomy
164.0	Malignant neoplasm of thymus, heart, and mediastinum; thymus
193	Malignant neoplasm of thyroid gland

A. 06.52, 193
B. 06.31, 193
C. 06.2, 164.0
D. 06.4, 193

Copyright © 2005, Elsevier Inc. All rights reserved.
CPT only © 2004. *Current Procedural Terminology, 2005, Professional Edition*, American Medical Association. All rights reserved.

34. Arrhythmia, elevation of ST segment and Q wave, and increased troponin level may be indicative of:
    A. cerebral vascular accident
    B. myocardial infarction
    C. respiratory failure
    D. atrial fibrillation

35. A 19-year-old male was admitted to the ASC for an abnormal finding on x-ray of the GI tract. The surgeon has determined that the patient may have a perforated appendicitis with abscess. The x-ray showed a dilated bowel in the midabdomen and pelvis and a loop in the sigmoid colon. The Pentax video sigmoidoscope was inserted without difficulty to 60 cm. Careful inspection in the mid-descending, distal descending, sigmoid, and rectum revealed no erythema, ulceration, exudate, friability, or other mucosal abnormalities. There were a few diverticula present. The mucosa was normal. No volvulus was noted. No diverticulitis and no obstructing lesion were seen. The patient tolerated the procedure well. The impression was that of a normal sigmoidoscopy to 60 cm. No obstruction or volvulus was noted; no appendicitis was noted. The mucosa was normal. The patient needs to have a small bowel obstruction ruled out. A small bowel series was recommended.

45330	Sigmoidoscopy, flexible; diagnostic, with or without collection of specimen(s) by brushing or washing (separate procedure)
45355	Colonoscopy, rigid or flexible, transabdominal via colostomy, single or multiple
45378	Colonoscopy, flexible, proximal to splenic flexure; diagnostic, with or without collection of specimen(s) by decompression (separate procedure)
45387	Colonoscopy, flexible, proximal to splenic flexure; with transendoscopic stent placement (includes predilation)
541	Appendicitis, unqualified
560.9	Intestinal obstruction without mention of hernia, unspecified intestinal obstruction
793.4	Nonspecific abnormal findings on radiological and other examination of body structure, gastrointestinal tract

A. 45355, 793.4, 541
B. 45330, 793.4
C. 45378, 793.4
D. 45387, 793.4, 560.9

Copyright © 2005, Elsevier Inc. All rights reserved.
CPT only © 2004. *Current Procedural Terminology, 2005, Professional Edition*, American Medical Association. All rights reserved.

36. The patient is brought to the ASC for a giant congenital nevus of the left pectoral region involving the left areola. The findings indicated a 7- to 4-cm giant congenital nevus (common nevus) involving about 50% of the areola on the left side. The surgeon performs an excision of the nevus along with a portion of areola of the left chest. Under general endotracheal anesthesia of plus 4 cc of 0.5% Xylocaine and 1 : 100,000 epinephrine, the procedure was begun. The patient's chest wall was prepped with Betadine scrub and solution and draped in a routine sterile fashion. 4 cc of 0.5% Xylocaine with 1 : 100,000 epinephrine were injected along the suture line, and the lesion was excised down to carpus fascia and included the complete dermis and a little subcutaneous fat. The bleeders were cauterized and the wound closed with subcuticular 3-0 Monocryl and three twists of 6-0 Prolene. One-half-inch Steri-Strips were applied, plus a clavicle strap for immobilization. The pathology report later indicated that the tissue was benign.

11446	Excision, other benign lesion including margins (unless listed elsewhere) face, ears, eyelids, nose, lips, mucous membrane; excised diameter 0.5 cm or less
19101	Biopsy of breast; percutaneous, needle core, not using imaging guidance (separate procedure)
21555	Excision tumor, soft tissue of neck or thorax; subcutaneous
173.5	Other malignant neoplasm of skin; skin of trunk, except scrotum
216.5	Benign neoplasm of skin; skin of trunk, except scrotum
239.2	Neoplasms of unspecified nature; bone, soft tissue, and skin
-LT	Left
-22	Unusual Procedural Service

A. 21555, 173.5
B. 21555-LT, 216.5
C. 19101, 239.2
D. 11446-22-LT, 216.5

Copyright © 2005, Elsevier Inc. All rights reserved.
CPT only © 2004. *Current Procedural Terminology, 2005, Professional Edition,* American Medical Association. All rights reserved.

37. This inpatient was admitted for repair of a frozen left shoulder. The surgeon is to perform an arthroscopic debridement and joint manipulation of the shoulder. The patient was anesthetized using general anesthetic. The left shoulder was prepped and draped in the usual fashion. A standard posterior arthroscopic portal was created, and the camera was introduced into the back of the joint. There was substantial inflammation throughout the entirety of the joint. Using a switch-stick technique, an anterior portal was created and the 7-mm cannula was then brought in from the front. Using a 4.0 double-biter resector, the synovium was then debrided throughout the entirety of the rotator cuff over the surface of the biceps and the anterior ligamentous structures as well as inferior ligamentous structures. With this completed, the joint was then thoroughly irrigated to remove any blood. The articular surfaces were inspected and were found to be normal. The arthroscopic portal was closed with absorbable sutures and Steri-Strips. The joint was then manipulated.

29806	Arthroscopy, shoulder, surgical; capsulorrhaphy
80.41	Incision and excision of joint structures; division of joint capsule, ligament, or cartilage; shoulder
80.1	Incision and excision of joint structures; other arthrotomy
80.81	Incision and excision of joint structures; other local excision or destruction of lesion of joint
726.0	Peripheral enthesopathies and allied syndromes; adhesive capsulitis of shoulder
726.10	Peripheral enthesopathies and allied syndromes; rotator cuff syndrome of shoulder and allied disorders; disorders of bursae and tendons in shoulder region, unspecified
-LT	Left

A. 29806-LT, 726.0
B. 80.81, 726.10
C. 80.41, 726.0
D. 80.1, 726.10

Copyright © 2005, Elsevier Inc. All rights reserved.
CPT only © 2004. *Current Procedural Terminology, 2005, Professional Edition,* American Medical Association. All rights reserved.

38. An 81-year-old woman is brought to the ASC for debridement and irrigation of infected wound, right shoulder. This patient had previously undergone an arthroscopic mini-open repair of a right rotator cuff tear, which was performed by the same physician who is again performing this procedure. At about the 4-week stage postoperatively, she developed drainage from the wound. This cultured positive for *Staphylococcus aureus*. She was then placed on oral antibiotics and did show some improvement, but there has been persistent drainage for the last 2 weeks without evidence of resolution. Because of the continuation of this problem, the decision was made to undertake the procedure. Under general anesthetic, the patient was laid in the beach-chair position on the operating table. The anterior 3 cm of the surgical wound was excised. There was fluid drainage from this area. A sinus tract was identified that went down to the area of the anterior acromial area. The edges of the sinus tract area were then fully debrided and then irrigated using a power lavage system and 4 L of normal saline. The soft tissues around the sinus tract were sutured.

10180	Incision and drainage, complex, postoperative wound infection
11000	Debridement of extensive eczematous or infected skin, up to 10% body surface
998.51	Other complications of procedures, NEC; postoperative infection; infected postoperative seroma
998.59	Other complications of procedures, NEC; postoperative infection; other postoperative infection
041.11	Staphylococcus aureus
-78	Return to the operating room for related procedure during the postoperative period
-RT	Right
-LT	Left

A. 10180-78-RT, 998.59, 041.11
B. 11000-78-LT, 998.59
C. 11000-78-LT, 998.51
D. 10180-78-LT, 998.51

Copyright © 2005, Elsevier Inc. All rights reserved.
CPT only © 2004. *Current Procedural Terminology, 2005, Professional Edition,* American Medical Association. All rights reserved.

39. The patient presents to the ASC for a kidney biopsy. The indications are chronic renal failure, hematuria, and proteinuria. The patient was placed in the prone position. The right kidney was visualized using ultrasound provided by radiology. The skin was prepped in the usual fashion. One-percent lidocaine was used for local anesthesia. Multiple core biopsies were obtained under real ultrasound guidance using an 18-gauge biopsy gun without difficulty. Multiple core biopsies were obtained and were sent for light electromicroscopy and immune fluorescence. He was sent back to the procedure area to be monitored in 6 hours with orders for repeat hemoglobin. The pathology report later indicated primary, renal cell adenocarcinoma.
Do not report the radiology service.

50200	Renal biopsy; percutaneous, by trocar or needle
189.0	Malignant neoplasm of kidney and other and unspecified urinary organs; kidney, except pelvis
189.1	Malignant neoplasm of kidney and other and unspecified urinary organs; renal pelvis
585	Chronic renal failure
599.7	Hematuria
791.0	Nonspecific findings on examination of urine, proteinuria
-RT	Right
-LT	Left

A. 50200-RT, 189.0, 585
B. 50200-RT, 189.1, 585, 599.7, 791.0
C 50200-LT, 189.1, 585, 599.7, 791.0
D. 50200-RT, 189.0, 585, 599.7, 791.0

40. This 2-year-old male child was brought to ASC for a circumcision due to recurrent balanitis and phimosis. The patient was given general mask anesthetic as well as caudal block for postoperative pain control. He was prepped and draped in the supine position, foreskin retracted, and adhesions broken down. Circumcision was performed using a dorsal slit technique. Hemostasis was achieved with judicious use of electrocautery and chromic ties. Prepuce was re-anastomosed to the penile skin using 5-0 chromic catgut. The pathology report later indicated benign penile tissue.

54160	Circumcision, surgical excision other than clamp, device or dorsal slit; newborn
54161	Circumcision, surgical excision other than clamp, device or dorsal slit; except newborn
605	Redundant prepuce and phimosis
607.1	Disorders of the penis, balanoposthitis

A. 54161, 605
B. 54160, 605, 607.1
C. 54160, 607.1
D. 54161, 605, 607.1

Copyright © 2005, Elsevier Inc. All rights reserved.
CPT only © 2004. *Current Procedural Terminology, 2005, Professional Edition,* American Medical Association. All rights reserved.

41. A 73-year-old woman was admitted for hypotension and respiratory failure. The woman was lifting a bag of dirt from a wheelbarrow in her back yard when she began to have some diaphoresis, and she did not feel well. Her husband brought her to the ED, where she was noted to have CHF/fluid overload with chest x-ray. She has been intubated and mechanically ventilated. Lasix 80 IV was given and a p.o. dose of Lasix 60 mg. was given. Her blood pressure is trending down and is now 60/40s. Dopamine drip has been started, and the nitroglycerin drip and saline infusion setup in the ED have been discontinued. At this time, the patient has congestive heart failure, pulmonary edema that has led to respiratory failure, and acute renal failure.

428.0	Heart failure, congestive heart failure, unspecified
458.9	Hypotension
518.81	Other diseases of the lung; acute respiratory failure
584.9	Acute renal failure, unspecified
780.8	Generalized hyperhidrosis, including diaphoresis

A. 458.9, 518.81, 428.0, 584.9
B. 518.81, 428.0, 584.9
C. 458.9, 518.81, 428.0, 584.9, 780.8
D. 518.81, 428.0, 584.9, 780.8

42. This 74-year-old man was admitted to the hospital after he presented for a Cardiolite stress test. Even before the test started, he began having retrosternal chest pain, became bradycardic after a sublingual nitroglycerin spray, and had to be given atropine. His heart rate was down to about 40. After the atropine, the heart rate returned to normal. Blood pressure was briefly down to the 90s and high 80s systolic, but then, after a fluid bolus, it returned to normal before admission. The record indicated that the patient was admitted for atrial fibrillation, cardiomyopathy, and to rule out myocardial infarction. The focus of the treatment was to bring the atrial fibrillation under control.

786.50	Chest pain
427.31	Cardiac dysrhythmias, atrial fibrillation and flutter
425.4	Cardiomyopathy, other primary cardiomyopathies, including NOS
410.9	Acute myocardial infarction, unspecified site
458.9	Hypotension

A. 786.50, 427.31, 425.4, 410.9, 458.9
B. 427.31, 425.4, 410.9
C. 427.31, 425.4, 410.9, 458.9
D. 427.31, 425.4

Copyright © 2005, Elsevier Inc. All rights reserved.
CPT only © 2004. *Current Procedural Terminology, 2005, Professional Edition,* American Medical Association. All rights reserved.

43. The 58-year-old patient originally came to the ED with severe back and abdominal pain. The patient was found to have a ruptured abdominal aortic aneurysm and was taken immediately to the operating room for surgery. The abdomen was entered through a mid-line incision. His abdomen was full of blood, and only after repeated attempts to control the bleeding could the hemorrhage be controlled by suture. The patient received 5351 cc of Cellsaver, 24,000 cc of crystalloid, 500 cc of albumin, 6978 cc of RBCs, 245 cc of platelets, 1051 cc of fresh frozen plasma, and 6000 cc of lactated Ringer's for treatment of acute blood loss anemia. The patient's incisions were partially closed, and the abdominal wound was left open. Steri-Drapes were placed within the abdominal wall, and then towels were placed over the Steri-Drapes, followed by Jackson-Pratt drains and then followed by adhesive Ioban drapes. This would allow for expansion of the abdomen resulting from the edema that occurred during surgery.

39.52	Repair of aneurysm, by suture
39.98	Control of hemorrhage, NOS, excludes that by suture
285.1	Acute posthemorrhagic anemia
441	Aortic aneurysm and dissection
441.3	Abdominal aneurysm, ruptured
998.11	Hemorrhage complicating a procedure

A. 39.98, 441.3, 285.1, 998.11
B. 39.52, 441.3, 998.11
C. 39.98, 441
D. 39.52, 441.3, 285.1, 998.11

44. A patient is admitted with appendicitis and scheduled for surgery. Before anesthesia can be administered, the patient has a cerebral thrombosis and the surgeon cancels the procedure. What would be the sequence of the codes to report this admission?
A. cerebral thrombosis, appendicitis, V code to report the surgical cancellation due to contraindication
B. appendicitis, cerebral thrombosis, V code to report the surgical cancellation due to contraindication
C. procedure code for appendicitis, V code to report the surgical cancellation due to contraindication, appendicitis, cerebral thrombosis
D. V code to report the surgical cancellation due to contraindication, appendicitis, cerebral thrombosis

45. Multiple fractures are sequenced in accordance with the _______?
A. location
B. severity
C. type
D. none of these

Copyright © 2005, Elsevier Inc. All rights reserved.
CPT only © 2004. *Current Procedural Terminology, 2005, Professional Edition*, American Medical Association. All rights reserved.

46. This patient is admitted for a hemodialysis treatment. The following Assessment/Plan is indicated in the record:

ASSESSMENT/PLAN:

1. Chronic renal failure/end-stage renal disease, secondary to the following:
   a. Status post right-sided nephrectomy in 1996 **(V45.73)**
   b. Left-sided renal artery stenosis/renal vascular hypertension (**403.91)**
   c. Diabetes II
   d. Diabetic nephropathy **(250.40, 583.81)**
   e. Coronary artery disease
2. Multiple electrolyte abnormalities related to problem chronic renal failure/end-stage renal disease
   a. Hyperphosphatemia. Continue Renagel and PhosLo (**275.3)**
   b. Hypocalcemia **(274.41)**
3. Hypothyroidism. Continue Synthroid **(244.9)**

   What would be the principal diagnosis?

A. 250.40
B. 403.91
C. V45.73
D. 583.81

47. The patient has end-stage renal disease and is admitted with acute peritonitis due to an infection of her peritoneal dialysis catheter. The patient is on chronic peritoneal dialysis. She was admitted with abdominal pain and cloudy dialysate. She was found to have alpha streptococcal peritonitis. She was given vancomycin, gentamicin, and Kefzol. The alpha Strep was sensitive to cephalosporins. She did well during her hospitalization and felt better. What would be the principal diagnosis?
A. complication of a catheter, specifically an infection
B. peritonitis
C. streptococcal infection
D. end-stage renal disease

48. The patient is a 30-year-old male who suffered a massive stroke 1 month ago. The patient presents to the outpatient radiology department of the hospital for a real-time imaging and Doppler analysis to assess the current status of his vessels. The clinical indications are noted to be previous stroke with right hemiparesis and aphasia. The medical documentation concluded that there was some stenosis on the right side. The left side implied occlusion distal to the area scanned. The diagnoses would be as follows:
A. 438.11 (Late, effect, with aphasia), 438.20 (Late, effect, cerebrovascular disease with hemiplegia/hemiparesis affecting unspecified side), 434.91 (Stroke)
B. 438.20 (Late, effect, cerebrovascular disease with hemiplegia/hemiparesis affecting unspecified side), 438.11 (Late, effect, with aphasia)
C. 434.91 (Stroke)
D. 434.91 (Stroke), 438.20 (Late, effect, cerebrovascular disease with hemiplegia/hemiparesis affecting unspecified side), 438.11 (Late, effect, with aphasia)

Copyright © 2005, Elsevier Inc. All rights reserved.
CPT only © 2004. *Current Procedural Terminology, 2005, Professional Edition,* American Medical Association. All rights reserved.

49. The patient is a 34-year-old, gravida 2, para 2, who has had multiple operations in the past for endometriosis after being admitted with endometriosis and resultant chronic pelvic pain. A total abdominal hysterectomy with bilateral salpingo-oophorectomy is performed. The uterus was found to be of normal size, but there were a lot of anterior cul-de-sac adhesions over the bladder and anterior surface of the uterus. There were some adhesions between the left tube and ovary and the posterior aspect of the left broad ligament. The pathology report later indicated that the uterus, bilateral tubes, and ovaries showed "endometriosis involving serous surface of the uterus, right ovary, and left ovary, adenomyosis, proliferating endometrium."

617.2	Endometriosis of fallopian tube
617.1	Endometriosis of ovary
617.3	Endometriosis, endometriosis of pelvic peritoneum
614.6	Pelvic peritoneal adhesions, female
625.9	Pelvic pain
68.4	Total abdominal hysterectomy
65.31	Unilateral oophorectomy, other unilateral oophorectomy
65.61	Bilateral salpingo-oophorectomy, other removal of both ovaries and tubes at same operative episode

A. 68.4, 65.61, 625.9, 617.3, 614.6
B. 68.4, 65.61, 617.3, 614.6
C. 68.4, 65.31, 617.2, 617.1
D. 68.4, 65.61, 617.3

Copyright © 2005, Elsevier Inc. All rights reserved.
CPT only © 2004. *Current Procedural Terminology, 2005, Professional Edition*, American Medical Association. All rights reserved.

50. The patient, an 85-year-old white female, presents to the ASC with the preoperative diagnosis of melena. The surgeon performs an esophagogastroduodenoscopy with biopsies. Two ulcers are seen in the stomach, one in the distal antrum measuring about 6 mm in diameter. It had a clean base and was biopsied. The second ulcer is present in the pyloric channel along the posterior wall and measures about 1 to 1.2 cm in diameter. It also had a clean base without any visible vessel or fresh or old blood. The physician noted the following directions in the patient's record: 1. Prilosec 20 mg daily for 8 weeks, 2. Review biopsies, 3. Discontinued nonsteroidal anti-inflammatory agents, which are being taken for gout. The pathology report later indicated "chronic active gastritis, mild to moderate, with mucosal atrophy. Organisms consistent with *Helicobacter pylori* are present."

43236	Upper gastrointestinal endoscopy including esophagus, stomach, and either the duodenum and/or jejunum as appropriate; diagnostic, with or without collection of specimen(s) by brushing or washing (separate procedure)
43239	Upper gastrointestinal endoscopy including esophagus, stomach, and either the duodenum and/or jejunum as appropriate; with biopsy, single or multiple
041.86	Helicobacter pylori
274.9	Gout, unspecified
531.40	Gastric ulcer, chronic or unspecified with hemorrhage, without mention of obstruction
535.1	Atrophic gastritis

A. 43236, 535.1, 274.9
B. 43239, 531.40, 041.86, 274.9
C. 43239, 535.1, 041.86, 274.9
D. 43239, 531.40, 041.86

Copyright © 2005, Elsevier Inc. All rights reserved.
CPT only © 2004. *Current Procedural Terminology, 2005, Professional Edition,* American Medical Association. All rights reserved.

51. The patient is a 23-month-old female with a history of left submandibular region mass. Over the past several months, the mass has been more superficial and appears to be an epidermal inclusion cyst. The patient presents to the ASC for excision of the branchial cleft cyst. The documentation indicated the following: The patient was placed under general anesthesia and endotracheally intubated without difficulty. The tenotomy scissors were then used to dissect down to the subcutaneous tissue, and a thin capsule was identified around sebaceous-appearing material. The cystlike mass was followed with the tenotomy scissors. The cyst was entered slightly superiorly, and thick sebaceous material extruded from the mass. The tenotomy scissors were used to dissect around the mass, taking care to stay close to the capsule but not entering into the cyst itself. Dissection was done medially, laterally, and inferiorly. Superiorly, the lesion appeared to extend medially and beneath the mandible. The cyst was followed gently. The cyst extended up inferior to the mandible, and by retracting with the stay stitch, it was removed in bulk. Upon examination of the wound, the lesion extended beneath the platysma down the medial aspect of the mandible. The patient tolerated the procedure well and was awakened from anesthesia.

The pathology report later indicated the following: Tissue with multiple caseating granuloma and acid-fast bacilli, highly consistent with tuberculosis.

42810	Excision of branchial cleft cyst, or vestige, confined to skin or subcutaneous tissue
42815	Excision of branchial cleft cyst, vestige, or fistula, extending beneath subcutaneous tissues, and/or into pharynx
017.25	Tuberculosis of other organs, peripheral lymph nodes
744.42	Branchial cleft cyst or fistula; branchial cleft cyst

A. 42810, 744.42, 017.25
B. 42810, 744.42
C. 42815, 744.42
D. 42815, 017.25

52. According to the UHDDS, the definition of a principal diagnosis is as follows:
A. condition established after study to occasion the admission of the patient to the hospital
B. the primary reason for the encounter
C. condition established after study to have caused this most recent admission
D. none of the above

Copyright © 2005, Elsevier Inc. All rights reserved.
CPT only © 2004. *Current Procedural Terminology, 2005, Professional Edition*, American Medical Association. All rights reserved.

53. A patient is admitted 2 months after a motor vehicle accident. The initial treatment of a fracture of the right femur has not been successful; she has a nonunion of the bones, which has given her pain on weight bearing. She is admitted for treatment of the fracture by means of open reduction and internal fixation, which will be followed with traction. During the procedure there is extensive hemorrhaging from the area, and the surgeon documents that the hemorrhage is finally brought under control. The patient is taken to the recovery area in stable condition. The patient was treated with 2 units PRBCs for acute blood loss.

285.1	Other and unspecified anemia; acute posthemorrhagic anemia
733.82	Malunion of fracture
905.4	Late effects, fracture, extremity lower
998.11	Hemorrhage, intraoperative or postoperative
79.15	Reduction of fracture and dislocation, closed reduction of fracture with internal fixation, femur
79.35	Reduction of fracture and dislocation; open reduction of fracture with internal fixation, femur

A. 79.15, 733.82, 285.1, 905.4, 998.11
B. 79.35, 733.82, 285.1, 905.4, 998.11
C. 79.35, 733.82, 285.1, 998.11
D. 79.35, 998.11, 733.82, 285.1, 905.4

54. This 60-year-old disabled female is admitted for marked congestion and respiratory distress. She is known to have mental retardation and frequent urinary tract and pulmonary infections. She has a recurrent epileptic disorder that is well controlled with Dilantin. On admission the vital signs indicate 101 F, 33 breaths per minute, 83 bpm, and bp of 120/70 mm Hg. Chest has bilateral crepitation that is diagnosed as bilateral staphylococcal pneumonia. The lab report indicates the patient has a urinary infection due to gram-negative bacteria. The patient is treated with intravenous vancomycin and Fortaz and shows marked improvement. The hospital course goes well, and the patient is discharged to the skilled nursing facility.

041.89	Bacterial infection in conditions classified elsewhere and of unspecified site; other specified bacterial infections; other gram-negative organisms
319	Unspecified mental retardation
345.90	Epilepsy, unspecified
482.40	Pneumonia, due to, staphylococcal, unspecified
482.49	Pneumonia, due to, other staphylococcal
518.82	Other diseases of the lung; other pulmonary insufficiency, NEC, including acute respiratory distress
599.0	Urinary tract infection, site not specified

A. 482.40, 518.82, 599.0, 041.89, 345.90
B. 518.82, 482.49, 319, 599.0, 041.89, 345.90
C. 482.49, 518.82, 319, 599.0, 041.89, 345.90
D. 518.82, 482.40, 319, 599.0, 041.89, 345.90

Copyright © 2005, Elsevier Inc. All rights reserved.
CPT only © 2004. *Current Procedural Terminology, 2005, Professional Edition*, American Medical Association. All rights reserved.

55. A patient, who underwent an elective abortion 5 days earlier, is admitted because of continued bleeding. A dilation and curettage is performed, resulting in removal of retained products of conception.

A. 634.11	Spontaneous abortion, complicated by delayed or excessive hemorrhage
B. 635.11	Legally induced abortion, complicated by delayed or excessive hemorrhage, incomplete
C. 638.1	Failed attempted abortion, complicated by delayed or excessive hemorrhage
D. 639	Complications following abortion and ectopic and molar pregnancies

56. A patient with advanced metastatic carcinoma of the breast is experiencing shortness of breath and is admitted to the hospital. She was dehydrated. The medical documentation indicates that the discharge diagnosis for this patient was uncontrolled pain and difficulty breathing that was secondary to widely metastatic breast carcinoma, dehydration, and uncontrolled type II diabetes. What would the principal diagnosis be?
A. malignant, primary, neoplasm of the breast
B. malignant, secondary, neoplasm of the breast
C. either A or B
D. uncontrolled type II diabetes

57. The patient is at 32 weeks' gestation and is admitted with severe bleeding with abdominal cramping. She is diagnosed with placenta previa, with indications of fetal distress. An emergency cesarean section is done. A viable male infant is delivered.

74.0	Classic cesarean section
74.99	Cesarean section of unspecified type
641.11	Pregnancy complicated by placenta previa
655.8	Other known or suspected fetal abnormality, NEC
656.31	Delivery, cesarean, with fetus in distress
V27.0	Outcome of delivery, single liveborn

A. 74.99, 641.11, 656.31, V27.0
B. 74.0, 641.11, 656.31
C. 74.0, 641.11, 655.8, V27.0
D. 74.99, 641.11, 656.31

Copyright © 2005, Elsevier Inc. All rights reserved.
CPT only © 2004. *Current Procedural Terminology, 2005, Professional Edition*, American Medical Association. All rights reserved.

58. Sally, a 19-year-old, was lighting a bonfire in the backyard when she sustained burns. The following burns were sustained and treated: third-degree burn—left upper arm (5%), second-degree burn—left upper arm (1%), first-degree burn—left anterior leg (9%). The codes for this diagnosis would be as follows:

943.33	Burn of upper limb, except wrist and hand, full-thickness skin loss [third degree NOS], upper arm
943.23	Burn of upper limb, except wrist and hand, blisters, epidermal loss [second degree], upper arm
945.10	Burn of lower limb, erythema [first degree], lower limb, unspecified site
948.00	Burns classified according to extent of body surface involved, <10 percent body surface, less than 10 percent involved in third degree
948.10	Burns classified according to extent of body surface involved, 10–19 percent body surface, less than 10 percent involved in third degree

A. 943.33, 943.23, 945.10, 948.10
B. 943.23, 945.10, 948.00
C. 943.33, 945.10, 948.10
D. 943.33, 943.23, 945.10

59. A 44-year-old female presented to the ED after she was injured on her farm, where she was treating a sick calf when a cow attacked her and stomped her. She was brought into the emergency room via ambulance complaining of an open right ankle dislocation and multiple abrasions. She also complained of some abrasions on her chin and under her left leg. Specifically, she denied loss of consciousness or headache. The toes were all dusky, she had a strong posterior tibial pulse, and the nurse thought she felt a faint dorsalis pedis. She had an abrasion under her left leg. She was given a tetanus shot and 1 g of Ancef. Immediately she was given parenteral fentanyl and Versed to allow for the reduction of the dislocation without difficulty. Postreduction film looked good. There was perhaps a subtle fracture noted only on the lateral projection. C-spine showed some degenerative change, but upon reexamination she was not tender in that area, but that may have been because she had such a severe distracting injury. Chest x-ray and left femur looked fine.

837.1	Dislocation of the foot, open dislocation, tarsal bone
837.4	Dislocation of the foot, open dislocation, metatarsal bone
910.0	Superficial injury of face, neck, and scalp except eye; abrasion or friction burn without mention of infection
910.8	Superficial injury of face, neck, and scalp except eye; other and unspecified superficial injury of face, neck, and scalp without mention of infection
916.0	Superficial injury of hip, thigh, leg, and ankle; abrasion or friction burn without mention of infection
916.8	Superficial injury of hip, thigh, leg, and ankle; other and unspecified injury of hip, thigh, leg, and ankle without mention of infection
E906.8	Attacked by an animal

A. Level 5, 837.1, 910.0, 916.0, E906.8
B. Level 4, 837.4, 910.0, 916.8
C. Level 5, 837.1, 910.0, 916.0
D. Level 5, 837.4, 910.8, 916.8

Copyright © 2005, Elsevier Inc. All rights reserved.
CPT only © 2004. *Current Procedural Terminology, 2005, Professional Edition*, American Medical Association. All rights reserved.

60. This payment status indicator indicates significant procedures for which payment is allowed under OPPS but to which multiple procedure reduction does not apply, such as nuclear medicine and CAT scan.
    A. J
    B. A
    C. N
    D. S

Copyright © 2005, Elsevier Inc. All rights reserved.
CPT only © 2004. *Current Procedural Terminology, 2005, Professional Edition*, American Medical Association. All rights reserved.

PART 2

Section A

1. CASE 1

   LOCATION: Hospital inpatient

   PREOPERATIVE DIAGNOSIS: Obstructed ventriculoperitoneal shunt.

   PROCEDURE PERFORMED: Revision of shunt. Replacement of ventricular valve and peritoneal end. Entire shunt replacement.

   PROCEDURE: Under general anesthesia, the patient's head, neck, and abdomen were prepped and draped in the usual manner. An incision was made over the previous site where the shunt had been inserted in the posterior right occipital area. This shunt was found to be nonfunctioning and was removed. The problem was that we could not get the ventricular catheter out without probably producing bleeding, so it was left inside. The peritoneal end of the shunt was then pulled out through the same incision. Having done this, I placed a new ventricular catheter into the ventricle. I then attached this to a medium-pressure bulb valve and secured this with 3-0 silk to the subcutaneous tissue. We then went to the abdomen and made an incision below the previous site, and we were able to trocar the peritoneal end of the shunt by making a stab wound in the neck and then connecting it up to the shunt. This was then connected to the shunt. Pumping on the shunt, we got fluid coming out the other end. I then inserted this end of the shunt into the abdomen by dividing the rectus fascia, splitting the muscle, and dividing the peritoneum and placing the shunt into the abdomen. One 2-0 chromic suture was used around the peritoneum. The wound was then closed with 2-0 Vicryl, 2-0 plain in the subcutaneous tissue, and surgical staples on the skin. The stab wound on the neck was closed with surgical staples. The head wound was closed with 2-0 Vicryl on the galea and surgical staples on the skin. A dressing was applied. The patient was discharged to the recovery room.

Copyright © 2005, Elsevier Inc. All rights reserved.
CPT only © 2004. *Current Procedural Terminology, 2005, Professional Edition*, American Medical Association. All rights reserved.

2. CASE 2

LOCATION: Inpatient hospital.

PREOPERATIVE DIAGNOSIS: Colitis, terminal ileitis, and possible appendicitis.

POSTOPERATIVE DIAGNOSIS: Acute appendicitis. No evidence of abscess or peritonitis. No pus in the abdomen.

PROCEDURE PERFORMED: Laparoscopic abdominal exploration, laparoscopic mobilization of the cecum converted to open appendectomy due to small serosal tear in the terminal ileum from a retraction injury.

SPECIMEN: Appendix.

ANESTHESIA: General endotracheal with 30 cc of Marcaine local augmentation.

PROCEDURE IN DETAIL: After good general endotracheal anesthesia, the patient was prepped and draped in the usual sterile fashion. A Foley and OT tube were both placed to decompress the stomach and also the bladder. A small infraumbilical incision was made, and under direct vision the fascia was nicked. The Veress needle was placed in the fascia, and the abdomen was insufflated to 16 Torr. After this, the fascial incision was lengthened, and a No.10 trocar was placed. The camera was placed through this, and the abdomen was inspected. The cecum was quite inflamed. The base of the appendix was noted. The appendix itself was stuck down to the cecum. The area of terminal ileum just adjacent to the cecum was inflamed. The cecum was mobilized, and the peritoneal reflection was taken down. This was done with hot scissors. Care was taken not to injure the bowel. The ovary was inspected and was normal. The appendix was felt to be quite friable, and there was a small serosal tear created with the Kitner while mobilizing the cecum. We were unable to determine laparoscopically whether this is just a serosal tear; additionally, the tissue was so friable that we were not confident that we would be able to close the stump of the appendix with an endoscopic stapler. Therefore the decision was made to open the abdomen. This was done with appendiceal incision. A Rocky-Davis incision was made after anesthetizing the area with Marcaine. The external oblique and transversus abdominis fascia was incised, and a muscle-sparing technique was applied. The peritoneum was entered, and the cecum was brought up into the wound. The base of the appendix was identified, and it was so friable that we could not simply tie off the base of the appendix and amputate the appendix distally. It was necessary to close the cecum where the appendix was attached and to divide the appendix off the cecum. This was done with running 3-0 Vicryl. After this, some imbricating 3-0 silk stitches were placed. Attention was then turned to the serosal injury. This indeed turned out to be just serosa. This was on the terminal ileum. The serosal injury was repaired with interrupted 3-0 silk. Next, the abdomen was irrigated, and pneumoperitoneum was sucked out. The pneumoperitoneum was released. The two ports, the No. 10 port and the No. 5 subport, were removed. The camera port was also removed. This was done prior to opening the abdomen. All the fascial stitches were used to close the umbilical port and also the left No. 10 port sites. The appendiceal wound was closed in layers with the peritoneum, and two layers of fascia were closed separately. The skin was closed with 4-0 Vicryl. Steri-Strips and sterile dressings were applied. The patient tolerated the procedure well, and sponge and needle counts were correct. She was extubated in the operating room and returned to the recovery room in good condition.

Copyright © 2005, Elsevier Inc. All rights reserved.
CPT only © 2004. *Current Procedural Terminology, 2005, Professional Edition,* American Medical Association. All rights reserved.

3. CASE 3

LOCATION: ASC

PREOPERATIVE DIAGNOSIS: Nasal obstruction with sleep apnea, septal deviation due to trauma, bilateral inferior turbinate hypertrophy, left middle turbinate hypertrophy, left concha bullosa.

POSTOPERATIVE DIAGNOSIS: Same.

PROCEDURE: Septoplasty, bilateral inferior turbinate reduction, and endoscopic excision of left concha bullosa.

PROCEDURE DESCRIPTION: Following informed consent from the patient, she was taken to the operating room and placed supine on the operating room table. The appropriate monitoring devices were placed on the patient, and general anesthesia was induced. She was orally intubated without difficulty. She was draped in the usual sterile fashion. The nose was packed bilaterally with Afrin-soaked gauze. The 0-degree endoscope was passed into the left nasal cavity after gauze removal. She was seen to have a left inferior septal spur somewhat anterior and a large left middle turbinate that was grossly widened. The concha bullosa was injected with approximately 0.5 cc of 1% Xylocaine with epinephrine. A sickle knife was used to incise through the base of the concha bullosa. Straight scissors were then used to further cut through the bony attachment of the concha bullosa to the middle turbinate. It was then removed in one thin section with the straight Wilde forceps. There was very little bleeding. I did repack the left osteomeatal complex with the Afrin-soaked gauze; after 2 minutes this was removed, and there was no bleeding.

The right and left nasal septums were each then injected with approximately 2 cc of lidocaine with epinephrine. The nasal septum was seen to be deviated superiorly on the right and left septal spur with some left posterior deviation as well. An incision was made at the anterior end of the right nasal septum. A mucoperichondrial and mucoperiosteal flap were then elevated. A 7 × 12 mm section of septal cartilage in the midportion of the cartilaginous septum was then removed. A mucoperichondrial and mucoperiosteal flap were then removed. A mucoperichondrial and mucoperiosteal flap were then elevated on the left nasal septum. Some of the bony vomer contributing to left posterior septal deviation was removed. No tear in the septum was created during this procedure. I did use an osteotome to remove the left septal spur with good result. Some of the superior, anterior, and right septal deviation was removed. However, I did not remove all of it since quite a bit of the right septal deviation was superior and did not contribute to any deviation of the inferior nasal septum on the right side. A small incision was made on the right nasal septum to allow for hematoma prevention. The inferior edges of both inferior turbinates were then cauterized with the needle point cautery. The butter knife was used to outfracture the inferior turbinates bilaterally. The nasopharynx was suctioned of blood. The anterior end of the nasal septal mucosa was reapproximated with 4-0 chromic catgut in an interrupted fashion. Doyle splints were then applied to the right and left nasal cavities bilaterally. They were sutured anteriorly with a 3-0 Ethilon suture tied on the left side. The patient was then allowed to recover from general anesthesia. She was transferred to the recovery room in good condition. She tolerated the procedure well. Estimated blood loss was less than 20 cc.

Copyright © 2005, Elsevier Inc. All rights reserved.
CPT only © 2004. *Current Procedural Terminology, 2005, Professional Edition*, American Medical Association. All rights reserved.

4. CASE 4

   LOCATION: ASC

   PREOPERATIVE DIAGNOSIS: Deviated septum.

   PROCEDURE PERFORMED:

   1. Septoplasty
   2. Resection of turbinates

   The patient was taken to the operating room and placed under general anesthesia. The fracture of the turbinates was first performed to do the septoplasty. Once this was done, the septoplasty was completed and the turbinates were placed back in their original position. The patient was taken to recovery in satisfactory condition. Code the procedure(s) and the diagnosis.

Copyright © 2005, Elsevier Inc. All rights reserved.
CPT only © 2004. *Current Procedural Terminology, 2005, Professional Edition,* American Medical Association. All rights reserved.

5. CASE 5

HISTORY AND PHYSICAL

LOCATION: Inpatient hospital

CHIEF COMPLAINT: Shortness of breath and back pain.

HISTORY OF PRESENT ILLNESS: This is a 90-year-old female with known history of coronary artery disease who was recently admitted on April 24 with a non-Q-wave myocardial infarction which was elected to be treated conservatively. Since that time the patient has felt relatively okay up until last night when the patient indicates she felt like she had increasing shortness of breath with pain in her chest which seemed to radiate into her back. The patient denied any associated diaphoresis or nausea which she had with her prior event. This pain came and went. It kind of resolved overnight. The patient's symptoms returned drastically this morning and subsequently the patient was unable to essentially move at home. She had her meals-on-wheels delivered and the delivery person called for the ambulance for her. Subsequently the patient presented to the emergency department.

In the emergency department, the patient received oxygen and nitroglycerin, which improved the patient's symptomatology.

Currently, patient denies any chest pain or chest pressure, or any nausea. The patient indicates she is currently not short of breath. The patient denies any increased swelling in her legs.

ALLERGIES: Sulfa.

PAST MEDICAL HISTORY:

1. Diabetes mellitus.
2. Glaucoma.
3. Coronary artery disease.
4. Hypertension.

MEDICATIONS:

1. Norvasc 5 mg daily.
2. Aspirin 81 mg daily.
3. Atenolol 50 mg daily.
4. Bumex 0.5 daily.
5. Plavix 75 mg daily.
6. Enalapril 40 mg daily.
7. Glyburide 2.5 mg daily.
8. Imdur 60 mg daily.
9. Xalatan eye drops.
10. Protonix 04 mg daily.
11. Timolol eye drops.

FAMILY HISTORY: Noncontributory.

REVIEW OF SYSTEMS: General, GI, cardiovascular, respiratory, ENT, eyes, neurologic, musculoskeletal, psych, endocrine performed. With the exception of those noted in the HPI and chronic paresthesias in patient's feet, otherwise unremarkable.

EXAMINATION: Vitals today: Temperature 36.4, pulse 65, respiratory rate 19, blood pressure 141/41, O2 sats 91% in room air. Cardiovascular: S1 and S2. No S3 or S4. Heart sounds are distant. Lungs: Bilateral breath sounds with crackles present. HEENT: Head is atraumatic. Extraocular movements are intact. Nonjaundiced sclera. Moist oral mucosal membranes. Neck is supple. Trachea is midline. The patient does have JVD. Abdomen is soft and nontender. Positive bowel sounds. No rebound tenderness or

Copyright © 2005, Elsevier Inc. All rights reserved.
CPT only © 2004. *Current Procedural Terminology, 2005, Professional Edition*, American Medical Association. All rights reserved.

guarding. No masses palpated. Extremities: Trace edema. Musculoskeletal: Patient moves all four extremities symmetrically and to command. Neurologic: Minimally decreased sensation to light touch in the lower extremities. Psych: Patient alert and oriented. Integument: No obvious petechia or purpura.
PA portable chest x-ray, which I visualized in the emergency department, shows pulmonary edema and no opacities.

LABORATORY DATA: Platelet count 162,000, white count 12.31, hemoglobin 9.4, BUN 41, sodium 139, potassium 4.9, chloride 102, bicarb 24.7, glucose 256, creatinine 1.4, calcium 8.3, CPK 27, troponin 0.07.

IMPRESSION:

1. Acute pulmonary edema.
2. Unstable angina.
3. Diabetes mellitus.

PLAN: At this point, we will admit the patient. The patient indicates that she wishes to be a code level II. Will place the patient on nitroglycerin at 5 mcg initial rate, titrating until chest is pain free or systolic pressure greater than 100. Provide the patient with Lovenox 1 mg/kg subcutaneously q. 12 hours. Will adjust dose for renal function as necessary. Keep the patient on aspirin. Keep the patient on beta blocker. Blood sugar checks q.i.d. Supplemental insulin scale. Continue the patient on glyburide. Serial cardiac enzymes. Obtain a UA and UC.

RADIOLOGY REPORT

EXAMINATION OF: Chest.

CLINICAL SYMPTOMS: Shortness of breath.

CHEST: 1:15 PM: Findings: Comparison is made with the portable chest of last month. Cardiac enlargement is unchanged given the difference in technique. Pulmonary vascularity is mildly elevated and has increased mildly since the previous study. No focal infiltrates. Slight fibrosis or atelectasis in the bases. Blunting of the right costophrenic angle is unchanged due to fluid or pleural thickening. No mediastinal widening.

PROGRESS REPORT

SUBJECTIVE: The patient indicates that she did have some chest discomfort last night, with some dyspnea. The patient received morphine, which improved her discomfort. The patient currently indicates that she is not short of breath. Her pain has resolved. The patient, however, feels fatigued at this point.

REVIEW OF SYSTEMS: General, gastrointestinal, cardiovascular, respiratory, and endocrine were performed, and with the exception of those noted in HPI, review was negative.

OBJECTIVE: Heart: Regular. No murmurs. Lungs: Bilateral breath sounds. No wheezes or rhonchi. Abdomen: Soft and nontender with positive bowel sounds. Extremities: No edema. Vitals: Pulse: 56. Blood Pressure: 97/43. Respiratory rate: 14. O2 sats: 96% on 4 liters. Psych: Alert and oriented.

IMPRESSION:

1. Non-Q-wave MI.
2. Pulmonary edema secondary to #1.
3. Diabetes mellitus.
4. Hypotension with history of hypertension.
5. Gastroesophageal reflux disease.
6. Overall poor prognosis.

Copyright © 2005, Elsevier Inc. All rights reserved.
CPT only © 2004. *Current Procedural Terminology, 2005, Professional Edition*, American Medical Association. All rights reserved.

PLAN: At this point, we did discuss with the patient the continued goal of conservative management as recommended by cardiology on admission. The patient is in agreement with this. Again, the patient has mild hypotension. We will decrease the patient's antihypertensive agents. We will continue the patient on her Imdur at 60 mg twice a day. We will obtain a basic metabolic panel today. We will continue the patient on her aspirin, beta blocker, and ACE inhibitor, although beta blocker needs to be at a lower dose. We will continue the patient on her Lovenox. We will obtain daily CBC and daily basic metabolic panel.

PROGRESS NOTE

SUBJECTIVE: The patient denies any chest pain, chest pressure, fever, chills, or nausea. The patient indicates she is feeling better today. The patient did have a hyperglycemic reaction this morning. However the patient indicates that this resolved.

REVIEW OF SYSTEMS: General, cardiovascular, respiratory, and endocrinology were performed. With the exception noted in the HPI, all are negative.

PHYSICAL EXAMINATION: VITALS: today: Temp is 36.1. Blood pressure is 105/42. Pulse is 71. Respiratory rate is 18. O2 sats are 97% on room air. Cardiovascular: S1 and S2. No S3, no S4. No murmurs, clicks, gallops, or rubs. Lungs: Bilateral breath sounds. No wheezes, rhonchi, or crackles. In general, a pleasant female lying comfortably in bed. The abdomen was soft and nontender. Positive bowel sounds. Psych: The patient is alert and oriented.

LABORATORY STUDIES: Blood sugars of 44, 120, 96, 88, and 102.

Reviewed nurse's and physical therapy notes. The patient refused physical therapy yesterday.

IMPRESSION:

1. Non-Q-wave MI.
2. Diabetes mellitus with moderate hypoglycemic reaction, currently improved.
3. Hypertension, improving.
4. Acute pulmonary edema, resolving.

PLAN: At this point, continue the patient on current diabetes mellitus medications. Continue the patient on current conservative therapy for her non-Q-wave MI and occupational and physical therapy. Have social service plan for discharge planning. It is possible that the patient may require nursing home placement given her poor functional status.

DISCHARGE SUMMARY

PRIMARY DIAGNOSES:

1. Acute myocardial infarction.
2. Pulmonary edema.
3. Coronary artery disease.
4. Diabetes mellitus.
5. Anemia.
6. Hypertension.
7. Gastroesophageal reflux disease.
8. Chronic renal failure.

HOSPITAL COURSE: The patient was admitted with acute pulmonary edema. Serial cardiac enzymes showed the patient to have a non-Q-wave myocardial infarction with a troponin of 0.85. The patient subsequently diuresed. The patient's Imdur was increased. The patient did exhibit some hypotension. The patient's antihypertensive dosage was reduced. The patient was also found to be anemic. The patient did consent to blood transfusion. The patient received 2 units packed red blood cells. The patient's symptoms did improve.

Copyright © 2005, Elsevier Inc. All rights reserved.
CPT only © 2004. *Current Procedural Terminology, 2005, Professional Edition*, American Medical Association. All rights reserved.

The patient was also noted to have chronic renal failure. The patient's renal failure was monitored, which essentially remained unchanged during hospital stay with some fluctuation. Creatinine 1.4 on admission and creatinine 1.6 with discharge.

EXAMINATION ON THE DAY OF DISCHARGE: Alert and oriented female. Heart is regular. No murmurs. Lungs: Fine breath founds. No wheezes or rhonchi. No crackles. Abdomen soft, nontender. Positive bowel sounds. Psychiatry: Patient alert and oriented.

The patient did have a hemoglobin of 9 upon discharge.

DISCHARGE MEDICATIONS:

1. Aspirin 81 mg a day.
2. Atenolol 25 mg daily.
3. Plavix 75 mg daily.
4. Lasix 20 mg twice a day.
5. Glyburide 2.5 mg daily.
6. Imdur 60 mg twice a day.
7. Xalatan eyedrops.
8. Protonix 40 mg daily.
9. Enalapril 20 mg daily.
10. Timolol eyedrops.

DISCHARGE INSTRUCTIONS: The patient is discharged home. Follow up with Dr. Green in 1 to 2 weeks with CBC. If the patient has any difficulties, she should return to the emergency department or contact Dr. Green's office.

6. CASE 6

   LOCATION: Hospital inpatient

   PREOPERATIVE DIAGNOSIS: Ventilator dependency, aspiration pneumonia.

   PROCEDURE PERFORMED: Tracheostomy.

   DESCRIPTION OF PROCEDURE: After consent was obtained, the patient was taken to the operating room and placed on the operating room table in the supine position. After an adequate level of general endotracheal anesthesia was obtained, the patient was positioned for tracheostomy. The patient's neck was prepped with Betadine and then draped in a sterile manner. A curvilinear incision was marked approximately a finger breadth above the sternal notch in any area just below the cricoid cartilage. This area was then infiltrated with 1% Xylocaine with 1 : 100,000 units of epinephrine. After several minutes, sharp dissection was carried down through the skin and subcutaneous tissue. The subcutaneous fat was removed down to the strap muscles. Strap muscles were divided in the midline and retracted laterally. The cricoid cartilage was then identified. The thyroid gland was divided in the midline with the Bovie, and then the two lobes were retracted laterally, exposing the anterior wall of the trachea. The space between the second and third tracheal rings was then identified. This was infiltrated with local solution. A cut was then made through the anterior wall. The endotracheal tube was then advanced superiorly. An inferior cut into the third tracheal ring was then done to make a flap. This was secured to the skin with 4-0 Vicryl suture. A No. 6 Shiley cuffed tracheostomy tube was then placed and secured to the skin with ties as well as the tracheostomy strap. The patient tolerated the procedure well and was taken to the critical care unit in stable condition. Report the procedure(s) and diagnosis.

Copyright © 2005, Elsevier Inc. All rights reserved.
CPT only © 2004. *Current Procedural Terminology, 2005, Professional Edition,* American Medical Association. All rights reserved.

7. CASE 7

   OPERATIVE REPORT

   LOCATION: Hospital Outpatient

   PROCEDURE: Excision of parotid tumor or gland or both.

   Once the patient was successfully under general anesthetic, Dr. Green, assisted by Dr. Smith, opened the area in which the parotid gland is located. After carefully inspecting the gland, the decision was made to excise the total gland because of the size of the tumor (5.0 cm). With careful dissection and preservation of the facial nerve, the parotid gland was removed. The wound was cleaned and closed, and the patient was brought to recovery in satisfactory condition.

8. CASE 8

   OPERATIVE REPORT

   LOCATION: ASC

   PREOPERATIVE DIAGNOSIS: Barrett's esophagus with severe dysplasia, possible carcinoma.

   POSTOPERATIVE DIAGNOSIS: Same.

   PROCEDURE PERFORMED: Exploratory laparotomy, biopsy of liver lesion, immobilization of stomach with pyloroplasty, and placement of feeding tube.

   OPERATIVE NOTE: With the patient under general anesthesia, the abdomen was prepped and draped in a sterile manner. Midline incision was made from the xiphoid to below the pubis. Sharp dissection was carried down into the peritoneal cavity, and hemostasis was maintained with electrocautery. We began by exploring the abdominal cavity. The liver was carefully palpated. The area that had been identified on CT was at the very apex of the right lobe of the liver. We could feel this area, and it did not have a thickened feel to it but was more consistent with an area of hemangioma. There was a small secondary lesion on the undersurface of the right lobe. A biopsy was taken, and it did return a diagnosis of hemangioma. The rest of the liver appeared normal, and in my opinion we did not need to proceed with anything further. We thus began with mobilization of the stomach, taking down the greater curvature vessels and preserving the gastroepiploica. We carried our dissection all the way up into the hiatal hernia, preserving the blood supply to the spleen and not injuring it. We were then able to detach the left gastric artery such that the stomach was tethered on its other vasculature but appeared completely viable. All these vessels were taken down with clamps and ligatures of 2-0 silk. We then circumferentially went around the esophagus and carried our dissection all the way back toward the pylorus. We then had the entire stomach freed up from the pylorus all the way up to the diaphragm. The stomach appeared viable with reasonable circulation. A Heineke-Mikulicz pyloroplasty then was performed to open the pylorus in one direction and close it in another using interrupted 3-0 silk sutures to complete the pyloroplasty. With this accomplished, we then picked up the jejunum approximated 40 or 50 cm beyond the ligament of Treitz and placed a red rubber feeding tube using a Witzel technique; this was a No. 18-2. The tube was attached to the skin and brought out through a separate stab incision. The abdominal cavity was then checked for hemostasis, and everything appeared to be intact. We then closed the incision using running 0 loop nylon. We closed the skin with staples. A sterile dressing was applied. Code the diagnosis and the biopsy of the liver lesion and pyloroplasty only.

Copyright © 2005, Elsevier Inc. All rights reserved.
CPT only © 2004. *Current Procedural Terminology, 2005, Professional Edition*, American Medical Association. All rights reserved.

9. CASE 9

   OPERATIVE REPORT

   LOCATION: Ambulatory Surgical Center

   PREOPERATIVE DIAGNOSIS: Upper gastrointestinal bleeding.

   POSTOPERATIVE DIAGNOSIS: Multiple serpiginous ulcers in the gastric antrum and body, not bleeding.

   FINDINGS: The video therapeutic double-channel endoscope was passed without difficulty into the oropharynx. The gastroesophageal junction was seen at 42 cm. Inspection of the esophagus revealed no erythema, ulceration, exudates, stricture, or other mucosal abnormalities. The stomach proper was entered. The endoscope was advanced to the second duodenum. Inspection of the second duodenum, first duodenum, duodenal bulb, and pylorus revealed no abnormalities. Retroflexion revealed no lesion along the cardia or lesser curvature. Inspection of the antrum, body, and fundus of the stomach revealed no abnormality except there were multiple serpiginous ulcerations in the gastric antrum and body. They were not bleeding. They had no recent stigmata of bleeding. Photographs and biopsies were obtained. The patient tolerated the procedure well.

10. CASE 10

    OPERATIVE REPORT

    LOCATION: Outpatient Surgery Center

    DIAGNOSIS: Large bladder neck obstruction.

    PROCEDURE PERFORMED: Cystoscopy and transurethral resection of the prostate.

    The patient is a 78-year-old male with obstructive symptoms and subsequent urinary retention. The patient underwent the usual spinal anesthetic, was put in the dorsolithotomy position, prepped, and draped in the usual fashion. Cystoscopic visualization showed a marked high-riding bladder. Median lobe enlargement was such that it was difficult even to get the cystoscope over. Inside the bladder, marked trabeculation was noted. No stones were present.

    The urethra was well-lubricated and dilated. The resectoscopic sheath was passed with the aid of obturator with some difficulty because of the median lobe. TURP of the median lobe was performed, getting several big loops of tissue, which helped to improve visualization. Anterior resection of the roof was carried out from the bladder neck. Bladder-wall resection was taken from 10 to 8 o'clock. This eliminated the rest of the median lobe tissue as well. The patient tolerated the procedure well. Code the procedure(s) performed and the diagnosis.

Copyright © 2005, Elsevier Inc. All rights reserved.
CPT only © 2004. *Current Procedural Terminology, 2005, Professional Edition*, American Medical Association. All rights reserved.

11. CASE 11

    LOCATION: Outpatient Surgery Center

    PREOPERATIVE DIAGNOSIS: Right inguinal hernia.

    POSTOPERATIVE DIAGNOSIS: Right direct and right indirect inguinal hernia.

    PROCEDURE: The patient was brought to the operating room and placed in a supine position on the operating table. After satisfactory general anesthesia had been induced, the patient's abdomen and groins were prepped and draped in a sterile manner. A short transverse incision was made over the right inguinal area. Subcutaneous tissue was divided sharply. Ties and cautery were used for hemostasis. The external oblique aponeurosis was identified and opened from above downward. The ilioinguinal nerve was identified and protected. The patient had a direct inguinal hernia about 1 cm superior and medial to the internal ring. It was properitoneal fat pushed through a very small opening of about 0.5 cm in size. We reduced this and closed the hole with interrupted Ethibond, which gave a solid closure without tension. We then dissected up the round ligament and ligated it distally. Proximally, we then separated the round ligament from a small sac. We ligated the round ligament from a small internal sac. We then closed the internal ring with Ethibond suture in a Bassini repair. This gave us a solid repair and fixed the hernias. We then irrigated the wound with neomycin. Final sponge and needle counts were taken; they were correct. We then closed the external oblique aponeurosis with Vicryl. Subcutaneous tissue was closed with chromic and skin with nylon. Blood loss during the procedure was minimal. The patient tolerated the procedure well and left for the recovery room in stable condition.

Copyright © 2005, Elsevier Inc. All rights reserved.
CPT only © 2004. *Current Procedural Terminology, 2005, Professional Edition,* American Medical Association. All rights reserved.

Section B

12. CASE 12

    LOCATION: Hospital Inpatient

    PREOPERATIVE DIAGNOSIS: Bleeding from splenic laceration with hemodynamic instability.

    POSTOPERATIVE DIAGNOSIS: Bleeding from splenic laceration with hemodynamic instability.

    PROCEDURE PERFORMED: Exploratory laparotomy and splenectomy.

    SPECIMEN: Spleen.

    OPERATIVE FINDINGS: There was a small grade 1 laceration of the left lobe of the liver that was not bleeding. There was a grade 4 laceration of the spleen with a large capsular hematoma that had ruptured, and there was active bleeding here. There were 1200 cc of blood in the abdomen. There was no other solid or hollow viscous injury. After good general endotracheal anesthesia, the patient was prepped and draped in the usual sterile fashion. A midline incision was made from the xiphoid process down to the umbilicus. The abdomen was entered, and the hemoperitoneum was released. This was evacuated, and the abdomen was packed off in four quadrants. We then inspected for bleeding. The liver was inspected, and there was a small amount of bleeding laceration of the edge of the left lobe. The bowel was run from the ligament of Treitz to the cecum, and no injury was noted. The ascending transverse and descending colon were inspected, as was the stomach, and no injures were noted. There was no retroperitoneal hematoma noted. The spleen itself, however, was bleeding. There was a grade 4 laceration with a subcapsular hematoma. The subcapsular hematoma had ruptured. It was quite enlarged. The spleen was taken down after blunt control was obtained at the hilum of the spleen. The splenic ligaments were divided with clamps and ties. After the spleen was fully mobilized and rotated towards the midline, the hilum was taken. Stick ties were used to secure the vessels at the hilum of the spleen, and it was divided. The organ was passed off as a specimen. Pelvic organs, including uterus and ovaries, were also inspected, and there was no injury here. The patient was then closed with running PDS and skin clips. She tolerated the procedure well.

13. CASE 13

    LOCATION: ASC

    PREOPERATIVE DIAGNOSIS: Granuloma, right inner cheek.

    POSTOPERATIVE DIAGNOSIS: Granuloma, right inner cheek.

    PROCEDURE PERFORMED: Excision of lesion from right buccal mucosa, likely benign.

    PROCEDURE IN DETAIL: After informed consent from the patient's parents was obtained, the patient was taken to the operating room and placed supine on the operating table. The appropriate monitoring devices were placed on the patient, and general anesthetic was induced. It was maintained by inhalation mask technique. The mouth was opened once the child was asleep. There was a 7 × 7 mm pedunculated lesion on the right anterior buccal mucosa. The lesion was excised by cutting through its base. It came out in one place. There was no bleeding. Great care was taken to be certain that there was no injury to the lips.

    The patient tolerated the procedure well. She was transferred to the recovery room in good condition.

Copyright © 2005, Elsevier Inc. All rights reserved.
CPT only © 2004. *Current Procedural Terminology, 2005, Professional Edition,* American Medical Association. All rights reserved.

14. CASE 14

LOCATION: Hospital Inpatient

PREOPERATIVE DIAGNOSIS: Myasthenia gravis.

POSTOPERATIVE DIAGNOSIS: Same.

PROCEDURE PERFORMED: Plasma exchange.

PHYSICIAN:

This is a 5′89″, 270-pound man who has increasing muscle weakness felt to be related to myasthenia gravis, and plasma exchange was elected. His hematocrit was 45.5. His platelets were 190,000. His total blood volume was 5769, and the calculated plasma volume was a little above 3 liters, about 3125 or so. I targeted him for 1 plasma volume exchange of 3 liters using 5% albumin with 1 amp of calcium gluconate/liter, and did a 1 to 1 exchange. He started it at 14:30 and completed the exchange by 16:00. He had no medical complications throughout. His pressures were stable. Cardiac rate was stable. During the exchange, he was aggressively hydrated with an IV because at the time I felt that he was still somewhat volume-contracted from his diarrhea. His pre lab reflected this, and post lab will be done. His final plasma value was 3575 on the machine. This was calculated from a 4297 total, minus the ACD-A of 722. The replacement volume was calculated at 3281 because there are not exactly 500 in each bottle of albumin; I was fairly close, and I was satisfied with this result. The patient will be reevaluated over the next 2 days with special attention paid to his renal status prior to continuing the next plasma exchange planned in 3 days, unless there are other problems that we have to deal with.

15. CASE 15

LOCATION: Outpatient Surgery Center

PROCEDURE NOTE: Jake is in for a vasectomy, having previously undergone counseling earlier today. Patient was placed in a supine position, and the scrotal area was shaved. Under sterile technique the scrotal area was prepped with Betadine, and the sterile drapes were applied. The right vas was localized and under sterile technique was infiltrated with 1% Xylocaine. The vas was externalized, and a 1.5-cm portion of the tube was removed. Proximal and distal stumps were doubly ligated with 4-0 silk. There was a small blood vessel in the skin that was oozing and was clamped. Attention was directed to the left side, where a similar procedure was performed. With hemostasis intact, the proximal and distal stumps on the left were retracted into the scrotum, and attention was directed to the right side, where there was slight oozing from the skin edge; with pressure this did resolve, and the proximal and distal stumps were retracted into the scrotum.

ASSESSMENT: Vasectomy.

PLAN: The patient had been given the postvasectomy instruction sheet, and bacitracin and a gauze dressing were applied. He is to apply antibiotics a couple of times a day with gauze and he was given an instruction sheet to have sperm counts done in 2 months time, and to take contraceptive precautions in the meantime.

Copyright © 2005, Elsevier Inc. All rights reserved.
CPT only © 2004. *Current Procedural Terminology, 2005, Professional Edition*, American Medical Association. All rights reserved.

16. CASE 16

LOCATION: Hospital Inpatient

PREOPERATIVE DIAGNOSIS: Right carotid stenosis.

POSTOPERATIVE DIAGNOSIS: Same.

PROCEDURE PERFORMED: Right carotid endarterectomy.

This case is monitored with EEGs. There were no changes at the clamping. The clamping time was 14 minutes.

PROCEDURE: Under general anesthesia, the patient was prepped and draped in the usual manner. The incision was made along the right side of the sternocleidomastoid. With sharp dissection, we got on to the common carotid artery. We then isolated the internal and external carotid arteries. We saw the hypoglossal nerve. We put ligaloops around these arteries. We then freed up the artery from its surrounding tissue. This was a high bifurcation. We had to go up higher so as to isolate a good portion of the internal carotid artery. This had not been done. I then placed the Farley Thompson retractor in so we would have adequate retraction. At this point in time, Dr. Allen came into the surgery to help me with the endarterectomy. We then gave the patient 5,000 units of heparin, waited 5 minutes, and placed the clamps on the internal common and external carotid arteries. The endarterectomy was done. The arterial base was cleaned out. There were no free fragments. We were able to nicely eliminate the plaque, which was quite stenotic and ulcerated. We then closed the artery with 5-0 Prolene. We utilized 5-0 Prolene starting at the distal end of the internal carotid artery, then at the proximal end at the common carotid artery, meeting in the middle, producing adequate back-bleeding, then closing the artery. We required two other sutures in the artery to stop some suture line bleeding. This was done. We then used Hemaseel on the arterial suture line. We then closed the wound in layers utilizing 2-0 chromic on the platysma with 2-0 plain in the subcutaneous tissue and 3-0 nylon interrupted mattress sutures on the skin. A dressing was applied. The patient was discharged to the recovery room in stable condition.

Copyright © 2005, Elsevier Inc. All rights reserved.
CPT only © 2004. *Current Procedural Terminology, 2005, Professional Edition,* American Medical Association. All rights reserved.

17. CASE 17

EMERGENCY DEPARTMENT REPORT

SUBJECTIVE: The patient is an 80-year-old male in acute respiratory distress. He is from the New York City area and was just about to take a train to go there today. He had sudden onset of shortness of breath and presents now because of it. He denies any chest pain or tightness. He has had no recent cough. He is bringing up frothy sputum as he arrives here.

PAST MEDICAL HISTORY:

Surgical:
1. Bypass surgery.
2. Angioplasty and stent.
3. Pacemaker.

Illnesses: The patient has a previous history of congestive heart failure and has been intubated in the past, most recently 4 months ago, with this same problem.

Family history, social history, and review of systems were not obtainable for this patient.

OBJECTIVE: This alert 80-year-old male appears to be in acute respiratory distress. Oxygen saturation is 72%. Blood pressure is 210/107. Respirations are 36. Pulse is 120. Telemetry shows a paced wide complexed rhythm. HEENT: Frothy pink sputum coming out of his mouth. Neck is supple without lymphadenopathy. His jugular veins are full. Respirations are labored. Lungs: Rales throughout. Heart: Rapid rate and rhythm. Abdomen: Soft and nontender with normal bowel sounds. Extremities: No peripheral edema is noted. No clubbing.

ASSESSMENT: Pulmonary edema.

PLAN: He was immediately given Lasix 80 mg IV, given Nitro spray, and started on a Nitro drip. We gave him a few minutes to try to turn around. He was on 100% oxygen. He did not turn around and, in fact, he looked worse. We then talked about intubation with him and his wife and proceeded with it. He was bagged. He was given Versed IV, and he then was given succinylcholine 100 mg IV. He was then intubated without difficulty with an 8.0 ET tube to 24 cm. Breath sounds were heard bilaterally. CO2 monitoring device confirmed placement. The patient was placed on the ventilator and transported to ICU in reasonably stable condition.

THORACIC MEDICINE/CRITICAL CARE CONSULTATION

I have been asked by Dr. Elhart to see the patient for ICU care. The patient was admitted with pulmonary edema, respiratory failure; he has chronic renal disease and is on Dr. Elhart's service—I would assume for the chronic renal disease as well as respiratory failure, but that was secondary. The patient looks like he had a myocardial infarction with elevated troponins, CK-MBs, CPKs, and CKs. His pulmonary edema has started to clear. He was adjusted on the ventilator this morning. The CPAP went from 6 o'clock to 8 o'clock, and then he got too short of breath and went back on the ventilator. Since then he has diuresed more, and I have him on CPAP at present. He is doing quite well, with a respiratory rate of 19 with good oxygenation. I think we have a fair chance of getting him extubated today.

The patient was visiting with relatives here in Manytown. He was trying to move some luggage, started to get diaphoretic, and did not feel well, and it started to become difficult to breathe. The wife felt he was gurgling, and he was sent to the emergency department, where he was found to be in pulmonary edema, intubated, and placed on a ventilator.

Copyright © 2005, Elsevier Inc. All rights reserved.
CPT only © 2004. *Current Procedural Terminology, 2005, Professional Edition*, American Medical Association. All rights reserved.

The patient is intubated and on a ventilator, so I do not have a good family history, social history, past medical history, past surgical history, or review of systems. I got some things from the chart and some things from his wife. The patient's wife is fairly sure that he had stenting of the LAD done last year. We will send for those records. He had a coronary artery bypass graft done before that. It sounds fairly extensive. It seems to have been in 1989. He had at least three grafts, and the cardiologist has this outlined pretty well and what was done at that point. He also had a pacemaker. He has a history of renal artery disease status post renal artery stenosis, history of hypertension, dyslipidemia, bradycardia, and chronic renal disease. He apparently has had some trouble with dye toxicity from an angiogram done a year ago and did not quite get over it. I guess there was partial clearing. It is difficult to tell without the records what went on.

PHYSICAL EXAMINATION: At the time I saw the patient, the physical examination reveals a patient who is alert, on a ventilator, and able to answer questions (yes and no, anyway). He certainly cannot verbalize it. HEENT: Benign. No blood was found in the posterior pharynx or the nose. Neck is supple. No JVD. Lungs actually show rales bilaterally but in the bases, not in the rest of the areas. Heart shows S1 and S2 are regular without an S3 or S4. There is a systolic murmur at the fourth interspace midclavicular line that is somewhat difficult to hear. It is somewhat vague and soft, but I think it is present. Abdomen is soft and benign without hepatosplenomegaly. Normal bowel sounds are present. No bruits heard in either flank; no masses palpable; nontender. Extremities show no edema, rashes, clubbing, cyanosis, or tremor. Lymphatic system: No nodes in the neck, clavicular, or axillary area.

IMPRESSION:

1. Acute myocardial infarction with acute pulmonary edema and acute respiratory failure.
2. Chronic renal failure. You can see that on today's material his BUN and creatinine levels are climbing. I am not sure what the plan is at this point. I am waiting for cardiology to come by, but I think I can get him extubated later this afternoon. I will check his sputum. He does have a fair amount to suction, and it is somewhat thick, so I will make sure he does not have an infection. He is already on Unasyn for any sort of aspiration that might have occurred, although it is not well documented. We will check a 24-hour urine for creatinine clearance, get the records from the Manytown hospital to see what actually was done there, and then check on his lab in the morning. I will wait for Dr. Elhart to come by before we make any other plans, but hopefully the patient will be extubated here shortly.

RADIOLOGY REPORT, CHEST

EXAMINATION OF: Chest.

CLINICAL SYMPTOMS: Follow-up pulmonary edema.

PORTABLE AP CHEST, 5:00 am: FINDINGS: Comparison is made with yesterday morning's portable AP chest. Sternotomy with mediastinal clips. The endotracheal tube and NG tube have been removed. No appreciable change in the heart size or pulmonary vascularity given the difference in technique. Lungs are clear.

RADIOLOGY REPORT, CHEST

EXAMINATION OF: Chest.

CLINICAL SYMPTOMS: Acute MI, pulmonary edema, acute respiratory failure, and renal disease.

Copyright © 2005, Elsevier Inc. All rights reserved.
CPT only © 2004. *Current Procedural Terminology, 2005, Professional Edition,* American Medical Association. All rights reserved.

PORTABLE CHEST X-RAY: FINDINGS: Endotracheal tube and NG tube are not significantly changed. The cardiac silhouette is upper normal to mildly prominent but stable. Mild interstitial prominence remains in the infrahilar areas, but no other significant interval change is noted.

THORACIC MEDICINE/CRITICAL CARE PROGRESS REPORT

This is a follow-up for this patient with acute respiratory failure. He was extubated yesterday. He apparently had a cardiac catheterization in the past, and his kidneys were bad enough that they thought he might need dialysis, but then he recovered; but he certainly recovered incompletely because BUN today is 72, creatinine 2.6, and creatinine clearance is pending. Interestingly enough, potassium is low at 2.8, so we will replace that with oral potassium. We will check his basic metabolic panel in the morning and transfer him to the floor on telemetry. He does not want anything done here. He wants to go home by train, which is probably not the best idea because there is no guarantee that what happened to him this time will not happen again.

PHYSICAL EXAMINATION: Chest: Clear. Chest x-ray looks pretty good, too. Heart: Regular rhythm. Abdomen: Benign. Extremities: No edema. No clubbing.

LABORATORY DATA: All in good shape. Sputum showed greater than 25 white cells, less 10 squamous. No bugs were seen, so it may be just inflammation rather than true infection.

MEDICATIONS: He is on Unasyn at this point. We stopped the Unasyn today and put him on Augmentin. There is some question about whether he aspirated on it, but I certainly do not see anything on x-ray right now.

He is going to be talking to Dr. Elhart later today to decide what to do about whether to discharge or have the study done here. The patient is really 4+ positive that he wants to go back home in case things go wrong with his kidneys. At least he is at home and can undergo the dialysis closer to home. He is most comfortable with the situation there as well as with his surroundings there, so we will leave that up to Dr. Elhart and the patient. But I still think it is a somewhat risky idea, so I imparted to the patient that particular idea. Otherwise, he can be discharged at cardiology's leisure.

DISCHARGE SUMMARY

The patient was admitted with pulmonary edema, respiratory failure, and chronic renal disease. The patient looked like he has had myocardial infarction with elevated troponins. The patient was extubated after the pulmonary edema (less than 96 hours). Discussions with the patient and his family indicated that he did not want anything further done. He wanted further cardiac care done at home. We arranged for him to be discharged, and he was discharged Tuesday. It was advised that he have a cardiac catheterization to determine the extent of his myocardial infarction and whether anything could be fixed, but this is on top of somebody with chronic renal disease who most likely would suffer from the toxic effects of the dye and would probably have some difficulty with renal failure post cardiac catheterization if everything went wrong. Please see my drug note that outlined the drugs the patient was on when he was sent home.

DISCHARGE DIAGNOSES:

1. Acute non-Q-wave myocardial infarction.
2. Congestive heart failure.
3. Pulmonary edema with acute respiratory failure.

Copyright © 2005, Elsevier Inc. All rights reserved.
CPT only © 2004. *Current Procedural Terminology, 2005, Professional Edition*, American Medical Association. All rights reserved.

18. CASE 18

HISTORY AND PHYSICIAL

LOCATION: Inpatient Hospital

CHIEF COMPLAINT: Cough and fever.

HISTORY OF PRESENT ILLNESS: This is a 67-year old man who was recently diagnosed with right lower lobe pneumonia. We attempted to treat him at home with oral antibiotics and rehydration; however, he has just not done that well. Last night, he began having more pleuritic pain on the right side, plus spiking fevers and sweats. When he came to the office today, he felt weak and dehydrated, and I felt it would be best to have him admitted to the hospital.

PAST MEDICAL HISTORY:

1. Chronic lymphocytic leukemia and an immunoglobin deficiency secondary to that. As a result, he has been susceptible to pneumococcal infections and has had repeated bouts of pneumonia in the past.
2. Chronic obstructive lung disease.
3. Diverticulosis coli.
4. Hypertension
5. Type 2 diabetes, which has recently required insulin.

CURRENT MEDICATIONS:

1. Insulin 75/25, 40 units twice a day.
2. Glucovance 5/500 1 b.i.d.
3. Ferrous sulfate 5 grains t.i.d.
4. Diovan HCT 160/12.5 once a day.
5. Aspirin 81 mg daily.
6. Vantin 200 mg twice a day.

He recently stopped taking Actos on my instructions.

ALLERGIES: Sulfa.

SOCIAL HISTORY: He lives with his wife. His daughter is a teacher at the local high school. He is not a smoker at the present time.

FAIMLY HISTORY: Nothing that pertains to the present problem.

REVIEW OF SYSTEMS: A complete review of systems today discloses no problems with bowel or urine. No pain in the abdomen. There has been a gradual weight loss over the last few months. He has not had any rash. No joint disease. No neurological symptoms. He has not been depressed. The remainder of his complete review of systems was negative.

PHYSICAL EXAMINATION: On physical exam, he was alert and oriented. Blood pressure: 134/60. Weight: 197 pounds, compared with 207 pounds about a year ago. He looked pale. He was not diaphoretic or febrile. Pulse was regular, but the rate was about 100. There was no abnormality of the head or neck. No palpable mass or lymphadenopathy in the neck. There was also no lymphadenopathy in any of the other major areas. There were rales at the right lung base but no signs of consolidation on percussion and auscultation. The heart had a regular sinus rhythm with tachycardia. His abdomen was soft and nontender. The spleen was very large. I could not tell if the liver was enlarged, too. Genitalia were normal. Rectal exam showed a benign symmetrical prostate gland. There was a fair amount of spasm when I did this exam. Some liquid brownish stool was present in the rectum, which was negative for occult blood. His extremities showed no edema. Pulses were present. There was no active joint or skin disease. No neurological deficits.

Copyright © 2005, Elsevier Inc. All rights reserved.
CPT only © 2004. *Current Procedural Terminology, 2005, Professional Edition*, American Medical Association. All rights reserved.

IMPRESSION:

1. Right lower lob pneumonia with pleurisy.
2. Chronic lymphocytic leukemia, with an immune deficiency as described above.
3. Hypertension.
4. Anemia of chronic disease.
5. Type 2 diabetes, recently converted to insulin.
6. Sulfa allergy.
7. Diverticulosis coli.

PLAN: We had blood cultures done 3 days ago. These came back negative. His white count is chronically elevated because of his CLL. The total count had actually dropped from 63,000 to 44,000 over the past week. He is anemic, with a hemoglobin of 9.9. Blood sugar was 317 earlier this week. Other labs were insignificant. Slightly low albumin of 3.1.

Will get him started on IV fluids and IV antibiotics. Respiratory therapy will also be called in to help with clearing his phlegm.

INFECTIOUS DISEASE CONSULTATION

IMPRESSION:

1. Nonresolving pneumonia due to probable *Streptococcus pneumoniae* pneumonia.
2. Immunoglobulin G deficiency secondary to #3.
3. Chronic lymphocytic leukemia.
4. Hypertension.
5. Chronic obstructive lung disease.
6. Diverticulosis.
7. Allergy to sulfa, manifested by hives.

RECOMMENDATIONS:

1. IV cefotaxime 2 grams every 8 hours.
2. Azithromycin 500 mg q 24.
3. Repeat sputum Gram's stain and culture.
4. Set up for a PICC.

HISTORY OF PRESENT ILLNESS: This is a 67-year-old gentleman who is known to have chronic lymphocytic leukemia and has had recurring pneumococcal pneumonias. He is also known to have an immune globulin deficiency.

Apparently, he was traveling back from New Mexico on October 20. He developed what appears to be a pneumococcal pneumonia and was empirically treated with a gatifloxacin. Although somewhat improved, he continued to have production of sputum. A chest x-ray was performed at that time and did disclose a new pneumonia. Repeat sputum was done and it did demonstrate pneumococcus and subsequently the patient was placed on cefpodoxime. A baseline trough level of his immune globulin was obtained last Friday, and it showed that his level was around 200. Over the last 3 to 5 days, he now has developed worsening fevers and chills and pleuritic chest pain. His temperature has been up to 101. He has not had any rigors. The severity of the pain is about a 3 to 4 out of 10. He says this is just like it was in New Mexico, just like it was a year ago when he was initially diagnosed with having an immune globulin deficiency. The duration of this particular exacerbation then has been going on since the 20th of October.

FAMILY HISTORY: His father died at age 79 of a cardiac condition. He also had diabetes. Mother died at age 83 of age-related conditions. He has one brother, who is in good health. There is no family history of or exposure to anyone with tuberculosis.

Copyright © 2005, Elsevier Inc. All rights reserved.
CPT only © 2004. *Current Procedural Terminology, 2005, Professional Edition*, American Medical Association. All rights reserved.

PAST MEDICAL HISTORY:

Medical: Significant for diabetes mellitus, hypertension, chronic obstructive lung disease, chronic lymphocytic leukemia, immune globulin deficiency, and history of diverticulosis. Operations: None.

MEDICATIONS: He has been on ACTOS, Glucovance, iron aspirin, and recently on cefpodoxime.

ALLERGIES: Sulfa manifested by hives.

REVIEW OF SYSTEMS: Complete and negative.

SOCIAL HISTORY: He is a married, retired teacher with six children. He quit smoking 20 years ago (20–25 packs year total). Sometimes drinks a beer and wine on weekends.

PHYSICAL EXAMINATION: His temperature is 100, pulse 94, blood pressure 130/60, weight 197 pounds. He appears rested, not in acute distress. HEENT: The TMs are clear bilaterally. The ear canals are normal. Conjunctivae were clear. I could not get a good red reflex on the right; there may be a cataract obscuring it. The left red reflex was normal. His nasal membranes and pharynx were clear. There is no cervical adenopathy. No thyroid tenderness. No carotid bruits. No supraclavicular adenopathy. Pulmonary: Reveals rales at the right lower quadrant. There are no secondary muscles of respiration. Cardiovascular: Regular, no thrills. Abdomen: Soft bowel sounds are noted. No guarding, no rigidity, no tenderness of the liver. No abdominal bruits. No groin adenopathy. Integument: No rashes or eruptions. Examination of the nail beds and finger pads shows no stigmata of endocarditis. Examination of wrists, elbows, knees, and ankles reveals no synovitis. Biceps, triceps, quads, and popliteal muscles were not tender.

LABORATORY DATA: Again, the immune globulin level is about 200, with a normal low of 600. Blood cultures were done about 2 weeks ago that remain negative. The culture done 2 weeks ago did grow out pneumococcus.

OPERATIVE REPORT

PREOPERATIVE DIAGNOSIS: Pneumonia.

POSTOPERATIVE DIAGNOSIS: Same.

PROCEDURE PERFORMED: Insertion of central venous peripheral catheter.

PICC INSERTED

INDICATION: Vascular access for IV antibiotics.

PROCEDURE: The patient was informed about the risks and benefits prior to the procedure, and consent was signed. The patient verbalizes an understanding of the risks and benefits, and he does accept.

The left medial vein was identified and cleansed with 70% isopropyl alcohol with 2% chlorhexidine gluconate. The area was then allowed to dry for 30 seconds. The area was then draped in a sterile fashion, and a tourniquet was applied. A 22-gauge IV catheter was placed successfully into the left median vein. Good flow of blood was observed. Subsequently, a guidewire was placed, and the 22-gauge IV catheter was removed. A small incision was made to facilitate the introducer and dilator, which were placed successfully. This guidewire was removed. The dilator was removed, and a polyurethane dual-lumen 5-French Per-Q-Cath catheter was placed without difficulty up to 0 cm. This catheter was trimmed to 52 cm. There was return of blood flow after the guidewire was removed. It was flushed with normal saline followed by heparin. The area was then dressed. Postprocedure chest x-ray has been obtained, checking for line placement.

Copyright © 2005, Elsevier Inc. All rights reserved.
CPT only © 2004. *Current Procedural Terminology, 2005, Professional Edition*, American Medical Association. All rights reserved.

RADIOLOGY REPORT

EXAMINATION OF: Chest.

CLINICAL SYMPTOMS: Right lower lobe pneumonia, pleurisy, PICC (peripherally inserted central catheter) line placement.

PORTABLE CHEST

FINDINGS: There is a large opacity with irregular margins located in the right and mid lung zone consistent with an infiltrate. A left-sided PICC line has been placed, and the tip is within the SVC near the right atrial margin. No pneumothorax. The left lung is clear.

INFECTIOUS DISEASE PROGRESS NOTE

This is day 3 of IV cefotaxime and azithromycin.

CHIEF COMPLAINT: Persistent pneumococcal pneumonia.

SUBJECTIVE: The patient is doing well. He has had no fevers or chills. He is breathing much better. His energy is much better. The illness has been going on for about 4 to 6 weeks.

REVIEW OF SYSTEMS: Pulmonary, cardiovascular, gastrointestinal, and genitourinary: Negative.

PAST MEDICAL HISTORY: Reviewed on previous consultation.

OBJECTIVE: He is afebrile. His T-maximum is 37.2, blood pressure 120/60, pulse around 90, and respiratory rate is 16. O2 sat is 96% on room air. He is resting comfortably. He is not in any distress. His pulmonary examination is clear. No secondary muscles of respiration. Cardiovascular: Regular. No thrills. Abdomen is soft. Bowel sounds are present. No guarding. No rigidity. No tenderness of the liver. Vascular access site is clean and intact. Good SKIN turgor.

In the LABORATORY, there is possibly a gram negative rod in rare amounts. No other pathogen.

IMPRESSION:

1. Nonresolving pneumonia due to *Streptococcus pneumoniae* pneumonia.
2. Immunoglobulin G deficiency secondary to #3.
3. Chronic lymphocytic leukemia.
4. Hypertension.
5. Chronic obstructive lung disease.
6. Diverticulosis.
7. Allergy to sulfa manifestated by hives.

PLANS:

1. We will set up the patient for ceftriaxone as an outpatient every 12 hours.
2. We will switch the azithromycin to 500 p.o. every day for 7 days.
3. We will follow up in a week.

DISCHARGE SUMMARY

DISCHARGE DIAGNOSES:

1. Right lower lobe pneumonia.
2. Immunodeficiency.
3. Chronic lymphocytic leukemia.
4. Hypertension.
5. Chronic obstructive pulmonary disease.
6. Diverticulosis coli.

Copyright © 2005, Elsevier Inc. All rights reserved.
CPT only © 2004. *Current Procedural Terminology, 2005, Professional Edition,* American Medical Association. All rights reserved.

HISTORY OF PRESENT ILLNESS. This 67-year-old man with a history of chronic lymphocytic leukemia was admitted to the hospital with right lower lobe pneumonia. This has been smoldering along for a couple weeks. He has had intermittent fevers and sweats and just felt so sick that he could not manage at home any longer. His examination showed rales at the right lung base, but otherwise he seemed to be quite well physically. His face was flushed. His pulse was rapid. There were no other physical findings.

His chest x-ray showed right middle lung pneumonia. There was no effusion, although the patient was having some symptoms of pleurisy. His electrocardiogram showed sinus tachycardia.

LABORATORY STUDIES: White count was quite elevated at 52,000. He was also anemic at 8.6 grams. Platelets were normal. Blood sugars fluctuated. Protime and PTT were normal. Urinalysis showed a few hyalin casts typical for dehydration. Two blood cultures were negative.

HOSPITAL COURSE: He was started on IV azithromycin and cefotaxime. He was also put on respiratory therapy. Aerosol treatments worked quite well for him. His blood sugars were high. He required his usual insulin dose plus supplemental NovoLog insulin for high sugars. He tended to be lower in the morning and higher throughout the day.

At the time of discharge, he had been afebrile. He was breathing easily and had oxygen saturations in the range of mid 90% level. There was little coughing and no general malaise. His appetite and activity were good. I felt he could continue with IV therapy at home.

DISCHARGE MEDICATIONS:

1. Aspirin 81 mg daily.
2. Diovan HCT 160/12.5 once a day.
3. NovoLog 70/30 insulin, 46 units in the morning and 40 units in the evening.
4. Glucovance 5/500, 1 b.i.d.
5. Tylenol p.r.n.
6. Aspirin p.r.n.
7. Zithromax 500 mg IV every 24 hours.
8. Claforan 2 gm IV every 8 hours.

FOLLOWUP: He will be coming back to see me for followup in about a week. In the meantime, I have asked home infusion therapy to follow him and supervise his IV therapy at his hometown facility.

Copyright © 2005, Elsevier Inc. All rights reserved.
CPT only © 2004. *Current Procedural Terminology, 2005, Professional Edition*, American Medical Association. All rights reserved.

19. CASE 19

ADMISSION HISTORY AND PHYSICAL

LOCATION: Inpatient Hospital

This patient is a 37-year-old Caucasian male who was involved in an accident. He was walking and fell onto a farm implement. He sustained three stab wounds. The patient was hospitalized for 2 days and then discharged. The patient began having distention, nausea, and vomiting today and, because of that, returned to the emergency department for evaluation. The patient also has a history of heavy drinking. The patient underwent evaluation which included an upper endoscopy, which showed some gastritis but no evidence of any definitive ulcer disease. His CT scan shows a small bowel obstruction consistent with a small neck of bowel caught in the lowermost stab wound that he sustained during his initial injury. The patient is now being admitted for exploratory laparotomy, reduction of small bowel obstruction with possible bowel resection with anastomosis, and possible appendectomy. The liver also will be examined at the same time.

PAST MEDICAL HISTORY:

OPERATIONS: None.

ILLNESSES: Hay fever.

MEDICATIONS: Chlor-Trimeton p.r.n.

ALLERGIES: Penicillin causes a rash.

REVIEW OF SYSTEMS: The patient does not smoke. He does drink. Neurologic: The patient denies any history of seizure disorder, headaches, or dizziness. Cardiac: No history of hypertension, myocardial infarction, or congenital heart disease. Pulmonary: No history of asthma or pneumonia. The patient does have hay fever. No history of hemoptysis. Gastrointestinal: The patient denies any diarrhea or constipation. No history of peptic ulcer disease. The patient has had nausea and vomiting. See present illness. GU: The patient denies any urgency, frequency, or dysuria. Hematologic: The patient has never received a blood transfusion. He denies any bleeding problems.

PHYSICAL EXAMINATION: The patient is a 37-year-old Caucasian male. Head: Eyes: Pupils are equal. Ears: TMS are normal. Nose within normal limits. Throat within normal limits. Neck is supple. No carotid bruits heard. Chest: Lungs are clear; no rales or rhonchi heard. Heart: Regular rhythm; no murmur. Abdomen: Normal bowel sounds. The patient has a soft mass palpable in the lowermost incision from his previous injury. No guarding or rebound tenderness.

IMPRESSION: Small bowel obstruction secondary to a piece of bowel caught in the patient's lowermost abdominal injury caused by a farm implement.

PLAN: The patient has been counseled for exploratory laparotomy, with possible bowel resection and possible appendectomy. He has consented to the surgery. The patient will be taken immediately to the operating room as soon as an operating room is available.

GASTROENTEROLOGY CONSULTATION

HISTORY OF PRESENT ILLNESS: This 37-year-old white male, who may be an alcoholic, was driving his vehicle at night and had a roll-over while he was trying to avoid hitting a deer. He was wearing his seat belt. He went out looking for help and then tripped over a farm implement, and was stabbed in the chest and abdomen. He was hospitalized, and CT scan showed some fluid in the peritoneal cavity around the liver and spleen but no injury to those organs. There was also a retroperitoneal bleed. The patient was stable when he left, but he was still continuing to have symptoms of lower abdominal discomfort, and anorexia, and has not had a bowel movement since

Copyright © 2005, Elsevier Inc. All rights reserved.
CPT only © 2004. *Current Procedural Terminology, 2005, Professional Edition,* American Medical Association. All rights reserved.

the above. Last night, he developed vomiting of coffee ground material. His urine was noted to be orange, and he has only urinated twice since yesterday. His wife also noted the onset of jaundice last evening.

On arrival to the emergency room, the patient's labs showed a BUN of 32, creatinine of 1.4, alkaline phosphatase of 145, bilirubin of 4.9, AST of 65, ALT of 106. We did not have baseline enzymes. His hemoglobin was 16.1, stable; white count was 8420.

PAST MEDICAL HISTORY: No high blood pressure, diabetes, kidney or cardiac disease.

ALLERGIES: Penicillin causes a rash.

SURGERIES: None.

PHYSICAL EXAM: Well-nourished male, in no acute distress. VITAL SIGNS are normal. ABDOMEN: No megaly or masses. There is some tenderness in the lower abdomen; it is distended. There is no rebound, rigidity, or guarding.

IMPRESSION: 37-year-old white male, who has some jaundice, elevated liver enzymes. He had an abdominal injury just a few days ago. We certainly need to be sure that he has not developed progression of that injury (i.e., bleeding from the liver or spleen), although his hemoglobin is stable and normal, and he is hemodynamically stable. The patient does drink excess alcohol, and he may well just be having some alcohol-related liver disease. The patient had coffee-ground emesis. We do an upper endoscopy to assess for that, for the presence of ulcers, and also for varices.

PLAN:

1. Upper endoscopy.
2. Follow liver enzymes.
3. CT scan to look for further injury to his biliary tract or liver.

CT REPORT

EXAMINATION OF: CT of abdomen and pelvis.

CLINICAL SYMPTOMS: Vomiting, small bowel obstruction status post trauma 4 days earlier.

CT OF ABDOMEN AND PELVIS: TECHNIQUE: The patient was scanned from the dome of the diaphragm through the symphysis pubis following the administration of intravenous contrast only. No oral contrast was administered due to the patient's known small bowel obstruction, as well as the urgent nature of the study.

FINDINGS: This examination is compared to a prior examination 3 days ago. The liver, spleen, pancreas, kidneys, and adrenal glands appear within normal limits. There is a small amount of fluid adjacent to the liver. There is also a small amount of fluid adjacent to the spleen. Scattered areas of mesenteric stranding are present. There is free fluid present within the pelvis. There is marked dilatation of a significant portion of small bowel. A portion of small bowel does appear to protrude through an area of the abdominal wall musculature within the right anterolateral aspect of the abdominal wall. That is seen just below the level of the iliac crest. That is best demonstrated on images 44 through 47. Bowel on one side of this hernia is dilated and, on the other side, decompressed. This is presumably the etiology of the small bowel obstruction. There is a small right-sided pleural effusion present. There is a drop of air seen on image 11, just posterior to the liver. It is very difficulty to say whether this is above or below the diaphragm. I feel this most likely related to a small area of aerated lung; however, I cannot exclude the possibility that this relates to a small area of pneumothorax or even a small amount of free intraperitoneal air. Close clinical correlation suggested. There is patchy opacity present within both lung bases. That could relate to either atelectasis or infiltrate.

Copyright © 2005, Elsevier Inc. All rights reserved.
CPT only © 2004. *Current Procedural Terminology, 2005, Professional Edition,* American Medical Association. All rights reserved.

IMPRESSION:

1. There is a hernia involving the anterior abdominal wall at the right anterolateral aspect. See above discussion.
2. There is dilatation of a large portion of the small bowel. Proximal to the obstruction, the bowel appears dilated and decompressed. The hernia is presumably the etiology of the small bowel obstruction.
3. Fluid identified within the abdomen as described above. This requires close clinical correlation.
4. Small amount of air noted posterior to the liver may be either above or below the diaphragm. This is felt to most likely relate to a small area of aerated lung; however, a small amount of pneumothorax or even pneumoperitoneum cannot be excluded.
5. Small right-sided pleural effusion with bibasilar pulmonary opacities.

Right psoas enlargement presumably related to hematoma is less prominent than in the previous study.

OPERATIVE REPORT

PREOPERATIVE DIAGNOSIS: Small bowel obstruction.

POSTOPERATIVE DIAGNOSIS: Same.

OPERATION PERFORMED. Release of small bowel obstruction; closure of right lower quadrant abdominal wall defect causing bowel obstruction.

ANESTHESIA: General anesthesia.

INDICATION FOR SURGERY: This is a 37-year-old Caucasian male who has a small bowel obstruction. The patient was found to have a loop of bowel incarcerated in a stab wound that he had in the right lower quadrant area. The wound occurred as a result of a fall. The patient was taken to the operating room for release of the small bowel obstruction.

DESCRIPTION OF OPERATION: The patient was prepped and draped in the usual manner. A midline abdominal incision was made, and the abdomen was entered. Blood was encountered in the abdomen. This was secondary to his previous accident. The right lower quadrant of the abdomen was examined, and a loop of small bowel ileum was found caught in the stab wound in the right lower quadrant area. The bowel was brought out and examined and appeared within normal limits and viable. It did not appear to have any type of necrosis. The small bowel was distended down to the point. The contents of the small bowel were then milked back up into the stomach so it could be aspirated from the stomach as the contents of the small bowel were irrigated. The liver was also examined. The liver and gallbladder appeared normal. The upper abdominal wound, which occurred at the same time as the lower abdominal wound, did not penetrate the abdominal wall. The right lower quadrant stab wound was then repaired. The skin wound was widened so the anterior fascia layer could be closed. After the incision was widened, the anterior fascia layer was closed with interrupted 0 Vicryl sutures. After this was completed, the posterior fascial layer and peritoneum were also repaired using interrupted 0 Vicryl sutures. The abdomen was thoroughly irrigated with at least 3 liters of normal saline.The small bowel was then returned to the abdomen, and the abdominal incision was closed. The incision was closed with a running looped #1 PDS suture. Subcutaneous tissues were irrigated, and the skin was closed with skin clips. The patient tolerated the operation and returned to recovery in stable condition.

DISCHARGE SUMMARY

REASON FOR HOSPITALIZATION: Abdominal puncture wound with herniation and small bowel obstruction.

Copyright © 2005, Elsevier Inc. All rights reserved.
CPT only © 2004. *Current Procedural Terminology, 2005, Professional Edition,* American Medical Association. All rights reserved.

SUMMARY OF HOSPITAL COURSE: The patient was admitted with small bowel obstruction. A release of the small bowel obstruction and closure of right lower quadrant abdominal wall defect were performed.

Patient had an episode of gout that resolved during this stay in the hospital.

The patient recovered and was discharged to home.

The patient was also diagnosed with *Helicobacter pylori* during his hospital stay.

INSTRUCTIONS TO PATIENT ON DISCHARGE: Activity: As tolerated. Diet: As tolerated.

DISCHARGE MEDICATIONS:

1. Metronidazole 500 mg 3 times daily for 10 days.
2. Protonix 40 mg twice daily for 10 days.
3. Pink bismuth 30 ml 4 times daily for 10 days.
4. Tetracycline 500 mg 4 times daily for 10 days.

FOLLOW UP with primary care physician at the clinic.

CONDITION AT DISCHARGE: Good.

DISCHARGE DIAGNOSIS: Small bowel obstruction secondary to traumatic hernia surgically repaired.

Copyright © 2005, Elsevier Inc. All rights reserved.
CPT only © 2004. *Current Procedural Terminology, 2005, Professional Edition,* American Medical Association. All rights reserved.

20. CASE 20

ADMISSION HISTORY AND PHYSICAL

LOCATION: Inpatient Hospital

REASON FOR ADMISSION: Pulmonary embolism.

HISTORY: This patient is a 56-year-old Caucasian gentleman who really has no significant past medical history. He was, however, diagnosed with some lumbar spinal cancer about 3 to 4 weeks ago. He is currently being considered for radiation and chemotherapy. He resides 50 miles south of here in Anytown and was here in town to attend a meeting. As he was walking out of the building where he had been attending a meeting, he had a near syncopal episode. The paramedics were subsequently called. He initially had refused to be brought into the hospital but was convinced otherwise by a physician who happened to be at the same meeting.

In the emergency department, he was noted to be very tachycardiac and hypoxic. He was started on continuous heparin for suspected pulmonary embolism. Bilateral lower extremity Doppler did reveal clots in the patient's lower extremities up to just above the level of the popliteal area.

On admission to the ICU, he really did not have any other specific complaints.

PAST MEDICAL HISTORY: Really unremarkable other than that stated in the history of present illness. He was recently diagnosed with spinal cancer. He also has a history of stool impaction secondary to the morphine that he was started on for his back pain.

MEDICATIONS: Morphine, unknown dose, for his back pain. He also takes several over-the-counter stool softeners.

ALLERGIES: He has no known drug allergies.

SOCIAL/FAMILY HISTORY: The patient's family/personal/social history cannot be obtained given the patient's current status (he is still acutely in respiratory distress).

REVIEW OF SYSTEMS: Also cannot be directly obtained from the patient given his acute respiratory distress; however, in speaking to the patient's wife, he really does not have any other constitutional symptoms. He has not had any recent fevers, chills, or night sweats. He did admit to being dyspneic right before he nearly passed out, but he denied any chest pain. He has been constipated, as per the history of present illness. He denies any changes in his bladder habits. He also denies any recent changes in his appetite or his weight. The rest of his systems were briefly reviewed with the patient's wife and were found to be essentially negative and unremarkable.

PHYSICAL EXAMINATION: He appeared to be in moderate respiratory distress. He was otherwise not in any acute pain. His blood pressure was 98/52, pulse rate around 126, and he was breathing about 26 to 30 per minute with very shallow respirations. His temperature was 36.3. Head/Neck: Showed pink palpebral conjunctivae with anicteric sclerae. He did not have any active nasal or ear discharge. Oropharynx was otherwise clear. He was on a nonrebreather mask during my exam. He was saturating about 77% on the nonrebreather initially. Currently, his saturations are up to 92%. Chest: Showed his lung fields to have some soft scattered rales. He also had some scattered wheezing, more prominent on the right side than on the left side. Otherwise, his chest expansion was symmetrical. Cardiac: Shows a tachycardic rate without any rubs. Abdomen: Showed it to be soft and nontender with normoactive bowel sounds. Extremities: Showed good and equal pulses peripherally without any significant edema. Both his hands and feet were warm to the touch.

LABORATORY DATA: A CBC showed fairly normal blood cell counts. A routine urinalysis was also likewise unremarkable. A comprehensive metabolic panel showed his glucose to be slightly elevated at 143 mg/dl. His albumin was low at 2.6 grams/dl; otherwise, the rest of his panel was within normal limits. His BUN was 15, his

Copyright © 2005, Elsevier Inc. All rights reserved.
CPT only © 2004. *Current Procedural Terminology, 2005, Professional Edition,* American Medical Association. All rights reserved.

creatinine was 0.9, and the rest of his electrolytes were within normal limits. A BNP was 84 picograms/ml. D-dimer test was more than 1000 SEU. His INR was 2.2 with a Protime of 17 seconds.

His chest x-ray showed some small infiltrates more prominent in the base of his lungs. His EKG showed sinus tachycardia with some nonspecific STT wave changes.

His lower extremity ultrasound showed clots extending from his lower thigh all the way up to his popliteal areas, and the left clot was noted to be fairly mobile. The clot on the right side was more chronic.

ASSESSMENT:

1. Venous thromboembolic disease with acute pulmonary embolism.
2. Spinal cancer.

PLAN:

1. Admit to the ICU.
2. Continue to anticoagulate the patient with unfractionated heparin adjusted to a therapeutic PTT.
3. Given the severity of the patient's pulmonary embolism and the fact that he still has a significant clot burden in his legs, will arrange for a temporary intravenous inferior vena cava filter placement tomorrow.

Total critical care time spent seeing the patient today and talking to the family was 120 minutes.

PROGRESS NOTE

The patient did well overnight. He was started on intravenous and fractionated heparin that was continuously adjusted to therapeutic PTT for his pulmonary embolism and venous thromboembolic disease.

This morning he said his breathing has been much better. Otherwise, he really does not have any other new complaints.

His past medical history, family history, and personal/social history have also been briefly reviewed.

His MEDICATIONS in the hospital have also been reviewed.

REVIEW OF SYSTEMS: He denies any fevers, chills, or night sweats overnight. His breathing is much better as per the HPI. He denies any chest pain. He is moving his bowels and is freely voiding without any difficulty. The rest of his systems were reviewed and found to be essentially negative and unremarkable.

PHYSICAL EXAMINATION: On examination he appeared to be fairly comfortable. He did not appear to be in any acute pain or distress. Blood pressure: 100/60. Pulse rate: 108. He was breathing about 22 to 24 breaths per minute and was saturating 94% to 96% on 2 liters per nasal cannula. Examination of his head and neck showed pink palpebral conjunctivae with anicteric sclerae. He did not have any active nasal or ear discharge. Oropharynx was otherwise clear. He was already on a nasal cannula; however, his saturation would still precipitously drop, requiring the placement of a 40% to 50% Venti mask. Exam of his chest showed his lung fields to be clear to auscultation, with only some occasional scattered rales and some soft wheezes, more prominent on the right side than the left. Cardiac exam showed a tachycardic rate without any rubs. Examination of his abdomen showed it to be soft and nontender with normoactive bowel sounds. Exam of his extremities showed good and equal pulses peripherally without any significant edema.

Copyright © 2005, Elsevier Inc. All rights reserved.
CPT only © 2004. *Current Procedural Terminology, 2005, Professional Edition,* American Medical Association. All rights reserved.

ASSESSMENT:

1. Acute hypoxic respiratory failure secondary to acute pulmonary embolism.
2. Venous thromboembolic disease with bilateral leg deep venous thrombosis.
3. Spinal cancer.

RECOMMENDATION AND PLAN:

1. The patient will get an inferior vena cava filter today.
2. Continue to anticoagulate the patient with heparin.
3. If the patient is stable after the placement of the filter, we should be able to transfer him out of the intensive care unit to the regular floor.

Total time spent managing the patient today and coordinating his care, including the placement of the inferior vena cava filter, was about 75 minutes.

CRITICAL CARE PROGRESS NOTE

The patient has had his temporary inferior vena cava filter placed yesterday. He currently is doing well. He has not had any further episodes of dyspnea.

His past medical history, family history, and social history remain unchanged.

His medications have also been reviewed and remain unchanged from yesterday.

REVIEW OF SYSTEMS: He denies any fever, chills, or night sweats. His breathing continues to improve every day. He denies any chest pain. He is moving his bowels and is freely voiding without any difficulty. The rest of his systems were reviewed and were found to be essentially negative, unremarkable, or noncontributory.

PHYSICAL EXAMINATION: He appears to be fairly comfortable. He was not in any acute pain or distress. His blood pressure was about 110/72 with a pulse rate of 94. He was breathing about 22 to 24 breaths per minute and was saturating 95% on 2 liters of oxygen via nasal cannula. Head/Neck: Showed pink palpebral conjunctivae with anicteric sclerae. He did not have any active nasal or ear discharge. His oropharynx is clear. Exam of his chest shows his lung fields to be clear to auscultation with only some occasional scattered rales, which are more prominent on the right side than on the left. However, even this was actually better than yesterday's exam. Cardiac: Regular rate and rhythm without any rubs. Examination of his abdomen showed it to be soft and nontender with normoactive bowel sounds. Exam of his extremities showed good and equal pulses peripherally without any significant edema.

ASSESSMENT:

1. Acute hypoxic respiratory failure secondary to acute pulmonary embolism, clinically improving.
2. Venous thromboembolic disease with bilateral leg deep venous thrombosis and pulmonary embolism, clinically stable.
3. Spinal cancer.

RECOMMENDATIONS/PLAN:

1. Continue the patient on anticoagulation.
2. Start the patient on heparin orally.
3. If the patient remains stable today, he should be able to be transferred out to the regular floor.

Total time spent seeing the patient today was 35 minutes.

CRITICAL CARE PROGRESS NOTE

The patient remained relatively stable overnight. However, he tried getting out of bed and inadvertently pulled on his Foley catheter. He did have a fair amount of hematuria afterwards. Repeated attempts to reinsert the Foley, unfortunately, failed. Otherwise, his respiratory function remains fairly stable.

Copyright © 2005, Elsevier Inc. All rights reserved.
CPT only © 2004. *Current Procedural Terminology, 2005, Professional Edition*, American Medical Association. All rights reserved.

Again, his past medical, family, and personal/social histories were briefly reviewed and remained unchanged.

MEDICATIONS: His medications also remained unchanged. We are still continuing to therapeutically anticoagulate him.

REVIEW OF SYSTEMS: He otherwise denies any fevers, chills, or night sweats. When asked about last night, he said that he was transiently confused but is currently, otherwise, awake, alert, and oriented. His breathing continues to improve. He has not had any chest pain. Prior to pulling out his Foley catheter, he had not had any problems with his bladder habits. He is also moving his bowels without any difficulty. The rest of his systems were reviewed and were found to be essentially negative and unremarkable.

PHYSICAL EXAMINATION: On examination, he appeared to be fairly comfortable. He was not in any acute pain or distress. His blood pressure was 106/70 with a pulse rate of 90. He was breathing about 18 to 20 breaths per minute. He was saturating more than 94% on 2 liters of oxygen via nasal cannula.

Exam of his head and neck showed pink palpebral conjunctivae with anicteric sclerae. He did not have any active nasal or ear discharge. Oropharynx was clear. His neck was supple and nontender. Exam of his chest showed his lung fields to be clear to auscultation bilaterally. Cardiac exam showed a regular rate and rhythm without any rubs. Exam of his abdomen showed it to be soft and nontender with normoactive bowel sounds. Exam of extremities showed good and equal pulses peripherally without any significant edema.

ASSESSMENT:

1. Acute hypoxic respiratory failure secondary to acute pulmonary embolism, clinically improving.
2. Venous thromboembolic disease with bilateral leg deep venous thrombosis and acute pulmonary embolism, clinically stable.
3. Spinal cancer.
4. Hematuria, atraumatic from the inadvertent removal of his catheter, rule out posterior urethral injury.

RECOMMENDATIONS AND PLAN:

1. Continue the patient on his anticoagulation.
2. Adjust his warfarin per INR.
3. Check a CBC every 8 hours.
4. We will try to reinsert a three-way Foley catheter and start continuous bladder irrigation.
5. Consult urology.

Total time spent seeing the patient today and coordinating his care, including coordinating his care with his consultants, was 12 minutes.

DISCHARGE SUMMARY

The patient is a 56-year-old gentleman who was admitted for an acute pulmonary embolism. The patient was promptly started on anticoagulation. Further assessment for venous thromboembolic disease did reveal deep venous thrombosis in both his legs. He subsequently had a temporary inferior vena cava filter placed because of his significant clot burden. His hospital course was complicated by a dramatic removal of his Foley catheter, leading to a posterior urethral injury and hematuria. Dr. Green was subsequently consulted for this.

Now overnight he remained fairly stable. His hematuria subsequently cleared. He does not have any other significant complaints.

Copyright © 2005, Elsevier Inc. All rights reserved.
CPT only © 2004. *Current Procedural Terminology, 2005, Professional Edition,* American Medical Association. All rights reserved.

His past medical/family history and personal and social histories have remained unchanged.

His medications have also been reviewed and remain unchanged.

On review of systems he denies any fever, chills, or night sweats overnight. His breathing continues to improve. He currently is able to ambulate without requiring oxygen. His bowel habits have otherwise remained unchanged. The rest of the systems were reviewed and were found to be essentially negative and unremarkable.

On physical examination he appeared to be fairly comfortable. He was not in any acute pain or distress. His blood pressure was 115/74 with a pulse rate of 88. He was saturating 96% to 97% on room air.

Examination of his head and neck showed pink palpebral conjunctiva with anicteric sclerae. He did not have any active nasal or ear discharge. Oropharynx was clear. The neck was supple and nontender. Examination of his chest shows lung fields to be clear to auscultation bilaterally. Cardiac exam showed a regular rate and rhythm without any rubs. Examination of his abdomen showed it to be soft and nontender, with normal active bowel sounds. Examination of his extremities showed good and equal pulses peripherally, without any significant edema. Exam of his external genitalia did not show any gross abnormality. He continues now to have a Foley catheter in place.

FINAL DIAGNOSES:

1. Acute hypoxic respiratory failure secondary to acute pulmonary embolism, clinically improving.
2. Venous thromboembolic disease with bilateral leg venous thrombosis and acute pulmonary embolism, clinically stable.
3. Spinal cancer.
4. Hematuria from traumatic removal of the Foley catheter.

RECOMMENDATION and PLAN:

1. Continue the patient on outpatient Lovenox and warfarin. The patient's Lovenox is to be discontinued once the patient's INR is therapeutic. Given the degree of his venous thromboembolic disease and his clot burden we would probably aim for an INR of 2.5.
2. Advised the patient to keep the Foley catheter in place for the next 5 to 7 days to avoid any urethral strictures. If, after removal of the catheter, the patient continues to experience some difficulty voiding, he was advised to follow up with his family practice physician.

DISCHARGE MEDICATIONS:

1. Morphine sulfate.
2. Lovenox
3. Warfarin.

The patient was instructed on how to take these medications and told to follow up with his primary care physician for further adjustments.

I have also spoken with his primary care physician and have given him an update of what has transpired during this current hospitalization. We also briefly discussed that because of his clot burden and his underlying spinal cancer, he will likely need to keep the inferior vena cava filter in place permanently. At that point, I also advised the patient to keep on chronic anticoagulation indefinitely.

Total time spent seeing and managing this patient today and coordinating his care, including discussing his discharge plans with his primary care provider, was a total of 120 minutes.

Copyright © 2005, Elsevier Inc. All rights reserved.
CPT only © 2004. *Current Procedural Terminology, 2005, Professional Edition,* American Medical Association. All rights reserved.

21. CASE 21

HISTORY AND PHYSICAL

REASON FOR ADMISSION: Renal failure, generalized edema, and coronary artery disease.

The patient is a 66-year-old male I was asked to see in consultation in the office today by his primary care physician for a rising creatinine level. The patient has been having progressive shortness of breath. A stress test was done, which was positive. This was followed by a cardiac catheterization, where the patient was found to have multivessel coronary artery disease including mid to right coronary artery, proximal LAD, and proximal circumflex with an ejection fraction of 66% without coarse regional motion abnormalities with normal systolic function without any mitral regurgitation. The patient was supposed to have bypass surgery today; however, because his creatinine has gone up from 1.8 mg/dl to 2.3 mg/dl, his bypass surgery has been postponed. His BUN is 48, sodium 136, potassium 4.6, chloride 97, bicarb 29, creatinine 2.3, and calcium 8.6. His white count was 6,000, with a hemoglobin of 11.5, MCV of 101.7, and platelets 192,000. He has a normal Protime and INR.

The patient states that he had a 24-hour urine collection in the past, but he does not recall the results of that. We tried to get a hold of the 24-hour urine taken by his primary care physician but were unsuccessful today.

The patient has been on Actos and recently was started on Crestor, which was switched from Lipitor 40 mg daily.

For the past few months, he has been having progressive shortness of breath. For the past week or so, he has been getting more leg swelling where he cannot even tie his shoes because of his increased abdominal girth. He has been having exertional dyspnea. He cannot even walk half a block. He denies any PND. He has no chest pain. He has never had any chest pain. He has no palpitations, but he complains of massive leg edema.

PAST MEDICAL HISTORY IS SIGNIFICANT FOR THE FOLLOWING:

1. Long-standing hypertension.
2. Type II diabetes mellitus, on Lantus and Humalog insulin.
3. Diabetic retinopathy.
4. Right eye blindness.
5. Congestive heart failure, but normal ejection fraction as mentioned.
6. Obesity.
7. Hyperlipidemia.
8. Questionable diabetic nephropathy (again, I do not have any urinalysis or 24-hour urine collection).
9. Hypothyroidism.

SOCIAL HISTORY: He is single. He has a girlfriend, who was with him today. He quit smoking in 1986. He uses alcohol occasionally. He is retired. He used to work as a store manager at Wal-Mart. He is a native of New York.

FAMILY HISTORY: Father died of unclear reasons. Mother died of a myocardial infarction at age 65. One sister with breast cancer. One sister with lung cancer. No kidney disease, dialysis, or kidney transplantation.

ALLERGIES: Questionable Vasotec.

CURRENT MEDICATIONS include the following:

1. Actos 15 mg daily.
2. Amitriptyline 50 mg daily.
3. Humalog 15 units t.i.d.

Copyright © 2005, Elsevier Inc. All rights reserved.
CPT only © 2004. *Current Procedural Terminology, 2005, Professional Edition,* American Medical Association. All rights reserved.

4. Lantus 56 units nightly.
5. Lisinopril 30 mg daily.
6. Multivitamins 1 daily.
7. Neurontin 300 mg 2 tabs b.i.d.
8. Prednisone eye drops.
9. Synthroid 0.075 mg daily.
10. Torsemide 20 mg 2 tabs b.i.d.
11. Crestor 10 mg daily.
12. Isosorbide mononitrate 30 mg daily.

REVIEW OF SYSTEMS: Constitutional: Generalized weakness with fatigue. Eyes: He wears glasses. He has right-sided blindness. ENT: Negative. Cardiovascular: As mentioned. Respiratory: Negative. Gastrointestinal: Negative, except for constipation. Genitourinary: Negative. Musculoskeletal: Chronic intermittent back pain. Skin: Negative. Neuro: Numbness and tingling in the fingers and toes. Psychiatry: Negative. Endocrine: He has diabetes and hypothyroidism. Hematology: Anemia from yesterday's labs.

EXAMINATION: The patient was short of breath but not in any distress. His temperature was 101.8 degrees. Respirations: 28 on room air. Pulse: 84/minute and regular. Weight 296 pounds. Blood pressure on the right side, 108/45 sitting and 108/50 standing. On the left, 108/56 standing. He has right-sided blindness. He has increased jugular venous pressure with positive hepatojugular reflux. Lungs had good air entry bilaterally, but he had a few crackles in the bases. He has abdominal wall and lower extremity edema. He has 1+ sacral edema. He had distinct heart sounds but no pericardial friction rub or murmurs. He did not have any carotid bruits.

His legs had palpable pulses, but 4+ edema in the lower extremities up to the thighs. No ulcerations. The patient was awake, alert, oriented ×3, without any focal neurological deficits. He had normal gait. He does have decreased sensations in his feet.

IMPRESSION:

1. Chronic renal failure with an estimated creatinine clearance of 13 ml/minute.
2. Acute renal failure possibly related to his cardiac catheterization. This patient could have thromboembolic disease.
3. Chronic renal failure could be related to the diabetic nephropathy but also could be related to hypertension or renal vascular disease; again, without knowing whether he has proteinuria or not, it is difficult to say. In any case, the patient does have generalized edema, and that edema needs to be taken care of. He is on a long-acting diuretic, and he probably would benefit from a shorter-acting diuretic.
4. Anemia of acute and chronic renal failure.
5. Slight macrocytosis.
6. Type II diabetes.
7. Severe coronary artery disease that would require bypass surgery.

PLAN:

1. The patient was admitted to telemetry.
2. He is code Level I.
3. We will make sure he has adequate intake output.
4. Fluid restriction 2 liters a day and also a salt restriction of 2 grams of sodium.
5. We will give him 2 mg of Bumex IV and start him at 0.125 mg an hour.
6. We will monitor his urine output hourly.
7. His surgery will be on hold until he is tuned up.
8. We will check potassium and magnesium every 6 hours and correct accordingly.
9. We will repeat his basic panel and CBC in the morning.
10. If his hemoglobin drops below 11, we will start him on Epo.

Copyright © 2005, Elsevier Inc. All rights reserved.
CPT only © 2004. *Current Procedural Terminology, 2005, Professional Edition*, American Medical Association. All rights reserved.

11. We will check iron studies and give him iron if need be.
12. Discontinue Crestor since his creatinine clearance is coming down.
13. Discontinue Actos since he has edema and it could be contributing to his massive edema and CHF symptoms.
14. Continue with his current insulin dose.

I had a long discussion with the patient about his renal function. I advised him that he might end up on dialysis either before or after his bypass surgery; however, he has severe coronary artery disease with a good ejection fraction, and he would benefit from bypass surgery. The patient understands that, and he agrees to dialysis if need be.

The option of what type of renal replacement therapy he would get will be discussed later.

The patient agrees to be admitted and diuresed. I discussed the case with Dr. Green on the phone, and he was in full agreement.

The total time I spent with this patient today was 65 minutes.

NEPHROLOGY/CRITICAL CARE PROGRESS NOTE

The patient is making good progress today as he made 1300 ml. Last night he had 32 and 850 output. His weight is 132–1/2 kg today, down from 133.4 kg yesterday. He has no complaints of chest pain or shortness of breath. He is awake, alert, oriented ×3 without any focal neurological deficits. His blood pressure is 124/57, temperature 36.9, heart rate in the low 70s per minute, respirations 18 per minute, and sats 94% on room air.

His lungs are clear. He has regular rate and rhythm. He has still sacral abdominal wall and low extremity edema, probably 2+.

His BUN today is 53, down from 57, sodium 139, potassium 4.4, chloride 101, bicarb 27, glucose 149, creatinine 2.2, down from 2.6.

His urinalysis on admission showed no protein. His microscopic examination showed no blood.

Magnesium today is elevated at 2.3.

IMPRESSION:

1. Chronic renal failure with estimated creatinine clearance of 30 ml/minutes.
2. Acute renal failure secondary to probably his cardiac cath and possibly atheroembolic disease, possible contrast nephropathy.
3. The patient does not have proteinuria, so it is unlikely that he has diabetic nephropathy. He could have renal artery stenosis or hypertensive nephrosclerosis. I think it is important to figure out what he has because if he does have renal stenosis, this probably would need to be fixed prior to his bypass surgery.
4. Generalized edema and congestive heart failure, probably precipitated by Actos.
5. Anemia of acute and chronic renal failure.
6. Type II diabetes.
7. Severe coronary artery disease which had required bypass surgery.

PLAN:

1. The patient will stay in the hospital for the time being.
2. Continue Bumex drip at 0.125 mg an hour.
3. Check spot urine protein and creatinine ratio.
4. Repeat labs in the morning to include BMP, CBC.
5. Renal ultrasound Monday morning because of the acute and chronic renal failure.
6. Will probably discharge him on Monday morning on oral Bumex.
7. The patient is already off Actos.
8. Will continue to monitor his potassium and magnesium every 6 hours and replace accordingly.

Copyright © 2005, Elsevier Inc. All rights reserved.
CPT only © 2004. *Current Procedural Terminology, 2005, Professional Edition*, American Medical Association. All rights reserved.

Discussed all of the above with the patient, including possible intervention on his renal arteries. He seems to understand and agree with the plan.

I discussed this case with the attending, and he was in agreement.

PROGRESS NOTE

The patient had no major events during the night. He is losing weight. He is diuresing very nicely. He had 341 in and 1000 out so far today. Yesterday he had 1461 in and 3750 out. He has no complaints of chest pain or shortness of breath. He appears euvolemic. He still has a little bit of edema in the lower extremities. His vitals are stable. His BUN is down to 41, sodium 140, potassium 4.2, chloride 101, bicarbonate 28.7, creatinine down to 1.7, and calcium 8.4.

His white count is 3.6 K , hemoglobin 11.1, platelets 214,000.

IMPRESSION:

1. Acute on top of chronic renal failure.
2. Generalized edema and congestive heart failure, probably precipitated by Actos, all improving.
3. The patient could have renovascular disease. If he does, it needs to be fixed prior to his bypass surgery.
4. Anemia due to acute and chronic renal failure.

PLAN:

1. The patient did not have a ride today, so he will stay here tonight and will be discharged home tomorrow.
2. We will do an ultrasound before he is discharged.
3. Repeat labs in the morning, including basic panel, magnesium, and CBC.
4. We will schedule a renal MRA as an outpatient.
5. Continue with Bumex for the time being. He will be discharged home on po Bumex. His lisinopril has been on hold and will continue to be on hold until renal MRA is done.

I discussed the above with the patient. He seems to understand and agrees with the plan.

DISCHARGE SUMMARY

DIAGNOSES:

1. Congestive heart failure and generalized edema.
2. Acute renal failure.
3. Chronic renal failure.
4. Severe coronary artery disease.

The patient is a 66-year-old male who is known to have coronary artery disease and was admitted because of generalized edema. The patient's creatinine has gone up to 2.3. He was found to have significant edema in bilateral lower extremities, thighs, and sacral area, and a few basilar crackles.

His Actos and Crestor were both discontinued. He was given Bumex and then started on Bumex for a couple of days. The patient did well. He had no major problems during his hospitalization. He had no chest pain. His edema significantly improved. He had no proteinuria, so he does not seem to have diabetic nephropathy.

The patient was discharged in good general condition; code level I. The patient's creatinine improved, going down to 1.7 on date of discharge.

Copyright © 2005, Elsevier Inc. All rights reserved.
CPT only © 2004. *Current Procedural Terminology, 2005, Professional Edition,* American Medical Association. All rights reserved.

DISCHARGE PLAN:

1. Patient will follow up with Dr. Green. He will follow up with me as well when the basic panel and CBC results are known.
2. He will continue on Bumex 2 mg daily, fluid restriction, and salt restriction. He is off Actos and Crestor.

DISCHARGE MEDICATIONS:

1. Amitriptyline 50 mg daily.
2. Humalog 15 units t.i.d. with meals.
3. Lantus 56 units nightly.
4. Lisinopril has been discontinued for the time being.
5. Multivitamin 1 daily.
6. Neurontin 300 mg, 2 tablets b.i.d.
7. Prednisone eye drops.
8. Synthroid 0.075 mg daily.
9. Torsemide discontinued.
10. Crestor discontinued.
11. Isosorbide mononitrate 30 mg daily.
12. Bumex 2 mg daily.

The patient agrees with all of the above.

Copyright © 2005, Elsevier Inc. All rights reserved.
CPT only © 2004. *Current Procedural Terminology, 2005, Professional Edition,* American Medical Association. All rights reserved.

ANSWERS WITH RATIONALES FOR FINAL EXAMINATION

PART 1

1. A 2-year-old child was brought to the outpatient radiology department at the hospital by his father for an ultrasound of child's heart. At the age of 10 months, he was diagnosed with a heart murmur due to ventricular septal defect. At age 11 months, the child developed congestive heart failure, and at that time the physician prescribed diuretics and digitalis.

745.4	Bulbus cordis anomalies and anomalies of cardiac septal closure, ventricular septal deviation
785.2	Symptoms involving cardiovascular system, undiagnosed cardiac murmurs
747.29	Other congenital anomalies of circulatory system, other anomalies of aorta, other congenital
779.8	Other specified conditions originating in the perinatal period, other specified conditions originating in the perinatal period

A. 745.4
B. 745.4, 785.2
C. 747.29, 745.4
D. 745.4, 779.29

Correct Answer: A. 745.4. This is the correct answer because the heart murmur is due to ventricular septal defect, which is reported with 745.4.

Rationale: B. 745.4, 785.2. This selection is incorrect. The murmur is not reported separately because the report indicates that the murmur was due to the ventricular septal defect and therefore reported as a part of 745.4.

C. 747.29, 745.4. This selection is incorrect because the 747.29 code represents a congenital defect of the aorta and this patient has a ventricular septal defect. The only code required is the 745.4.

D. 745.4, 779.29. This is incorrect because the 779.29 code is not necessary: All conditions that this child has are related to the ventricular septal defect and reported with 745.4.

Copyright © 2005, Elsevier Inc. All rights reserved.
CPT only © 2004. *Current Procedural Terminology, 2005, Professional Edition*, American Medical Association. All rights reserved.

2. A patient is admitted to the hospital for bacterial endocarditis due to AIDS:

042	Human Immunodeficiency virus (HIV) disease
421.0	Acute and subacute bacterial endocarditis
421.1	Acute and subacute infective endocarditis in diseases classified elsewhere
421.9	Acute endocarditis, unspecified

A. 421.0, 042
B. 042, 421.9
C. 421.1, 042
D. 042, 421.0

Correct Answer: D. This correctly identifies AIDS with 042 and bacterial endocarditis with 421.0. AIDS is sequenced first according to the Official Guidelines for Coding and Reporting, Section 1, C1, 2.

Rationale: A. 042, the code for AIDS, should be sequenced first, not second; 421.0 reports bacterial endocarditis. See the Official Guidelines for Coding and Reporting, Section 1, C1, 2.

B. 042 is correct and sequenced correctly. However, 421.9 reports acute unspecified endocarditis as the cause, whereas the question identified bacterial endocarditis. See the Official Guidelines for Coding and Reporting, Section 1, C1, 2.

C. The code for AIDS should be sequenced first, not second; 421.1 reports infective endocarditis, not endocarditis. See the Official Guidelines for Coding and Reporting, Section 1, C1, 2.

3. The system that edits outpatient claims data to identify errors and returns a series of edit flags is known as:
A. APC
B. CCI
C. OCE
D. PPS

Correct Answer: C. The term OCE stands for the Outpatient Claim Edits and is a software system used by CMS to edit claims to identify errors and return an edit flag for each error on a claim.

Rationale: A. APC, Ambulatory Patient Classification, groups services that are alike clinically and in the resource required to provide service.

B. CCI, Correct Coding Initiative, promotes national correct coding methodologies and controls improper coding, which could lead to inappropriate payment of Part B claims.

D. PPS, Prospective Payment System, is a system that pays a fixed amount for patients discharged in a treatment category or Diagnosis Related Group (DRG).

Copyright © 2005, Elsevier Inc. All rights reserved.
CPT only © 2004. *Current Procedural Terminology, 2005, Professional Edition*, American Medical Association. All rights reserved.

4. Female patient is admitted to the hospital for bilateral radical mastectomy. Final diagnosis is carcinoma of upper-outer quadrant of the breast.

85.42	Bilateral simple mastectomy
85.45	Unilateral radical mastectomy
85.46	Bilateral radical mastectomy
174.4	Malignant neoplasm of the female breast upper-outer quadrant
174.5	Malignant neoplasm of the female breast lower-outer quadrant
198.81	Secondary malignant neoplasm of the breast

A. 85.46, 174.4
B. 85.42, 174.5
C. 85.45, 174.4
D. 85.46, 198.81

Correct Answer:* A. *85.46 correctly reports a bilateral radical mastectomy; the diagnosis of breast cancer is correctly reported with 174.4, which indicates a malignant neoplasm of the female breast upper-outer quadrant.

Rationale: B. *85.42 reports a bilateral simple mastectomy, whereas the procedure performed is stated as radical. 174.5 is the diagnosis of malignant neoplasm of the female breast lower-outer quadrant rather than the upper-outer quadrant.*

C. *85.45 reports a unilateral radical mastectomy. This code would be incorrect because the procedure performed is stated as bilateral. The diagnosis code is correct.*

D. *85.46 is the correct procedure code. However, 198.81 is the diagnosis of a secondary malignant neoplasm of the breast. The stated diagnosis is a malignant neoplasm of the female breast upper-outer quadrant without any secondary neoplasm noted.*

Copyright © 2005, Elsevier Inc. All rights reserved.
CPT only © 2004. *Current Procedural Terminology, 2005, Professional Edition,* American Medical Association. All rights reserved.

5. A 26-year-old patient is seen in the ED with wrist pain received when he fell from a dirt bike. The patient is in apparent pain, and the wrist has begun to swell. He is unable to flex the wrist. The patient reports that he did strike his head on a log as a result of the fall. He denies any loss of consciousness. The ED physician ordered skull and wrist x-rays. The x-rays show no fracture of the skull but a small fracture of the wrist. The ED staff splinted the wrist. The physician prescribes acetaminophen with codeine, PO 325 mg q4h. The patient was discharged to home.

733.12	Pathologic fracture of distal radius and ulna, wrist NOS
814.00	Fracture of carpal bones, closed, unspecified, wrist NOS

A. Level 1, 733.12
B. Level 2, 814.00
C. Level 4, 814.00
D. Level 4, 733.12

Correct Answer: C. Level 4, 814.00. This choice is correct because the ED physician ordered x-rays of the wrist (Level 4, point 1) and prescribed acetaminophen with codeine (Level 3, point 4), placing this service at a Level 4. The diagnosis is a closed fracture (indicated by fifth digit 0) of the wrist.

Rationale: A. Level 2, 733.12 is incorrect because a Level 2 ED service does not contain either the x-rays of the wrist and skull (Level 4, point 1) or the prescribed acetaminophen with codeine (Level 3, point 4). The diagnosis is also incorrect because it reports a pathological injury (nontraumatic, spontaneous) and this was a traumatic injury reported with 814.00.

B. Level 2, 814.00. In this choice, the diagnosis is correct but the level is incorrect. It should be Level 3, based on the fact that the ED physician ordered an x-ray of the wrist (Level 3, point 4) and prescribed acetaminophen with codeine (Level 3, point 4).

D. Level 4, 733.12. In this choice, the level is correct but the diagnosis is incorrect because it reports a pathological injury (nontraumatic, spontaneous), whereas this was a traumatic injury reported with 814.00.

Copyright © 2005, Elsevier Inc. All rights reserved.
CPT only © 2004. *Current Procedural Terminology, 2005, Professional Edition,* American Medical Association. All rights reserved.

6. Patient fell, struck his head, and was brought to the ED. He denies any loss of consciousness. He has significant bruising on the left side of his body and complains of pain under his left arm. A series of x-rays were ordered in addition to an MRI. Examination and review of the MRI and x-rays reveal a closed fracture of the skull, with extradural hemorrhage, and fracture of two ribs. Review of the medical record reveals hypertension. Patient is admitted to inpatient observation. Report the ED service, but not the radiology service:

803.21	Skull fracture, closed with subarachnoid, subdural and extradural hemorrhage
807.02	Fracture, closed, two ribs
852.41	Extradural hemorrhage following injury without mention of open intracranial wound, no loss of consciousness
853.01	Other and unspecified intracranial hemorrhage following injury, without mention of open intracranial wound, no loss of consciousness

A. Level 4, 807.02, 803.21
B. Level 4, 803.21, 807.02
C. Level 3, 853.01, 852.41, 807.02
D. either A or B

Correct Answer: B. ***Level 4, 803.21, 807.02. In this correct answer, the skull fracture is sequenced before the rib fracture. ICD-9-CM guideline C17 B4 states multiple fractures are sequenced in accordance with the severity of the fracture. The skull fracture is considered more severe than the closed rib fracture, so it is the principal diagnosis. 803.21 is the correct code because codes 852.41 and 853.01 exclude intracranial injury with skull fracture. See excludes note at beginning of 850 codes.***

Rationale: A. *Level 4, 807.02, 803.21. The level is correct, but the diagnoses are in the wrong sequence. Rib fractures (807.02) are considered less severe than the skull fracture (803.21); the former is considered a secondary diagnosis and sequenced after the principal diagnosis.*

C. *Level 3, 853.01, 852.41, 807.02. In this incorrect selection, the level should have been Level 4 because x-rays and an MRI were ordered (Level 4, point 1 and 2). 853.01 reports an unspecified intracranial hemorrhage, but there is no documentation of this injury. The diagnosis code 852.41 is incorrect because it does not include an extradural hemorrhage due to a skull fracture (See excludes note at beginning of 850 codes). 807.02 is correct to report the rib fracture.*

D. *Either A or B. In this choice, only choice B is correct. For choice A Level 4, 807.02, 803.21, the level is correct, but the diagnoses are in the wrong sequence. Rib fractures (807.02) are considered less severe than the skull fracture (803.21) and would be sequenced second and considered a secondary diagnosis.*

Copyright © 2005, Elsevier Inc. All rights reserved.
CPT only © 2004. *Current Procedural Terminology, 2005, Professional Edition,* American Medical Association. All rights reserved.

7. A patient is admitted to the hospital with carcinoma of the prostate. The surgeon performed a bilateral pelvic lymphadenectomy with frozen section, radical retropubic prostatectomy, and plastic repair of the bladder neck using an open approach. The procedure was performed with spinal anesthetic. The pathology report later indicated T4a adenocarcinoma of the prostate.

40.29	Simple excision of other lymphatic structure, includes simple lymphadenectomy
57.85	Cystourethroplasty and plastic repair of bladder neck
60.69	Other prostatectomy, by any approach
60.5	Radical prostatectomy, by any approach
185	Malignant neoplasm of prostate

A. 60.69, 40.29, 57.85, 185
B. 60.5, 57.85, 185
C. 60.5, 57.85, 40.29, 185
D. 60.69, 57.85, 185

Correct Answer: C. 60.5, 57.85, 40.29, 185. The report indicated the procedures were a lymphadenectomy (40.29), radical prostatectomy (60.5), and plastic repair of the bladder neck (57.85). The diagnosis is primary, malignant neoplasm of the prostate reported with 185.

Rationale: A. 60.69, 40.29, 57.85, 185. This selection has only one incorrect code, that for the radical prostatectomy (60.5), not other prostatectomy (60.69).

B. 60.5, 57.85, 185. This selection is correct except it is missing the report of the lymphadenectomy with 40.29.

D. 60.69, 57.85, 185. This selection is incorrect because it reports an "Other prostatectomy" when the documentation indicates "Radical prostatectomy." Also missing is the lymphadenectomy (40.29).

Copyright © 2005, Elsevier Inc. All rights reserved.
CPT only © 2004. *Current Procedural Terminology, 2005, Professional Edition,* American Medical Association. All rights reserved.

8. A 28-week pregnant woman is seen in the ED for a fracture of the right ankle, which is not affecting the pregnancy. Patient also complains of constant radiating pain down the left leg, which, after examination, is determined to be related to the pregnancy. The correct coding sequence is:
   A. pregnancy related code, ankle fracture, leg pain
   B. ankle fracture, pregnancy related code, leg pain
   C. ankle fracture, leg pain, pregnancy related code
   D. leg pain, ankle fracture, pregnancy related code

Correct Answer: B. ***This is the correct sequence. The ankle fracture is the primary reason for the patient's visit to the ED. According to the Official Guidelines for Coding and Reporting, C11, 1 and 2, unless the physician states the encounter is incidental to the pregnancy, the codes from Chapter 11, Complications of Pregnancy, Childbirth, and the Puerperium should be sequenced first. In this case, the physician stated the right ankle fracture was not affecting the pregnancy, but the left leg radiating pain was affecting the pregnancy. The physician states that the leg pain was related to the pregnancy, so it is correct to report a code from this classification; a code would then be reported to indicate what the complication was (leg pain).***

Rationale: A. *This choice is incorrect because the ankle fracture, not the pregnancy, is the primary reason for the ED visit.*

C. *Although the ankle fracture is the primary reason for the ED visit, the sequencing of the two remaining codes is incorrect. According to the Official Guidelines for Coding and Reporting, C11, 1 and 2, unless the physician states the encounter is incidental to the pregnancy, the codes from Chapter 11, Complications of Pregnancy, Childbirth, and the Puerperium should be sequenced first. In this case, the physician stated the right ankle fracture was not affecting the pregnancy, but the left leg radiating pain was affecting the pregnancy. The physician states that the leg pain was related to the pregnancy, so it is correct to report a code from this classification; a code would then be reported to indicate what the complication was (leg pain).*

D. *This choice is incorrect because the leg pain is not the primary reason for the ED visit. Rather, the primary reason for the visit is the ankle fracture, followed by a pregnancy-related code to report a condition was complicating pregnancy and a code to indicate what the complication was (leg pain).*

Copyright © 2005, Elsevier Inc. All rights reserved.
CPT only © 2004. *Current Procedural Terminology, 2005, Professional Edition*, American Medical Association. All rights reserved.

9. Patient is admitted to the hospital for congestive heart failure, hypertensive heart disease, and hypertensive renal disease. The coder assigns:
   A. congestive heart failure and hypertensive renal disease
   B. combination code for hypertensive heart and renal disease
   C. hypertensive heart disease, hypertensive renal disease
   D. combination code for hypertensive heart and renal disease and congestive heart failure

Correct Answer: D. ***The sequencing for this choice is correct per ICD-9-CM guideline Section I C7, 4, which directs the coder to assign codes from the combination category for hypertensive heart and renal disease and then assign an additional code to identify the type of heart failure (in this case, congestive heart failure).***

Rationale: A. *Sequencing the congestive heart failure first is incorrect based on the ICD-9-CM guideline Section I C7, 4, which directs the coder to assign a code from the combination category for hypertensive heart and renal disease and then assign an additional code to identify the type of heart failure (in this case, congestive heart failure).*

B. *Although the combination code is correct to report the hypertensive heart and renal disease, a code to report the congestive heart failure is missing.*

C. *ICD-9-CM guidelines direct the coder to report the hypertensive heart disease and hypertensive renal disease with a combination code, not, as in this choice, where the hypertensive heart disease is reported first followed by the hypertensive renal disease. In addition, this choice is missing the code for the congestive heart failure.*

Copyright © 2005, Elsevier Inc. All rights reserved.
CPT only © 2004. *Current Procedural Terminology, 2005, Professional Edition,* American Medical Association. All rights reserved.

10. A 10-year-old boy presents to the ED for injuries caused by falling off his bike. All wounds were superficial. He has a 2-cm wound to his nose and a 1-cm wound to his cheek. He also has a 2.5-cm wound to his elbow. All injuries were simple repair by means of suture. Acetaminophen was administered, 325 mg. The patient's mother was advised to give the child acetaminophen if needed for pain. Directions for care of the wounds were given with follow-up with the child's pediatrician in 10 days. What would the code(s) be to report the wound repair?

12001	Simple repair of superficial wounds of scalp, neck, axillae, external genitalia, trunk and\or extremities (including hands and feet); 2.5 cm or less
12002	Simple repair of superficial wounds of scalp, neck, axillae, external genitalia, trunk and\or extremities (including hands and feet); 2.6 cm to 7.5 cm
12011	Simple repair of superficial wounds of face, ears, eyelids, nose, lips and\or mucous membranes; 2.5 cm or less
12013	Simple repair of superficial wounds of face, ears, eyelids, nose, lips and\or mucous membranes; 2.6 cm to 5.0 cm

A. Level 2, 12002
B. Level 2, 12013, 12001
C. Level 1, 12013, 12002
D. Level 1, 12011, 12002

Correct Answer: B. ***Level 2 is correct because this patient was given an over-the-counter medicine (acetaminophen) and provided simple discharge information. 12013 describes a simple repair of superficial wounds to the face or nose (2.6 to 5.0 cm), and the superficial wounds to this patient were a 2-cm wound to the nose and a 1-cm wound to the cheek; so you add those two superficial wounds together (3 cm) before you choose the correct code (12013). 12001 describes the simple repair of superficial wounds to extremities (2.5 cm or smaller), and this patient's wound was a superficial wound to the elbow with a length of 2.5 cm. NOTE: Be certain always to add the lengths of repairs together for each group of anatomical sites of the same complexity.***

Rationale: A. *Level 2 is correct because this patient was given an over-the-counter medicine (acetaminophen) and provided simple discharge information. 12011 is not correct because it is for simple repair of superficial wounds of the face or nose (2.5 cm or smaller), and the patient had a 2-cm repair of the nose and a 1-cm repair of the cheek (nose and face); these are added together (3 cm) before the correct code is chosen. Because 12011 is for wounds smaller than 2.5 cm, it is not the correct code. 12001 is the correct code because it describes simple repair of superficial wounds to extremities (2.5 cm or smaller), and this patient's wound was a superficial wound to the elbow with a length of 2.5 cm.*

C. *Level 1 is incorrect because this patient was given an over-the-counter medicine (acetaminophen) and provided simple discharge information as reported with Level 2. 12013 is correct for the first code because it describes a simple repair of superficial wounds to the face or nose (2.6 to 5.0 cm), and the superficial wounds to the patient were a 2-cm wound to the nose and a 1-cm wound to the cheek; so you add those two superficial wounds together*

Copyright © 2005, Elsevier Inc. All rights reserved.
CPT only © 2004. *Current Procedural Terminology, 2005, Professional Edition,* American Medical Association. All rights reserved.

(3 cm) before you choose the correct code (12013). 12002 is not correct, however, because it describes a simple repair of superficial wound of extremities 2.6 cm to 7.5 cm, and the patient's elbow wound was 2.5 cm.

D. Level 1 is incorrect because this patient was given an over-the-counter medicine (acetaminophen) and provided simple discharge information as reported with Level 2. 12011 is not correct because it is for simple repair of superficial wounds of the face or nose (2.5 cm or smaller), and the patient had a 2-cm repair of the nose and a 1-cm repair of the cheek (nose and face), which are added together (3 cm) before the correct code is chosen. Because 12011 is for wounds smaller than 2.5 cm, it is not the correct code. 12002 is not correct for the elbow repair because 12002 is a simple repair of superficial wounds of extremities 2.6 to 7.5cm, and the patient's elbow wound was 2.5 cm.

11. Patient presents to the ASC for incisional biopsy of both breasts.

19102	Biopsy of breast; percutaneous, needle core, using imaging guidance
19101	Biopsy of breast; open incisional
19125	Excision of breast lesion identified by preoperative placement of radiological marker, open, single lesion
-50	Bilateral Procedure
-LT	Left
-RT	Right

A. 19102-50
B. 19101-RT, 19101-LT
C. 19101-50
D. 19125-RT, 19125-LT

Correct Answer: B. 19101 is for an open biopsy of the breast. -RT and -LT are used to report that the procedure was bilateral.

Rationale: A. 19102-50 is for a percutaneous biopsy of breast, not an open biopsy.

C. 19101-50 is for an open biopsy of the breast, and modifiers -RT and -LT are the most specific and should be reported rather than -50.

D. 19125-RT, 19125-LT describes an excision of breast lesion identified by preoperative placement of radiological marker, open, single lesion. The procedure documented is a biopsy, not an excision of a lesion. The documentation did not indicate the placement of a radiological marker.

Copyright © 2005, Elsevier Inc. All rights reserved.
CPT only © 2004. *Current Procedural Terminology, 2005, Professional Edition*, American Medical Association. All rights reserved.

12. A patient with ovarian cancer is admitted to the hospital to receive chemotherapy. The patient develops uncontrolled nausea and vomiting. The principal diagnosis is:
    A. uncontrolled nausea
    B. ovarian cancer
    C. chemotherapy
    D. vomiting

Correct Answer: C. ***Chemotherapy. This is the correct choice because, according to the ICD-9-CM guideline Section I, C2, E3, when a patient is admitted for chemotherapy and develops complications such as nausea and vomiting, the principal or first-listed diagnosis is the chemotherapy (V58.1).***

Rationale: A. & D. *Uncontrolled nausea and vomiting are complications of the chemotherapy, the primary reason for admission, and as such are listed as secondary diagnoses, not the primary diagnosis.*

B. *ICD-9-CM guideline Section I, C2, E2 states that if the patient admission is solely for the chemotherapy, the therapy is the first-listed or principal diagnosis.*

13. Marsha presents to the ASC after having an abnormal shoulder x-ray in the clinic yesterday. The physician does a diagnostic arthroscopy and performs a limited debridement of the shoulder joint.

29805	Arthroscopy, shoulder, diagnostic, with or without synovial biopsy (separate procedure)
29822	Arthroscopy, shoulder, surgical; debridement, limited
29823	; debridement, extensive

A. 29805
B. 29823
C. 29822, 29805
D. 29822

Correct Answer: D. ***29822 Arthroscopy, shoulder, surgical; debridement, limited, which is the service provided.***

Rationale: A. *29805 is used to report a diagnostic arthroscopy, and although the procedure began as a diagnostic procedure, the surgeon performed a surgical procedure; as such, only the surgical procedure is reported. The diagnostic procedure is bundled into the surgical procedure.*

B. *29823 is used to report arthroscopy with extensive debridement, and there was only a limited debridement performed.*

C. *This choice includes the code for arthroscopy with limited debridement (29822) and a code (29805) for the diagnostic arthroscopy, which is always included in a surgical arthroscopy (CPT guideline prior to endoscopy/arthroscopy section contains this information).*

Copyright © 2005, Elsevier Inc. All rights reserved.
CPT only © 2004. *Current Procedural Terminology, 2005, Professional Edition,* American Medical Association. All rights reserved.

14. Cole comes into the ED today with his mother after falling from the top bunk bed where he and his brother were wrestling. He is having pain in his left lower leg and is unable to bear weight on it. He also complains of a headache and nausea. Cole was taken to the x-ray department for views of the ankle and skull. After the physician talks with the radiologist regarding the diagnosis of ankle fracture and probable concussion, a walking short leg cast is applied from just below his knee to his toes. The patient is admitted to observation. What is the principal diagnosis reported by the hospital for the admission?
    A. ankle fracture
    B. concussion
    C. headache
    D. headache and nausea

Correct Answer: B. ***Concussion is the diagnosis, which, after study, is the physician's reason for admission. Inpatient settings report possible diagnoses as indicated in the guideline, Section II, H, which states to code the possible diagnosis "as if it existed or was established."***

Rationale: A. *Ankle fracture is the reason for cast application.*

C. & D. *Headache and nausea are both symptoms of the possible concussion; however, inpatient diagnostic coding rules allow for coding of probable conditions as if they are established.*

15. A 17-year-old male is admitted to the hospital for a tonsillectomy and possible adenoidectomy due to chronic tonsillitis. On inspection, the adenoids were found not to be inflamed; a tonsillectomy was performed:

474.00	Chronic tonsillitis
474.02	Chronic tonsillitis and adenoiditis
474.10	Hypertrophy of tonsils with adenoids
28.2	Tonsillectomy without adenoidectomy
28.3	Tonsillectomy with adenoidectomy

    A. 28.2, 474.00
    B. 28.2, 474.02
    C. 28.3, 474.10
    D. 28.3, 474.00

Correct Answer: A. ***28.2 is a tonsillectomy without adenoidectomy, as indicated in the statement of the procedure. 474.00 (chronic tonsillitis) is the correct diagnosis code.***

Rationale: B. *28.2 is a tonsillectomy without adenoidectomy, as indicated in the statement of the procedure. However, 474.02 is the diagnosis for chronic tonsillitis and chronic adenoiditis; the patient had only chronic tonsillitis*

C. *28.3 is a tonsillectomy with adenoidectomy; the case indicated a tonsillectomy, not an adenoidectomy. 474.10 is the diagnosis for hypertrophy of tonsils and adenoids, but the patient had chronic tonsillitis.*

D. *28.3 is a tonsillectomy with adenoidectomy; the case indicated a tonsillectomy, not an adenoidectomy. 474.00 (chronic tonsillitis) is the correct diagnosis code.*

Copyright © 2005, Elsevier Inc. All rights reserved.
CPT only © 2004. *Current Procedural Terminology, 2005, Professional Edition,* American Medical Association. All rights reserved.

16. A 62-year-old female presents to ASC for a sigmoidoscopy. The physician inserts a flexible scope into the patient's rectum and determines the rectum is clear of any polyps. The scope is advanced to the sigmoid colon, and three polyps are found. Using the snare technique, the polyps are removed. The remainder of the colon is free of polyps. The scope is withdrawn.

153.3	Malignant neoplasm of sigmoid colon
153.9	Malignant neoplasm of colon, unspecified
211.3	Benign neoplasm of colon
44110	Excision of one or more lesions of small or large intestine not requiring anastomosis, exteriorization, or fistulization; single enterotomy
44111	Excision of one or more lesions of small or large intestine not requiring anastomosis, exteriorization, or fistulization; multiple enterotomies
45383	Colonoscopy, flexible, proximal to splenic flexure; with ablation of tumor(s), polyp(s), or other lesion(s) not amenable to removal by hot biopsy forceps, bipolar cautery or snare technique
45338	Sigmoidoscopy, flexible; with removal of tumor(s), polyp(s), or other lesion(s) by snare technique

A. 45383, 211.3
B. 44110, 153.9
C. 45338, 211.3
D. 44111, 153.3

Correct Answer: C. 45338, 211.3. 45338 is a flexible sigmoidoscopy with snare removal of polyp(s). 211.3 is the correct code for polyps of the sigmoid colon.

Rationale: A. 45383 is a colonoscopy with removal of polyp(s) that cannot be removed with a snare. Snare is the technique used to remove the polyps in this case. 211.3 is the correct diagnosis code.

B. 44110 describes removal of lesion(s) through an abdominal incision and then incision into the colon (colotomy), but the procedure described in the case is removal by means of a scope. 153.9 is the code for malignant neoplasm, colon. The report does not state that the polyps were malignant.

D. 44111 is removal of a lesion(s) through an abdominal incision and then incision into the colon (colotomy), but the procedure described in the case was removal by means of a scope. 153.3 is the code for malignant neoplasm, sigmoid colon. This code is also incorrect; the report says nothing about a malignancy.

Copyright © 2005, Elsevier Inc. All rights reserved.
CPT only © 2004. *Current Procedural Terminology, 2005, Professional Edition,* American Medical Association. All rights reserved.

17. Margie, a 62-year-old female, presents to the ED with complaints of chest pain and shortness of breath. She has been experiencing these symptoms for the last 2 hours. The ED physician requests a portable two-view chest x-ray, various laboratory studies, and an ultrasound. It is decided to admit the patient to the hospital. The cardiologist will assume care for this patient. Report the ED services.

786	Symptoms involving respiratory system and other chest symptoms
786.05	Shortness of breath
786.50	Chest pain, unspecified

A. Level 4, 786.50, 786
B. Level 4, 786.50, 786.05
C. Level 5, 786, 786.05
D. Level 5, 786.50, 786.05

Correct Answer: D. Level 5, 786.50, 786.05. This choice correctly reports the level as Level 5 because the patient was admitted (Level 5, point 8). The diagnosis codes are 786.50 for chest pain and 786.05 for shortness of breath.

Rationale: A. Level 4, 786.50, 786. This choice is not correct because the ED service was a Level 5, not Level 4. See Level 5, point 8, which indicates hospital admission. Even though the x-rays of one area (chest) are Level 3 and the ultrasound is Level 4, this patient was admitted and therefore is a Level 5. 786.50 is the correct diagnosis code for chest pain, but 786 needs all five digits to be correct. Always code to the furthest specificity, which means do not use a three-digit code if a four-digit code is available, and do not use a four-digit code if a five-digit one is available.

B. Level 4, 786.50, 786.05. This choice is not correct because the ED service was a Level 5, not Level 4. See Level 5, point 8, which indicates hospital admission. Even though the x-rays of one area (chest) are Level 3 and the ultrasound is Level 4, this patient was admitted and therefore is a Level 5. 786.50 and 786.05 are the correct diagnoses codes.

C. Level 5, 786, 786.05. The level for this choice is correct at a Level 5, as is the diagnosis for the SOB (shortness of breath, 786.05). 786 is not correct for the chest pains because a five-digit code is available. Always code to the furthest specificity, which means do not use a three-digit code if a four-digit code is available, and do not use a four-digit code if a five-digit one is available.

Copyright © 2005, Elsevier Inc. All rights reserved.
CPT only © 2004. *Current Procedural Terminology, 2005, Professional Edition,* American Medical Association. All rights reserved.

18. The physician lists the final diagnosis as cough and high fever for this inpatient. Physician documentation states possible acute bronchitis versus pneumonia. The following diagnoses codes are assigned:

466.0	Acute bronchitis
486	Pneumonia, organism unspecified
780.6	Fever
786.2	Cough

A. 466.0, 780.6
B. 780.6, 786.2, 486, 466.0
C. 486, 466.0
D. 786.2, 780.6

Correct Answer: B. ***780.6, 786.2, 486, 466.0. 780.6, Fever, 786.2, Cough, 486 Pneumonia, organism unspecified, and 466.0, Acute bronchitis. ICD-9-CM guideline section II A states that codes for signs and symptoms are not to used as a principal diagnosis when a related definitive diagnosis has been established. In this case, a definitive diagnosis of either pneumonia or acute bronchitis has not been established; therefore it is correct to sequence the signs and symptoms of fever and cough first (see Section II, E). ICD-9-CM guideline Section II, H states to code "probable," "suspected," "likely," questionable," "possible," or "still to be ruled out" conditions as if they existed. Therefore pneumonia and acute bronchitis are also assigned.***

Rationale: A. & C. *are both incorrect because a definitive diagnosis of acute bronchitis or pneumonia has not yet been reached.*

D. *Although 786.2, Cough, and 780.6, Fever, are correct as the principal diagnosis per the ICD-9-CM guidelines, this choice does not include the "probable," "suspected," "likely," "questionable," "possible," or "still to be ruled out" conditions of pneumonia and acute bronchitis.*

Copyright © 2005, Elsevier Inc. All rights reserved.
CPT only © 2004. *Current Procedural Terminology, 2005, Professional Edition,* American Medical Association. All rights reserved.

19. This 70-year-old male is taken to the ED with severe chest pain. While the ED physician is attempting to stabilize the patient, the patient's pressures drop and he goes into cardiac arrest. Cardiopulmonary resuscitation is performed on the patient, and his pressure returns to normal. The ED physician and staff spent 90 minutes providing services to this patient. He is transferred to the intensive care unit in critical condition.

92950	Cardiopulmonary resuscitation (e.g., in cardiac arrest)
92960	Cardioversion, elective, electrical conversion of arrhythmia; external
92970	Cardioassist-method of circulatory assist; internal
99291	Critical care, 30–74 minutes
99292	each additional 30 minutes
786.50	Chest pain
427.5	Cardiac arrest

A. 92950, 427.5
B. 92970, 427.5, 786.50
C. 99291, 92950, 427.5
D. 99291, 99292, 92950, 427.5, 786.50

Correct Answer: C. ***99291, 92950, 427.5. The ED physician and staff spent 90 minutes providing care to this patient, so the critical care code 99291 is correct. EDs report only 99291 no matter the time spent in care of the patient. 92950 correctly reports only the cardiopulmonary resuscitation. 427.5 is the code for cardiac arrest.***

Rationale: A. *92950, 427.5. This choice is incorrect because the report of the critical care is missing. 92950 is correct, however, for the cardiopulmonary resuscitation. 427.5 is coded correctly.*

B. *92970, 427.5, 786.50 is incorrect because the 92970 is used to report cardioassist method of circulatory assist, internal, and was not specified in the case. Also missing is the critical care service. 427.5 is the correct diagnosis for cardiac arrest. It is incorrect to report the chest pain in addition to the cardiac arrest.*

D. *99291, 99292, 92950, 427.5, 786.50 is correct except for the reporting of the chest pain (786.50), which is not reported separately because it would be included in the more definitive diagnosis as cardiac arrest, and the second critical care code, as EDs report only 99291.*

20. This modifier indicates that an outpatient procedure was converted to an inpatient status due to an unexpected occurrence during a scheduled outpatient procedure:
A. -58
B. -73
C. -CA
D. -74

Correct Answer: C. ***-CA is the modifier that indicates that a procedure that began in the outpatient setting was transferred to the inpatient setting. This modifier is assigned only to inpatient procedures.***

Rationale: A. *-58 indicates a staged or related procedure or service by the same physician during the postoperative period.*

B. *-73 indicates a discontinued outpatient hospital/ambulatory surgery center procedure prior to the administration of anesthesia.*

D. *-74 indicates a discontinued outpatient hospital/ambulatory surgery center procedure after the administration of anesthesia.*

Copyright © 2005, Elsevier Inc. All rights reserved.
CPT only © 2004. *Current Procedural Terminology, 2005, Professional Edition*, American Medical Association. All rights reserved.

21. A 51-year-old male patient had surgery to remove two separate carbuncles of the left axilla. Pathology report indicated staphylococcal infection. Report the diagnoses.

680.3	Carbuncle and Furuncle Upper arm and forearm, Axilla, Shoulder
041.10	Staphylococcus, unspecified
041.19	Other staphylococcus
041.09	Other streptococcus

A. 680.3, 041.10
B. 680.3, 041.09
C. 680.3, 041.19
D. 041.09, 680.3

Correct Answer: A. The carbuncle is listed first using 680.3, and the cause of the infection (staphylococcal, unspecified, 041.10) is listed second.

Rationale: B. 041.09 is the code used to report streptococcus, not staphylococcus; 680.9 is for a site that is not specified.

C. 041.19 is used to report other staphylococcus, which means other than staphylococcus not specified and not S. aureus. *680.3 is correct for the carbuncle.*

D. 041.09 is used to report other staphylococcus, but again, 680.9 is for a site that is not specified.

Copyright © 2005, Elsevier Inc. All rights reserved.
CPT only © 2004. *Current Procedural Terminology, 2005, Professional Edition*, American Medical Association. All rights reserved.

22. Richard, a 34-year-old male, was transferred to the ASC from the ED. He had fallen from a 4-foot scaffolding and hit his lower leg on the bottom rung of the support, fracturing his tibial shaft. The fracture sites were secured by means of percutaneous fixation.

27750	Closed treatment of tibial shaft fracture (with or without fibular fracture); without manipulation
27752	; with manipulation, with or without skeletal traction
27756	Percutaneous skeletal fixation of tibial shaft fracture (with or without fibular fracture) (e.g., pins or screws)
823.20	Shaft, closed tibia alone
823.30	Shaft, open tibia alone

A. 27750, 823.30
B. 27756, 823.30
C. 27752, 823.20
D. 27756, 823.20

Correct Answer: D. 27756 describes the treatment of a tibial shaft fracture with percutaneous fixation, which is the service provided in this scenario. 823.20 is the correct diagnosis for this patient. ICD-9-CM guidelines for coding of fractures not specified as open or closed stipulate that they be coded as closed.

Rationale: A. 27750 is used for the closed treatment of a tibial fracture without manipulation as in this service; however, it does include the percutaneous fixation that was performed. 823.30 is a documented open shaft fracture of the tibia. ICD-9-CM guidelines indicate that a fracture not specified as open or closed is to be reported as a closed fracture.

B. 27756 is the correct procedure code. 823.30 is a documented open shaft fracture of the fibula with the tibia. ICD-9-CM guidelines indicate that a fracture not specified as open or closed is to be reported as a closed fracture.

C. 27752 is used for closed treatment with manipulation of a tibial fracture with or without skeletal traction. 823.20 is the correct diagnosis.

Copyright © 2005, Elsevier Inc. All rights reserved.
CPT only © 2004. *Current Procedural Terminology, 2005, Professional Edition*, American Medical Association. All rights reserved.

23. Procedure performed is an endoscopic ethmoidectomy total with an endoscopic maxillary antrostomy with removal of maxillary tissue due to chronic sinusitis. Surgery was performed at ASC, located within the hospital. Code the procedure(s) and diagnosis.

31200	Ethmoidectomy; intranasal, anterior
31225	Maxillectomy; without orbital exenteration
31254	Nasal/sinus endoscopy, surgical; with ethmoidectomy, partial (anterior)
31255	Nasal/sinus endoscopy, surgical; with ethmoidectomy, total (anterior and posterior)
31256	Nasal/sinus endoscopy, surgical, with maxillary antrostomy;
31267	Nasal/sinus endoscopy, surgical, with maxillary antrostomy; with removal of tissue from maxillary sinus
461.9	Acute sinusitis, unspecified
473.9	Unspecified sinusitis (chronic)
-51	Multiple procedure

A. 31254, 31256-51, 473.9
B. 31255, 31267-51, 461.9
C. 31255, 31267-51, 473.9
D. 31200, 31225-51, 473.9

Correct Answer: C. ***31255, nasal/sinus endoscopy, surgical; with ethmoidectomy, total; 31267-51, nasal/sinus endoscopy, surgical, with maxillary antrostomy, with removal of tissue from maxillary sinus; the -51 modifier shows that a multiple procedure was performed. 473.9, chronic sinusitis, correctly describes the stated diagnosis.***

Rationale: A. *31254 is for a nasal/sinus endoscopy, surgical, but with only a partial ethmoidectomy; the question indicated a total ethmoidectomy. 31256-51 is for a surgical nasal/sinus endoscopy, with maxillary antrostomy without maxillary sinus tissue removal; 473.9, chronic sinusitis, is the correct diagnosis.*

B. *31255, nasal/sinus endoscopy with total ethmoidectomy is the correct code. 31267-51, nasal/sinus endoscopy with maxillary antrostomy with -51 modifier is the correct code; 461.9 acute sinusitis is incorrect. The operative report states that the patient suffers from chronic sinusitis, 473.9.*

D. *31200 is for ethmoidectomy, intranasal, anterior; 31225-51 is for maxillectomy without orbital exenteration, and 473.9 chronic sinusitis is the correct diagnosis.*

Copyright © 2005, Elsevier Inc. All rights reserved.
CPT only © 2004. *Current Procedural Terminology, 2005, Professional Edition*, American Medical Association. All rights reserved.

24. A 65-year-old gentleman is an inpatient who underwent left total hip arthroplasty and developed urinary retention. He has had several trials of voiding with both alpha blockade and bethanechol. The patient was given a spinal anesthetic, prepped, and draped in the lithotomy position. A 28 French resectoscope was passed under direct vision. Again, the prostate showed irregular ingrowth and obstruction. The bladder shows mild to moderate trabeculation. The prostate was thoroughly resected, chips evacuated from the bladder, and hemostasis achieved. A 22 French three-way catheter was inserted into the bladder and placed at continuous bladder irrigation. There was a large piece of tissue acting as a ball valve. A transurethral resection of the prostate was performed. The medical record indicates recurrent prostatic hyperplasia.

57.32	Other cystoscopy, transurethral cystoscopy
57.33	Closed (transurethral) biopsy of bladder
60.21	Transurethral (ultrasound) guided laser induced prostatectomy, TULIP
60.29	Other transurethral prostatectomy, TURP
601.8	Other specified inflammatory diseases of the prostate
600.91	Hyperplasia of prostate with urinary obstruction

A. 60.29, 57.32, 600.91
B. 60.21, 57.33, 600.91
C. 57.32, 60.29, 601.8
D. 60.29, 600.91

Correct Answer: A. 60.29, 57.32, 600.91. This choice correctly reports the services of a transurethral resection of the prostate (TURP) with 60.29 and transurethral cystoscopy with 57.32. The diagnosis of hyperplasia of the prostate with urinary retention is reported with 600.91.

Rationale: B. 60.21, 57.33, 600.91. Both procedures are incorrectly reported on this choice. The procedure was a transurethral resection of the prostate (TURP, 60.29), not one with ultrasound guidance (60.21), and transurethral cystoscopy (57.32), not a closed transurethral biopsy of the bladder (57.33).

C. 57.32, 60.29, 601.8. This choice is incorrect because the diagnosis is not other specified inflammatory diseases of the prostate but rather hyperplasia of the prostate with urinary obstruction.

D. 60.29, 600.91. This choice is correct except that it is missing the procedure code to report that this was a transurethral cystoscopy (57.32).

Copyright © 2005, Elsevier Inc. All rights reserved.
CPT only © 2004. *Current Procedural Terminology, 2005, Professional Edition*, American Medical Association. All rights reserved.

25. Susan was admitted to the hospital for dysfunctional uterine bleeding. She was taken to the operating room, where the bladder was straight catheterized. A weighted speculum was placed in the vagina. The anterior lip of the cervix was grasped with a single tooth tenaculum. Kevorkian curet was then used to obtain endocervical curetting. The uterus was then sounded to a depth of 6 cm. The cervical os was then serially dilated to allow passage of the hysteroscope. The hysteroscope was then passed, and uterine contents were examined, documented, and photographed. No evidence of polyps or fibroids were found. A fractional dilation and curettage was accomplished when a sharp curet was used to thoroughly sample endometrial cavity, with return of a moderate amount of tissue. The tenaculum was removed from the cervix, and the tenaculum site was oversewn with 3-0 chromic figure-of-eight sutures.

68.16	Closed biopsy of the uterus
69.09	Dilation and curettage of the uterus, other dilation and curettage
626.2	Disorders of menstruation and other abnormal bleeding from female genital tract, excessive or frequent menstruation
626.8	Disorders of menstruation and other abnormal bleeding from female genital tract, other, dysfunctional or functional uterine hemorrhage NOS

A. 68.16, 626.8
B. 68.16, 69.09, 626.8
C. 69.09, 626.8
D. 69.09, 626.2

Correct Answer: B. 68.16, 69.09, 626.8. This choice is correct because it reports the closed biopsy (68.16), dilation and curettage (69.09), and the diagnosis as dysfunctional uterine bleeding (626.8).

Rationale: A. 68.16, 626.8. This choice is incorrect because it does not report the dilation and curettage (69.09).

C. 69.09, 626.8. This choice is incorrect because it does not report the closed biopsy (68.16).

D. 69.09, 626.2. This choice is incorrect because it does not report the closed biopsy (68.16), nor does it report the diagnosis correctly as dysfunctional uterine bleeding (626.8); rather, it reports excessive or frequent menstruation (626.2). The report specified dysfunctional uterine bleeding.

Copyright © 2005, Elsevier Inc. All rights reserved.
CPT only © 2004. *Current Procedural Terminology, 2005, Professional Edition,* American Medical Association. All rights reserved.

26. A 16-year-old female with history of chronic renal failure due to cytomegalovirus infection and a failed kidney transplant was admitted to the hospital for her second transplant. The patient has an established AV fistula and received hemodialysis during the hospital stay prior to the transplant procedure. The failed kidney was removed and replaced with a donor organ. Postoperatively the donor organ was fully functional. The hospital course was without further complication, and the patient was subsequently discharged.

078.5	Cytomegalovirus disease
996.81	Complications of transplanted organ, kidney
586	Renal failure, unspecified
585	Chronic renal failure
55.53	Complete nephrectomy, removal of transplanted or rejected kidney
55.69	Transplant of kidney, other kidney transplant
39.95	Hemodialysis

A. 585, 996.81, 078.5, 55.53, 55.69, 39.95
B. 996.81, 078.5, 55.53, 55.69
C. 586, 996.81, 078.5, 55.53, 55.69, 39.95
D. 996.81, 078.5, 585, 55.53, 55.69, 39.95

Correct Answer: D. 996.81, 078.5, 585, 55.53, 55.69, 39.95. In this correct choice, 996.81 correctly reports the complication first because according to the guidelines, Section II, G: "When the admission is for treatment of a complication resulting from surgery of other medical care, the complication code is sequenced as the principal diagnosis. If the complication is classified to the 996-999 series, an additional code for the specific complication may be assigned." The complication is, therefore, listed first followed by 078.5 to report the cytomegalovirus disease, which lead to the complication. The diagnoses also stated chronic renal failure reported with 585. The procedures performed were nephrectomy (55.53), kidney transplant (55.69), and hemodialysis (39.95).

Rationale: A. 585, 996.81, 078.5, 55.53, 55.69, 39.95. In this response the codes are correct, but the principal diagnosis should have been the reason for the admission, which was a complication of the transplanted kidney (996.81) and as such listed first.

B. 996.81, 078.5, 55.53, 55.69. In this response the chronic renal failure code (585) and the hemodialysis treatment (39.95) are missing.

C. 586, 996.81, 078.5, 55.53, 55.69, 39.95. In this response the principal diagnosis should have been the reason for the admission, which was a complication of the transplanted kidney (996.81) and as such listed first. Also, 586 reports renal failure, and this patient had chronic renal failure (585).

Copyright © 2005, Elsevier Inc. All rights reserved.
CPT only © 2004. *Current Procedural Terminology, 2005, Professional Edition*, American Medical Association. All rights reserved.

27. A 21-year-old male patient is brought to the ED by ambulance. He is unresponsive, with tachycardia and tachypnea. He fell from scaffolding at work, approximately 40 feet. He has sustained multiple skull fractures and severe head trauma and has been unconscious about 20 minutes now. The ED physician placed an endotracheal tube for intubation and inserted a temporary central venous catheter (non-tunneled and centrally inserted). The ED physician had to hand bag the patient for 10 minutes until the neurologist arrived in the ED to assume care of this critically injured patient. The ED physician spent a total of 80 minutes caring for this patient.

99291	Critical care E/M, first 30–74 minutes
99292	each additional 30 minutes
31500	Intubation, endotracheal, emergency procedure
36556	Insertion of non-tunneled centrally inserted central venous catheter, over 5
36558	Insertion of tunneled centrally inserted central venous catheter, without subcutaneous port or pump, over 5
803.46	Other and unqualified skull fractures, closed with intracranial injury of other and unspecified nature, with loss of consciousness of unspecified duration
803.42	Other and unqualified skull fractures, closed with intracranial injury of other and unspecified nature, with brief [less than one hour] loss of consciousness

A. Level 5, 31500, 36556, 803.46
B. 99291, 31500, 36556, 803.46
C. 99291, 99292 × 2, 803.42
D. Level 5, 99291, 99292, 803.42

Correct Answer: B. ***99291, 31500, 36556, 803.46. According to the acuity sheet, major trauma care is point 3 under the column Critical Care. This means that the levels of care under the Critical Care column are to be reported with critical care code 99291. The diagnosis is a skull fracture with intracranial injury of an unspecified nature and has resulted in the patient having been and continuing to be unconscious. The report of the endotracheal intubation and insertion of the central venous line are correctly coded because these services are not listed as being included in the critical care codes and as such are reported separately. The diagnosis is that of a closed skull fracture that resulted in intracranial injury and from which the patient is unconscious, meaning it is unknown at this time how long the patient will be unconscious.***

Rationale: A. *Level 5, 31500, 36556, 803.46. This answer is incorrect because, according to the acuity sheet, major trauma care is point 3 under the column Critical Care. This means that the levels of care under the Critical Care column are to be reported with critical care code 99291. The endotracheal intubation and insertion of the central venous line are correctly coded because these services are not listed as being included in the critical care codes and as such are reported separately. The diagnosis is that of a closed skull fracture that resulted in intracranial injury and from which the patient is unconscious, meaning it is unknown at this time how long the patient will be unconscious.*

Copyright © 2005, Elsevier Inc. All rights reserved.
CPT only © 2004. *Current Procedural Terminology, 2005, Professional Edition*, American Medical Association. All rights reserved.

C. *99291, 99292 × 2, 803.42. The use of the critical care codes is correct, but 99292 is only used once. Missing is the report for the endotracheal intubation and insertion of the central venous line; these services are not listed as being included in the critical care codes and as such are reported separately. The diagnosis is incorrect because the patient had been unconscious 20 minutes when he was brought to the ED, but he continues to be unconscious, and it is unknown how long he will be unconscious. So, at the end of the ED service, which you are reporting, the status of the consciousness of the patient is not known.*

D. *Level 5, 99291, 99292, 803.42. This answer is incorrect because, according to the acuity sheet, major trauma care is point 3 under the column Critical Care. This means that the levels of care under the Critical Care column are to be reported with critical care code 99291. You would not report Level 5 and the critical care codes unless there were other services provided to the patient that were indicated within the report.*

The diagnosis is incorrect because the patient had been unconscious 20 minutes when he was brought to the ED, but he continues to be unconscious, and it is unknown how long he will be unconscious. So, at the end of the ED service, which you are reporting, the status of the consciousness of the patient is not known.

Copyright © 2005, Elsevier Inc. All rights reserved.
CPT only © 2004. *Current Procedural Terminology, 2005, Professional Edition*, American Medical Association. All rights reserved.

28. A patient is seen in the ASC for multiple colon polyps and diverticulosis. A flexible colonoscopy is inserted. A polyp was removed from the colon with a snare. A lesion was also noted on the cecum and was biopsied with a hot biopsy forceps. Another lesion was noted in the anal canal and biopsied. Areas of diverticulosis were noted and inspected. The pathology report later indicated that the lesion in the cecum was a benign polyp, the anal canal polyp a benign adenomatous polyp, and the polyp in the colon was benign.

45380	Colonoscopy, flexible, proximal to splenic flexure; with biopsy, single or multiple
45384	Colonoscopy, flexible, proximal to splenic flexure; with removal of tumor(s), polyp(s), or other lesions(s) by, hot biopsy forceps or bipolar cautery
45385	Colonoscopy, flexible, proximal to splenic flexure; with removal of tumor(s), polyp(s), or other lesions(s) by, snare technique
211.3	Benign neoplasm of other parts of digestive system, colon, including cecum and large intestine NOS
211.4	Benign neoplasm of other parts of digestive system, rectum and anal canal
211.9	Benign neoplasm of other parts of digestive system, other unspecified site
562.10	Diverticulosis of colon without mention of hemorrhage
-59	Distinct procedural service
-51	Multiple procedures

A. 45385, 211.3, 211.4, 562.10
B. 45380-59, 211.3, 211.4, 562.10
C. 45385, 45380-59, 211.3, 211.4, 562.10
D. 45385, 45384-51, 45380-51, 211.3, 211.9, 562.10

Correct Answer: C. ***45385, 45380-59, 211.3, 211.4, and 562.10. This choice correctly reports the flexible colonoscopy for removal of a polyp by snare (45385), biopsy of the cecum lesion with hot biopsy forceps (45380), and anal canal lesion biopsied (45380). Code 45380 would only be used once as the code description includes "biopsies." Modifier -59 indicates a distinct procedure. The diagnoses are benign neoplasm of adenomatous polyp cecum and colon (211.3) and benign neoplasm of the anal canal (211.4). The diverticulosis is reported with 562.10.***

Rationale: A. *45385, 211.3, 211.4, 562.10. This choice is incorrect because it does not report 45380 for the biopsy of the cecum and anal canal. 45380 would require -59 to indicate that it was a distinct procedure. All other codes are correct for this choice.*

B. *45380-59, 211.3, 211.4, 562.10. The only code missing from this choice is 45385 to indicate the flexible colonoscopy for removal of a polyp by snare.*

D. *45385, 45384-51, 45380-51, 211.3, 211.9, 562.10. In this choice, modifier -51 is incorrectly used when -59 should have been used to indicate distinct procedure. All other codes in this selection are correct except 45384, because the report states the lesion in the cecum was biopsied, and because the entire lesion was not removed, 45384 is incorrect.*

Copyright © 2005, Elsevier Inc. All rights reserved.
CPT only © 2004. *Current Procedural Terminology, 2005, Professional Edition*, American Medical Association. All rights reserved.

29. The patient presents to the ASC for removal of a 2.5-cm basal cell carcinoma from his chin and a 1.5-cm basal cell carcinoma of the nose. The surgeon excises the areas of carcinoma and repairs the areas with split-thickness skin grafts.

11643	Excision, malignant lesion including margins, face, ears, eyelids, nose, lips; excised diameter, 2.1-3.0 cm
15120	Split graft, face, scalp, eyelids, mouth, neck, ears, orbits, genitalia, hands, feet and/or multiple digits; first 100 sq cm or less, or one percent of body area of infants and children
173.3	Other malignant neoplasm of skin, skin of other and unspecified parts of the face, including cheek, chin, eyebrow, forehead, nose, temple
216.3	Benign neoplasm of skin, skin of other and unspecified parts of face, including cheek, eyebrow, nose, temple

A. 15120, 11643, 173.3
B. 15120, 11643 × 2, 173.3
C. 15120, 11643 × 2, 216.3
D. 15120, 11643, 216.3

Correct Answer: A. ***15120, 11643, 173.3. This answer correctly reports the split graft, and because this graft is only for 16 sq cm (2.5 + 1.5 = 4 cm and then 4 × 4 = 16 sq cm), with 15120. The excision of the malignant lesion is correctly reported with 11643, and because the code description includes both the location of the neoplasms removed (chin and nose), 11643 is reported only once. The diagnosis is that of a malignant neoplasm (basal cell carcinoma) of the skin (173.3).***

Rationale: B. *15120, 11643 × 2, 173.3. This choice is incorrect because the excision of the malignant lesion is correctly reported with 11643 only one time because the code description includes both locations of the neoplasms removed (chin and nose).*

C. *15120, 11643 × 2, 216.3. This choice is incorrect because the excision of the malignant lesion is correctly reported with 11643 only one time because the code description includes both locations of the neoplasms removed (chin and nose). Also, the diagnosis is incorrect because a malignant neoplasm was removed, not a benign neoplasm.*

D. *15120, 11643, 216.3. This choice is incorrect because the diagnosis is incorrect. A malignant neoplasm was removed, not a benign neoplasm.*

Copyright © 2005, Elsevier Inc. All rights reserved.
CPT only © 2004. *Current Procedural Terminology, 2005, Professional Edition*, American Medical Association. All rights reserved.

30. A 6-year-old is brought to the ASC for removal of an impacted PE tube and placement of a new PE tube. General anesthesia was administered, and a 3.5-mm speculum was inserted into the right ear. The speculum was removed and inserted in the left ear. The impacted PE tube was then removed. There was some granulation tissue around this site. A new site was created posteriorly within some tympanosclerotic plaque. A new PE tube was inserted.

69405	Eustachian tube catheterization, transtympanic
69424	Ventilating tube removal requiring general anesthesia
69436	Tympanostomy (requiring insertion of ventilation tube), general anesthesia
388.8	Other disorders of the ear
996.59	Mechanical complication of other specified prosthetic device, implant, and graft; due to other implant and internal device not elsewhere classifiable
-LT	Left

A. 69424 × 2, 996.59
B. 69405-LT, 996.59
C. 69424, 388.8
D. 69424-LT, 69436-LT, 996.59

Correct Answer: D. 69424-LT, 69436-LT, 996.59. This answer is correct because it reports the removal of the ventilation tube (pressure equalizing tube or PE tube, 69424) from the left ear (-LT) and the insertion of a new tube (69436) in the left ear (-LT). The diagnosis is a complication of an internally implanted device (996.59).

Rationale: A. 69424 × 2, 996.59. This is incorrect because only one tube was removed, not two.

B. 69405-LT, 996.59. This is incorrect because this was not a Eustachian tube catheterization; rather, it was the removal of a previously placed tube and insertion of a new tube.

C. 69424, 388.8. This is incorrect because it does not report the removal of the previously placed tube. Also, the diagnosis is the complication of the tube, not another disorder of the ear.

Copyright © 2005, Elsevier Inc. All rights reserved.
CPT only © 2004. *Current Procedural Terminology, 2005, Professional Edition,* American Medical Association. All rights reserved.

31. This outpatient was brought to the ASC for a section of the flexor retinaculum for carpal tunnel syndrome of the left hand. Under Bier block anesthesia and under tourniquet, the patient's left hand was prepped and draped in the usual manner. An incision was made in a curvilinear fashion over the flexor crease. The border of the flexor retinaculum was localized. It was cut along the ulnar side in its entirety up to the mid-palm area. The wound was then sutured in one layer with 4-0 nylon interrupted mattress sutures. A dressing was applied. The patient was then discharged to the recovery room. He has meds at home that he will be able to take for pain.

64716	Neuroplasty and/or transposition; cranial nerve (specify)
64772	Decompression; unspecified nerve(s) (specify)
64726	Decompression; unspecified nerve(s) (specify), plantar digital nerve
354.0	Mononeuritis of upper limb and mononeuritis multiplex, carpal tunnel syndrome
354.5	Mononeuritis multiplex, combination of a single condition classifiable to 354 or 355
-LT	Left
-RT	Right

A. 64772, 354.5
B. 64726-RT, 354.0
C. 64716-LT, 354.5
D. 64772-LT, 354.0

Correct Answer: D. 64772-LT, 354.0. The procedure was a decompression for carpal tunnel syndrome, correctly reported with 64772. The diagnosis was carpal tunnel syndrome, correctly reported with 354.0.

Rationale: A. 64772, 354.5. This choice is correct for the service code but incorrect for the diagnosis but missing -LT. 354.5 reports mononeuritis multiplex, which is neuritis (inflammation of the nerve) and the condition in this report was carpal tunnel syndrome (entrapment of the medial nerve).

B. 64726-RT, 354.0. This choice has the correct diagnosis code but the incorrect service code and -RT modifier to indicate right rather than left with -LT. 64726 is a decompression of the plantar digital nerve, and this report was for the decompression of the medial nerve (carpal tunnel syndrome is the entrapment of the medial nerve).

C. 64716-LT, 354.5. In this choice, both the service code, 64716, and the diagnosis code, 354.5, are incorrect. 64716 reports a plastic repair of the cranial nerve, and in this case the medial nerve was decompressed. 354.5 reports mononeuritis multiplex, which is neuritis (inflammation of the nerve), and the condition in this report was carpal tunnel syndrome (entrapment of the medial nerve).

Copyright © 2005, Elsevier Inc. All rights reserved.
CPT only © 2004. *Current Procedural Terminology, 2005, Professional Edition*, American Medical Association. All rights reserved.

32. The patient presents to the ASC with a herniated disk. The surgeon performs a hemilaminectomy at L4-5 and L5-S1. The lower back area was opened; after decompression of the nerve roots, the interspace at L4-5 disk was excised. Next, the interspace at L5-S1 disk was excised.

63030	Laminotomy (hemilaminectomy), with decompression of nerve root(s), including partial facetectomy, foraminotomy and/or excision of herniated intervertebral disk, one interspace; lumbar
63035	Laminotomy (hemilaminectomy), with decompression of nerve root(s), including partial facetectomy, foraminotomy and/or excision of herniated intervertebral disk; each additional interspace, cervical or lumbar (list separately in addition to code for primary procedure)
63040	Laminotomy (hemilaminectomy), with decompression of nerve root(s), including partial facetectomy, foraminotomy and/or excision of herniated intervertebral disc, reexploration, single interspace; cervical
63045	Laminectomy, facetectomy and foraminotomy (unilateral or bilateral with decompression of spinal cord, cauda equina and/or nerve root(s), e.g., spinal or lateral recess stenosis), single vertebral segment; cervical
63043	each additional cervical interspace (list separately in addition to code for primary condition)
63048	each additional segment, cervical, thoracici, or lumbar (list separately in addition to code for primary condition)
722.10	Intervertebral disc disorders, displacement of thoracic or lumbar intervertebral disc without myelopathy, lumbar intervertebral disc without myelopathy
722.2	Displacement of intervertebral disc, site unspecified, without myelopathy
839.00	Other, multiple, and ill-defined dislocations; cervical vertebra, closed; cervical vertebra, unspecified

A. 63045, 63048, 722.2
B. 63040, 63043, 839.00
C. 63030, 63035, 722.10
D. 63040, 63043, 722.10

Correct Answer: C. ***63030 reports one lumbar interspace (L4-5) repair, 63035 reports each additional lumbar interspace (L5-S1) repair, and 722.10 is used to report displacement of a lumbar intervertebral disk.***

Rationale: A. *63045 reports one cervical interspace repair, and 63048 reports each additional cervical interspace repair, but the case indicated repair of lumbar interspaces. 722.2 is the displacement of an intervertebral disk with an unspecified site, but the site is known in the case as L5-S1 and L4-5.*

B. *63040 reports repair of a cervical interspace, and 63043 reports each additional cervical interspace, but the repair was of the lumbar interspaces. 839.00 is cervical dislocation of the spine, not displacement of a lumbar intervertebral disk.*

D. *63040 reports repair of a cervical interspace, and 63043 reports each additional cervical interspace, but the case indicated lumbar interspace repair, not cervical. The diagnosis code 722.10 is correctly used to report displacement of a lumbar intervertebral disk, the condition in this case.*

Copyright © 2005, Elsevier Inc. All rights reserved.
CPT only © 2004. *Current Procedural Terminology, 2005, Professional Edition,* American Medical Association. All rights reserved.

33. The patient was admitted for a malignant tumor of the thyroid. The surgeon performs a total thyroidectomy. The patient was prepped and draped. The neck area was opened. With careful radical dissection of the neck completed, one could visualize the size of the tumor. The decision was made to do a total thyroidectomy. The pathology report later indicated that the tumor was malignant.

06.2	Operations on thyroid and parathyroid glands, unilateral thyroid lobectomy
06.31	Operations on thyroid and parathyroid glands, other partial thyroidectomy, excision of lesion of thyroid gland
06.4	Operations on thyroid and parathyroid glands, complete thyroidectomy
06.52	Operations on thyroid and parathyroid glands, substernal thyroidectomy, complete substernal thyroidectomy
164.0	Malignant neoplasm of thymus, heart, and mediastinum; thymus
193	Malignant neoplasm of thyroid gland

A. 06.52, 193
B. 06.31, 193
C. 06.2, 164.0
D. 06.4, 193

Correct Answer: D. 06.4, 193. 06.4 is used to report a complete thyroidectomy. 193 is the code for malignant neoplasm of the thyroid gland.

Rationale: A. 06.52, 193. 06.52 is used to report a complete substernal thyroidectomy, and in this procedure the neck area was accessed, not the sternum. 193 is the correct diagnosis code.

B. 06.31, 193. 06.31 reports an excision of a lesion of the thyroid, not the total removal of the thyroid as was performed in this case. 193 is the correct diagnosis code.

C. 06.2, 164.0. 06.2 reports a unilateral (one side) thyroid lobectomy where only one lobe of the thyroid is removed (hemithyroidectomy). 164.0 is the code for malignant neoplasm of the thymus gland, which is incorrect. The report stated thyroid.

34. Arrhythmia, elevation of ST segment and Q wave, and increased troponin level may be indicative of:
A. cerebral vascular accident
B. myocardial infarction
C. respiratory failure
D. atrial fibrillation

Correct Answer: B. Myocardial infarction.

Rationale: A. Cerebral vascular symptoms include paralysis, weakness, speech defect, and aphasia.

C. Hypoxemia, inadequate gas exchange, and rapid respirations are symptoms of respiratory failure

D. Atrial fibrillation is characterized by rapid, random contractions of the atria, which cause irregular ventricular beats.

Copyright © 2005, Elsevier Inc. All rights reserved.
CPT only © 2004. *Current Procedural Terminology, 2005, Professional Edition,* American Medical Association. All rights reserved.

35. A 19-year-old male was admitted to the ASC for an abnormal finding on x-ray of the GI tract. The surgeon has determined that the patient may have a perforated appendicitis with abscess. The x-ray showed a dilated bowel in the midabdomen and pelvis and a loop in the sigmoid colon. The Pentax video sigmoidoscope was inserted without difficulty to 60 cm. Careful inspection in the mid-descending, distal descending, sigmoid, and rectum revealed no erythema, ulceration, exudate, friability, or other mucosal abnormalities. There were a few diverticula present. The mucosa was normal. No volvulus was noted. No diverticulitis and no obstructing lesion were seen. The patient tolerated the procedure well. The impression was that of a normal sigmoidoscopy to 60 cm. No obstruction or volvulus was noted; no appendicitis was noted. The mucosa was normal. The patient needs to have a small bowel obstruction ruled out. A small bowel series was recommended.

45330	Sigmoidoscopy, flexible; diagnostic, with or without collection of specimen(s) by brushing or washing (separate procedure)
45355	Colonoscopy, rigid or flexible, transabdominal via colostomy, single or multiple
45378	Colonoscopy, flexible, proximal to splenic flexure; diagnostic, with or without collection of specimen(s) by decompression (separate procedure)
45387	Colonoscopy, flexible, proximal to splenic flexure; with transendoscopic stent placement (includes predilation)
541	Appendicitis, unqualified
560.9	Intestinal obstruction without mention of hernia, unspecified intestinal obstruction
793.4	Nonspecific abnormal findings on radiological and other examination of body structure, gastrointestinal tract

A. 45355, 793.4, 541
B. 45330, 793.4
C. 45378, 793.4
D. 45387, 793.4, 560.9

Correct Answer: B. ***45330, 793.4. This is a diagnostic sigmoidoscopy, not a diagnostic colonoscopy, because the description of a sigmoidoscopy in the CPT manual (preceding 45300) includes not only the sigmoid colon but also the descending colon. The diagnosis code is located in the Index as "Abnormal, radiological examination" (793.4) because the procedure did not diagnose any condition that the physician repaired. The physician suspects that the patient may have a small bowel obstruction, as indicated in the report, but this is not a confirmed diagnosis.***

Copyright © 2005, Elsevier Inc. All rights reserved.
CPT only © 2004. *Current Procedural Terminology, 2005, Professional Edition,* American Medical Association. All rights reserved.

Rationale: A. *45355, 793.4, 541. This selection is incorrect because 45355 is for a colonoscopy, and the description of a sigmoidoscopy in the CPT manual (preceding 45300) includes not only the sigmoid colon but also the descending colon. The report indicated that the mid-descending, distal descending, sigmoid, and rectum were inspected, which is included in 45330. The diagnosis for the appendicitis (541) is not reported because this is an outpatient setting and suspected conditions are not reported; also, at the end of the report the physician indicates that no appendicitis was found, so that condition had been ruled out.*

C. *45378, 793.4. This selection is incorrect because 45378 is for a colonoscopy, and the description of a sigmoidoscopy in the CPT manual (preceding 45300) includes not only the sigmoid colon but also the descending colon. The report indicated that the mid-descending, distal descending, sigmoid, and rectum were inspected, which is included in 45330. The diagnosis is correct.*

D. *45387, 793.4, 560.9. This selection is incorrect because 45378 is for a colonoscopy, and the description of a sigmoidoscopy in the CPT manual (preceding 45300) includes not only the sigmoid colon but also the descending colon. The report indicated that the mid-descending, distal descending, sigmoid and rectum were inspected, which is included in 45330. 793.4 is correct, but 560.9 is incorrect because it reports a bowel obstruction, and this service was provided in the outpatient setting, which means that the "rule out" diagnosis of bowel obstruction is not reported.*

Copyright © 2005, Elsevier Inc. All rights reserved.
CPT only © 2004. *Current Procedural Terminology, 2005, Professional Edition*, American Medical Association. All rights reserved.

36. The patient is brought to the ASC for a giant congenital nevus of the left pectoral region involving the left areola. The findings indicated a 7- to 4-cm giant congenital nevus (common nevus) involving about 50% of the areola on the left side. The surgeon performs an excision of the nevus along with a portion of areola of the left chest. Under general endotracheal anesthesia of plus 4 cc of 0.5% Xylocaine and 1 : 100,000 epinephrine, the procedure was begun. The patient's chest wall was prepped with Betadine scrub and solution and draped in a routine sterile fashion. 4 cc of 0.5% Xylocaine with 1 : 100,000 epinephrine were injected along the suture line, and the lesion was excised down to carpus fascia and included the complete dermis and a little subcutaneous fat. The bleeders were cauterized and the wound closed with subcuticular 3-0 Monocryl and three twists of 6-0 Prolene. One-half-inch Steri-Strips were applied, plus a clavicle strap for immobilization. The pathology report later indicated that the tissue was benign.

11446	Excision, other benign lesion including margins (unless listed elsewhere) face, ears, eyelids, nose, lips, mucous membrane; excised diameter 0.5 cm or less
19101	Biopsy of breast; percutaneous, needle core, not using imaging guidance (separate procedure)
21555	Excision tumor, soft tissue of neck or thorax; subcutaneous
173.5	Other malignant neoplasm of skin; skin of trunk, except scrotum
216.5	Benign neoplasm of skin; skin of trunk, except scrotum
239.2	Neoplasms of unspecified nature; bone, soft tissue, and skin
-LT	Left
-22	Unusual Procedural Service

A. 21555, 173.5
B. 21555-LT, 216.5
C. 19101, 239.2
D. 11446-22-LT, 216.5

Correct Answer: B. 21555-LT, 216.5. The surgeon removed a neoplasm of the skin of the thorax, involving the subcutaneous tissue or the deep soft tissues, which is reported with 21555. Code 21556 is for the deep subfascial plane or intramuscular area. This report indicates "down to the . . . fascia" and not into or below the fascia. The diagnosis is a benign neoplasm of the skin of the chest, which is reported with 216.5.

Rationale: A. 21555, 173.5. This choice is incorrect because, although the CPT code is correct, the report specified left side and as such requires -LT. The diagnosis is also incorrect because 173.5 reports a malignant neoplasm of the chest and this neoplasm was stated to be benign; as such, it should have been reported with 216.5.

C. 19101, 239.2. This selection is incorrect because 19101 reports an open breast biopsy rather than the removal of a neoplasm from the skin of the thorax. 239.2 incorrectly reports uncertain behavior of a neoplasm, but this neoplasm is known to be benign and would be reported with 216.5.

D. 11446-22-LT, 216.5. This selection is incorrect because 11446 indicates the excision of a benign lesion over 4.0 cm; this procedure was not a skin procedure but a musculoskeletal procedure based on the depth of the excision. Modifier -22, Unusual Procedural Service, is not reported in the ASC setting. 216.5 is correct to report a benign neoplasm of the skin of the chest.

Copyright © 2005, Elsevier Inc. All rights reserved.
CPT only © 2004. *Current Procedural Terminology, 2005, Professional Edition,* American Medical Association. All rights reserved.

37. This inpatient was admitted for repair of a frozen left shoulder. The surgeon is to perform an arthroscopic debridement and joint manipulation of the shoulder. The patient was anesthetized using general anesthetic. The left shoulder was prepped and draped in the usual fashion. A standard posterior arthroscopic portal was created, and the camera was introduced into the back of the joint. There was substantial inflammation throughout the entirety of the joint. Using a switch-stick technique, an anterior portal was created and the 7-mm cannula was then brought in from the front. Using a 4.0 double-biter resector, the synovium was then debrided throughout the entirety of the rotator cuff over the surface of the biceps and the anterior ligamentous structures as well as inferior ligamentous structures. With this completed, the joint was then thoroughly irrigated to remove any blood. The articular surfaces were inspected and were found to be normal. The arthroscopic portal was closed with absorbable sutures and Steri-Strips. The joint was then manipulated.

29806	Arthroscopy, shoulder, surgical; capsulorrhaphy
80.41	Incision and excision of joint structures; division of joint capsule, ligament, or cartilage; shoulder
80.1	Incision and excision of joint structures; other arthrotomy
80.81	Incision and excision of joint structures; other local excision or destruction of lesion of joint
726.0	Peripheral enthesopathies and allied syndromes; adhesive capsulitis of shoulder
726.10	Peripheral enthesopathies and allied syndromes; rotator cuff syndrome of shoulder and allied disorders; disorders of bursae and tendons in shoulder region, unspecified
-LT	Left

A. 29806-LT, 726.0
B. 80.81, 726.10
C. 80.41, 726.0
D. 80.1, 726.10

Correct Answer: C. 80.41, 726.0. The service is a joint release of the left shoulder, reported with 80.41. The manipulation is part of the procedure and is not reported separately. The arthroscopy is the approach and is not coded separately. The diagnosis is frozen shoulder and is reported with 726.0.

Rationale: A. 29806-LT, 726.0. This selection is incorrect because this is an inpatient, and inpatient surgical procedures are reported with Volume 3 codes (80.41). The diagnosis code is correct.

B. 80.81, 726.10. This choice is incorrect because this report did not indicate the excision or destruction of a lesion of the joint (80.81); rather, it described the removal of joint structures. The diagnosis code (726.10) is also incorrect because this report did not specify the rotator cuff.

D. 80.1, 726.10. This choice is incorrect because this was not just an arthrotomy but the removal of joint structure from the joint, reported with 80.41. The diagnosis code is incorrect because this report did not specify the rotator cuff.

Copyright © 2005, Elsevier Inc. All rights reserved.
CPT only © 2004. *Current Procedural Terminology, 2005, Professional Edition*, American Medical Association. All rights reserved.

38. An 81-year-old woman is brought to the ASC for debridement and irrigation of infected wound, right shoulder. This patient had previously undergone an arthroscopic mini-open repair of a right rotator cuff tear, which was performed by the same physician who is again performing this procedure. At about the 4-week stage postoperatively, she developed drainage from the wound. This cultured positive for *Staphylococcus aureus*. She was then placed on oral antibiotics and did show some improvement, but there has been persistent drainage for the last 2 weeks without evidence of resolution. Because of the continuation of this problem, the decision was made to undertake the procedure. Under general anesthetic, the patient was laid in the beach-chair position on the operating table. The anterior 3 cm of the surgical wound was excised. There was fluid drainage from this area. A sinus tract was identified that went down to the area of the anterior acromial area. The edges of the sinus tract area were then fully debrided and then irrigated using a power lavage system and 4 L of normal saline. The soft tissues around the sinus tract were sutured.

10180	Incision and drainage, complex, postoperative wound infection
11000	Debridement of extensive eczematous or infected skin, up to 10% body surface
998.51	Other complications of procedures, NEC; postoperative infection; infected postoperative seroma
998.59	Other complications of procedures, NEC; postoperative infection; other postoperative infection
041.11	Staphylococcus aureus
-78	Return to the operating room for related procedure during the postoperative period
-RT	Right
-LT	Left

A. 10180-78-RT, 998.59, 041.11
B. 11000-78-LT, 998.59
C. 11000-78-LT, 998.51
D. 10180-78-LT, 998.51

Correct Answer: A. ***10180-78-RT, 998.59, 041.11. The code description for 10180 is specifically assigned to postoperative wound infection, so it is incorrect to assign a debridement code to this service even though the Procedure Performed section of the report indicates that the service was a "Debridement and irrigation of infected wound, right shoulder." Modifier -78 is added to indicate a return to the operating room within the postoperative period by the same physician that performed the first service, and modifier -RT is added to indicate the right side. 041.11 is reported to indicate that the postoperative infection (998.59) was Staphylococcus aureus.***

Copyright © 2005, Elsevier Inc. All rights reserved.
CPT only © 2004. *Current Procedural Terminology, 2005, Professional Edition*, American Medical Association. All rights reserved.

Rationale: *B. 11000-78-LT, 998.59. This choice is incorrect because this was not a debridement but an incision and drainage that should have been reported with 10180. The diagnosis code is correct. Missing is also 041.11 to identify the infection as Staphylococcus aureus.*

C. 11000-78-LT, 998.51. This choice is incorrect because this was not a debridement but an incision and drainage that should have been reported with 10180. The diagnosis code is incorrect because 998.51 reports infected seroma, which is a tumorlike collection of serum in the tissues, and this report did not indicate that condition. Missing is also 041.11 to identify the infection as Staphylococcus aureus.

D. 10180-78-LT, 998.51. The service code is correct in this choice, but the diagnosis code is incorrect because 998.51 reports infected seroma, which is a tumorlike collection of serum in the tissues, and this report did not indicate that condition. Missing is also 041.11 to identify the infection as Staphylococcus aureus.

39. The patient presents to the ASC for a kidney biopsy. The indications are chronic renal failure, hematuria, and proteinuria. The patient was placed in the prone position. The right kidney was visualized using ultrasound provided by radiology. The skin was prepped in the usual fashion. One-percent lidocaine was used for local anesthesia. Multiple core biopsies were obtained under real ultrasound guidance using an 18-gauge biopsy gun without difficulty. Multiple core biopsies were obtained and were sent for light electromicroscopy and immune fluorescence. He was sent back to the procedure area to be monitored in 6 hours with orders for repeat hemoglobin. The pathology report later indicated primary, renal cell adenocarcinoma.
Do not report the radiology service.

50200	Renal biopsy; percutaneous, by trocar or needle
189.0	Malignant neoplasm of kidney and other and unspecified urinary organs; kidney, except pelvis
189.1	Malignant neoplasm of kidney and other and unspecified urinary organs; renal pelvis
585	Chronic renal failure
599.7	Hematuria
791.0	Nonspecific findings on examination of urine, proteinuria
-RT	Right
-LT	Left

A. 50200-RT, 189.0, 585
B. 50200-RT, 189.1, 585, 599.7, 791.0
C. 50200-LT, 189.1, 585, 599.7, 791.0
D. 50200-RT, 189.0, 585, 599.7, 791.0

Correct Answer: A. 50200-RT, 189.0, 585. The service is a kidney biopsy by means of a percutaneous biopsy needle and reported with 50200. The diagnosis is as stated in the pathology report, as primary neoplasm of the kidney, reported with 189.0. Although CRF (chronic renal failure) is often a complication of many other diseases, it is usually still coded (585). The symptom codes for the hematuria and proteinuria are not coded because they are symptoms of the CRF.

Copyright © 2005, Elsevier Inc. All rights reserved.
CPT only © 2004. *Current Procedural Terminology, 2005, Professional Edition,* American Medical Association. All rights reserved.

Rationale: B. *50200-RT, 189.1, 585, 599.7, 791.0. This choice is incorrect because the report does not indicate malignant neoplasm was of the renal pelvis as reported with 189.1; rather, it was the location of kidney, except pelvis. The hematuria (599.7) and proteinuria (791.0) are not reported because they are symptoms of the chronic renal failure.*

C. *50200-LT, 50200-RT, 189.1, 585, 599.7, 791.0. This choice is incorrect because this was only the right kidney (50200-RT). The report does not indicate the renal pelvis, as reported with 189.1; rather, it was the location of kidney, except pelvis. The hematuria (599.7) and proteinuria (791.0) are not reported because they are symptoms of the chronic renal failure.*

D. *50200-RT, 189.0, 585, 599.7, 791.0. This choice is incorrect. The hematuria (599.7) and proteinuria (791.0) are not reported because they are symptoms of the chronic renal failure.*

40. This 2-year-old male child was brought to ASC for a circumcision due to recurrent balanitis and phimosis. The patient was given general mask anesthetic as well as caudal block for postoperative pain control. He was prepped and draped in the supine position, foreskin retracted, and adhesions broken down. Circumcision was performed using a dorsal slit technique. Hemostasis was achieved with judicious use of electrocautery and chromic ties. Prepuce was re-anastomosed to the penile skin using 5-0 chromic catgut. The pathology report later indicated benign penile tissue.

54160	Circumcision, surgical excision other than clamp, device or dorsal slit; newborn
54161	Circumcision, surgical excision other than clamp, device or dorsal slit; except newborn
605	Redundant prepuce and phimosis
607.1	Disorders of the penis, balanoposthitis

A. 54161, 605
B. 54160, 605, 607.1
C. 54160, 607.1
D. 54161, 605, 607.1

Correct Answer:* D. *54161, 605, 607.1. The service was a circumcision of other than a newborn by means of excision and reported with 54161. The diagnoses are as stated on the postoperative diagnosis as balanitis (607.1) and phimosis (605).

Rationale: A. *54161, 605. This choice is incorrect because the balanoposthitis was not reported.*

B. *54160, 605, 607.1. This choice is incorrect because the procedure was not performed on a newborn.*

C. *54160, 607.1. This choice is incorrect because the procedure was not performed on a newborn. Also missing from this choice is the 605 code to report the phimosis.*

Copyright © 2005, Elsevier Inc. All rights reserved.
CPT only © 2004. *Current Procedural Terminology, 2005, Professional Edition,* American Medical Association. All rights reserved.

41. A 73-year-old woman was admitted for hypotension and respiratory failure. The woman was lifting a bag of dirt from a wheelbarrow in her back yard when she began to have some diaphoresis, and she did not feel well. Her husband brought her to the ED, where she was noted to have CHF/fluid overload with chest x-ray. She has been intubated and mechanically ventilated. Lasix 80 IV was given and a p.o. dose of Lasix 60 mg. was given. Her blood pressure is trending down and is now 60/40s. Dopamine drip has been started, and the nitroglycerin drip and saline infusion setup in the ED have been discontinued. At this time, the patient has congestive heart failure, pulmonary edema that has led to respiratory failure, and acute renal failure.

428.0	Heart failure, congestive heart failure, unspecified
458.9	Hypotension
518.81	Other diseases of the lung; acute respiratory failure
584.9	Acute renal failure, unspecified
780.8	Generalized hyperhidrosis, including diaphoresis

A. 458.9, 518.81, 428.0, 584.9
B. 518.81, 428.0, 584.9
C. 458.9, 518.81, 428.0, 584.9, 780.8
D. 518.81, 428.0, 584.9, 780.8

Correct Answer: A. 458.9, 518.81, 428.0, 584.9. The hypotension is not stated in the last line of the report but is the most prominent feature at this time. As such, it is the principal diagnosis and listed first. The respiratory failure is reported with 518.81. The congestive heart failure is reported with 428.0, and the acute renal failure is reported with 584.9

Rationale: B. 518.81, 428.0, 584.9. This choice is incorrect because the hypotension should have been listed as the principal diagnosis.

C. 458.9, 518.81, 428.0, 584.9, 780.8. This choice is incorrect because the diaphoresis (780.8) is not reported separately because it is a symptom of the heart failure.

D. 518.81, 428.0, 584.9, 780.8. This choice is incorrect because the hypotension should have been listed as the principal diagnosis. Also, the diaphoresis (780.8) is not reported separately because it is a symptom of the heart failure.

Copyright © 2005, Elsevier Inc. All rights reserved.
CPT only © 2004. *Current Procedural Terminology, 2005, Professional Edition,* American Medical Association. All rights reserved.

42. This 74-year-old man was admitted to the hospital after he presented for a Cardiolite stress test. Even before the test started, he began having retrosternal chest pain, became bradycardic after a sublingual nitroglycerin spray, and had to be given atropine. His heart rate was down to about 40. After the atropine, the heart rate returned to normal. Blood pressure was briefly down to the 90s and high 80s systolic, but then, after a fluid bolus, it returned to normal before admission. The record indicated that the patient was admitted for atrial fibrillation, cardiomyopathy, and to rule out myocardial infarction. The focus of the treatment was to bring the atrial fibrillation under control.

786.50	Chest pain
427.31	Cardiac dysrhythmias, atrial fibrillation and flutter
425.4	Cardiomyopathy, other primary cardiomyopathies, including NOS
410.9	Acute myocardial infarction, unspecified site
458.9	Hypotension

A. 786.50, 427.31, 425.4, 410.9, 458.9
B. 427.31, 425.4, 410.9
C. 427.31, 425.4, 410.9, 458.9
D. 427.31, 425.4

Correct Answer: B. 427.31, 425.4, 410.9. The record indicated that the patient was admitted for atrial fibrillation, cardiomyopathy, and to rule out myocardial infarction, and these are the diagnoses that are to be reported for this patient.

Rationale: A. 786.50, 427.31, 425.4, 410.9, 458.9. This selection is incorrect because the symptom of chest pain (786.50) is not reported: Chest pain is a symptom of the heart condition. The episode of hypotension (458.9) was prior to the admission.

C. 427.31, 425.4, 410.9, 458.9. This selection is incorrect because the episode of hypotension (458.9) was prior to the admission.

D. 427.31, 425.4. This selection is incorrect because the acute myocardial infarction (410.9) was not reported.

Copyright © 2005, Elsevier Inc. All rights reserved.
CPT only © 2004. *Current Procedural Terminology, 2005, Professional Edition,* American Medical Association. All rights reserved.

43. 58-year-old patient originally came to the ED with severe back and abdominal pain. The patient was found to have a ruptured abdominal aortic aneurysm and was taken immediately to the operating room for surgery. Through abdomen was entered through a mid-line incision. His abdomen was full of blood, and only after repeated attempts to control the bleeding could the hemorrhage be controlled by suture. The patient received 5351 cc of Cellsaver, 24,000 cc of crystalloid, 500 cc of albumin, 6978 cc of RBCs, 245 cc of platelets, 1051 cc of fresh frozen plasma, and 6000 cc of lactated Ringer's for treatment of acute blood loss anemia. The patient's incisions were partially closed, and the abdominal wound was left open. Steri-Drapes were placed within the abdominal wall, and then towels were placed over the Steri-Drapes, followed by Jackson-Pratt drains and then followed by adhesive Ioban drapes. This would allow for expansion of the abdomen resulting from the edema that occurred during surgery.

39.52	Repair of aneurysm, by suture
39.98	Control of hemorrhage, NOS, excludes that by suture
285.1	Acute posthemorrhagic anemia
441	Aortic aneurysm and dissection
441.3	Abdominal aneurysm, ruptured
998.11	Hemorrhage complicating a procedure

A. 39.98, 441.3, 285.1, 998.11
B. 39.52, 441.3, 998.11
C. 39.98, 441.3
D. 39.52, 441.3, 998.11, 285.1

Correct Answer: D. 39.52, 441.3, 998.11, 285.1. This selection is correct because it reports the suture repair of an aneurysm (39.52) for the surgical procedure. The first-listed diagnosis is the ruptured abdominal aneurysm, as that was the reason the patient presented to the ED. The blood loss is reported, as it was documented to be significant and complicated the surgical procedure. The complication code is reported (998.11) followed by the type of complication, which was acute anemia due to blood loss (285.1).

Rationale: A. 39.98, 441, 285.1, 998.11. This selection is incorrect because this choice excludes control of hemorrhage that is accomplished by means of suture; this report indicated that the hemorrhage was controlled with suture. This selection is also incorrect as the complication code (998.11) should have been sequenced before the complication code of acute blood loss anemia (285.1).

B. 39.52, 441.3, 998.11. This choice is incorrect because the anemia (285.1) is a result of the hemorrhage and would therefore need to be reported following 998.11.

C. 39.98, 441.3. This selection is incorrect because this choice excludes control of hemorrhage that is accomplished by means of suture; this report indicated that the hemorrhage was controlled with suture. Also missing from this choice is the acute posthemorrhagic anemia due to excessive blood loss (285.11) and the code to report hemorrhage that complicated the procedure (998.11).

Copyright © 2005, Elsevier Inc. All rights reserved.
CPT only © 2004. *Current Procedural Terminology, 2005, Professional Edition,* American Medical Association. All rights reserved.

44. A patient is admitted with appendicitis and scheduled for surgery. Before anesthesia can be administered, the patient has a cerebral thrombosis and the surgeon cancels the procedure. What would be the sequence of the codes to report this admission?
    A. cerebral thrombosis, appendicitis, V code to report the surgical cancellation due to contraindication
    B. appendicitis, cerebral thrombosis, V code to report the surgical cancellation due to contraindication
    C. procedure code for appendicitis, V code to report the surgical cancellation due to contraindication, appendicitis, cerebral thrombosis
    D. V code to report the surgical cancellation due to contraindication, appendicitis, cerebral thrombosis

Correct Answer: B. Appendicitis, cerebral thrombosis, V code to report the surgical cancellation due to contraindication. The reason for admission was appendicitis, and, as such, appendicitis is reported as the principal diagnosis. The cerebral thrombosis is listed as a secondary diagnosis, with the reason for the surgical cancellation added to indicate why the procedure was not carried out.

Rationale: A. Cerebral thrombosis, appendicitis, V code to report the surgical cancellation due to contraindication. This is an incorrect choice because the reason for admission was not the cerebral thrombosis but rather the appendicitis.

C. Procedure code for appendicitis, V code to report the surgical cancellation due to contraindication, appendicitis, cerebral thrombosis. This is an incorrect choice because the reason for admission was the appendicitis, and that code should be listed first. No procedure code is listed because no procedure was performed.

D. V code to report the surgical cancellation due to contraindication, appendicitis, cerebral thrombosis. This is an incorrect choice because a V code is never a principal diagnosis in the inpatient setting.

45. Multiple fractures are sequenced in accordance with the _______?
    A. location
    B. severity
    C. type
    D. none of these

Correct Answer: B. Severity. According to Official Coding and Reporting Guidelines, Section I, B, 4, multiple fractures are sequenced in accordance with the severity of the fracture, and the physician should be asked to list the fracture diagnoses in order of severity.

Rationale: A. Location. This selection is incorrect because, according to the Official Coding and Reporting Guidelines, Section I, B, 4, multiple fractures are sequenced in accordance with the severity of the fracture, and the physician should be asked to list the fracture diagnoses in order of severity.

C. Type. This selection is incorrect because, according to the Official Coding and Reporting Guidelines, Section I, B, 4, multiple fractures are sequenced in accordance with the severity of the fracture, and the physician should be asked to list the fracture diagnoses in order of severity.

D. None of these. This selection is incorrect because, according to the Official Coding and Reporting Guidelines, Section I, B, 4, multiple fractures are sequenced in accordance with the severity of the fracture, and the physician should be asked to list the fracture diagnoses in order of severity.

Copyright © 2005, Elsevier Inc. All rights reserved.
CPT only © 2004. *Current Procedural Terminology, 2005, Professional Edition*, American Medical Association. All rights reserved.

46. This patient is admitted for a hemodialysis treatment. The following Assessment/Plan is indicated in the record:

ASSESSMENT/PLAN:

1. Chronic renal failure/end-stage renal disease, secondary to the following:
   a. Status post right-sided nephrectomy in 1996 **(V45.73)**
   b. Left-sided renal artery stenosis/renal vascular hypertension (**403.91)**
   c. Diabetes II
   d. Diabetic nephropathy **(250.40, 583.81)**
   e. Coronary artery disease
2. Multiple electrolyte abnormalities related to problem chronic renal failure/end-stage renal disease
   a. Hyperphosphatemia. Continue Renagel and PhosLo (**275.3)**
   b. Hypocalcemia **(274.41**)
3. Hypothyroidism. Continue Synthroid (**244.9**)

   What would be the principal diagnosis?

A. 250.40
B. 403.91
C. V45.73
D. 583.81

Correct Answer: B. ***403.91. According to the Official Guidelines for Coding and Reporting, Section 1, C7, 3, the coder is to assign a code from 403 hypertensive renal disease when conditions classified to 585–587 are present. This means that the chronic renal failure is reported when 403.91 is assigned. Because this patient was admitted for hemodialysis, the first-listed code is 403.91.***

Rationale: A. *250.40. This choice is incorrect because the diabetic nephropathy is not the principal condition; rather, the left-sided renal artery stenosis/renal vascular hypertension is reported first (403.91) because this was the principal reason the patient was admitted. According to the Official Guidelines for Coding and Reporting, Section 1, C7, 3, the coder is to assign a code from 403 hypertensive renal disease when conditions classified to 585–587 are present. This means that the chronic renal failure is reported when 403.91 is assigned. Because this patient was admitted for hemodialysis, the first-listed code is 403.91.*

C. *V45.73. This choice is incorrect because a V code is never a principal diagnosis in an inpatient setting.*

D. *583.81. This choice is incorrect because 403.91 must be sequenced first. The patient was admitted for hemodialysis, which means 403.91 would be listed first.*

Copyright © 2005, Elsevier Inc. All rights reserved.
CPT only © 2004. *Current Procedural Terminology, 2005, Professional Edition,* American Medical Association. All rights reserved.

47. The patient has end-stage renal disease and is admitted with acute peritonitis due to an infection of her peritoneal dialysis catheter. The patient is on chronic peritoneal dialysis. She was admitted with abdominal pain and cloudy dialysate. She was found to have alpha streptococcal peritonitis. She was given vancomycin, gentamicin, and Kefzol. The alpha Strep was sensitive to cephalosporins. She did well during her hospitalization and felt better. What would be the principal diagnosis?
   A. complication of a catheter, specifically an infection
   B. peritonitis
   C. streptococcal infection
   D. end-stage renal disease

Correct Answer: A. ***Complication of a catheter, specifically an infection. This is correct because it is the primary reason the patient was admitted to the hospital.***

Rationale: B. *Peritonitis. This is an incorrect answer because it is not the principal reason the patient was admitted. Rather, the patient was admitted because of a complication of the peritoneal dialysis catheter.*

C. *Streptococcal infection. This is an incorrect answer because it is not the principal reason the patient was admitted. Rather, the patient was admitted because of a complication of the peritoneal dialysis catheter.*

D. *End-stage renal disease. This is an incorrect answer because it is not the principal reason the patient was admitted. Rather, the patient was admitted because of a complication of the peritoneal dialysis catheter.*

48. The patient is a 30-year-old male who suffered a massive stroke 1 month ago. The patient presents to the outpatient radiology department of the hospital for a real-time imaging and Doppler analysis to assess the current status of his vessels. The clinical indications are noted to be previous stroke with right hemiparesis and aphasia. The medical documentation concluded that there was some stenosis on the right side. The left side implied occlusion distal to the area scanned. The diagnoses would be as follows:
   A. 438.11 (Late, effect, with aphasia), 438.20 (Late, effect, cerebrovascular disease with hemiplegia/hemiparesis affecting unspecified side), 434.91 (Stroke)
   B. 438.20 (Late, effect, cerebrovascular disease with hemiplegia/hemiparesis affecting unspecified side), 438.11 (Late, effect, with aphasia)
   C. 434.91 (Stroke)
   D. 434.91 (Stroke), 438.20 (Late, effect, cerebrovascular disease with hemiplegia/hemiparesis affecting unspecified side), 438.11 (Late, effect, with aphasia)

Correct Answer: B. ***438.20 (Late, effect, cerebrovascular disease with hemiplegia/hemiparesis affecting unspecified side), 438.11 (Late, effect, with aphasia). This is the correct answer because the service was specifically to assess the late effects of the stroke.***

Rationale: A. *438.11 (Late, effect, with aphasia), 438.20 (Late, effect, cerebrovascular disease with hemiplegia/hemiparesis affecting unspecified side), 434.91 (Stroke). This is an incorrect choice because a current stroke is not reported; only the late effects of the stroke that are present are reported.*

C. *434.91 (Stroke). This is an incorrect choice because a current stroke is not reported; only the late effects of the stroke that are present are reported.*

D. *434.91 (Stroke), 438.20 (Late, effect, cerebrovascular disease with hemiplegia/hemiparesis affecting unspecified side), 438.11 (Late, effect, with aphasia). This is an incorrect choice because a current stroke is not reported; only the late effects of the stroke that are present are reported.*

Copyright © 2005, Elsevier Inc. All rights reserved.
CPT only © 2004. *Current Procedural Terminology, 2005, Professional Edition*, American Medical Association. All rights reserved.

49. The patient is a 34-year-old, gravida 2, para 2, who has had multiple operations in the past for endometriosis after being admitted with endometriosis and resultant chronic pelvic pain. A total abdominal hysterectomy with bilateral salpingo-oophorectomy is performed. The uterus was found to be of normal size, but there were a lot of anterior cul-de-sac adhesions over the bladder and anterior surface of the uterus. There were some adhesions between the left tube and ovary and the posterior aspect of the left broad ligament. The pathology report later indicated that the uterus, bilateral tubes, and ovaries showed "endometriosis involving serous surface of the uterus, right ovary, and left ovary. Adenomyosis, proliferating endometrium."

617.2	Endometriosis of fallopian tube
617.1	Endometriosis of ovary
617.3	Endometriosis, endometriosis of pelvic peritoneum
614.6	Pelvic peritoneal adhesions, female
625.9	Pelvic pain
68.4	Total abdominal hysterectomy
65.31	Unilateral oophorectomy, other unilateral oophorectomy
65.61	Bilateral salpingo-oophorectomy, other removal of both ovaries and tubes at same operative episode

A. 68.4, 65.61, 625.9, 617.3, 614.6
B. 68.4, 65.61, 617.3, 614.6
C. 68.4, 65.31, 617.2, 617.1
D. 68.4, 65.61, 617.3

Correct Answer: B. 68.4, 65.61, 617.3, 614.6. This is the correct selection because it reports the procedures as total abdominal hysterectomy (68.4) and bilateral salpingo-oophorectomy with the removal of both ovaries and tubes at same operative episode (65.61). The diagnoses are endometriosis of the pelvic peritoneum (617.3) and pelvic peritoneal adhesions (614.6).

Rationale: A. 68.4, 65.61, 625.9, 617.3, 614.6. This selection is incorrect because it reports the pelvic pain (625.9), which is a symptom of endometriosis is not reported separately.

C. 68.4, 65.31, 617.2, 617.1. This selection is incorrect because it reports a unilateral oophorectomy (65.31) rather than the bilateral salpingo-oophorectomy with the removal of both ovaries and tubes at same operative episode (65.61).

D. 68.4, 65.61, 617.3. This selection is incorrect because it does not report the pelvic peritoneal adhesions (614.6).

Copyright © 2005, Elsevier Inc. All rights reserved.
CPT only © 2004. *Current Procedural Terminology, 2005, Professional Edition,* American Medical Association. All rights reserved.

50. The patient, an 85-year-old white female, presents to the ASC with the preoperative diagnosis of melena. The surgeon performs an esophagogastroduodenoscopy with biopsies. Two ulcers are seen in the stomach, one in the distal antrum measuring about 6 mm in diameter. It had a clean base and was biopsied. The second ulcer is present in the pyloric channel along the posterior wall and measures about 1 to 1.2 cm in diameter. It also had a clean base without any visible vessel or fresh or old blood. The physician noted the following directions in the patient's record: 1. Prilosec 20 mg daily for 8 weeks, 2. Review biopsies, 3. Discontinued nonsteroidal anti-inflammatory agents, which are being taken for gout. The pathology report later indicated "chronic active gastritis, mild to moderate, with mucosal atrophy. Organisms consistent with *Helicobacter pylori* are present."

43236	Upper gastrointestinal endoscopy including esophagus, stomach, and either the duodenum and/or jejunum as appropriate; diagnostic, with or without collection of specimen(s) by brushing or washing (separate procedure)
43239	Upper gastrointestinal endoscopy including esophagus, stomach, and either the duodenum and/or jejunum as appropriate; with biopsy, single or multiple
041.86	Helicobacter pylori
274.9	Gout, unspecified
531.40	Gastric ulcer, chronic or unspecified with hemorrhage, without mention of obstruction
535.1	Atrophic gastritis

A. 43236, 535.1, 274.9
B. 43239, 531.40, 041.86, 274.9
C. 43239, 535.1, 041.86, 274.9
D. 43239, 531.40, 041.86

Correct Answer: C. ***43239, 535.1, 041.86, 274.9. In this correct answer, the procedure is the upper GI endoscopy with biopsy (43239), and the diagnoses are atrophic gastritis (535.1),*** **Helicobacter pylori** ***(041.86), and 274.9 unspecified gout (because the gout medication is being discontinued).***

Rationale: A. *43236, 535.1, 041.86, 274.9. This selection is incorrect because the CPT code description does not indicate that biopsies were performed. Also, the* Helicobacter pylori *(041.86) was not reported.*

B. *43239, 531.40, 041.86, 274.9. This selection is incorrect because 531.40 reports stomach ulcer, but the pathology report stated atrophic gastritis (535.1).*

D. *43239, 531.40, 041.86. This selection is incorrect because 531.40 reports stomach ulcer, but the pathology report stated atrophic gastritis (535.1). Also, the gout should have been reported with 274.9 (unspecified gout) because the gout medication is being discontinued.*

Copyright © 2005, Elsevier Inc. All rights reserved.
CPT only © 2004. *Current Procedural Terminology, 2005, Professional Edition*, American Medical Association. All rights reserved.

51. The patient is a 23-month-old female with a history of left submandibular region mass. Over the past several months, the mass has been more superficial and appears to be an epidermal inclusion cyst. The patient presents to the ASC for excision of the branchial cleft cyst. The documentation indicated the following: The patient was placed under general anesthesia and endotracheally intubated without difficulty. The tenotomy scissors were then used to dissect down to the subcutaneous tissue, and a thin capsule was identified around sebaceous-appearing material. The cystlike mass was followed with the tenotomy scissors. The cyst was entered slightly superiorly, and thick sebaceous material extruded from the mass. The tenotomy scissors were used to dissect around the mass, taking care to stay close to the capsule but not entering into the cyst itself. Dissection was done medially, laterally, and inferiorly. Superiorly, the lesion appeared to extend medially and beneath the mandible. The cyst was followed gently. The cyst extended up inferior to the mandible, and by retracting with the stay stitch, it was removed in bulk. Upon examination of the wound, the lesion extended beneath the platysma down the medial aspect of the mandible. The patient tolerated the procedure well and was awakened from anesthesia.

 The pathology report later indicated the following: Tissue with multiple caseating granuloma and acid-fast bacilli, highly consistent with tuberculosis.

42810	Excision of branchial cleft cyst, or vestige, confined to skin or subcutaneous tissue
42815	Excision of branchial cleft cyst, vestige, or fistula, extending beneath subcutaneous tissues, and/or into pharynx
017.25	Tuberculosis of other organs, peripheral lymph nodes
744.42	Branchial cleft cyst or fistula; branchial cleft cyst

A. 42810, 744.42, 017.25
B. 42810, 744.42
C. 42815, 744.42
D. 42815, 017.25

Correct Answer: D. ***42815, 017.25. In this correct choice, 42815 is reported to indicate that the tissue extended beneath the subcutaneous tissue. The pathology report indicated a more definitive diagnosis than the branchial cleft cyst—that of tuberculosis, reported with 017.25.***

Rationale: A. *42810, 744.42, 017.25. This choice is incorrect because the procedure was not confined to the skin or subcutaneous tissue; rather, it extended beneath the subcutaneous tissue and therefore is reported with 42815. Also, this selection reports the branchial cleft cyst, and the pathology report indicated a more definitive diagnosis, that of tuberculosis reported with 017.25.*

B. *42810, 744.42. This choice is incorrect because the procedure was not confined to the skin or subcutaneous tissue, rather, it extended beneath the subcutaneous tissue and therefore, reported with 42815. Also, this selection reports the branchial cleft cyst and the pathology report indicated a more definitive diagnosis, that of tuberculosis reported with 017.25.*

C. *42815, 744.42. This selection is incorrect because the pathology report indicated a more definitive diagnosis, that of of tuberculosis reported with 017.25.*

Copyright © 2005, Elsevier Inc. All rights reserved.
CPT only © 2004. *Current Procedural Terminology, 2005, Professional Edition,* American Medical Association. All rights reserved.

52. According to the UHDDS, the definition of a principal diagnosis is as follows:
    A. condition established after study to occasion the admission of the patient to the hospital
    B. the primary reason for the encounter
    C. condition established after study to have caused this most recent admission
    D. none of the above

Correct Answer: A. Condition established after study to occasion the admission of the patient to the hospital

Rationale: B. The primary reason for the encounter. This selection is incorrect because it is not the UHDDS definition of a principal diagnosis.

C. Condition established after study to have caused this most recent admission. This selection is incorrect because it is not the UHDDS definition of a principal diagnosis.

D. None of the above. This selection is incorrect because Choice A is the UHDDS definition of a principal diagnosis.

Copyright © 2005, Elsevier Inc. All rights reserved.
CPT only © 2004. *Current Procedural Terminology, 2005, Professional Edition*, American Medical Association. All rights reserved.

53. A patient is admitted 2 months after a motor vehicle accident. The initial treatment of a fracture of the right femur has not been successful; she has a nonunion of the bones, which has given her pain on weight bearing. She is admitted for treatment of the fracture by means of open reduction and internal fixation, which will be followed with traction. During the procedure there is extensive hemorrhaging from the area, and the surgeon documents that the hemorrhage is finally brought under control. The patient is taken to the recovery area in stable condition. The patient was treated with 2 units PRBCs for acute blood loss.

285.1	Other and unspecified anemia; acute posthemorrhagic anemia
733.82	Malunion of fracture
905.4	Late effects, fracture, extremity lower
998.11	Hemorrhage, intraoperative or postoperative
79.15	Reduction of fracture and dislocation, closed reduction of fracture with internal fixation, femur
79.35	Reduction of fracture and dislocation; open reduction of fracture with internal fixation, femur

A. 79.15, 733.82, 285.1, 905.4, 998.11
B. 79.35, 733.82, 998.11, 285.1, 905.4
C. 79.35, 733.82, 285.1, 998.11
D. 79.35, 998.11, 733.82, 285.1, 905.4

Correct Answer: B. 79.35, 733.82, 998.11 285.1, 905.4. This choice correctly indicates the procedure as an open reduction of a fractured femur with internal fixation (79.35). The diagnoses are stated as malunion of a fracture with 733.82, which is the principal diagnosis. 998.11 reports an intraoperative hemorrhage and 285.1 identifies the anemia due to blood loss, 905.4 reports the late effects of the fracture of the lower extremity.

Rationale: A. 79.15, 733.82, 285.1, 905.4, 998.11. This selection is incorrect because the procedure was not a closed procedure, as indicated by 79.15, but rather an open procedure, reported with 79.35. This selection is also incorrect, as the complication code (998.11) should have been sequenced before the complication of acute blood loss anemia (285.1).

C. 79.35, 733.82, 285.1, 998.11. This selection is incorrect because it is missing the report of this condition as a late effect of a previous fracture. This selection is also incorrect, as the complication code (998.11) should have been sequenced before the complication of acute blood loss anemia (285.1).

D. 79.35, 998.11, 733.82, 285.1, 905.4. This selection is incorrect because the late effect code 998.11 is listed first as the principal diagnosis. The reason for this service is the malunion of the fracture, reported with 733.82. This selection is also incorrect, as the complication code (998.11) should have been sequenced before the complication of acute blood loss anemia (285.1).

Copyright © 2005, Elsevier Inc. All rights reserved.
CPT only © 2004. *Current Procedural Terminology, 2005, Professional Edition*, American Medical Association. All rights reserved.

54. This 60-year-old disabled female is admitted for marked congestion and respiratory distress. She is known to have mental retardation and frequent urinary tract and pulmonary infections. She has a recurrent epileptic disorder that is well controlled with Dilantin. On admission the vital signs indicate 101 F, 33 breaths per minute, 83 bpm, and bp of 120/70 mm Hg. Chest has bilateral crepitation that is diagnosed as bilateral staphylococcal pneumonia. The lab report indicates the patient has a urinary infection due to gram-negative bacteria. The patient is treated with intravenous vancomycin and Fortaz and shows marked improvement. The hospital course goes well, and the patient is discharged to the skilled nursing facility.

041.89	Bacterial infection in conditions classified elsewhere and of unspecified site; other specified bacterial infections; other gram-negative organisms
319	Unspecified mental retardation
345.90	Epilepsy, unspecified
482.40	Pneumonia, due to, staphylococcal, unspecified
482.49	Pneumonia, due to, other staphylococcal
518.82	Other diseases of the lung; other pulmonary insufficiency, NEC, including acute respiratory distress
599.0	Urinary tract infection, site not specified

A. 482.40, 518.82, 599.0, 041.89, 345.90
B. 518.82, 482.49, 319, 599.0, 041.89, 345.90
C. 482.49, 518.82, 319, 599.0, 041.89, 345.90
D. 518.82, 482.40, 319, 599.0, 041.89, 345,90

Correct Answer: D. 518.82, 482.40, 319, 599.0, 041.89, 345.90. This selection is correct because it lists as the principal diagnosis the respiratory distress (518.82), followed by the pneumonia (482.40), unspecified mental retardation (319), urinary tract infection (599.0, site unspecified), other gram-negative organism (041.89), and epilepsy (345.90).

Rationale: A. 482.40, 518.82, 599.0, 041.89, 345.90. This selection is incorrect because the principal diagnosis should be the respiratory distress (518.82), followed by the pneumonia (482.40), unspecified mental retardation (319, which is missing in this selection), urinary tract infection (599.0, site unspecified), other gram-negative organism (041.89), and epilepsy (345.90).

B. 518.82, 482.49, 319, 599.0, 041.89, 345.90. This selection is incorrect because pneumonia due to unspecified staphylococcal infection is reported with 482.40.

C. 482.49, 518.82, 319, 599.0, 041.89, 345.90. This selection is incorrect because the principal diagnosis should be the respiratory distress (518.82), followed by the pneumonia (482.40), unspecified mental retardation (319), urinary tract infection (599.0, site unspecified), other gram-negative organism (041.89), and epilepsy (345.90, which is missing from this selection).

Copyright © 2005, Elsevier Inc. All rights reserved.
CPT only © 2004. *Current Procedural Terminology, 2005, Professional Edition*, American Medical Association. All rights reserved.

55. A patient, who underwent an elective abortion 5 days earlier, is admitted because of continued bleeding. A dilation and curettage is performed, resulting in removal of retained products of conception.

A. 634.11	Spontaneous abortion, complicated by delayed or excessive hemorrhage
B. 635.11	Legally induced abortion, complicated by delayed or excessive hemorrhage, incomplete
C. 638.1	Failed attempted abortion, complicated by delayed or excessive hemorrhage
D. 639	Complications following abortion and ectopic and molar pregnancies

Correct Answer: **B.** ***635.11 Legally induced abortion, complicated by delayed or excessive hemorrhage, incomplete. This is the correct choice because the abortion was previously performed, but hemorrhage occurs from this initial incomplete abortion, as shown by the POC (products of conception) that remained. The initial abortion was incomplete.***

Rationale: A. *634.11 Spontaneous abortion, complicated by delayed or excessive hemorrhage. This is an incorrect choice because the abortion was previously performed, and then hemorrhage occurs from the initial incomplete abortion, as shown by the POC (products of conception) that remained. The D&C was conducted to remove the POC.*

C. *638.1 Failed attempted abortion, complicated by delayed or excessive hemorrhage. This is an incorrect choice because the abortion was previously performed, and then hemorrhage occurs from the initial incomplete abortion, as shown by the POC (products of conception) that remained. The D&C was conducted to remove the POC.*

D. *639 Complications following abortion and ectopic and molar pregnancies. This is an incorrect choice because the abortion that was previously performed was incomplete, as shown by the POC (products of conception) that remained. The D&C was conducted to remove the POC.*

56. A patient with advanced metastatic carcinoma of the breast is experiencing shortness of breath and is admitted to the hospital. She was dehydrated. The medical documentation indicates that the discharge diagnosis for this patient was uncontrolled pain and difficulty breathing that was secondary to widely metastatic breast carcinoma, dehydration, and uncontrolled type II diabetes. What would the principal diagnosis be?
A. malignant, primary, neoplasm of the breast
B. malignant, secondary, neoplasm of the breast
C. either A or B
D. uncontrolled type II diabetes

Correct Answer: **B.** ***Malignant, secondary, neoplasm of the breast. The patient was admitted because she was experiencing shortness of breath that was later diagnosed as due to the widely metastatic breast cancer.***

Rationale: A. *Malignant, primary, neoplasm of the breast. This is not the correct answer: The patient was admitted because she was experiencing shortness of breath that was later diagnosed as due to the widely metastatic breast cancer.*

C. *Either A or B. Only B is the correct choice. Choice A is not the correct answer because the patient was admitted because she was experiencing shortness of breath that was later diagnosed as due to the widely metastatic breast cancer.*

D. *Uncontrolled type II diabetes. This is not the correct answer because the patient was admitted because she was experiencing shortness of breath that was later diagnosed as due to the widely metastatic breast cancer.*

Copyright © 2005, Elsevier Inc. All rights reserved.
CPT only © 2004. *Current Procedural Terminology, 2005, Professional Edition*, American Medical Association. All rights reserved.

57. The patient is at 32 weeks' gestation and is admitted with severe bleeding with abdominal cramping. She is diagnosed with placenta previa, with indications of fetal distress. An emergency cesarean section is done. A viable male infant is delivered.

74.0	Classic cesarean section
74.99	Cesarean section of unspecified type
641.11	Pregnancy complicated by placenta previa
655.8	Other known or suspected fetal abnormality, NEC
656.31	Delivery, cesarean, with fetus in distress
V27.0	Outcome of delivery, single liveborn

A. 74.99, 641.11, 656.31, V27.0
B. 74.0, 641.11, 656.31
C. 74.0, 641.11, 655.8, V27.0
D. 74.99, 641.11, 656.31

Correct Answer: A. 74.99, 641.11, 656.31, V27.0. This is the correct answer because it reports the cesarean section (74.99) with the principal diagnosis of pregnancy complicated by placenta previa (641.11), with secondary diagnoses of a cesarean delivery in which the fetus was in distress (656.31) and an outcome of delivery of a single liveborn (V27.0).

Rationale: B. 74.0, 641.11, 656.31. This is an incorrect choice because the cesarean delivery is reported with a code to indicate that a classic cesarean section was performed, but the report does not indicate the type of cesarean, so the correct code should report an unspecified type of cesarean section (74.99). The outcome of delivery reported was also not reported (V27.0).

C. 74.0, 641.11, 655.8, V27.0. This is an incorrect choice because the procedure is reported with a code to indicate that classic cesarean section was performed, but the report does not indicate the type of cesarean, so the correct code should report an unspecified type of cesarean section (74.99). Also, the fetal distress is incorrectly reported as a known or suspected fetal abnormality, but no indication was stated as to any fetal abnormality, only that the fetus was in distress when it was delivered.

D. 74.99, 641.11, 656.31. This choice is incorrect because the outcome of delivery of a single liveborn is missing (V27.0).

Copyright © 2005, Elsevier Inc. All rights reserved.
CPT only © 2004. *Current Procedural Terminology, 2005, Professional Edition*, American Medical Association. All rights reserved.

58. Sally, a 19-year-old, was lighting a bonfire in the backyard when she sustained burns. The following burns were sustained and treated: third-degree burn—left upper arm (5%), second-degree burn—left upper arm (1%), first-degree burn—left anterior leg (9%). The codes for this diagnosis would be as follows:

943.33	Burn of upper limb, except wrist and hand, full-thickness skin loss [third degree NOS], upper arm
943.23	Burn of upper limb, except wrist and hand, blisters, epidermal loss [second degree], upper arm
945.10	Burn of lower limb, erythema [first degree], lower limb, unspecified site
948.00	Burns classified according to extent of body surface involved, <10 percent body surface, less than 10 percent involved in third degree
948.10	Burns classified according to extent of body surface involved, 10–19 percent body surface, less than 10 percent involved in third degree

A. 943.33, 943.23, 945.10, 948.10
B. 943.23, 945.10, 948.00
C. 943.33, 945.10, 948.10
D. 943.33, 943.23, 945.10

Correct Answer: C. 943.33, 945.10, 948.10. This selection correctly reports the third-degree burn to the arm with 943.33 and is correctly listed first as the principal diagnosis because it is the most severe burn according to the Official Guidelines for Coding and Reporting, Section I, C17, C, 1. 945.10 correctly reports the first-degree burn of the leg and is sequenced second. 948.10 correctly reports the percentage of body surface involved in the burn as 15% (fourth digit 1), with 5% involved in third-degree burn (fifth digit 0). No E codes are reported because, according to the guidelines for the AHIMA certification (available on the AHIMA website), the only E codes that are to be reported are those for medications correctly prescribed and correctly taken.

Rationale: A. 943.33, 943.23, 945.10, 948.10. This choice is incorrect because it reports the second-degree burn of the upper arm, which should not be reported because there is a more severe third-degree burn of that area that was reported. All other codes in this choice are correct.

B. 943.23, 945.10, 948.00. This choice is incorrect because the second-degree burn (943.23) was reported rather than the third-degree burn of that same area (943.33). Also, 948.00 indicates that less than 10% of the body was involved in the burn, whereas 15% of the body was involved.

D. 943.33, 943.23, 945.10. This choice is incorrect because the second-degree burn (943.23) was reported along with the third-degree burn of that same area (943.33). According to Official Guidelines for Coding and Reporting, Section I, C17, C, only the highest level of burn of the same area is to be reported. Also missing from this selection is the code to report the total body surface involved in the burn and the percentage of body surface in the burn (948.10).

Copyright © 2005, Elsevier Inc. All rights reserved.
CPT only © 2004. *Current Procedural Terminology, 2005, Professional Edition*, American Medical Association. All rights reserved.

59. A 44-year-old female presented to the ED after she was injured on her farm, where she was treating a sick calf when a cow attacked her and stomped her. She was brought into the emergency room via ambulance complaining of an open right ankle dislocation and multiple abrasions. She also complained of some abrasions on her chin and under her left leg. Specifically, she denied loss of consciousness or headache. The toes were all dusky, she had a strong posterior tibial pulse, and the nurse thought she felt a faint dorsalis pedis. She had an abrasion under her left leg. She was given a tetanus shot and 1 g of Ancef. Immediately she was given parenteral fentanyl and Versed to allow for the reduction of the dislocation without difficulty. Postreduction film looked good. There was perhaps a subtle fracture noted only on the lateral projection. C-spine showed some degenerative change, but upon reexamination she was not tender in that area, but that may have been because she had such a severe distracting injury. Chest x-ray and left femur looked fine.

837.1	Dislocation of the foot, open dislocation, tarsal bone
837.4	Dislocation of the foot, open dislocation, metatarsal bone
910.0	Superficial injury of face, neck, and scalp except eye; abrasion or friction burn without mention of infection
910.8	Superficial injury of face, neck, and scalp except eye; other and unspecified superficial injury of face, neck, and scalp without mention of infection
916.0	Superficial injury of hip, thigh, leg, and ankle; abrasion or friction burn without mention of infection
916.8	Superficial injury of hip, thigh, leg, and ankle; other and unspecified injury of hip, thigh, leg, and ankle without mention of infection
E906.8	Attacked by an animal

A. Level 5, 837.1, 910.0, 916.0, E906.8
B. Level 4, 837.4, 910.0, 916.8
C. Level 5, 837.1, 910.0, 916.0
D. Level 5, 837.4, 910.8, 916.8

Correct Answer: C. ***Level 5, 837.1, 910.0, 916.0. This is the correct answer because it correctly indicates the Level 5 ED service based on the fracture dislocation reduction (Level 5, point 11). The diagnoses codes are correct, with the open ankle dislocation (837.1) listed as the principal diagnosis, followed by the code to report the superficial injury to the chin (910.0) and the superficial injury to the leg (916.0).***

Copyright © 2005, Elsevier Inc. All rights reserved.
CPT only © 2004. *Current Procedural Terminology, 2005, Professional Edition,* American Medical Association. All rights reserved.

Rationale: A. *Level 5, 837.1, 910.0, 916.0, E906.8. This choice is incorrect because no E codes should have been reported. According to the guidelines for the AHIMA certification (available on AHIMA website), the only E codes that are to be reported are those for medications correctly prescribed and correctly taken.*

B. *Level 4, 837.4, 910.0, 916.8. This choice is incorrect because the correct ED level is Level 5 service based on the fracture dislocation reduction (Level 5, point 11). Also incorrect is the 837.4 code, which reports the metatarsal bone rather than the ankle bone or tarsal bone. Also incorrect is 916.8, which reports other and unspecified injuries when it is known that the injury was an abrasion; therefore the fourth digit of 0 is more specific.*

D. *Level 5, 837.4, 910.8, 916.8. The level in this choice is correct. The diagnosis code to report the open ankle dislocation is not 837.4 (metatarsal bone) but rather 837.1. Also, incorrect are 910.8 and 916.8. 910.0 the fourth digit of 8 is for other and unspecified superficial injury. We know that the injury was an abrasion; therefore the fourth digit of 0 is more specific. 916.0 the fourth digit of 8 is for other and unspecified superficial injury. We know that the injury was an abrasion; therefore, the fourth digit of 0 is more specific.*

60. This payment status indicator indicates significant procedures for which payment is allowed under OPPS but to which multiple procedure reduction does not apply, such as nuclear medicine and CAT scan.
A. J
B. A
C. N
D. S

Correct Answer: D. S. This payment status indicator indicates significant procedures for which payment is allowed under OPPS but to which multiple procedure reduction does not apply, such as nuclear medicine and CAT scan.

Rationale: A. *J. This choice is incorrect because J indicates new drug/biological pass-through items. S is the payment status indicator indicating significant procedures for which payment is allowed under OPPS but to which multiple procedure reduction does not apply, such as nuclear medicine and CAT scan.*

B. *A. This choice is incorrect because A indicates that services are paid under some other method, such as a fee schedule or occupational therapy. S is the payment status indicator indicating significant procedures for which payment is allowed under OPPS but to which multiple procedure reduction does not apply, such as nuclear medicine and CAT scan.*

C. *N. This choice is incorrect because N indicates services are incidental with payment packaged into the APC grouper. S is the payment status indicator indicating significant procedures for which payment is allowed under OPPS but to which multiple procedure reduction does not apply, such as nuclear medicine and CAT scan.*

Copyright © 2005, Elsevier Inc. All rights reserved.
CPT only © 2004. *Current Procedural Terminology, 2005, Professional Edition*, American Medical Association. All rights reserved.

PART 2

Section A

1. CASE 1

LOCATION: Hospital inpatient

PREOPERATIVE DIAGNOSIS: Obstructed ventriculoperitoneal shunt.

PROCEDURE PERFORMED: Revision of shunt. Replacement of ventricular valve and peritoneal end. Entire shunt replacement.

PROCEDURE: Under general anesthesia, the patient's head, neck, and abdomen were prepped and draped in the usual manner. An incision was made over the previous site where the shunt had been inserted in the posterior right occipital area. This shunt was found to be nonfunctioning and was removed. The problem was that we could not get the ventricular catheter out without probably producing bleeding, so it was left inside. The peritoneal end of the shunt was then pulled out through the same incision. Having done this, I placed a new ventricular catheter into the ventricle. I then attached this to a medium-pressure bulb valve and secured this with 3-0 silk to the subcutaneous tissue. We then went to the abdomen and made an incision below the previous site, and we were able to trocar the peritoneal end of the shunt by making a stab wound in the neck and then connecting it up to the shunt. This was then connected to the shunt. Pumping on the shunt, we got fluid coming out the other end. I then inserted this end of the shunt into the abdomen by dividing the rectus fascia, splitting the muscle, and dividing the peritoneum and placing the shunt into the abdomen. One 2-0 chromic suture was used around the peritoneum. The wound was then closed with 2-0 Vicryl, 2-0 plain in the subcutaneous tissue, and surgical staples on the skin. The stab wound on the neck was closed with surgical staples. The head wound was closed with 2-0 Vicryl on the galea and surgical staples on the skin. A dressing was applied. The patient was discharged to the recovery room.

Correct Answer and Rationale: ***02.42 Replacement of ventriculoperitoneal shunt at ventricular site and 54.95 indicates incision of the peritoneum for revision of ventriculoperitoneal shunt at peritoneal site. 996.2 is mechanical complication of a nervous system device, implant (ventricular shunt).***

Copyright © 2005, Elsevier Inc. All rights reserved.
CPT only © 2004. *Current Procedural Terminology, 2005, Professional Edition,* American Medical Association. All rights reserved.

2. CASE 2

LOCATION: Inpatient hospital

PREOPERATIVE DIAGNOSIS: Colitis, terminal ileitis, and possible appendicitis.

POSTOPERATIVE DIAGNOSIS: Acute appendicitis. No evidence of abscess or peritonitis. No pus in the abdomen.

PROCEDURE PERFORMED: Laparoscopic abdominal exploration, laparoscopic mobilization of the cecum converted to open appendectomy due to small serosal tear in the terminal ileum from a retraction injury.

SPECIMEN: Appendix.

ANESTHESIA: General endotracheal with 30 cc of Marcaine local augmentation.

PROCEDURE IN DETAIL: After good general endotracheal anesthesia, the patient was prepped and draped in the usual sterile fashion. A Foley and OT tube were both placed to decompress the stomach and also the bladder. A small infraumbilical incision was made, and under direct vision the fascia was nicked. The Veress needle was placed in the fascia, and the abdomen was insufflated to 16 Torr. After this, the fascial incision was lengthened, and a No.10 trocar was placed. The camera was placed through this, and the abdomen was inspected. The cecum was quite inflamed. The base of the appendix was noted. The appendix itself was stuck down to the cecum. The area of terminal ileum just adjacent to the cecum was inflamed. The cecum was mobilized, and the peritoneal reflection was taken down. This was done with hot scissors. Care was taken not to injure the bowel. The ovary was inspected and was normal. The appendix was felt to be quite friable, and there was a small serosal tear created with the Kitner while mobilizing the cecum. We were unable to determine laparoscopically whether this is just a serosal tear; additionally, the tissue was so friable that we were not confident that we would be able to close the stump of the appendix with an endoscopic stapler. Therefore the decision was made to open the abdomen. This was done with appendiceal incision. A Rocky-Davis incision was made after anesthetizing the area with Marcaine. The external oblique and transversus abdominis fascia was incised, and a muscle-sparing technique was applied. The peritoneum was entered, and the cecum was brought up into the wound. The base of the appendix was identified, and it was so friable that we could not simply tie off the base of the appendix and amputate the appendix distally. It was necessary to close the cecum where the appendix was attached and to divide the appendix off the cecum. This was done with running 3-0 Vicryl. After this, some imbricating 3-0 silk stitches were placed. Attention was then turned to the serosal injury. This indeed turned out to be just serosa. This was on the terminal ileum. The serosal injury was repaired with interrupted 3-0 silk. Next, the abdomen was irrigated, and pneumoperitoneum was sucked out. The pneumoperitoneum was released. The two ports, the No. 10 port and the No. 5 subport, were removed. The camera port was also removed. This was done prior to opening the abdomen. All the fascial stitches were used to close the umbilical port and also the left No. 10 port sites. The appendiceal wound was closed in layers with the peritoneum, and two layers of fascia were closed separately. The skin was closed with 4-0 Vicryl. Steri-Strips and sterile dressings were applied. The patient tolerated the procedure well, and sponge and needle counts were correct. She was extubated in the operating room and returned to the recovery room in good condition.

Copyright © 2005, Elsevier Inc. All rights reserved.
CPT only © 2004. *Current Procedural Terminology, 2005, Professional Edition*, American Medical Association. All rights reserved.

Correct Answer: ***47.2 reports the appendectomy for this inpatient. 540.9 indicates acute appendicitis without mention of abscess or peritonitis. 998.2 reports the complication of an accidental puncture or laceration during this surgery. 863.29 identifies the injured area as the ileum. Although this procedure began as a laparoscopic procedure, the surgeon decided to open the abdomen because of a tear in the serosal surface. V64.4 indicates that this procedure began laparoscopically and was converted to an open procedure.***

3. CASE 3

LOCATION: ASC

PREOPERATIVE DIAGNOSIS: Nasal obstruction with sleep apnea, septal deviation due to trauma, bilateral inferior turbinate hypertrophy, left middle turbinate hypertrophy, left concha bullosa.

POSTOPERATIVE DIAGNOSIS: Same.

PROCEDURE: Septoplasty, bilateral inferior turbinate reduction, and endoscopic excision of left concha bullosa.

PROCEDURE DESCRIPTION: Following informed consent from the patient, she was taken to the operating room and placed supine on the operating room table. The appropriate monitoring devices were placed on the patient, and general anesthesia was induced. She was orally intubated without difficulty. She was draped in the usual sterile fashion. The nose was packed bilaterally with Afrin-soaked gauze. The 0-degree endoscope was passed into the left nasal cavity after gauze removal. She was seen to have a left inferior septal spur somewhat anterior and a large left middle turbinate that was grossly widened. The concha bullosa was injected with approximately 0.5 cc of 1% Xylocaine with epinephrine. A sickle knife was used to incise through the base of the concha bullosa. Straight scissors were then used to further cut through the bony attachment of the concha bullosa to the middle turbinate. It was then removed in one thin section with the straight Wilde forceps. There was very little bleeding. I did repack the left osteomeatal complex with the Afrin-soaked gauze; after 2 minutes this was removed, and there was no bleeding.

The right and left nasal septums were each then injected with approximately 2 cc of lidocaine with epinephrine. The nasal septum was seen to be deviated superiorly on the right and left septal spur with some left posterior deviation as well. An incision was made at the anterior end of the right nasal septum. A mucoperichondrial and mucoperiosteal flap were then elevated. A 7 × 12 mm section of septal cartilage in the midportion of the cartilaginous septum was then removed. A mucoperichondrial and mucoperiosteal flap were then removed. A mucoperichondrial and mucoperiosteal flap were then elevated on the left nasal septum. Some of the bony vomer contributing to left posterior septal deviation was removed. No tear in the septum was created during this procedure. I did use an osteotome to remove the left septal spur with good result. Some of the superior, anterior, and right septal deviation was removed. However, I did not remove all of it since quite a bit of the right septal deviation was superior and did not contribute to any deviation of the inferior nasal septum on the right side. A small incision was made on the right nasal septum to allow for hematoma prevention. The inferior edges of both inferior turbinates were then cauterized with the needle point cautery. The butter knife was used to outfracture the inferior turbinates bilaterally. The nasopharynx was suctioned of blood. The anterior end of the nasal septal mucosa was reapproximated with 4-0 chromic catgut in an interrupted fashion. Doyle splints were

Copyright © 2005, Elsevier Inc. All rights reserved.
CPT only © 2004. *Current Procedural Terminology, 2005, Professional Edition*, American Medical Association. All rights reserved.

then applied to the right and left nasal cavities bilaterally. They were sutured anteriorly with a 3-0 Ethilon suture tied on the left side. The patient was then allowed to recover from general anesthesia. She was transferred to the recovery room in good condition. She tolerated the procedure well. Estimated blood loss was less than 20 cc.

Correct Answer and Rationale: ***Procedures performed are 30520 Septoplasty. There is no code for inferior turbinate mucosal reduction, but the note below 30140 Submucous resection turbinate, partial or complete, any method directs you to code 30140-52 for the reduction of turbinates. The correct code for the tonsillectomy performed on a person over 12 years of age is 42826. The diagnosis codes supporting these services are 780.57 Other and unspecified sleep apnea, 470 deviated nasal septum. Because the septal deviation is due to a traumatic injury to the patient's nose, the acquired rather than the congenital code for this condition is correct. Additional diagnoses are hypertrophy of the turbinates, 478.0 and the tonsils 474.11.***

4. CASE 4

   LOCATION: ASC

   PREOPERATIVE DIAGNOSIS: Deviated septum.

   PROCEDURE PERFORMED:

   1. Septoplasty
   2. Resection of turbinates

   The patient was taken to the operating room and placed under general anesthesia. The fracture of the turbinates was first performed to do the septoplasty. Once this was done, the septoplasty was completed and the turbinates were placed back in their original position. The patient was taken to recovery in satisfactory condition. Code the procedure(s) and the diagnosis.

Correct Answer and Rationale: ***30520 indicates septoplasty and 30140-52, submucous resection of turbinate with the -52 modifier showing a reduced service. (See parenthetical note following 30140 in the CPT manual.) Both the septoplasty and the removal of the turbinate must be reported to describe completely the service provided. The diagnosis code 470 indicates a deviation of the septum.***

Copyright © 2005, Elsevier Inc. All rights reserved.
CPT only © 2004. *Current Procedural Terminology, 2005, Professional Edition*, American Medical Association. All rights reserved.

5. CASE 5

HISTORY AND PHYSICAL

LOCATION: Inpatient hospital

CHIEF COMPLAINT: Shortness of breath and back pain.

HISTORY OF PRESENT ILLNESS: This is a 90-year-old female with known history of coronary artery disease who was recently admitted on April 24 with a non-Q-wave myocardial infarction which was elected to be treated conservatively. Since that time the patient has felt relatively okay up until last night when the patient indicates she felt like she had increasing shortness of breath with pain in her chest which seemed to radiate into her back. The patient denied any associated diaphoresis or nausea which she had with her prior event. This pain came and went. It kind of resolved overnight. The patient's symptoms returned drastically this morning and subsequently the patient was unable to essentially move at home. She had her meals-on-wheels delivered and the delivery person called for the ambulance for her. Subsequently the patient presented to the emergency department.

In the emergency department, the patient received oxygen and nitroglycerin, which improved the patient's symptomatology.

Currently, patient denies any chest pain or chest pressure, or any nausea. The patient indicates she is currently not short of breath. The patient denies any increased swelling in her legs.

ALLERGIES: Sulfa.

PAST MEDICAL HISTORY:

1. Diabetes mellitus.
2. Glaucoma.
3. Coronary artery disease.
4. Hypertension.

MEDICATIONS:

1. Norvasc 5 mg daily.
2. Aspirin 81 mg daily.
3. Atenolol 50 mg daily.
4. Bumex 0.5 daily.
5. Plavix 75 mg daily.
6. Enalapril 40 mg daily.
7. Glyburide 2.5 mg daily.
8. Imdur 60 mg daily.
9. Xalatan eye drops.
10. Protonix 04 mg daily.
11. Timolol eye drops.

FAMILY HISTORY: Noncontributory.

REVIEW OF SYSTEMS: General, GI, cardiovascular, respiratory, ENT, eyes, neurologic, musculoskeletal, psych, endocrine performed. With the exception of those noted in the HPI and chronic paresthesias in patient's feet, otherwise unremarkable.

EXAMINATION: Vitals today: Temperature 36.4, pulse 65, respiratory rate 19, blood pressure 141/41, O2 sats 91% in room air. Cardiovascular: S1 and S2. No S3 or S4. Heart sounds are distant. Lungs: Bilateral breath sounds with crackles present. HEENT: Head is atraumatic. Extraocular movements are intact. Nonjaundiced sclera. Moist oral mucosal membranes. Neck is supple. Trachea is midline. The patient does have JVD. Abdomen is soft and nontender. Positive bowel sounds. No rebound tenderness or

Copyright © 2005, Elsevier Inc. All rights reserved.
CPT only © 2004. *Current Procedural Terminology, 2005, Professional Edition*, American Medical Association. All rights reserved.

guarding. No masses palpated. Extremities: Trace edema. Musculoskeletal: Patient moves all four extremities symmetrically and to command. Neurologic: Minimally decreased sensation to light touch in the lower extremities. Psych: Patient alert and oriented. Integument: No obvious petechia or purpura.

PA portable chest x-ray, which I visualized in the emergency department, shows pulmonary edema and no opacities.

LABORATORY DATA: Platelet count 162,000, white count 12.31, hemoglobin 9.4, BUN 41, sodium 139, potassium 4.9, chloride 102, bicarb 24.7, glucose 256, creatinine 1.4, calcium 8.3, CPK 27, troponin 0.07.

IMPRESSION:

1. Acute pulmonary edema.
2. Unstable angina.
3. Diabetes mellitus.

PLAN: At this point, we will admit the patient. The patient indicates that she wishes to be a code level II. Will place the patient on nitroglycerin at 5 mcg initial rate, titrating until chest is pain free or systolic pressure greater than 100. Provide the patient with Lovenox 1 mg/kg subcutaneously q. 12 hours. Will adjust dose for renal function as necessary. Keep the patient on aspirin. Keep the patient on beta blocker. Blood sugar checks q.i.d. Supplemental insulin scale. Continue the patient on glyburide. Serial cardiac enzymes. Obtain a UA and UC.

RADIOLOGY REPORT

EXAMINATION OF: Chest.

CLINICAL SYMPTOMS: Shortness of breath.

CHEST: 1:15 PM: Findings: Comparison is made with the portable chest of last month. Cardiac enlargement is unchanged given the difference in technique. Pulmonary vascularity is mildly elevated and has increased mildly since the previous study. No focal infiltrates. Slight fibrosis or atelectasis in the bases. Blunting of the right costophrenic angle is unchanged due to fluid or pleural thickening. No mediastinal widening.

PROGRESS REPORT

SUBJECTIVE: The patient indicates that she did have some chest discomfort last night, with some dyspnea. The patient received morphine, which improved her discomfort. The patient currently indicates that she is not short of breath. Her pain has resolved. The patient, however, feels fatigued at this point.

REVIEW OF SYSTEMS: General, gastrointestinal, cardiovascular, respiratory, and endocrine were performed, and with the exception of those noted in HPI, review was negative.

OBJECTIVE: Heart: Regular. No murmurs. Lungs: Bilateral breath sounds. No wheezes or rhonchi. Abdomen: Soft and nontender with positive bowel sounds. Extremities: No edema. Vitals: Pulse: 56. Blood Pressure: 97/43. Respiratory rate: 14. O2 sats: 96% on 4 liters. Psych: Alert and oriented.

IMPRESSION:

1. Non-Q-wave MI.
2. Pulmonary edema secondary to #1.
3. Diabetes mellitus.
4. Hypotension with history of hypertension.
5. Gastroesophageal reflux disease.
6. Overall poor prognosis.

Copyright © 2005, Elsevier Inc. All rights reserved.
CPT only © 2004. *Current Procedural Terminology, 2005, Professional Edition,* American Medical Association. All rights reserved.

PLAN: At this point, we did discuss with the patient the continued goal of conservative management as recommended by cardiology on admission. The patient is in agreement with this. Again, the patient has mild hypotension. We will decrease the patient's antihypertensive agents. We will continue the patient on her Imdur at 60 mg twice a day. We will obtain a basic metabolic panel today. We will continue the patient on her aspirin, beta blocker, and ACE inhibitor, although beta blocker needs to be at a lower dose. We will continue the patient on her Lovenox. We will obtain daily CBC and daily basic metabolic panel.

PROGRESS NOTE

SUBJECTIVE: The patient denies any chest pain, chest pressure, fever, chills, or nausea. The patient indicates she is feeling better today. The patient did have a hyperglycemic reaction this morning. However the patient indicates that this resolved.

REVIEW OF SYSTEMS: General, cardiovascular, respiratory, and endocrinology were performed. With the exception noted in the HPI, all are negative.

PHYSICAL EXAMINATION: VITALS: today: Temp is 36.1. Blood pressure is 105/42. Pulse is 71. Respiratory rate is 18. O2 sats are 97% on room air. Cardiovascular: S1 and S2. No S3, no S4. No murmurs, clicks, gallops, or rubs. Lungs: Bilateral breath sounds. No wheezes, rhonchi, or crackles. In general, a pleasant female lying comfortably in bed. The abdomen was soft and nontender. Positive bowel sounds. Psych: The patient is alert and oriented.

LABORATORY STUDIES: Blood sugars of 44, 120, 96, 88, and 102.

Reviewed nurse's and physical therapy notes. The patient refused physical therapy yesterday.

IMPRESSION:

1. Non-Q-wave MI.
2. Diabetes mellitus with moderate hypoglycemic reaction, currently improved.
3. Hypertension, improving.
4. Acute pulmonary edema, resolving.

PLAN: At this point, continue the patient on current diabetes mellitus medications. Continue the patient on current conservative therapy for her non-Q-wave MI and occupational and physical therapy. Have social service plan for discharge planning. It is possible that the patient may require nursing home placement given her poor functional status.

DISCHARGE SUMMARY

PRIMARY DIAGNOSES:

1. Acute myocardial infarction.
2. Pulmonary edema.
3. Coronary artery disease.
4. Diabetes mellitus.
5. Anemia.
6. Hypertension.
7. Gastroesophageal reflux disease.
8. Chronic renal failure.

Copyright © 2005, Elsevier Inc. All rights reserved.
CPT only © 2004. *Current Procedural Terminology, 2005, Professional Edition,* American Medical Association. All rights reserved.

HOSPITAL COURSE: The patient was admitted with acute pulmonary edema. Serial cardiac enzymes showed the patient to have a non-Q-wave myocardial infarction with a troponin of 0.85. The patient subsequently diuresed. The patient's Imdur was increased. The patient did exhibit some hypotension. The patient's antihypertensive dosage was reduced. The patient was also found to be anemic. The patient did consent to blood transfusion. The patient received 2 units packed red blood cells. The patient's symptoms did improve.
The patient was also noted to have chronic renal failure. The patient's renal failure was monitored, which essentially remained unchanged during hospital stay with some fluctuation. Creatinine 1.4 on admission and creatinine 1.6 with discharge.

EXAMINATION ON THE DAY OF DISCHARGE: Alert and oriented female. Heart is regular. No murmurs. Lungs: Fine breath founds. No wheezes or rhonchi. No crackles. Abdomen soft, nontender. Positive bowel sounds. Psychiatry: Patient alert and oriented.

The patient did have a hemoglobin of 9 upon discharge.

DISCHARGE MEDICATIONS:

1. Aspirin 81 mg a day.
2. Atenolol 25 mg daily.
3. Plavix 75 mg daily.
4. Lasix 20 mg twice a day.
5. Glyburide 2.5 mg daily.
6. Imdur 60 mg twice a day.
7. Xalatan eyedrops.
8. Protonix 40 mg daily.
9. Enalapril 20 mg daily.
10. Timolol eyedrops.

DISCHARGE INSTRUCTIONS: The patient is discharged home. Follow up with Dr. Green in 1 to 2 weeks with CBC. If the patient has any difficulties, she should return to the emergency department or contact Dr. Green's office.

Correct Answer and Rationale: ***99.04 identifies the transfusion of packed cells the patient received prior to discharge. The principal diagnosis is 410.70 Acute myocardial infarction. Additional diagnoses include 518.4 acute pulmonary edema, 414.9 Chronic ischemic heart disease, unspecified, 414.01 coronary artery disease, 250.00 Diabetes mellitus type II, not stated as uncontrolled, 285.9 anemia (this is also the supporting diagnosis for the transfusion), 401.9 unspecified hypertension, 530.81 Gastroesophageal reflux disease. Hypertension and chronic renal failure are coded 403.91, even though the physician doesn't link these two conditions together, ICD-9-CM presumes a relationship between renal disease and hypertension, unless the physician specifically states that the renal failure is not due to hypertension. (Note this presumption does not include acute renal failure) see Official Coding and Reporting Guidelines C7, 2 regarding end-stage renal disease.***

Copyright © 2005, Elsevier Inc. All rights reserved.
CPT only © 2004. *Current Procedural Terminology, 2005, Professional Edition*, American Medical Association. All rights reserved.

6. CASE 6

   LOCATION: Hospital inpatient

   PREOPERATIVE DIAGNOSIS: Ventilator dependency, aspiration pneumonia.

   PROCEDURE PERFORMED: Tracheostomy.

   DESCRIPTION OF PROCEDURE: After consent was obtained, the patient was taken to the operating room and placed on the operating room table in the supine position. After an adequate level of general endotracheal anesthesia was obtained, the patient was positioned for tracheostomy. The patient's neck was prepped with Betadine and then draped in a sterile manner. A curvilinear incision was marked approximately a finger breadth above the sternal notch in any area just below the cricoid cartilage. This area was then infiltrated with 1% Xylocaine with 1:100,000 units of epinephrine. After several minutes, sharp dissection was carried down through the skin and subcutaneous tissue. The subcutaneous fat was removed down to the strap muscles. Strap muscles were divided in the midline and retracted laterally. The cricoid cartilage was then identified. The thyroid gland was divided in the midline with the Bovie, and then the two lobes were retracted laterally, exposing the anterior wall of the trachea. The space between the second and third tracheal rings was then identified. This was infiltrated with local solution. A cut was then made through the anterior wall. The endotracheal tube was then advanced superiorly. An inferior cut into the third tracheal ring was then done to make a flap. This was secured to the skin with 4-0 Vicryl suture. A No. 6 Shiley cuffed tracheostomy tube was then placed and secured to the skin with ties as well as the tracheostomy strap. The patient tolerated the procedure well and was taken to the critical care unit in stable condition. Report the procedure(s) and diagnosis.

Correct Answer and Rationale: ***31.1 reports a tracheostomy for assistance in breathing. 507.0 is the correct diagnosis for aspiration pneumonia.***

7. CASE 7

   OPERATIVE REPORT

   LOCATION: Hospital Outpatient

   PROCEDURE: Excision of parotid tumor or gland or both.

   Once the patient was successfully under general anesthetic, Dr. Green, assisted by Dr. Smith, opened the area in which the parotid gland is located. After carefully inspecting the gland, the decision was made to excise the total gland because of the size of the tumor (5.0 cm). With careful dissection and preservation of the facial nerve, the parotid gland was removed. The wound was cleaned and closed, and the patient was brought to recovery in satisfactory condition.

Correct Answer and Rationale: ***42420 is used to report the total excision of the parotid gland with dissection and preservation of the facial nerve. The cleaning and closure are included in the surgical package for 42420. 239.0 indicates a neoplasm, parotid unspecified. The procedure does not specify whether the tumor is malignant or benign.***

Copyright © 2005, Elsevier Inc. All rights reserved.
CPT only © 2004. *Current Procedural Terminology, 2005, Professional Edition,* American Medical Association. All rights reserved.

8. CASE 8

OPERATIVE REPORT

LOCATION: ASC

PREOPERATIVE DIAGNOSIS: Barrett's esophagus with severe dysplasia, possible carcinoma.

POSTOPERATIVE DIAGNOSIS: Same.

PROCEDURE PERFORMED: Exploratory laparotomy, biopsy of liver lesion, immobilization of stomach with pyloroplasty, and placement of feeding tube.

OPERATIVE NOTE: With the patient under general anesthesia, the abdomen was prepped and draped in a sterile manner. Midline incision was made from the xiphoid to below the pubis. Sharp dissection was carried down into the peritoneal cavity, and hemostasis was maintained with electrocautery. We began by exploring the abdominal cavity. The liver was carefully palpated. The area that had been identified on CT was at the very apex of the right lobe of the liver. We could feel this area, and it did not have a thickened feel to it but was more consistent with an area of hemangioma. There was a small secondary lesion on the undersurface of the right lobe. A biopsy was taken, and it did return a diagnosis of hemangioma. The rest of the liver appeared normal, and in my opinion we did not need to proceed with anything further. We thus began with mobilization of the stomach, taking down the greater curvature vessels and preserving the gastroepiploica. We carried our dissection all the way up into the hiatal hernia, preserving the blood supply to the spleen and not injuring it. We were then able to detach the left gastric artery such that the stomach was tethered on its other vasculature but appeared completely viable. All these vessels were taken down with clamps and ligatures of 2-0 silk. We then circumferentially went around the esophagus and carried our dissection all the way back toward the pylorus. We then had the entire stomach freed up from the pylorus all the way up to the diaphragm. The stomach appeared viable with reasonable circulation. A Heineke-Mikulicz pyloroplasty then was performed to open the pylorus in one direction and close it in another using interrupted 3-0 silk sutures to complete the pyloroplasty. With this accomplished, we then picked up the jejunum approximated 40 or 50 cm beyond the ligament of Treitz and placed a red rubber feeding tube using a Witzel technique; this was a No. 18-2. The tube was attached to the skin and brought out through a separate stab incision. The abdominal cavity was then checked for hemostasis, and everything appeared to be intact. We then closed the incision using running 0 loop nylon. We closed the skin with staples. A sterile dressing was applied. Code the diagnoses and the biopsy of the liver lesion and pyloroplasty only.

Correct Answer and Rationale: ***43800 is used to report a pyloroplasty, and 47001 is correct to report a liver biopsy. 530.2 is the correct ICD-9-CM code for reporting Barrett's esophagus, and 228.09 reports the hemangioma of other sites (Liver)***

Copyright © 2005, Elsevier Inc. All rights reserved.
CPT only © 2004. *Current Procedural Terminology, 2005, Professional Edition*, American Medical Association. All rights reserved.

9. CASE 9

OPERATIVE REPORT

LOCATION: Ambulatory Surgical Center

PREOPERATIVE DIAGNOSIS: Upper gastrointestinal bleeding.

POSTOPERATIVE DIAGNOSIS: Multiple serpiginous ulcers in the gastric antrum and body, not bleeding.

FINDINGS: The video therapeutic double-channel endoscope was passed without difficulty into the oropharynx. The gastroesophageal junction was seen at 42 cm. Inspection of the esophagus revealed no erythema, ulceration, exudates, stricture, or other mucosal abnormalities. The stomach proper was entered. The endoscope was advanced to the second duodenum. Inspection of the second duodenum, first duodenum, duodenal bulb, and pylorus revealed no abnormalities. Retroflexion revealed no lesion along the cardia or lesser curvature. Inspection of the antrum, body, and fundus of the stomach revealed no abnormality except there were multiple serpiginous ulcerations in the gastric antrum and body. They were not bleeding. They had no recent stigmata of bleeding. Photographs and biopsies were obtained. The patient tolerated the procedure well.

Correct Answer and Rationale: ***43239 describes an upper gastrointestinal endoscopy to the furthest extent of the duodenum, with multiple biopsies obtained. 531.90 is assigned for a gastric ulcer without mention of acute or chronic status and no mention of hemorrhage or perforation. The fifth digit 0 is assigned to indicate without mention of obstruction.***

10. CASE 10

OPERATIVE REPORT

LOCATION: Outpatient Surgery Center

DIAGNOSIS: Large bladder neck obstruction.

PROCEDURE PERFORMED: Cystoscopy and transurethral resection of the prostate.

The patient is a 78-year-old male with obstructive symptoms and subsequent urinary retention. The patient underwent the usual spinal anesthetic, was put in the dorsolithotomy position, prepped, and draped in the usual fashion. Cystoscopic visualization showed a marked high-riding bladder. Median lobe enlargement was such that it was difficult even to get the cystoscope over. Inside the bladder, marked trabeculation was noted. No stones were present.

The urethra was well-lubricated and dilated. The resectoscopic sheath was passed with the aid of obturator with some difficulty because of the median lobe. TURP of the median lobe was performed, getting several big loops of tissue, which helped to improve visualization. Anterior resection of the roof was carried out from the bladder neck. Bladder-wall resection was taken from 10 to 8 o'clock. This eliminated the rest of the median lobe tissue as well. The patient tolerated the procedure well. Code the procedure(s) performed and the diagnosis.

Correct Answer and Rationale: ***52450 reports the transurethral incision of the prostate. 52000-59 reports the cystourethroscopy, done independently of the main procedure with modifier -59. 596.0 is for obstruction bladder neck (acquired).***

Copyright © 2005, Elsevier Inc. All rights reserved.
CPT only © 2004. *Current Procedural Terminology, 2005, Professional Edition*, American Medical Association. All rights reserved.

11. CASE 11

LOCATION: Outpatient Surgery Center

PREOPERATIVE DIAGNOSIS: Right inguinal hernia.

POSTOPERATIVE DIAGNOSIS: Right direct and right indirect inguinal hernia.

PROCEDURE: The patient was brought to the operating room and placed in a supine position on the operating table. After satisfactory general anesthesia had been induced, the patient's abdomen and groins were prepped and draped in a sterile manner. A short transverse incision was made over the right inguinal area. Subcutaneous tissue was divided sharply. Ties and cautery were used for hemostasis. The external oblique aponeurosis was identified and opened from above downward. The ilioinguinal nerve was identified and protected. The patient had a direct inguinal hernia about 1 cm superior and medial to the internal ring. It was properitoneal fat pushed through a very small opening of about 0.5 cm in size. We reduced this and closed the hole with interrupted Ethibond, which gave a solid closure without tension. We then dissected up the round ligament and ligated it distally. Proximally, we then separated the round ligament from a small sac. We ligated the round ligament from a small internal sac. We then closed the internal ring with Ethibond suture in a Bassini repair. This gave us a solid repair and fixed the hernias. We then irrigated the wound with neomycin. Final sponge and needle counts were taken; they were correct. We then closed the external oblique aponeurosis with Vicryl. Subcutaneous tissue was closed with chromic and skin with nylon. Blood loss during the procedure was minimal. The patient tolerated the procedure well and left for the recovery room in stable condition.

Correct Answer and Rationale: ***49505 reports the repair of a reducible initial inguinal hernia in a patient age 5 or over. 550.90 describes the inguinal hernia repair, without mention of obstruction or gangrene unilateral.***

Copyright © 2005, Elsevier Inc. All rights reserved.
CPT only © 2004. *Current Procedural Terminology, 2005, Professional Edition*, American Medical Association. All rights reserved.

Section B

12. CASE 12

    LOCATION: Hospital Inpatient

    PREOPERATIVE DIAGNOSIS: Bleeding from splenic laceration with hemodynamic instability.

    POSTOPERATIVE DIAGNOSIS: Bleeding from splenic laceration with hemodynamic instability.

    PROCEDURE PERFORMED: Exploratory laparotomy and splenectomy.

    SPECIMEN: Spleen.

    OPERATIVE FINDINGS: There was a small grade 1 laceration of the left lobe of the liver that was not bleeding. There was a grade 4 laceration of the spleen with a large capsular hematoma that had ruptured, and there was active bleeding here. There were 1200 cc of blood in the abdomen. There was no other solid or hollow viscous injury. After good general endotracheal anesthesia, the patient was prepped and draped in the usual sterile fashion. A midline incision was made from the xiphoid process down to the umbilicus. The abdomen was entered, and the hemoperitoneum was released.This was evacuated, and the abdomen was packed off in four quadrants. We then inspected for bleeding. The liver was inspected, and there was a small amount of bleeding laceration of the edge of the left lobe. The bowel was run from the ligament of Treitz to the cecum, and no injury was noted. The ascending transverse and descending colon were inspected, as was the stomach, and no injures were noted. There was no retroperitoneal hematoma noted. The spleen itself, however, was bleeding. There was a grade 4 laceration with a subcapsular hematoma. The subcapsular hematoma had ruptured. It was quite enlarged. The spleen was taken down after blunt control was obtained at the hilum of the spleen. The splenic ligaments were divided with clamps and ties. After the spleen was fully mobilized and rotated towards the midline, the hilum was taken. Stick ties were used to secure the vessels at the hilum of the spleen, and it was divided. The organ was passed off as a specimen. Pelvic organs, including uterus and ovaries, were also inspected, and there was no injury here. The patient was then closed with running PDS and skin clips. She tolerated the procedure well.

Correct Answer and Rationale: ***41.5 Total removal of the spleen or Splenectomy. When referencing this procedure by laparotomy, you are instructed to "omit code." This indicates that the approach is bundled into the procedure and only the 41.5 code is needed for the total removal of the spleen. 865.02 identifies an injury to the spleen with rupture of capsule (subcapsular rupture).***

Copyright © 2005, Elsevier Inc. All rights reserved.
CPT only © 2004. *Current Procedural Terminology, 2005, Professional Edition*, American Medical Association. All rights reserved.

13. CASE 13

LOCATION: ASC

PREOPERATIVE DIAGNOSIS: Granuloma, right inner cheek.

POSTOPERATIVE DIAGNOSIS: Granuloma, right inner cheek.

PROCEDURE PERFORMED: Excision of lesion from right buccal mucosa, likely benign.

PROCEDURE IN DETAIL: After informed consent from the patient's parents was obtained, the patient was taken to the operating room and placed supine on the operating table. The appropriate monitoring devices were placed on the patient, and general anesthetic was induced. It was maintained by inhalation mask technique. The mouth was opened once the child was asleep. There was a 7 × 7 mm pedunculated lesion on the right anterior buccal mucosa. The lesion was excised by cutting through its base. It came out in one place. There was no bleeding. Great care was taken to be certain that there was no injury to the lips.

The patient tolerated the procedure well. She was transferred to the recovery room in good condition.

Correct Answer and Rationale: ***40810 describes the excision of a lesion of the vestibule of the mouth. This would not be considered destruction because the lesion was removed in one piece. 528.9 Other and unspecified diseases of the oral soft tissues. The alphabetic index to locate the code for granuloma of the inner cheek (oral mucosa) refers you to code 528.9, which is for unspecified diseases of the oral soft tissues and the correct code for this case.***

Copyright © 2005, Elsevier Inc. All rights reserved.
CPT only © 2004. *Current Procedural Terminology, 2005, Professional Edition*, American Medical Association. All rights reserved.

14. CASE 14

LOCATION: Hospital Inpatient

PREOPERATIVE DIAGNOSIS: Myasthenia gravis.

POSTOPERATIVE DIAGNOSIS: Same.

PROCEDURE PERFORMED: Plasma exchange.

This is a 5′9″, 270-pound man who has increasing muscle weakness felt to be related to myasthenia gravis, and plasma exchange was elected. His hematocrit was 45.5. His platelets were 190,000. His total blood volume was 5769, and the calculated plasma volume was a little above 3 liters, about 3125 or so. I targeted him for 1 plasma volume exchange of 3 liters using 5% albumin with 1 amp of calcium gluconate/liter, and did a 1 to 1 exchange. He started it at 14:30 and completed the exchange by 16:00. He had no medical complications throughout. His pressures were stable. Cardiac rate was stable. During the exchange, he was aggressively hydrated with an IV because at the time I felt that he was still somewhat volume-contracted from his diarrhea. His pre lab reflected this, and post lab will be done. His final plasma value was 3575 on the machine. This was calculated from a 4297 total, minus the ACD-A of 722. The replacement volume was calculated at 3281 because there are not exactly 500 in each bottle of albumin; I was fairly close, and I was satisfied with this result. The patient will be reevaluated over the next 2 days with special attention paid to his renal status prior to continuing the next plasma exchange planned in 3 days, unless there are other problems that we have to deal with.

Correct Answer and Rationale: ***99.01 reports plasma exchange transfusion. 358.00 reports myasthenia, gravis***

Copyright © 2005, Elsevier Inc. All rights reserved.
CPT only © 2004. *Current Procedural Terminology, 2005, Professional Edition,* American Medical Association. All rights reserved.

15. CASE 15

LOCATION: Outpatient Surgery Center

PROCEDURE NOTE: Jake is in for a vasectomy, having previously undergone counseling earlier today. Patient was placed in a supine position, and the scrotal area was shaved. Under sterile technique the scrotal area was prepped with Betadine, and the sterile drapes were applied. The right vas was localized and under sterile technique was infiltrated with 1% Xylocaine. The vas was externalized, and a 1.5-cm portion of the tube was removed. Proximal and distal stumps were doubly ligated with 4-0 silk. There was a small blood vessel in the skin that was oozing and was clamped. Attention was directed to the left side, where a similar procedure was performed. With hemostasis intact, the proximal and distal stumps on the left were retracted into the scrotum, and attention was directed to the right side, where there was slight oozing from the skin edge; with pressure this did resolve, and the proximal and distal stumps were retracted into the scrotum.

ASSESSMENT: Vasectomy.

PLAN: The patient had been given the postvasectomy instruction sheet, and bacitracin and a gauze dressing were applied. He is to apply antibiotics a couple of times a day with gauze and he was given an instruction sheet to have sperm counts done in 2 months time, and to take contraceptive precautions in the meantime.

Correct Answer and Rationale: ***55250 reports a unilateral or bilateral vasectomy, including postoperative semen examination. V25.2 describes an encounter for contraceptive management, sterilization and correctly supports this service.***

Copyright © 2005, Elsevier Inc. All rights reserved.
CPT only © 2004. *Current Procedural Terminology, 2005, Professional Edition,* American Medical Association. All rights reserved.

16. CASE 16

    LOCATION: Hospital Inpatient

    PREOPERATIVE DIAGNOSIS: Right carotid stenosis.

    POSTOPERATIVE DIAGNOSIS: Same.

    PROCEDURE PERFORMED: Right carotid endarterectomy.

    This case is monitored with EEGs. There were no changes at the clamping. The clamping time was 14 minutes.

    PROCEDURE: Under general anesthesia, the patient was prepped and draped in the usual manner. The incision was made along the right side of the sternocleidomastoid. With sharp dissection, we got on to the common carotid artery. We then isolated the internal and external carotid arteries. We saw the hypoglossal nerve. We put ligaloops around these arteries. We then freed up the artery from its surrounding tissue. This was a high bifurcation. We had to go up higher so as to isolate a good portion of the internal carotid artery. This had not been done. I then placed the Farley Thompson retractor in so we would have adequate retraction. At this point in time, Dr. Allen came into the surgery to help me with the endarterectomy. We then gave the patient 5,000 units of heparin, waited 5 minutes, and placed the clamps on the internal common and external carotid arteries. The endarterectomy was done. The arterial base was cleaned out. There were no free fragments. We were able to nicely eliminate the plaque, which was quite stenotic and ulcerated. We then closed the artery with 5-0 Prolene. We utilized 5-0 Prolene starting at the distal end of the internal carotid artery, then at the proximal end at the common carotid artery, meeting in the middle, producing adequate back-bleeding, then closing the artery. We required two other sutures in the artery to stop some suture line bleeding. This was done. We then used Hemaseel on the arterial suture line. We then closed the wound in layers utilizing 2-0 chromic on the platysma with 2-0 plain in the subcutaneous tissue and 3-0 nylon interrupted mattress sutures on the skin. A dressing was applied. The patient was discharged to the recovery room in stable condition.

Correct Answer and Rationale: ***36.03 describes a thromboendarterectomy of the carotid artery with patch graft. 433.10 indicates an occlusion and stenosis of the carotid artery without mention of cerebral infarction.***

Copyright © 2005, Elsevier Inc. All rights reserved.
CPT only © 2004. *Current Procedural Terminology, 2005, Professional Edition*, American Medical Association. All rights reserved.

17. CASE 17

EMERGENCY DEPARTMENT REPORT

SUBJECTIVE: The patient is an 80-year-old male in acute respiratory distress. He is from the New York City area and was just about to take a train to go there today. He had sudden onset of shortness of breath and presents now because of it. He denies any chest pain or tightness. He has had no recent cough. He is bringing up frothy sputum as he arrives here.

PAST MEDICAL HISTORY:

Surgical:

1. Bypass surgery.
2. Angioplasty and stent.
3. Pacemaker.

Illnesses: The patient has a previous history of congestive heart failure and has been intubated in the past, most recently 4 months ago, with this same problem.

Family history, social history, and review of systems were not obtainable for this patient.

OBJECTIVE: This alert 80-year-old male appears to be in acute respiratory distress. Oxygen saturation is 72%. Blood pressure is 210/107. Respirations are 36. Pulse is 120. Telemetry shows a paced wide complexed rhythm. HEENT: Frothy pink sputum coming out of his mouth. Neck is supple without lymphadenopathy. His jugular veins are full. Respirations are labored. Lungs: Rales throughout. Heart: Rapid rate and rhythm. Abdomen: Soft and nontender with normal bowel sounds. Extremities: No peripheral edema is noted. No clubbing.

ASSESSMENT: Pulmonary edema.

PLAN: He was immediately given Lasix 80 mg IV, given Nitro spray, and started on a Nitro drip. We gave him a few minutes to try to turn around. He was on 100% oxygen. He did not turn around and, in fact, he looked worse. We then talked about intubation with him and his wife and proceeded with it. He was bagged. He was given Versed IV, and he then was given succinylcholine 100 mg IV. He was then intubated without difficulty with an 8.0 ET tube to 24 cm. Breath sounds were heard bilaterally. CO2 monitoring device confirmed placement. The patient was placed on the ventilator and transported to ICU in reasonably stable condition.

THORACIC MEDICINE/CRITICAL CARE CONSULTATION

I have been asked by Dr. Elhart to see the patient for ICU care. The patient was admitted with pulmonary edema, respiratory failure; he has chronic renal disease and is on Dr. Elhart's service—I would assume for the chronic renal disease as well as respiratory failure, but that was secondary. The patient looks like he had a myocardial infarction with elevated troponins, CK-MBs, CPKs, and CKs. His pulmonary edema has started to clear. He was adjusted on the ventilator this morning. The CPAP went from 6 o'clock to 8 o'clock, and then he got too short of breath and went back on the ventilator. Since then he has diuresed more, and I have him on CPAP at present. He is doing quite well, with a respiratory rate of 19 with good oxygenation. I think we have a fair chance of getting him extubated today.

The patient was visiting with relatives here in Manytown. He was trying to move some luggage, started to get diaphoretic, and did not feel well, and it started to become difficult to breathe. The wife felt he was gurgling, and he was sent to the emergency department, where he was found to be in pulmonary edema, intubated, and placed on a ventilator.

Copyright © 2005, Elsevier Inc. All rights reserved.
CPT only © 2004. *Current Procedural Terminology, 2005, Professional Edition*, American Medical Association. All rights reserved.

The patient is intubated and on a ventilator, so I do not have a good family history, social history, past medical history, past surgical history, or review of systems. I got some things from the chart and some things from his wife. The patient's wife is fairly sure that he had stenting of the LAD done last year. We will send for those records. He had a coronary artery bypass graft done before that. It sounds fairly extensive. It seems to have been in 1989. He had at least three grafts, and the cardiologist has this outlined pretty well and what was done at that point. He also had a pacemaker. He has a history of renal artery disease status post renal artery stenosis, history of hypertension, dyslipidemia, bradycardia, and chronic renal disease. He apparently has had some trouble with dye toxicity from an angiogram done a year ago and did not quite get over it. I guess there was partial clearing. It is difficult to tell without the records what went on.

PHYSICAL EXAMINATION: At the time I saw the patient, the physical examination reveals a patient who is alert, on a ventilator, and able to answer questions (yes and no, anyway). He certainly cannot verbalize it. HEENT: Benign. No blood was found in the posterior pharynx or the nose. Neck is supple. No JVD. Lungs actually show rales bilaterally but in the bases, not in the rest of the areas. Heart shows S1 and S2 are regular without an S3 or S4. There is a systolic murmur at the fourth interspace midclavicular line that is somewhat difficult to hear. It is somewhat vague and soft, but I think it is present. Abdomen is soft and benign without hepatosplenomegaly. Normal bowel sounds are present. No bruits heard in either flank; no masses palpable; nontender. Extremities show no edema, rashes, clubbing, cyanosis, or tremor. Lymphatic system: No nodes in the neck, clavicular, or axillary area.

IMPRESSION:

1. Acute myocardial infarction with acute pulmonary edema and acute respiratory failure.
2. Chronic renal failure. You can see that on today's material his BUN and creatinine levels are climbing. I am not sure what the plan is at this point. I am waiting for cardiology to come by, but I think I can get him extubated later this afternoon. I will check his sputum. He does have a fair amount to suction, and it is somewhat thick, so I will make sure he does not have an infection. He is already on Unasyn for any sort of aspiration that might have occurred, although it is not well documented. We will check a 24-hour urine for creatinine clearance, get the records from the Manytown hospital to see what actually was done there, and then check on his lab in the morning. I will wait for Dr. Elhart to come by before we make any other plans, but hopefully the patient will be extubated here shortly.

RADIOLOGY REPORT, CHEST

EXAMINATION OF: Chest.

CLINICAL SYMPTOMS: Follow-up pulmonary edema.

PORTABLE AP CHEST, 5:00 am: FINDINGS: Comparison is made with yesterday morning's portable AP chest. Sternotomy with mediastinal clips. The endotracheal tube and NG tube have been removed. No appreciable change in the heart size or pulmonary vascularity given the difference in technique. Lungs are clear.

RADIOLOGY REPORT, CHEST

EXAMINATION OF: Chest.

CLINICAL SYMPTOMS: Acute MI, pulmonary edema, acute respiratory failure, and renal disease.

PORTABLE CHEST X-RAY: FINDINGS: Endotracheal tube and NG tube are not significantly changed. The cardiac silhouette is upper normal to mildly prominent but stable. Mild interstitial prominence remains in the infrahilar areas, but no other significant interval change is noted.

Copyright © 2005, Elsevier Inc. All rights reserved.
CPT only © 2004. *Current Procedural Terminology, 2005, Professional Edition,* American Medical Association. All rights reserved.

THORACIC MEDICINE/CRITICAL CARE PROGRESS REPORT

This is a follow-up for this patient with acute respiratory failure. He was extubated yesterday. He apparently had a cardiac catheterization in the past, and his kidneys were bad enough that they thought he might need dialysis, but then he recovered; but he certainly recovered incompletely because BUN today is 72, creatinine 2.6, and creatinine clearance is pending. Interestingly enough, potassium is low at 2.8, so we will replace that with oral potassium. We will check his basic metabolic panel in the morning and transfer him to the floor on telemetry. He does not want anything done here. He wants to go home by train, which is probably not the best idea because there is no guarantee that what happened to him this time will not happen again.

PHYSICAL EXAMINATION: Chest: Clear. Chest x-ray looks pretty good, too. Heart: Regular rhythm. Abdomen: Benign. Extremities: No edema. No clubbing.

LABORATORY DATA: All in good shape. Sputum showed greater than 25 white cells, less 10 squamous. No bugs were seen, so it may be just inflammation rather than true infection.

MEDICATIONS: He is on Unasyn at this point. We stopped the Unasyn today and put him on Augmentin. There is some question about whether he aspirated on it, but I certainly do not see anything on x-ray right now.

He is going to be talking to Dr. Elhart later today to decide what to do about whether to discharge or have the study done here. The patient is really 4+ positive that he wants to go back home in case things go wrong with his kidneys. At least he is at home and can undergo the dialysis closer to home. He is most comfortable with the situation there as well as with his surroundings there, so we will leave that up to Dr. Elhart and the patient. But I still think it is a somewhat risky idea, so I imparted to the patient that particular idea. Otherwise, he can be discharged at cardiology's leisure.

DISCHARGE SUMMARY

The patient was admitted with pulmonary edema, respiratory failure, and chronic renal disease. The patient looked like he has had myocardial infarction with elevated troponins. The patient was extubated after the pulmonary edema (less than 96 hours). Discussions with the patient and his family indicated that he did not want anything further done. He wanted further cardiac care done at home. We arranged for him to be discharged, and he was discharged Tuesday. It was advised that he have a cardiac catheterization to determine the extent of his myocardial infarction and whether anything could be fixed, but this is on top of somebody with chronic renal disease who most likely would suffer from the toxic effects of the dye and would probably have some difficulty with renal failure post cardiac catheterization if everything went wrong. Please see my drug note that outlined the drugs the patient was on when he was sent home.

DISCHARGE DIAGNOSES:

1. Acute non-Q-wave myocardial infarction.
2. Congestive heart failure.
3. Pulmonary edema with acute respiratory failure.

Correct Answer and Rationale: ***Procedure code for the nonoperative intubation of the nasopharyngeal airway is 96.01, mechanical ventilation, continuous, less than 96 hours is 96.71. The principal diagnosis is 410.71 acute myocardial infarction. Additional diagnoses include 428.0 congestive heart failure with acute pulmonary edema (combined left and right heart), 585 chronic renal failure, and acute respiratory failure (518.81).***

Copyright © 2005, Elsevier Inc. All rights reserved.
CPT only © 2004. *Current Procedural Terminology, 2005, Professional Edition,* American Medical Association. All rights reserved.

18. CASE 18

HISTORY AND PHYSICIAL

LOCATION: Inpatient Hospital

CHIEF COMPLAINT: Cough and fever.

HISTORY OF PRESENT ILLNESS: This is a 67-year old man who was recently diagnosed with right lower lobe pneumonia. We attempted to treat him at home with oral antibiotics and rehydration; however, he has just not done that well. Last night, he began having more pleuritic pain on the right side, plus spiking fevers and sweats. When he came to the office today, he felt weak and dehydrated, and I felt it would be best to have him admitted to the hospital.

PAST MEDICAL HISTORY:

1. Chronic lymphocytic leukemia and an immunoglobin deficiency secondary to that. As a result, he has been susceptible to pneumococcal infections and has had repeated bouts of pneumonia in the past.
2. Chronic obstructive lung disease.
3. Diverticulosis coli.
4. Hypertension
5. Type 2 diabetes, which has recently required insulin.

CURRENT MEDICATIONS:

1. Insulin 75/25, 40 units twice a day.
2. Glucovance 5/500 1 b.i.d.
3. Ferrous sulfate 5 grains t.i.d.
4. Diovan HCT 160/12.5 once a day.
5. Aspirin 81 mg daily.
6. Vantin 200 mg twice a day.

He recently stopped taking Actos on my instructions.

ALLERGIES: Sulfa.

SOCIAL HISTORY: He lives with his wife. His daughter is a teacher at the local high school. He is not a smoker at the present time.

FAIMLY HISTORY: Nothing that pertains to the present problem.

REVIEW OF SYSTEMS: A complete review of systems today discloses no problems with bowel or urine. No pain in the abdomen. There has been a gradual weight loss over the last few months. He has not had any rash. No joint disease. No neurological symptoms. He has not been depressed. The remainder of his complete review of systems was negative.

PHYSICAL EXAMINATION: On physical exam, he was alert and oriented. Blood pressure: 134/60. Weight: 197 pounds, compared with 207 pounds about a year ago. He looked pale. He was not diaphoretic or febrile. Pulse was regular, but the rate was about 100. There was no abnormality of the head or neck. No palpable mass or lymphadenopathy in the neck. There was also no lymphadenopathy in any of the other major areas. There were rales at the right lung base but no signs of consolidation on percussion and auscultation. The heart had a regular sinus rhythm with tachycardia. His abdomen was soft and nontender. The spleen was very large. I could not tell if the liver was enlarged, too. Genitalia were normal. Rectal exam showed a benign symmetrical prostate gland. There was a fair amount of spasm when I did this exam. Some liquid brownish stool was present in the rectum, which was negative for occult blood. His extremities showed no edema. Pulses were present. There was no active joint or skin disease. No neurological deficits.

Copyright © 2005, Elsevier Inc. All rights reserved.
CPT only © 2004. *Current Procedural Terminology, 2005, Professional Edition*, American Medical Association. All rights reserved.

IMPRESSION:

1. Right lower lob pneumonia with pleurisy.
2. Chronic lymphocytic leukemia, with an immune deficiency as described above.
3. Hypertension.
4. Anemia of chronic disease.
5. Type 2 diabetes, recently converted to insulin.
6. Sulfa allergy.
7. Diverticulosis coli.

PLAN: We had blood cultures done 3 days ago. These came back negative. His white count is chronically elevated because of his CLL. The total count had actually dropped from 63,000 to 44,000 over the past week. He is anemic, with a hemoglobin of 9.9. Blood sugar was 317 earlier this week. Other labs were insignificant. Slightly low albumin of 3.1.

Will get him started on IV fluids and IV antibiotics. Respiratory therapy will also be called in to help with clearing his phlegm.

INFECTIOUS DISEASE CONSULTATION

IMPRESSION:

1. Nonresolving pneumonia due to probable *Streptococcus pneumoniae* pneumonia.
2. Immunoglobulin G deficiency secondary to #3.
3. Chronic lymphocytic leukemia.
4. Hypertension.
5. Chronic obstructive lung disease.
6. Diverticulosis.
7. Allergy to sulfa, manifested by hives.

RECOMMENDATIONS:

1. IV cefotaxime 2 grams every 8 hours.
2. Azithromycin 500 mg q 24.
3. Repeat sputum Gram's stain and culture.
4. Set up for a PICC.

HISTORY OF PRESENT ILLNESS: This is a 67-year-old gentleman who is known to have chronic lymphocytic leukemia and has had recurring pneumococcal pneumonias. He is also known to have an immune globulin deficiency.

Apparently, he was traveling back from New Mexico on October 20. He developed what appears to be a pneumococcal pneumonia and was empirically treated with a gatifloxacin. Although somewhat improved, he continued to have production of sputum. A chest x-ray was performed at that time and did disclose a new pneumonia. Repeat sputum was done and it did demonstrate pneumococcus and subsequently the patient was placed on cefpodoxime. A baseline trough level of his immune globulin was obtained last Friday, and it showed that his level was around 200. Over the last 3 to 5 days, he now has developed worsening fevers and chills and pleuritic chest pain. His temperature has been up to 101. He has not had any rigors. The severity of the pain is about a 3 to 4 out of 10. He says this is just like it was in New Mexico, just like it was a year ago when he was initially diagnosed with having an immune globulin deficiency. The duration of this particular exacerbation then has been going on since the 20th of October.

FAMILY HISTORY: His father died at age 79 of a cardiac condition. He also had diabetes. Mother died at age 83 of age-related conditions. He has one brother, who is in good health. There is no family history of or exposure to anyone with tuberculosis.

Copyright © 2005, Elsevier Inc. All rights reserved.
CPT only © 2004. *Current Procedural Terminology, 2005, Professional Edition,* American Medical Association. All rights reserved.

PAST MEDICAL HISTORY:

Medical: Significant for diabetes mellitus, hypertension, chronic obstructive lung disease, chronic lymphocytic leukemia, immune globulin deficiency, and history of diverticulosis. Operations: None.

MEDICATIONS: He has been on ACTOS, Glucovance, iron aspirin, and recently on cefpodoxime.

ALLERGIES: Sulfa manifested by hives.

REVIEW OF SYSTEMS: Complete and negative.

SOCIAL HISTORY: He is a married, retired teacher with six children. He quit smoking 20 years ago (20–25 packs year total). Sometimes drinks a beer and wine on weekends.

PHYSICAL EXAMINATION: His temperature is 100, pulse 94, blood pressure 130/60, weight 197 pounds. He appears rested, not in acute distress. HEENT: The TMs are clear bilaterally. The ear canals are normal. Conjunctivae were clear. I could not get a good red reflex on the right; there may be a cataract obscuring it. The left red reflex was normal. His nasal membranes and pharynx were clear. There is no cervical adenopathy. No thyroid tenderness. No carotid bruits. No supraclavicular adenopathy. Pulmonary: Reveals rales at the right lower quadrant. There are no secondary muscles of respiration. Cardiovascular: Regular, no thrills. Abdomen: Soft bowel sounds are noted. No guarding, no rigidity, no tenderness of the liver. No abdominal bruits. No groin adenopathy. Integument: No rashes or eruptions. Examination of the nail beds and finger pads shows no stigmata of endocarditis. Examination of wrists, elbows, knees, and ankles reveals no synovitis. Biceps, triceps, quads, and popliteal muscles were not tender.

LABORATORY DATA: Again, the immune globulin level is about 200, with a normal low of 600. Blood cultures were done about 2 weeks ago that remain negative. The culture done 2 weeks ago did grow out pneumococcus.

OPERATIVE REPORT

PREOPERATIVE DIAGNOSIS: Pneumonia.

POSTOPERATIVE DIAGNOSIS: Same.

PROCEDURE PERFORMED: Insertion of central venous peripheral catheter.

PICC INSERTED

INDICATION: Vascular access for IV antibiotics.

PROCEDURE: The patient was informed about the risks and benefits prior to the procedure, and consent was signed. The patient verbalizes an understanding of the risks and benefits, and he does accept.

The left medial vein was identified and cleansed with 70% isopropyl alcohol with 2% chlorhexidine gluconate. The area was then allowed to dry for 30 seconds. The area was then draped in a sterile fashion, and a tourniquet was applied. A 22-gauge IV catheter was placed successfully into the left median vein. Good flow of blood was observed. Subsequently, a guidewire was placed, and the 22-gauge IV catheter was removed. A small incision was made to facilitate the introducer and dilator, which were placed successfully. This guidewire was removed. The dilator was removed, and a polyurethane dual-lumen 5-French Per-Q-Cath catheter was placed without difficulty up to 0 cm. This catheter was trimmed to 52 cm. There was return of blood flow after the guidewire was removed. It was flushed with normal saline followed by heparin. The area was then dressed. Postprocedure chest x-ray has been obtained, checking for line placement.

Copyright © 2005, Elsevier Inc. All rights reserved.
CPT only © 2004. *Current Procedural Terminology, 2005, Professional Edition*, American Medical Association. All rights reserved.

RADIOLOGY REPORT

EXAMINATION OF: Chest.

CLINICAL SYMPTOMS: Right lower lobe pneumonia, pleurisy, PICC (peripherally inserted central catheter) line placement.

PORTABLE CHEST

FINDINGS: There is a large opacity with irregular margins located in the right and mid lung zone consistent with an infiltrate. A left-sided PICC line has been placed, and the tip is within the SVC near the right atrial margin. No pneumothorax. The left lung is clear.

INFECTIOUS DISEASE PROGRESS NOTE

This is day 3 of IV cefotaxime and azithromycin.

CHIEF COMPLAINT: Persistent pneumococcal pneumonia.

SUBJECTIVE: The patient is doing well. He has had no fevers or chills. He is breathing much better. His energy is much better. The illness has been going on for about 4 to 6 weeks.

REVIEW OF SYSTEMS: Pulmonary, cardiovascular, gastrointestinal, and genitourinary: Negative.

PAST MEDICAL HISTORY: Reviewed on previous consultation.

OBJECTIVE: He is afebrile. His T-maximum is 37.2, blood pressure 120/60, pulse around 90, and respiratory rate is 16. O2 sat is 96% on room air. He is resting comfortably. He is not in any distress. His pulmonary examination is clear. No secondary muscles of respiration. Cardiovascular: Regular. No thrills. Abdomen is soft. Bowel sounds are present. No guarding. No rigidity. No tenderness of the liver. Vascular access site is clean and intact. Good SKIN turgor.

In the LABORATORY, there is possibly a gram negative rod in rare amounts. No other pathogen.

IMPRESSION:

1. Nonresolving pneumonia due to *Streptococcus pneumoniae* pneumonia.
2. Immunoglobulin G deficiency secondary to #3.
3. Chronic lymphocytic leukemia.
4. Hypertension.
5. Chronic obstructive lung disease.
6. Diverticulosis.
7. Allergy to sulfa manifestated by hives.

PLANS:

1. We will set up the patient for ceftriaxone as an outpatient every 12 hours.
2. We will switch the azithromycin to 500 p.o. every day for 7 days.
3. We will follow up in a week.

DISCHARGE SUMMARY

DISCHARGE DIAGNOSES:

1. Right lower lobe pneumonia.
2. Immunodeficiency.
3. Chronic lymphocytic leukemia.
4. Hypertension.
5. Chronic obstructive pulmonary disease.
6. Diverticulosis coli.

Copyright © 2005, Elsevier Inc. All rights reserved.
CPT only © 2004. *Current Procedural Terminology, 2005, Professional Edition*, American Medical Association. All rights reserved.

HISTORY OF PRESENT ILLNESS. This 67-year-old man with a history of chronic lymphocytic leukemia was admitted to the hospital with right lower lobe pneumonia. This has been smoldering along for a couple weeks. He has had intermittent fevers and sweats and just felt so sick that he could not manage at home any longer. His examination showed rales at the right lung base, but otherwise he seemed to be quite well physically. His face was flushed. His pulse was rapid. There were no other physical findings.

His chest x-ray showed right middle lung pneumonia. There was no effusion, although the patient was having some symptoms of pleurisy. His electrocardiogram showed sinus tachycardia.

LABORATORY STUDIES: White count was quite elevated at 52,000. He was also anemic at 8.6 grams. Platelets were normal. Blood sugars fluctuated. Protime and PTT were normal. Urinalysis showed a few hyalin casts typical for dehydration. Two blood cultures were negative.

HOSPITAL COURSE: He was started on IV azithromycin and cefotaxime. He was also put on respiratory therapy. Aerosol treatments worked quite well for him. His blood sugars were high. He required his usual insulin dose plus supplemental NovoLog insulin for high sugars. He tended to be lower in the morning and higher throughout the day.

At the time of discharge, he had been afebrile. He was breathing easily and had oxygen saturations in the range of mid 90% level. There was little coughing and no general malaise. His appetite and activity were good. I felt he could continue with IV therapy at home.

DISCHARGE MEDICATIONS:

1. Aspirin 81 mg daily.
2. Diovan HCT 160/12.5 once a day.
3. NovoLog 70/30 insulin, 46 units in the morning and 40 units in the evening.
4. Glucovance 5/500, 1 b.i.d.
5. Tylenol p.r.n.
6. Aspirin p.r.n.
7. Zithromax 500 mg IV every 24 hours.
8. Claforan 2 gm IV every 8 hours.

FOLLOWUP: He will be coming back to see me for followup in about a week. In the meantime, I have asked home infusion therapy to follow him and supervise his IV therapy at his hometown facility.

Correct Answer and Rationale: ***38.93 Is coded for the insertion of a central venous peripheral catheter (PICC). The principal diagnosis is 481 Pneumococcal pneumonia; additional diagnoses include 279.00 Hypogammaglobulinemia, unspecified. This code is chosen because of the below-normal levels of immune globulin. 204.10 Chronic lymphocytic leukemia, 401.9 Unspecified Hypertension, 496 COPD, 562.10 Diverticulosis coli, and 250.00 Diabetes type II, not stated as uncontrolled.***

Copyright © 2005, Elsevier Inc. All rights reserved.
CPT only © 2004. *Current Procedural Terminology, 2005, Professional Edition*, American Medical Association. All rights reserved.

19. CASE 19

ADMISSION HISTORY AND PHYSICAL

LOCATION: Inpatient Hospital

This patient is a 37-year-old Caucasian male who was involved in an accident. He was walking and fell onto a farm implement. He sustained three stab wounds. The patient was hospitalized for 2 days and then discharged. The patient began having distention, nausea, and vomiting today and, because of that, returned to the emergency department for evaluation. The patient also has a history of heavy drinking. The patient underwent evaluation which included an upper endoscopy, which showed some gastritis but no evidence of any definitive ulcer disease. His CT scan shows a small bowel obstruction consistent with a small neck of bowel caught in the lowermost stab wound that he sustained during his initial injury. The patient is now being admitted for exploratory laparotomy, reduction of small bowel obstruction with possible bowel resection with anastomosis, and possible appendectomy. The liver also will be examined at the same time.

PAST MEDICAL HISTORY:

OPERATIONS: None.

ILLNESSES: Hay fever.

MEDICATIONS: Chlor-Trimeton p.r.n.

ALLERGIES: Penicillin causes a rash.

REVIEW OF SYSTEMS: The patient does not smoke. He does drink. Neurologic: The patient denies any history of seizure disorder, headaches, or dizziness. Cardiac: No history of hypertension, myocardial infarction, or congenital heart disease. Pulmonary: No history of asthma or pneumonia. The patient does have hay fever. No history of hemoptysis. Gastrointestinal: The patient denies any diarrhea or constipation. No history of peptic ulcer disease. The patient has had nausea and vomiting. See present illness. GU: The patient denies any urgency, frequency, or dysuria. Hematologic: The patient has never received a blood transfusion. He denies any bleeding problems.

PHYSICAL EXAMINATION: The patient is a 37-year-old Caucasian male. Head: Eyes: Pupils are equal. Ears: TMS are normal. Nose within normal limits. Throat within normal limits. Neck is supple. No carotid bruits heard. Chest: Lungs are clear; no rales or rhonchi heard. Heart: Regular rhythm; no murmur. Abdomen: Normal bowel sounds. The patient has a soft mass palpable in the lowermost incision from his previous injury. No guarding or rebound tenderness.

IMPRESSION: Small bowel obstruction secondary to a piece of bowel caught in the patient's lowermost abdominal injury caused by a farm implement.

PLAN: The patient has been counseled for exploratory laparotomy, with possible bowel resection and possible appendectomy. He has consented to the surgery. The patient will be taken immediately to the operating room as soon as an operating room is available.

GASTROENTEROLOGY CONSULTATION

HISTORY OF PRESENT ILLNESS: This 37-year-old white male, who may be an alcoholic, was driving his vehicle at night and had a roll-over while he was trying to avoid hitting a deer. He was wearing his seat belt. He went out looking for help and then tripped over a farm implement, and was stabbed in the chest and abdomen. He was hospitalized, and CT scan showed some fluid in the peritoneal cavity around the liver and spleen but no injury to those organs. There was also a retroperitoneal bleed. The patient was stable when he left, but he was still continuing to have symptoms of

Copyright © 2005, Elsevier Inc. All rights reserved.
CPT only © 2004. *Current Procedural Terminology, 2005, Professional Edition*, American Medical Association. All rights reserved.

lower abdominal discomfort, and anorexia, and has not had a bowel movement since the above. Last night, he developed vomiting of coffee ground material. His urine was noted to be orange, and he has only urinated twice since yesterday. His wife also noted the onset of jaundice last evening.

On arrival to the emergency room, the patient's labs showed a BUN of 32, creatinine of 1.4, alkaline phosphatase of 145, bilirubin of 4.9, AST of 65, ALT of 106. We did not have baseline enzymes. His hemoglobin was 16.1, stable; white count was 8420.

PAST MEDICAL HISTORY: No high blood pressure, diabetes, kidney or cardiac disease.

ALLERGIES: Penicillin causes a rash.

SURGERIES: None.

PHYSICAL EXAM: Well-nourished male, in no acute distress. VITAL SIGNS are normal. ABDOMEN: No megaly or masses. There is some tenderness in the lower abdomen; it is distended. There is no rebound, rigidity, or guarding.

IMPRESSION: 37-year-old white male, who has some jaundice, elevated liver enzymes. He had an abdominal injury just a few days ago. We certainly need to be sure that he has not developed progression of that injury (i.e., bleeding from the liver or spleen), although his hemoglobin is stable and normal, and he is hemodynamically stable. The patient does drink excess alcohol, and he may well just be having some alcohol-related liver disease. The patient had coffee-ground emesis. We do an upper endoscopy to assess for that, for the presence of ulcers, and also for varices.

PLAN:

1. Upper endoscopy.
2. Follow liver enzymes.
3. CT scan to look for further injury to his biliary tract or liver.

CT REPORT

EXAMINATION OF: CT of abdomen and pelvis.

CLINICAL SYMPTOMS: Vomiting, small bowel obstruction status post trauma 4 days earlier.

CT OF ABDOMEN AND PELVIS: TECHNIQUE: The patient was scanned from the dome of the diaphragm through the symphysis pubis following the administration of intravenous contrast only. No oral contrast was administered due to the patient's known small bowel obstruction, as well as the urgent nature of the study.

FINDINGS: This examination is compared to a prior examination 3 days ago. The liver, spleen, pancreas, kidneys, and adrenal glands appear within normal limits. There is a small amount of fluid adjacent to the liver. There is also a small amount of fluid adjacent to the spleen. Scattered areas of mesenteric stranding are present. There is free fluid present within the pelvis. There is marked dilatation of a significant portion of small bowel. A portion of small bowel does appear to protrude through an area of the abdominal wall musculature within the right anterolateral aspect of the abdominal wall. That is seen just below the level of the iliac crest. That is best demonstrated on images 44 through 47. Bowel on one side of this hernia is dilated and, on the other side, decompressed. This is presumably the etiology of the small bowel obstruction. There is a small right-sided pleural effusion present. There is a drop of air seen on image 11, just posterior to the liver. It is very difficulty to say whether this is above or below the diaphragm. I feel this most likely related to a small area of aerated lung; however, I cannot exclude the possibility that this relates to a small area of pneumothorax or even a small amount of free intraperitoneal air. Close clinical correlation suggested. There is patchy opacity present within both lung bases. That could relate to either atelectasis or infiltrate.

Copyright © 2005, Elsevier Inc. All rights reserved.
CPT only © 2004. *Current Procedural Terminology, 2005, Professional Edition*, American Medical Association. All rights reserved.

IMPRESSION:

1. There is a hernia involving the anterior abdominal wall at the right anterolateral aspect. See above discussion.
2. There is dilatation of a large portion of the small bowel. Proximal to the obstruction, the bowel appears dilated and decompressed. The hernia is presumably the etiology of the small bowel obstruction.
3. Fluid identified within the abdomen as described above. This requires close clinical correlation.
4. Small amount of air noted posterior to the liver may be either above or below the diaphragm. This is felt to most likely relate to a small area of aerated lung; however, a small amount of pneumothorax or even pneumoperitoneum cannot be excluded.
5. Small right-sided pleural effusion with bibasilar pulmonary opacities.

Right psoas enlargement presumably related to hematoma is less prominent than in the previous study.

OPERATIVE REPORT

PREOPERATIVE DIAGNOSIS: Small bowel obstruction.

POSTOPERATIVE DIAGNOSIS: Same.

OPERATION PERFORMED. Release of small bowel obstruction; closure of right lower quadrant abdominal wall defect causing bowel obstruction.

ANESTHESIA: General anesthesia.

INDICATION FOR SURGERY: This is a 37-year-old Caucasian male who has a small bowel obstruction. The patient was found to have a loop of bowel incarcerated in a stab wound that he had in the right lower quadrant area. The wound occurred as a result of a fall. The patient was taken to the operating room for release of the small bowel obstruction.

DESCRIPTION OF OPERATION: The patient was prepped and draped in the usual manner. A midline abdominal incision was made, and the abdomen was entered. Blood was encountered in the abdomen. This was secondary to his previous accident. The right lower quadrant of the abdomen was examined, and a loop of small bowel ileum was found caught in the stab wound in the right lower quadrant area. The bowel was brought out and examined and appeared within normal limits and viable. It did not appear to have any type of necrosis. The small bowel was distended down to the point. The contents of the small bowel were then milked back up into the stomach so it could be aspirated from the stomach as the contents of the small bowel were irrigated. The liver was also examined. The liver and gallbladder appeared normal. The upper abdominal wound, which occurred at the same time as the lower abdominal wound, did not penetrate the abdominal wall. The right lower quadrant stab wound was then repaired. The skin wound was widened so the anterior fascia layer could be closed. After the incision was widened, the anterior fascia layer was closed with interrupted 0 Vicryl sutures. After this was completed, the posterior fascial layer and peritoneum were also repaired using interrupted 0 Vicryl sutures. The abdomen was thoroughly irrigated with at least 3 liters of normal saline. The small bowel was then returned to the abdomen, and the abdominal incision was closed. The incision was closed with a running looped #1 PDS suture. Subcutaneous tissues were irrigated, and the skin was closed with skin clips. The patient tolerated the operation and returned to recovery in stable condition.

DISCHARGE SUMMARY

REASON FOR HOSPITALIZATION: Abdominal puncture wound with herniation and small bowel obstruction.

Copyright © 2005, Elsevier Inc. All rights reserved.
CPT only © 2004. *Current Procedural Terminology, 2005, Professional Edition*, American Medical Association. All rights reserved.

SUMMARY OF HOSPITAL COURSE: The patient was admitted with small bowel obstruction. A release of the small bowel obstruction and closure of right lower quadrant abdominal wall defect were performed.

Patient had an episode of gout that resolved during this stay in the hospital.

The patient recovered and was discharged to home.

The patient was also diagnosed with *Helicobacter pylori* during his hospital stay.

INSTRUCTIONS TO PATIENT ON DISCHARGE: Activity: As tolerated. Diet: As tolerated.

DISCHARGE MEDICATIONS:

1. Metronidazole 500 mg 3 times daily for 10 days.
2. Protonix 40 mg twice daily for 10 days.
3. Pink bismuth 30 ml 4 times daily for 10 days.
4. Tetracycline 500 mg 4 times daily for 10 days.

FOLLOW UP with primary care physician at the clinic.

CONDITION AT DISCHARGE: Good.

DISCHARGE DIAGNOSIS: SMALL BOWEL OBSTRUCTION SECONDARY TO TRAUMATIC HERNIA SURGICALLY REPAIRED.

Correct Answer and Rationale: ***54.63 reports the suture of the abdominal wall. 552.8 Hernia of other specified sites with obstruction. (Alphabetical index obstruction, intestine with hernia—see also hernia by site with obstruction). 906.0—late effect of open wound of head, neck, and trunk. 305.0 reports alcohol abuse.***

20. CASE 20

ADMISSION HISTORY AND PHYSICAL

LOCATION: Inpatient Hospital

REASON FOR ADMISSION: Pulmonary embolism.

HISTORY: This patient is a 56-year-old Caucasian gentleman who really has no significant past medical history. He was, however, diagnosed with some lumbar spinal cancer about 3 to 4 weeks ago. He is currently being considered for radiation and chemotherapy. He resides 50 miles south of here in Anytown and was here in town to attend a meeting. As he was walking out of the building where he had been attending a meeting, he had a near syncopal episode. The paramedics were subsequently called. He initially had refused to be brought into the hospital but was convinced otherwise by a physician who happened to be at the same meeting.

In the emergency department, he was noted to be very tachycardiac and hypoxic. He was started on continuous heparin for suspected pulmonary embolism. Bilateral lower extremity Doppler did reveal clots in the patient's lower extremities up to just above the level of the popliteal area.

On admission to the ICU, he really did not have any other specific complaints.

PAST MEDICAL HISTORY: Really unremarkable other than that stated in the history of present illness. He was recently diagnosed with spinal cancer. He also has a history of stool impaction secondary to the morphine that he was started on for his back pain.

Copyright © 2005, Elsevier Inc. All rights reserved.
CPT only © 2004. *Current Procedural Terminology, 2005, Professional Edition*, American Medical Association. All rights reserved.

MEDICATIONS: Morphine, unknown dose, for his back pain. He also takes several over-the-counter stool softeners.

ALLERGIES: He has no known drug allergies.

SOCIAL/FAMILY HISTORY: The patient's family/personal/social history cannot be obtained given the patient's current status (he is still acutely in respiratory distress).

REVIEW OF SYSTEMS: Also cannot be directly obtained from the patient given his acute respiratory distress; however, in speaking to the patient's wife, he really does not have any other constitutional symptoms. He has not had any recent fevers, chills, or night sweats. He did admit to being dyspneic right before he nearly passed out, but he denied any chest pain. He has been constipated, as per the history of present illness. He denies any changes in his bladder habits. He also denies any recent changes in his appetite or his weight. The rest of his systems were briefly reviewed with the patient's wife and were found to be essentially negative and unremarkable.

PHYSICAL EXAMINATION: He appeared to be in moderate respiratory distress. He was otherwise not in any acute pain. His blood pressure was 98/52, pulse rate around 126, and he was breathing about 26 to 30 per minute with very shallow respirations. His temperature was 36.3. Head/Neck: Showed pink palpebral conjunctivae with anicteric sclerae. He did not have any active nasal or ear discharge. Oropharynx was otherwise clear. He was on a nonrebreather mask during my exam. He was saturating about 77% on the nonrebreather initially. Currently, his saturations are up to 92%. Chest: Showed his lung fields to have some soft scattered rales. He also had some scattered wheezing, more prominent on the right side than on the left side. Otherwise, his chest expansion was symmetrical. Cardiac: Shows a tachycardic rate without any rubs. Abdomen: Showed it to be soft and nontender with normoactive bowel sounds. Extremities: Showed good and equal pulses peripherally without any significant edema. Both his hands and feet were warm to the touch.

LABORATORY DATA: A CBC showed fairly normal blood cell counts. A routine urinalysis was also likewise unremarkable. A comprehensive metabolic panel showed his glucose to be slightly elevated at 143 mg/dl. His albumin was low at 2.6 grams/dl; otherwise, the rest of his panel was within normal limits. His BUN was 15, his creatinine was 0.9, and the rest of his electrolytes were within normal limits. A BNP was 84 picograms/ml. D-dimer test was more than 1000 SEU. His INR was 2.2 with a Protime of 17 seconds.

His chest x-ray showed some small infiltrates more prominent in the base of his lungs. His EKG showed sinus tachycardia with some nonspecific STT wave changes.

His lower extremity ultrasound showed clots extending from his lower thigh all the way up to his popliteal areas, and the left clot was noted to be fairly mobile. The clot on the right side was more chronic.

ASSESSMENT:

1. Venous thromboembolic disease with acute pulmonary embolism.
2. Spinal cancer.

PLAN:

1. Admit to the ICU.
2. Continue to anticoagulate the patient with unfractionated heparin adjusted to a therapeutic PTT.
3. Given the severity of the patient's pulmonary embolism and the fact that he still has a significant clot burden in his legs, will arrange for a temporary intravenous inferior vena cava filter placement tomorrow.

Copyright © 2005, Elsevier Inc. All rights reserved.
CPT only © 2004. *Current Procedural Terminology, 2005, Professional Edition*, American Medical Association. All rights reserved.

Total critical care time spent seeing the patient today and talking to the family was 120 minutes.

PROGRESS NOTE

The patient did well overnight. He was started on intravenous and fractionated heparin that was continuously adjusted to therapeutic PTT for his pulmonary embolism and venous thromboembolic disease.

This morning he said his breathing has been much better. Otherwise, he really does not have any other new complaints.

His past medical history, family history, and personal/social history have also been briefly reviewed.

His MEDICATIONS in the hospital have also been reviewed.

REVIEW OF SYSTEMS: He denies any fevers, chills, or night sweats overnight. His breathing is much better as per the HPI. He denies any chest pain. He is moving his bowels and is freely voiding without any difficulty. The rest of his systems were reviewed and found to be essentially negative and unremarkable.

PHYSICAL EXAMINATION: On examination he appeared to be fairly comfortable. He did not appear to be in any acute pain or distress. Blood pressure: 100/60. Pulse rate: 108. He was breathing about 22 to 24 breaths per minute and was saturating 94% to 96% on 2 liters per nasal cannula. Examination of his head and neck showed pink palpebral conjunctivae with anicteric sclerae. He did not have any active nasal or ear discharge. Oropharynx was otherwise clear. He was already on a nasal cannula; however, his saturation would still precipitously drop, requiring the placement of a 40% to 50% Venti mask. Exam of his chest showed his lung fields to be clear to auscultation, with only some occasional scattered rales and some soft wheezes, more prominent on the right side than the left. Cardiac exam showed a tachycardic rate without any rubs. Examination of his abdomen showed it to be soft and nontender with normoactive bowel sounds. Exam of his extremities showed good and equal pulses peripherally without any significant edema.

ASSESSMENT:

1. Acute hypoxic respiratory failure secondary to acute pulmonary embolism.
2. Venous thromboembolic disease with bilateral leg deep venous thrombosis.
3. Spinal cancer.

RECOMMENDATION AND PLAN:

1. The patient will get an inferior vena cava filter today.
2. Continue to anticoagulate the patient with heparin.
3. If the patient is stable after the placement of the filter, we should be able to transfer him out of the intensive care unit to the regular floor.

Total time spent managing the patient today and coordinating his care, including the placement of the inferior vena cava filter, was about 75 minutes.

CRITICAL CARE PROGRESS NOTE

The patient has had his temporary inferior vena cava filter placed yesterday. He currently is doing well. He has not had any further episodes of dyspnea.

His past medical history, family history, and social history remain unchanged.

His medications have also been reviewed and remain unchanged from yesterday.

Copyright © 2005, Elsevier Inc. All rights reserved.
CPT only © 2004. *Current Procedural Terminology, 2005, Professional Edition,* American Medical Association. All rights reserved.

REVIEW OF SYSTEMS: He denies any fever, chills, or night sweats. His breathing continues to improve every day. He denies any chest pain. He is moving his bowels and is freely voiding without any difficulty. The rest of his systems were reviewed and were found to be essentially negative, unremarkable, or noncontributory.

PHYSICAL EXAMINATION: He appears to be fairly comfortable. He was not in any acute pain or distress. His blood pressure was about 110/72 with a pulse rate of 94. He was breathing about 22 to 24 breaths per minute and was saturating 95% on 2 liters of oxygen via nasal cannula. Head/Neck: Showed pink palpebral conjunctivae with anicteric sclerae. He did not have any active nasal or ear discharge. His oropharynx is clear. Exam of his chest shows his lung fields to be clear to auscultation with only some occasional scattered rales, which are more prominent on the right side than on the left. However, even this was actually better than yesterday's exam. Cardiac: Regular rate and rhythm without any rubs. Examination of his abdomen showed it to be soft and nontender with normoactive bowel sounds. Exam of his extremities showed good and equal pulses peripherally without any significant edema.

ASSESSMENT:

1. Acute hypoxic respiratory failure secondary to acute pulmonary embolism, clinically improving.
2. Venous thromboembolic disease with bilateral leg deep venous thrombosis and pulmonary embolism, clinically stable.
3. Spinal cancer.

RECOMMENDATIONS/PLAN:

1. Continue the patient on anticoagulation.
2. Start the patient on heparin orally.
3. If the patient remains stable today, he should be able to be transferred out to the regular floor.

Total time spent seeing the patient today was 35 minutes.

CRITICAL CARE PROGRESS NOTE

The patient remained relatively stable overnight. However, he tried getting out of bed and inadvertently pulled on his Foley catheter. He did have a fair amount of hematuria afterwards. Repeated attempts to reinsert the Foley, unfortunately, failed. Otherwise, his respiratory function remains fairly stable.

Again, his past medical, family, and personal/social histories were briefly reviewed and remained unchanged.

MEDICATIONS: His medications also remained unchanged. We are still continuing to therapeutically anticoagulate him.

REVIEW OF SYSTEMS: He otherwise denies any fevers, chills, or night sweats. When asked about last night, he said that he was transiently confused but is currently, otherwise, awake, alert, and oriented. His breathing continues to improve. He has not had any chest pain. Prior to pulling out his Foley catheter, he had not had any problems with his bladder habits. He is also moving his bowels without any difficulty. The rest of his systems were reviewed and were found to be essentially negative and unremarkable.

PHYSICAL EXAMINATION: On examination, he appeared to be fairly comfortable. He was not in any acute pain or distress. His blood pressure was 106/70 with a pulse rate of 90. He was breathing about 18 to 20 breaths per minute. He was saturating more than 94% on 2 liters of oxygen via nasal cannula.

Copyright © 2005, Elsevier Inc. All rights reserved.
CPT only © 2004. *Current Procedural Terminology, 2005, Professional Edition*, American Medical Association. All rights reserved.

Exam of his head and neck showed pink palpebral conjunctivae with anicteric sclerae. He did not have any active nasal or ear discharge. Oropharynx was clear. His neck was supple and nontender. Exam of his chest showed his lung fields to be clear to auscultation bilaterally. Cardiac exam showed a regular rate and rhythm without any rubs. Exam of his abdomen showed it to be soft and nontender with normoactive bowel sounds. Exam of extremities showed good and equal pulses peripherally without any significant edema.

ASSESSMENT:

1. Acute hypoxic respiratory failure secondary to acute pulmonary embolism, clinically improving.
2. Venous thromboembolic disease with bilateral leg deep venous thrombosis and acute pulmonary embolism, clinically stable.
3. Spinal cancer.
4. Hematuria, atraumatic from the inadvertent removal of his catheter, rule out posterior urethral injury.

RECOMMENDATIONS AND PLAN:

1. Continue the patient on his anticoagulation.
2. Adjust his warfarin per INR.
3. Check a CBC every 8 hours.
4. We will try to reinsert a three-way Foley catheter and start continuous bladder irrigation.
5. Consult urology.

Total time spent seeing the patient today and coordinating his care, including coordinating his care with his consultants, was 12 minutes.

DISCHARGE SUMMARY

The patient is a 56-year-old gentleman who was admitted for an acute pulmonary embolism. The patient was promptly started on anticoagulation. Further assessment for venous thromboembolic disease did reveal deep venous thrombosis in both his legs. He subsequently had a temporary inferior vena cava filter placed because of his significant clot burden. His hospital course was complicated by a dramatic removal of his Foley catheter, leading to a posterior urethral injury and hematuria. Dr. Green was subsequently consulted for this.

Now overnight he remained fairly stable. His hematuria subsequently cleared. He does not have any other significant complaints.

His past medical/family history and personal and social histories have remained unchanged.

His medications have also been reviewed and remain unchanged.

On review of systems he denies any fever, chills, or night sweats overnight. His breathing continues to improve. He currently is able to ambulate without requiring oxygen. His bowel habits have otherwise remained unchanged. The rest of the systems were reviewed and were found to be essentially negative and unremarkable.

On physical examination he appeared to be fairly comfortable. He was not in any acute pain or distress. His blood pressure was 115/74 with a pulse rate of 88. He was saturating 96% to 97% on room air.

Copyright © 2005, Elsevier Inc. All rights reserved.
CPT only © 2004. *Current Procedural Terminology, 2005, Professional Edition*, American Medical Association. All rights reserved.

Examination of his head and neck showed pink palpebral conjunctiva with anicteric sclerae. He did not have any active nasal or ear discharge. Oropharynx was clear. The neck was supple and nontender. Examination of his chest shows lung fields to be clear to auscultation bilaterally. Cardiac exam showed a regular rate and rhythm without any rubs. Examination of his abdomen showed it to be soft and nontender, with normal active bowel sounds. Examination of his extremities showed good and equal pulses peripherally, without any significant edema. Exam of his external genitalia did not show any gross abnormality. He continues now to have a Foley catheter in place.

FINAL DIAGNOSES:

1. Acute hypoxic respiratory failure secondary to acute pulmonary embolism, clinically improving.
2. Venous thromboembolic disease with bilateral leg venous thrombosis and acute pulmonary embolism, clinically stable.
3. Spinal cancer.
4. Hematuria from traumatic removal of the Foley catheter.

RECOMMENDATION and PLAN:

1. Continue the patient on outpatient Lovenox and warfarin. The patient's Lovenox is to be discontinued once the patient's INR is therapeutic. Given the degree of his venous thromboembolic disease and his clot burden we would probably aim for an INR of 2.5.
2. Advised the patient to keep the Foley catheter in place for the next 5 to 7 days to avoid any urethral strictures. If, after removal of the catheter, the patient continues to experience some difficulty voiding, he was advised to follow up with his family practice physician.

DISCHARGE MEDICATIONS:

1. Morphine sulfate.
2. Lovenox
3. Warfarin.

The patient was instructed on how to take these medications and told to follow up with his primary care physician for further adjustments.

I have also spoken with his primary care physician and have given him an update of what has transpired during this current hospitalization. We also briefly discussed that because of his clot burden and his underlying spinal cancer, he will likely need to keep the inferior vena cava filter in place permanently. At that point, I also advised the patient to keep on chronic anticoagulation indefinitely.

Total time spent seeing and managing this patient today and coordinating his care, including discussing his discharge plans with his primary care provider, was a total of 120 minutes.

Correct Answer and Rationale:

415.19 reports acute pulmonary embolism.
518.81 reports acute respiratory failure.
453.8 reports venous thrombosis of the legs.
170.2 reports lumbar spinal cancer.
599.7 reports hematuria.
996.70 reports a complication of a bladder catheter.

Copyright © 2005, Elsevier Inc. All rights reserved.
CPT only © 2004. *Current Procedural Terminology, 2005, Professional Edition,* American Medical Association. All rights reserved.

21. CASE 21

HISTORY AND PHYSICAL

REASON FOR ADMISSION: Renal failure, generalized edema, and coronary artery disease.

The patient is a 66-year-old male I was asked to see in consultation in the office today by his primary care physician for a rising creatinine level. The patient has been having progressive shortness of breath. A stress test was done, which was positive. This was followed by a cardiac catheterization, where the patient was found to have multivessel coronary artery disease including mid to right coronary artery, proximal LAD, and proximal circumflex with an ejection fraction of 66% without coarse regional motion abnormalities with normal systolic function without any mitral regurgitation. The patient was supposed to have bypass surgery today; however, because his creatinine has gone up from 1.8 mg/dl to 2.3 mg/dl, his bypass surgery has been postponed. His BUN is 48, sodium 136, potassium 4.6, chloride 97, bicarb 29, creatinine 2.3, and calcium 8.6. His white count was 6,000, with a hemoglobin of 11.5, MCV of 101.7, and platelets 192,000. He has a normal Protime and INR.

The patient states that he had a 24-hour urine collection in the past, but he does not recall the results of that. We tried to get a hold of the 24-hour urine taken by his primary care physician but were unsuccessful today.

The patient has been on Actos and recently was started on Crestor, which was switched from Lipitor 40 mg daily.

For the past few months, he has been having progressive shortness of breath. For the past week or so, he has been getting more leg swelling where he cannot even tie his shoes because of his increased abdominal girth. He has been having exertional dyspnea. He cannot even walk half a block. He denies any PND. He has no chest pain. He has never had any chest pain. He has no palpitations, but he complains of massive leg edema.

PAST MEDICAL HISTORY IS SIGNIFICANT FOR THE FOLLOWING:

1. Long-standing hypertension.
2. Type II diabetes mellitus, on Lantus and Humalog insulin.
3. Diabetic retinopathy.
4. Right eye blindness.
5. Congestive heart failure, but normal ejection fraction as mentioned.
6. Obesity.
7. Hyperlipidemia.
8. Questionable diabetic nephropathy (again, I do not have any urinalysis or 24-hour urine collection).
9. Hypothyroidism.

SOCIAL HISTORY: He is single. He has a girlfriend, who was with him today. He quit smoking in 1986. He uses alcohol occasionally. He is retired. He used to work as a store manager at Wal-Mart. He is a native of New York.

FAMILY HISTORY: Father died of unclear reasons. Mother died of a myocardial infarction at age 65. One sister with breast cancer. One sister with lung cancer. No kidney disease, dialysis, or kidney transplantation.

ALLERGIES: Questionable Vasotec.

CURRENT MEDICATIONS include the following:

1. Actos 15 mg daily.
2. Amitriptyline 50 mg daily.
3. Humalog 15 units t.i.d.

Copyright © 2005, Elsevier Inc. All rights reserved.
CPT only © 2004. *Current Procedural Terminology, 2005, Professional Edition*, American Medical Association. All rights reserved.

4. Lantus 56 units nightly.
5. Lisinopril 30 mg daily.
6. Multivitamins 1 daily.
7. Neurontin 300 mg 2 tabs b.i.d.
8. Prednisone eye drops.
9. Synthroid 0.075 mg daily.
10. Torsemide 20 mg 2 tabs b.i.d.
11. Crestor 10 mg daily.
12. Isosorbide mononitrate 30 mg daily.

REVIEW OF SYSTEMS: Constitutional: Generalized weakness with fatigue. Eyes: He wears glasses. He has right-sided blindness. ENT: Negative. Cardiovascular: As mentioned. Respiratory: Negative. Gastrointestinal: Negative, except for constipation. Genitourinary: Negative. Musculoskeletal: Chronic intermittent back pain. Skin: Negative. Neuro: Numbness and tingling in the fingers and toes. Psychiatry: Negative. Endocrine: He has diabetes and hypothyroidism. Hematology: Anemia from yesterday's labs.

EXAMINATION: The patient was short of breath but not in any distress. His temperature was 101.8 degrees. Respirations: 28 on room air. Pulse: 84/minute and regular. Weight 296 pounds. Blood pressure on the right side, 108/45 sitting and 108/50 standing. On the left, 108/56 standing. He has right-sided blindness. He has increased jugular venous pressure with positive hepatojugular reflux. Lungs had good air entry bilaterally, but he had a few crackles in the bases. He has abdominal wall and lower extremity edema. He has 1+ sacral edema. He had distinct heart sounds but no pericardial friction rub or murmurs. He did not have any carotid bruits.

His legs had palpable pulses, but 4+ edema in the lower extremities up to the thighs. No ulcerations. The patient was awake, alert, oriented x 3, without any focal neurological deficits. He had normal gait. He does have decreased sensations in his feet.

IMPRESSION:

1. Chronic renal failure with an estimated creatinine clearance of 13 ml/minute.
2. Acute renal failure possibly related to his cardiac catheterization. This patient could have thromboembolic disease.
3. Chronic renal failure could be related to the diabetic nephropathy but also could be related to hypertension or renal vascular disease; again, without knowing whether he has proteinuria or not, it is difficult to say. In any case, the patient does have generalized edema, and that edema needs to be taken care of. He is on a long-acting diuretic, and he probably would benefit from a shorter-acting diuretic.
4. Anemia of acute and chronic renal failure.
5. Slight macrocytosis.
6. Type II diabetes.
7. Severe coronary artery disease that would require bypass surgery.

PLAN:

1. The patient was admitted to telemetry.
2. He is code Level I.
3. We will make sure he has adequate intake output.
4. Fluid restriction 2 liters a day and also a salt restriction of 2 grams of sodium.
5. We will give him 2 mg of Bumex IV and start him at 0.125 mg an hour.
6. We will monitor his urine output hourly.
7. His surgery will be on hold until he is tuned up.
8. We will check potassium and magnesium every 6 hours and correct accordingly.
9. We will repeat his basic panel and CBC in the morning.
10. If his hemoglobin drops below 11, we will start him on Epo.

Copyright © 2005, Elsevier Inc. All rights reserved.
CPT only © 2004. *Current Procedural Terminology, 2005, Professional Edition,* American Medical Association. All rights reserved.

11. We will check iron studies and give him iron if need be.
12. Discontinue Crestor since his creatinine clearance is coming down.
13. Discontinue Actos since he has edema and it could be contributing to his massive edema and CHF symptoms.
14. Continue with his current insulin dose.

I had a long discussion with the patient about his renal function. I advised him that he might end up on dialysis either before or after his bypass surgery; however, he has severe coronary artery disease with a good ejection fraction, and he would benefit from bypass surgery. The patient understands that, and he agrees to dialysis if need be.

The option of what type of renal replacement therapy he would get will be discussed later.

The patient agrees to be admitted and diuresed. I discussed the case with Dr. Green on the phone, and he was in full agreement.

The total time I spent with this patient today was 65 minutes.

NEPHROLOGY/CRITICAL CARE PROGRESS NOTE

The patient is making good progress today as he made 1300 ml. Last night he had 32 and 850 output. His weight is 132–1/2 kg today, down from 133.4 kg yesterday. He has no complaints of chest pain or shortness of breath. He is awake, alert, oriented x 3 without any focal neurological deficits. His blood pressure is 124/57, temperature 36.9, heart rate in the low 70s per minute, respirations 18 per minute, and sats 94% on room air.

His lungs are clear. He has regular rate and rhythm. He has still sacral abdominal wall and low extremity edema, probably 2+.

His BUN today is 53, down from 57, sodium 139, potassium 4.4, chloride 101, bicarb 27, glucose 149, creatinine 2.2, down from 2.6.

His urinalysis on admission showed no protein. His microscopic examination showed no blood.

Magnesium today is elevated at 2.3.

IMPRESSION:

1. Chronic renal failure with estimated creatinine clearance of 30 ml/minutes.
2. Acute renal failure secondary to probably his cardiac cath and possibly atheroembolic disease, possible contrast nephropathy.
3. The patient does not have proteinuria, so it is unlikely that he has diabetic nephropathy. He could have renal artery stenosis or hypertensive nephrosclerosis. I think it is important to figure out what he has because if he does have renal stenosis, this probably would need to be fixed prior to his bypass surgery.
4. Generalized edema and congestive heart failure, probably precipitated by Actos.
5. Anemia of acute and chronic renal failure.
6. Type II diabetes.
7. Severe coronary artery disease which had required bypass surgery.

PLAN:

1. The patient will stay in the hospital for the time being.
2. Continue Bumex drip at 0.125 mg an hour.
3. Check spot urine protein and creatinine ratio.
4. Repeat labs in the morning to include BMP, CBC.
5. Renal ultrasound Monday morning because of the acute and chronic renal failure.
6. Will probably discharge him on Monday morning on oral Bumex.
7. The patient is already off Actos.
8. Will continue to monitor his potassium and magnesium every 6 hours and replace accordingly.

Copyright © 2005, Elsevier Inc. All rights reserved.
CPT only © 2004. *Current Procedural Terminology, 2005, Professional Edition*, American Medical Association. All rights reserved.

Discussed all of the above with the patient, including possible intervention on his renal arteries. He seems to understand and agree with the plan.

I discussed this case with the attending, and he was in agreement.

PROGRESS NOTE

The patient had no major events during the night. He is losing weight. He is diuresing very nicely. He had 341 in and 1000 out so far today. Yesterday he had 1461 in and 3750 out. He has no complaints of chest pain or shortness of breath. He appears euvolemic. He still has a little bit of edema in the lower extremities. His vitals are stable. His BUN is down to 41, sodium 140, potassium 4.2, chloride 101, bicarbonate 28.7, creatinine down to 1.7, and calcium 8.4.

His white count is 3.6 K, hemoglobin 11.1, platelets 214,000.

IMPRESSION:

1. Acute on top of chronic renal failure.
2. Generalized edema and congestive heart failure, probably precipitated by Actos, all improving.
3. The patient could have renovascular disease. If he does, it needs to be fixed prior to his bypass surgery.
4. Anemia due to acute and chronic renal failure.

PLAN:

1. The patient did not have a ride today, so he will stay here tonight and will be discharged home tomorrow.
2. We will do an ultrasound before he is discharged.
3. Repeat labs in the morning, including basic panel, magnesium, and CBC.
4. We will schedule a renal MRA as an outpatient.
5. Continue with Bumex for the time being. He will be discharged home on po Bumex. His lisinopril has been on hold and will continue to be on hold until renal MRA is done.

I discussed the above with the patient. He seems to understand and agrees with the plan.

DISCHARGE SUMMARY

DIAGNOSES:

1. Congestive heart failure and generalized edema.
2. Acute renal failure.
3. Chronic renal failure.
4. Severe coronary artery disease.

The patient is a 66-year-old male who is known to have coronary artery disease and was admitted because of generalized edema. The patient's creatinine has gone up to 2.3. He was found to have significant edema in bilateral lower extremities, thighs, and sacral area, and a few basilar crackles.

His Actos and Crestor were both discontinued. He was given Bumex and then started on Bumex for a couple of days. The patient did well. He had no major problems during his hospitalization. He had no chest pain. His edema significantly improved. He had no proteinuria, so he does not seem to have diabetic nephropathy.

The patient was discharged in good general condition; code level I. The patient's creatinine improved, going down to 1.7 on date of discharge.

Copyright © 2005, Elsevier Inc. All rights reserved.
CPT only © 2004. *Current Procedural Terminology, 2005, Professional Edition*, American Medical Association. All rights reserved.

DISCHARGE PLAN:

1. Patient will follow up with Dr. Green. He will follow up with me as well when the basic panel and CBC results are known.
2. He will continue on Bumex 2 mg daily, fluid restriction, and salt restriction. He is off Actos and Crestor.

DISCHARGE MEDICATIONS:

1. Amitriptyline 50 mg daily.
2. Humalog 15 units t.i.d. with meals.
3. Lantus 56 units nightly.
4. Lisinopril has been discontinued for the time being.
5. Multivitamin 1 daily.
6. Neurontin 300 mg, 2 tablets b.i.d.
7. Prednisone eye drops.
8. Synthroid 0.075 mg daily.
9. Torsemide discontinued.
10. Crestor discontinued.
11. Isosorbide mononitrate 30 mg daily.
12. Bumex 2 mg daily.

The patient agrees with all of the above.

Correct Answer and Rationale:

428.0 reports the congestive heart failure. CHF is not stated as due to hypertension; per coding guidelines a cause and effect relationship between hypertension and heart disease cannot be assumed (see Coding Clinic 4989 2nd Quarter).
401.9 reports the hypertension
584.9 reports acute renal failure.
585 reports chronic renal failure.
414.00 reports severe coronary artery disease.
250.02 reports Type II diabetes.

Copyright © 2005, Elsevier Inc. All rights reserved.
CPT only © 2004. *Current Procedural Terminology, 2005, Professional Edition*, American Medical Association. All rights reserved.

Appendix A

ICD-9-CM Official Guidelines for Coding and Reporting

Effective October 1, 2003

The Centers for Medicare and Medicaid Services (CMS) formerly the Health Care Financing Administration (HCFA) and the National Center for Health Statistics (NCHS), two departments within the Department of Health and Human Services (DHHS) present the following guidelines for coding and reporting using the International Classification of Diseases, 9th Revision, Clinical Modification (ICD-9-CM). These guidelines should be used as a companion document to the official version of the ICD-9-CM as published on CD-ROM.

These guidelines for coding and reporting have been developed and approved by the Cooperating Parties for ICD-9-CM: the American Hospital Association, the American Health Information Management Association, CMS, and the NCHS. These guidelines, published by the Department of Health and Human Services have also appeared in the Coding Clinic for ICD-9-CM, published by the American Hospital Association.

These guidelines have been developed to assist the user in coding and reporting in situations where the ICD-9-CM does not provide direction. Coding and sequencing instructions in volumes I, II, and III of ICD-9-CM take precedence over any guidelines. The conventions, general guidelines and chapter-specific guidelines apply to the proper use of ICD-9-CM, regardless of the health care setting. A joint effort between the attending physician and coder is essential to achieve complete and accurate documentation, code assignment, and reporting of diagnoses and procedures. These guidelines have been developed and approved by the Cooperating Parties to assist both the physician and the coder in identifying those diagnoses that are to be reported. The importance of consistent, complete documentation in the medical record cannot be overemphasized. Without such documentation the application of all coding guidelines is a difficult, if not impossible, task.

These guidelines are not exhaustive. The cooperating parties are continuing to conduct reviews of these guidelines and develop new guidelines as needed. Users of the ICD-9-CM should be aware that only guidelines approved by the cooperating parties are official. Revision of these guidelines and new guidelines will be published by the U.S. Department of Health and Human Services when they are approved by the cooperating parties. The term "admitted" is used generally to mean a health care encounter in any setting.

The guidelines have been reorganized into several new sections including an enhanced introduction that provides more detail about the structure and conventions of the classification usually found in the classification itself. The other new section, General Guidelines, brings together overarching guidelines that were previously found throughout the various sections of the guidelines. The new format of the guidelines also includes a resequencing of the disease-specific guidelines. They are sequenced in the same order as they appear in the tabular list chapters (Infectious and Parasitic diseases, Neoplasms, etc.)

These changes will make it easier for coders, experienced and beginners, to more easily find the specific portion of the coding guideline information they seek.

Table of Contents

Copyright © 2005, Elsevier Inc. All rights reserved.
CPT only © 2004. *Current Procedural Terminology, 2005, Professional Edition*, American Medical Association. All rights reserved.

C. Chapter-specific Guidelines

- C1. Infectious and Parasitic diseases
  - A. Human Immunodeficiency Virus (HIV) Infections
    - Asymptomatic HIV Infection
    - Confirmed Cases of HIV Infection/Illness
    - HIV Infection in Pregnancy, Childbirth and the Puerperium
    - Inconclusive Lab Test for HIV
    - Previously Diagnosed HIV-related Illness
    - Selection and Sequencing of HIV Code
    - Testing for HIV
  - B. Septicemia, Systemic Inflammatory Response Syndrome (SIRS), Sepsis, Severe Sepsis, and Septic Shock
- C2. Neoplasms
- C3. Endocrine, Nutritional, and Metabolic Diseases and Immunity Disorders
  - Reserved for future guidelines expansion
- C4. Diseases of Blood and Blood Forming Organs
  - Reserved for future guideline expansion
- C5. Mental Disorders
  - Reserved for future guideline expansion
- C6. Diseases of Nervous System and Sense Organs
  - Reserved for future guideline expansion
- C7. Diseases of Circulatory System
  - A. Hypertension
    - Controlled Hypertension
    - Elevated Blood Pressure
    - Essential Hypertension
    - Hypertension with Heart Disease
    - Hypertensive Cerebrovascular Disease
    - Hypertensive Heart and Renal Disease
    - Hypertensive Renal Disease with Chronic Renal Failure
    - Hypertensive Retinopathy
    - Secondary Hypertension
    - Transient Hypertension
    - Uncontrolled Hypertension
  - B. Late Effect of Cerebrovascular Accident
- C8. Diseases of Respiratory System
  - Reserved for future guideline expansion

Copyright © 2005, Elsevier Inc. All rights reserved.
CPT only © 2004. *Current Procedural Terminology, 2005, Professional Edition*, American Medical Association. All rights reserved.

Copyright © 2005, Elsevier Inc. All rights reserved.
CPT only © 2004. *Current Procedural Terminology, 2005, Professional Edition*, American Medical Association. All rights reserved.

Coding of Injuries

Coding of Burns

Coding of Debridement of Wound, Infection or Burn

Coding of Adverse Effects, Poisoning and Toxic Effects

C18. Supplemental Classification of Factors Influencing Health Status and Contact with Health Service (V-Codes)

1. Contact/Exposure
2. Inoculations and vaccinations
3. Status
4. History (of)
5. Screening
6. Observation
7. Aftercare
8. Follow-up
9. Donor
10. Counseling
11. Obstetrics
12. Newborn, infant and child
13. Routine and administrative examinations
14. Miscellaneous V codes
15. Nonspecific V codes

C19. Supplemental Classification of External Causes of Injury and Poisoning

Child and Adult Abuse

General Coding guidelines

Late effects

Misadventures and complications of care

Multiple external causes

Place of occurrence

Poisonings and adverse effects of drugs

Terrorism

Undetermined cause

Unknown intent

Section II Selection of Principal Diagnosis(es) for Inpatient, Short-term, Acute Care, and Long Term Care Hospital Records

Complications of Surgery and Other Medical Care

Original Treatment Plan Not Carried Out

Symptoms, Signs, and Ill-defined Conditions

Copyright © 2005, Elsevier Inc. All rights reserved.
CPT only © 2004. *Current Procedural Terminology, 2005, Professional Edition*, American Medical Association. All rights reserved.

Symptom Followed by Contrasting/Comparative Diagnoses

Two or More Comparative or Contrasting Conditions

Two or More Equally Meet Definition

Two or More Interrelated Conditions

Uncertain Diagnosis

Section III Reporting Additional Diagnoses for Inpatient, Short-term, Acute Care, and Long Term Care Hospital Records

Abnormal Findings

General Rules

Previous Conditions

Uncertain Diagnosis

Section IV Diagnostic Coding and Reporting Guidelines for Outpatient Services

SECTION I CONVENTIONS, GENERAL CODING GUIDELINES AND CHAPTER-SPECIFIC GUIDELINES

The conventions, general guidelines and chapter-specific guidelines are applicable to all health care settings unless otherwise indicated.

A. Conventions for the ICD-9-CM

The conventions for the ICD-9-CM are the general rules for use of the classification independent of the guidelines. These conventions are incorporated within the index and tabular of the ICD-9-CM as instructional notes. The conventions are as follows:

1. Format: The ICD-9-CM uses an indented format for ease in reference
2. Abbreviations

a. Index Abbreviations

NEC "Not elsewhere classifiable"

This abbreviation in the index represents "other specified" When a specific code is not available for a condition the index directs the coder to the "other specified" code in the tabular.

b. Tabular Abbreviations

NEC "Not elsewhere classifiable"

This abbreviation in the tabular represents "other specified" When a specific code is not available for a condition the tabular includes an NEC entry under a code to identify the code as the "other specified" code. (see "Other" codes)

NOS "Not otherwise specified" This abbreviation is the equivalent of unspecified. (see "Unspecified" codes)

3. Punctuation

[ ] Brackets are used in the tabular list to enclose synonyms, alternative wording or explanatory phrases. Brackets are used in the index to identify manifestation codes. (see etiology/manifestations)

( ) Parentheses are used in both the index and tabular to enclose supplementary words which may be present or absent in the statement of a

Copyright © 2005, Elsevier Inc. All rights reserved.
CPT only © 2004. *Current Procedural Terminology, 2005, Professional Edition*, American Medical Association. All rights reserved.

disease or procedure without affecting the code number to which it is assigned. The terms within the parentheses are referred to as nonessential modifiers.

: Colons are used in the Tabular list after an incomplete term which needs one or more of the modifiers following the colon to make it assignable to a given category.

4. Includes and Excludes Notes and Inclusion terms

Includes: This note appears immediately under a three-digit code title to further define, or give examples of, the content of the category.

Excludes: An excludes note under a code indicate that the terms excluded from the code are to be coded elsewhere. In some cases the codes for the excluded terms should not be used in conjunction with the code from which it is excluded. An example of this is a congenital condition excluded from an acquired form of the same condition. The congenital and acquired codes should not be used together. In other cases, the excluded terms may be used together with an excluded code. An example of this is when fractures of different bones are coded to different codes. Both codes may be used together if both types of fractures are present.

Inclusion terms: List of terms are included under certain four and five digit codes. These terms are the conditions for which that code number is to be used. The terms may be synonyms of the code title, or, in the case of "other specified" codes, the terms are a list of the various conditions assigned to that code. The inclusion terms are not necessarily exhaustive. Additional terms found only in the index may also be assigned to a code.

5. Other and Unspecified codes

a. "Other" codes

Codes titled "other" or "other specified" (usually a code with a 4th digit 8 or fifth-digit 9 for diagnosis codes) are for use when the information in the medical record provides detail for which a specific code does not exist. Index entries with NEC in the line designate "other" codes in the tabular. These index entries represent specific disease entities for which no specific code exists so the term is included within an "other" code.

b. "Unspecified" codes

Codes (usually a code with a 4th digit 9 or 5th digit 0 for diagnosis codes) titled "unspecified" are for use when the information in the medical record is insufficient to assign a more specific code.

6. Etiology/manifestation convention ("code first", "use additional code" and "in diseases classified elsewhere" notes)

Certain conditions have both an underlying etiology and multiple body system manifestations due to the underlying etiology. For such conditions the ICD-9-CM has a coding convention that requires the underlying condition be sequenced first followed by the manifestation. Wherever such a combination exists there is a "use additional code" note at the etiology code, and a "code first" note at the manifestation code. These instructional notes indicate the proper sequencing order of the codes, etiology followed by manifestation.

Copyright © 2005, Elsevier Inc. All rights reserved.
CPT only © 2004. *Current Procedural Terminology, 2005, Professional Edition*, American Medical Association. All rights reserved.

In most cases the manifestation codes will have in the code title, "in diseases classified elsewhere." Codes with this title are a component of the etiology/manifestation convention. The code title indicates that it is a manifestation code. "In diseases classified elsewhere" codes are never permitted to be used as first listed or principal diagnosis codes. They must be used in conjunction with an underlying condition code and they must be listed following the underlying condition.

There are manifestation codes that do not have "in diseases classified elsewhere" in the title. For such codes a "use additional code" note will still be present and the rules for sequencing apply.

In addition to the notes in the tabular, these conditions also have a specific index entry structure. In the index both conditions are listed together with the etiology code first followed by the manifestation codes in brackets. The code in brackets is always to be sequenced second.

The most commonly used etiology/manifestation combinations are the codes for Diabetes mellitus, category 250. For each code under category 250 there is a use additional code note for the manifestation that is specific for that particular diabetic manifestation. Should a patient have more than one manifestation of diabetes more than one code from category 250 may be used with as many manifestation codes as are needed to fully describe the patient's complete diabetic condition. The 250 diabetes codes should be sequenced first, followed by the manifestation codes.

"Code first" and "Use additional code" notes are also used as sequencing rules in the classification for certain codes that are not part of an etiology/manifestation combination. See-Other multiple coding for a single condition in the General Guidelines section.

B. General Coding Guidelines

1. Use of Both Alphabetic Index and Tabular List

   Use both the Alphabetic Index and the Tabular List when locating and assigning a code. Reliance on only the Alphabetic Index or the Tabular List leads to errors in code assignments and less specificity in code selection.

2. Locate each term in the Alphabetic Index and verify the code selected in the Tabular List. Read and be guided by instructional notations that appear in both the Alphabetic Index and the Tabular List.

3. Level of Detail in Coding

   Diagnosis and procedure codes are to be used at their highest number of digits available.

   ICD-9-CM diagnosis codes are composed of codes with 3, 4, or 5 digits. Codes with three digits are included in ICD-9-CM as the heading of a category of codes that may be further subdivided by the use of fourth and/or fifth digits, which provide greater detail.

   A three-digit code is to be used only if it is not further subdivided. Where fourth-digit subcategories and/or fifth-digit subclassifications are provided, they must be assigned. A code is invalid if it has not been coded to the full number of digits required for that code. For example, Acute myocardial infarction, code 410, has fourth digits that describe the location of the infarction (e.g., 410.2, Of inferolateral wall), and fifth digits that identify the episode of care. It would be incorrect to report a code in category 410 without a fourth and fifth digit.

   ICD-9-CM Volume 3 procedure codes are composed of codes with either 3 or 4 digits. Codes with two digits are included in ICD-9-CM as the heading of a category of codes that may be further subdivided by the use of third and/or fourth digits, which provide greater detail.

Copyright © 2005, Elsevier Inc. All rights reserved.
CPT only © 2004. *Current Procedural Terminology, 2005, Professional Edition,* American Medical Association. All rights reserved.

4. The appropriate code or codes from 001.0 through V83.89 must be used to identify diagnoses, symptoms, conditions, problems, complaints or other reason(s) for the encounter/visit.

5. The selection of codes 001.0 through 999.9 will frequently be used to describe the reason for the admission/encounter. These codes are from the section of ICD-9-CM for the classification of diseases and injuries (e.g., infectious and parasitic diseases; neoplasms; symptoms, signs, and ill-defined conditions, etc.).

6. Codes that describe symptoms and signs, as opposed to diagnoses, are acceptable for reporting purposes when a related definitive diagnosis has not been established (confirmed) by the physician. Chapter 16 of ICD-9-CM, Symptoms, Signs, and Ill-defined conditions (codes 780.0–799.9) contain many, but not all codes for symptoms.

7. Conditions that are an integral part of a disease process

   Signs and symptoms that are integral to the disease process should not be assigned as additional codes.

8. Conditions that are not an integral part of a disease process

   Additional signs and symptoms that may not be associated routinely with a disease process should be coded when present.

9. Multiple coding for a single condition

   In addition to the etiology/manifestation convention that requires two codes to fully describe a single condition that affects multiple body systems, there are other single conditions that also require more than one code. "Use additional code" notes are found in the tabular at codes that are not part of an etiology/manifestation pair where a secondary code is useful to fully describe a condition. The sequencing rule is the same, "use additional code" indicates that a secondary code should be added.

   For example, for infections that are not included in chapter 1, a secondary code from category 041, Bacterial infection in conditions classified elsewhere and of unspecified site, may be required to identify the bacterial organism causing the infection. A "use additional code" note will normally be found at the infection code indicates a need for the organism code to be added as a secondary code.

   "Code first" notes are also under certain codes that are not specifically manifestation codes but may be due to an underlying cause. When a "code first" note is present and an underlying condition is present the underlying condition should be sequenced first.

   "Code, if applicable, any causal condition first", notes indicate that this code may be assigned as a principal diagnosis when the causal condition is unknown or not applicable. If a causal condition is known, then the code for that condition should be sequenced as the principal or first-listed diagnosis.

   Multiple codes may be needed for late effects, complication codes and obstetric codes to more fully describe a condition. See the specific guidelines for these conditions for further instruction.

10. Acute and Chronic Conditions

    If the same condition is described as both acute (subacute) and chronic, and separate subentries exist in the Alphabetic Index at the same indentation level, code both and sequence the acute (subacute) code first.

Copyright © 2005, Elsevier Inc. All rights reserved.
CPT only © 2004. *Current Procedural Terminology, 2005, Professional Edition*, American Medical Association. All rights reserved.

11. Combination Code

A combination code is a single code used to classify:
two diagnoses, or
A diagnosis with an associated secondary process (manifestation)
A diagnosis with an associated complication

Combination codes are identified by referring to subterm entries in the Alphabetic Index and by reading the inclusion and exclusion notes in the Tabular List.

Assign only the combination code when that code fully identifies the diagnostic conditions involved or when the Alphabetic Index so directs. Multiple coding should not be used when the classification provides a combination code that clearly identifies all of the elements documented in the diagnosis. When the combination code lacks necessary specificity in describing the manifestation or complication, an additional code may be used as a secondary code.

12. Late Effects

A late effect is the residual effect (condition produced) after the acute phase of an illness or injury has terminated. There is no time limit on when a late effect code can be used. The residual may be apparent early, such as in cerebrovascular accident cases, or it may occur months or years later, such as that due to a previous injury. Coding of late effects generally requires two codes sequenced in the following order: The condition or nature of the late effect is sequenced first. The late effect code is sequenced second.

An exception to the above guidelines are those instances where the code for late effect is followed by a manifestation code identified in the Tabular List and title, or the late effect code has been expanded (at the fourth and fifth-digit levels) to include the manifestation(s). The code for the acute phase of an illness or injury that led to the late effect is never used with a code for the late effect.

13. Impending or Threatened Condition

Code any condition described at the time of discharge as "impending" or "threatened" as follows:

If it did occur, code as confirmed diagnosis.

If it did not occur, reference the Alphabetic Index to determine if the condition has a subentry term for "impending" or "threatened" and also reference main term entries for "Impending" and for "Threatened."

If the subterms are listed, assign the given code.

If the subterms are not listed, code the existing underlying condition(s) and not the condition described as impending or threatened.

C. Chapter-Specific Coding Guidelines

In addition to general coding guidelines, there are guidelines for specific diagnoses and/or conditions in the classification. Unless otherwise indicated, these guidelines apply to all health care settings.

C1. Infectious and Parasitic Diseases

A. Human Immunodeficiency Virus (HIV) Infections

1. Code only confirmed cases of HIV infection/illness. This is an exception to the hospital inpatient guideline Section II, H.

   In this context, "confirmation" does not require documentation of positive serology or culture for HIV; the physician's diagnostic

Copyright © 2005, Elsevier Inc. All rights reserved.
CPT only © 2004. *Current Procedural Terminology, 2005, Professional Edition*, American Medical Association. All rights reserved.

statement that the patient is HIV positive, or has an HIV-related illness is sufficient.

2. Selection and sequencing

    a. If a patient is admitted for an HIV-related condition, the principal diagnosis should be 042, followed by additional diagnosis codes for all reported HIV-related conditions.

    b. If a patient with HIV disease is admitted for an unrelated condition (such as a traumatic injury), the code for the unrelated condition (e.g., the nature of injury code) should be the principal diagnosis. Other diagnoses would be 042 followed by additional diagnosis codes for all reported HIV-related conditions.

    c. Whether the patient is newly diagnosed or has had previous admissions/encounters for HIV conditions is irrelevant to the sequencing decision.

    d. V08 Asymptomatic human immunodeficiency virus [HIV] infection, is to be applied when the patient without any documentation of symptoms is listed as being "HIV positive," "known HIV," "HIV test positive," or similar terminology. Do not use this code if the term "AIDS" is used or if the patient is treated for any HIV-related illness or is described as having any condition(s) resulting from his/her HIV positive status; use 042 in these cases.

    e. Patients with inconclusive HIV serology, but no definitive diagnosis or manifestations of the illness, may be assigned code 795.71, Inconclusive serologic test for Human Immunodeficiency Virus [HIV]

    f. Previously diagnosed HIV-related illness

       Patients with any known prior diagnosis of an HIV-related illness should be coded to 042. Once a patient had developed an HIV-related illness, the patient should always be assigned code 042 on every subsequent admission/encounter. Patients previously diagnosed with any HIV illness (042) should never be assigned to 795.71 or V08.

    g. HIV Infection in Pregnancy, Childbirth and the Puerperium

       During pregnancy, childbirth or the puerperium, a patient admitted (or presenting for a health care encounter) because of an HIV-related illness should receive a principal diagnosis of 647.6X, Other specified infectious and parasitic diseases in the mother classifiable elsewhere, but complicating the pregnancy, childbirth or the puerperium, followed by 042 and the code(s) for the HIV-related illness(es). Codes from Chapter 15 always take sequencing priority.

       Patients with asymptomatic HIV infection status admitted (or presenting for a health care encounter) during pregnancy, childbirth, or the puerperium should receive codes of 647.6X and V08.

    h. Encounters for Testing for HIV

       If a patient is being seen to determine his/her HIV status, use code V73.89, Screening for other specified viral disease. Use code V69.8,

Copyright © 2005, Elsevier Inc. All rights reserved.
CPT only © 2004. *Current Procedural Terminology, 2005, Professional Edition*, American Medical Association. All rights reserved.

Other problems related to lifestyle, as a secondary code if an asymptomatic patient is in a known high risk group for HIV. Should a patient with signs or symptoms of illness, or a confirmed HIV related diagnosis be tested for HIV, code the signs and symptoms or the diagnosis. An additional counseling code V65.44 may be used if counseling is provided during the encounter for the test.

When a patient returns to be informed of his/her HIV test results use code V65.44, HIV counseling, if the results of the test are negative.

If the results are positive but the patient is asymptomatic use code V08, Asymptomatic HIV infection. If the results are positive and the patient is symptomatic use code 042, HIV infection, with codes for the HIV related symptoms or diagnosis. The HIV counseling code may also be used if counseling is provided for patients with positive test results.

B. Septicemia, Systemic Inflammatory Response Syndrome (SIRS), Sepsis, Severe Sepsis, and Septic Shock

1. In most cases, it will be a code from category 038, Septicemia, that will be used in conjunction with a code from subcategory 995.9.
   a. If the documentation in the record states streptococcal sepsis, codes 038.0 and code 995.91 should be used, in that sequence.
   b. If the documentation states streptococcal septicemia, only code 038.0 should be assigned, however, the physician should be queried whether the patient has sepsis, an infection with SIRS.
   c. Either the term sepsis or SIRS must be documented, to assign a code from subcategory 995.9.

2. If the terms sepsis, severe sepsis, or SIRS are used with an underlying infection other than septicemia, such as pneumonia, cellulitis or a nonspecified urinary tract infection, code 038.9 should be assigned first, then code 995.91, followed by the code for the initial infection. The use of the terms sepsis or SIRS indicates that the patient's infection has advanced to the point of a systemic infection so the systemic infection should be sequenced before the localized infection. The instructional note under subcategory 995.9 instructs to assign the underlying condition first.

   Note: The term urosepsis is a nonspecific term. If that is the only term documented then only code 599.0 should be assigned based on the default for the term in the ICD-9-CM index, in addition to the code for the causal organism if known.

3. For patients with severe sepsis, the code for the systemic infection (038.x) or trauma should be sequenced first, followed by either code 995.92, Systemic inflammatory response syndrome due to infectious process with organ dysfunction, or code 995.94, Systemic inflammatory response syndrome due to noninfectious process with organ dysfunction. Codes for the specific organ dysfunctions should also be assigned.

4. If septic shock is documented, it is necessary to code first the initiating systemic infection or trauma, then either code 995.92 or 995.94, followed by code 785.52, Septic shock.

Copyright © 2005, Elsevier Inc. All rights reserved.
CPT only © 2004. *Current Procedural Terminology, 2005, Professional Edition*, American Medical Association. All rights reserved.

5. Sepsis and septic shock associated with abortion, ectopic pregnancy, and molar pregnancy are classified to category codes in Chapter 11 (630–639).
6. Negative or inconclusive blood cultures do not preclude a diagnosis of septicemia or sepsis in patients with clinical evidence of the condition, however, the physician should be queried.

C2. Neoplasms

Chapter 2 of the ICD-9-CM contains the code for most benign and all malignant neoplasms. Certain benign neoplasms, such as prostatic adenomas, may be found in the specific body system chapters. To properly code a neoplasm it is necessary to determine from the record if the neoplasm is benign, in-situ, malignant, or of uncertain histologic behavior. If malignant, any secondary (metastatic) sites should also be determined.

The neoplasm table in the Alphabetic Index should be referenced first. If the histological term is documented, that term should be referenced first, rather than going immediately to the Neoplasm Table, in order to determine which column in the Neoplasm Table is appropriate. For example, if the documentation indicates "adenoma," refer to the term in the Alphabetic Index to review the entries under this term and the instructional note to "see also neoplasm, by site, benign." The table provides the proper code based on the type of neoplasm and the site. It is important to select the proper column in the table that corresponds to the type of neoplasm. The tabular should then be referenced to verify that the correct code has been selected from the table and that a more specific site code does not exist.

A. If the treatment is directed at the malignancy, designate the malignancy as the principal diagnosis.

B. When a patient is admitted because of a primary neoplasm with metastasis and treatment is directed toward the secondary site only, the secondary neoplasm is designated as the principal diagnosis even though the primary malignancy is still present.

C. Coding and sequencing of complications associated with the malignant neoplasm or with the therapy thereof are subject to the following guidelines:

1. When admission/encounter is for management of an anemia associated with the malignancy, and the treatment is only for anemia, the anemia is designated as the principal diagnosis and is followed by the appropriate code(s) for the malignancy.

2. When the admission/encounter is for management of an anemia associated with chemotherapy or radiotherapy and the only treatment is for the anemia, the anemia is sequenced first followed by the appropriate code(s) for the malignancy.

3. When the admission/encounter is for management of dehydration due to the malignancy or the therapy, or a combination of both, and only the dehydration is being treated (intravenous rehydration), the dehydration is sequenced first, followed by the code(s) for the malignancy.

Copyright © 2005, Elsevier Inc. All rights reserved.
CPT only © 2004. *Current Procedural Terminology, 2005, Professional Edition,* American Medical Association. All rights reserved.

4. When the admission/encounter is for treatment of a complication resulting from a surgical procedure performed for the treatment of an intestinal malignancy, designate the complication as the principal or first-listed diagnosis if treatment is directed at resolving the complication.

D. When a primary malignancy has been previously excised or eradicated from its site and there is no further treatment directed to that site and there is no evidence of any existing primary malignancy, a code from category V10, Personal history of malignant neoplasm, should be used to indicate the former site of the malignancy. Any mention of extension, invasion, or metastasis to another site is coded as a secondary malignant neoplasm to that site. The secondary site may be the principal or first-listed with the V10 code used as a secondary code.

E. Admissions/Encounters involving chemotherapy and radiation therapy

1. When an episode of care involves the surgical removal of a neoplasm, primary or secondary site, followed by chemotherapy or radiation treatment, the neoplasm code should be assigned as principal or first-listed diagnosis. When an episode of inpatient care involves surgical removal of a primary site or secondary site malignancy followed by adjunct chemotherapy or radiotherapy, code the malignancy as the principal or first-listed diagnosis, using codes in the 140-198 series or where appropriate in the 200-203 series.

2. If a patient admission/encounter is solely for the administration of chemotherapy or radiation therapy code V58.0, Encounter for radiation therapy, or V58.1, Encounter for chemotherapy, should be the first-listed or principal diagnosis. If a patient receives both chemotherapy and radiation therapy both codes should be listed, in either order of sequence.

3. When a patient is admitted for the purpose of radiotherapy or chemotherapy and develops complications such as uncontrolled nausea and vomiting or dehydration, the principal or first-listed diagnosis is V58.0, Encounter for radiotherapy, or V58.1, Encounter for chemotherapy.

F. When the reason for admission/encounter is to determine the extent of the malignancy, or for a procedure such as paracentesis or thoracentesis, the primary malignancy or appropriate metastatic site is designated as the principal or first-listed diagnosis, even though chemotherapy or radiotherapy is administered.

G. Symptoms, signs, and ill-defined conditions listed in Chapter 16 characteristic of, or associated with, an existing primary or secondary site malignancy cannot be used to replace the malignancy as principal or

Copyright © 2005, Elsevier Inc. All rights reserved.
CPT only © 2004. *Current Procedural Terminology, 2005, Professional Edition,* American Medical Association. All rights reserved.

first-listed diagnosis, regardless of the number of admissions or encounters for treatment and care of the neoplasm.

C3. Endocrine, Nutritional, and Metabolic Diseases and Immunity Disorders

Reserved for future guideline expansion

C4. Diseases of Blood and Blood Forming Organs

Reserved for future guideline expansion

C5. Mental Disorders

Reserved for future guideline expansion

C6. Diseases of Nervous System and Sense Organs

Reserved for future guideline expansion

C7. Diseases of Circulatory System

A. Hypertension

The Hypertension Table, found under the main term, "Hypertension", in the Alphabetic Index, contains a complete listing of all conditions due to or associated with hypertension and classifies them according to malignant, benign, and unspecified.

1. Hypertension, Essential, or NOS Assign hypertension (arterial) (essential) (primary) (systemic) (NOS) to category code 401 with the appropriate fourth digit to indicate malignant (.0), benign (.1), or unspecified (.9). Do not use either .0 malignant or .1 benign unless medical record documentation supports such a designation.

2. Hypertension with Heart Disease

Heart conditions (425.8, 429.0-429.3, 429.8, 429.9) are assigned to a code from category 402 when a causal relationship is stated (due to hypertension) or implied (hypertensive). Use an additional code from category 428 to identify the type of heart failure in those patients with heart failure. More than one code from category 428 may be assigned if the patient has systolic or diastolic failure and congestive heart failure.

The same heart conditions (425.8, 428, 429.0-429.3, 429.8, 429.9) with hypertension, but without a stated causal relationship, are coded separately. Sequence according to the circumstances of the admission/encounter.

3. Hypertensive Renal Disease with Chronic Renal Failure

Assign codes from category 403, Hypertensive renal disease, when conditions classified to categories 585-587 are present. Unlike hypertension with heart disease, ICD-9-CM presumes a cause-and-effect relationship and classifies renal failure with hypertension as hypertensive renal disease.

Copyright © 2005, Elsevier Inc. All rights reserved.
CPT only © 2004. *Current Procedural Terminology, 2005, Professional Edition,* American Medical Association. All rights reserved.

4. Hypertensive Heart and Renal Disease

   Assign codes from combination category 404, Hypertensive heart and renal disease, when both hypertensive renal disease and hypertensive heart disease are stated in the diagnosis. Assume a relationship between the hypertension and the renal disease, whether or not the condition is so designated. Assign an additional code from category 428, to identify the type of heart failure. More than one code from category 428 may be assigned if the patient has systolic or diastolic failure and congestive heart failure.

5. Hypertensive Cerebrovascular Disease

   First assign codes from 430-438, Cerebrovascular disease, then the appropriate hypertension code from categories 401-405.

6. Hypertensive Retinopathy

   Two codes are necessary to identify the condition. First assign the code from subcategory 362.11, Hypertensive retinopathy, then the appropriate code from categories 401-405 to indicate the type of hypertension.

7. Hypertension, Secondary

   Two codes are required: one to identify the underlying etiology and one from category 405 to identify the hypertension. Sequencing of codes is determined by the reason for admission/encounter.

8. Hypertension, Transient

   Assign code 796.2, Elevated blood pressure reading without diagnosis of hypertension, unless patient has an established diagnosis of hypertension. Assign code 642.3x for transient hypertension of pregnancy.

9. Hypertension, Controlled

   Assign appropriate code from categories 401-405. This diagnostic statement usually refers to an existing state of hypertension under control by therapy.

10. Hypertension, Uncontrolled

    Uncontrolled hypertension may refer to untreated hypertension or hypertension not responding to current therapeutic regimen. In either case, assign the appropriate code from categories 401-405 to designate the stage and type of hypertension. Code to the type of hypertension.

11. Elevated Blood Pressure

    For a statement of elevated blood pressure without further specificity, assign code 796.2, Elevated blood pressure reading without diagnosis of hypertension, rather than a code from category 401.

B. Late Effects of Cerebrovascular Disease

Category 438 is used to indicate conditions classifiable to categories 430-437 as the causes of late effects (neurologic deficits), themselves classified elsewhere. These "late effects" include neurologic deficits that persist after initial onset of conditions classifiable to 430-437. The neurologic deficits caused by cerebrovascular disease may be present from

Copyright © 2005, Elsevier Inc. All rights reserved.
CPT only © 2004. *Current Procedural Terminology, 2005, Professional Edition*, American Medical Association. All rights reserved.

the onset or may arise at any time after the onset of the condition classifiable to 430-437.

Codes from category 438 may be assigned on a health care record with codes from 430-437, if the patient has a current cerebrovascular accident (CVA) and deficits from an old CVA. Assign code V12.59 (and not a code from category 438) as an additional code for history of cerebrovascular disease when no neurologic deficits are present.

C8. Diseases of Respiratory System

Reserved for future guideline expansion

C9. Diseases of Digestive System

Reserved for future guideline expansion

C10. Diseases of Genitourinary System

Reserved for future guideline expansion

C11. Complications of Pregnancy, Childbirth, and the Puerperium

A. General Rules for Obstetric Cases

1. Obstetric cases require codes from chapter 11, codes in the range 630-677, Complications of Pregnancy, Childbirth, and the Puerperium. Should the physician document that the pregnancy is incidental to the encounter, then code V22.2 should be used in place of any chapter 11 codes. It is the physician's responsibility to state that the condition being treated is not affecting the pregnancy.
2. Chapter 11 codes have sequencing priority over codes from other chapters. Additional codes from other chapters may be used in conjunction with chapter 11 codes to further specify conditions. For example, sepsis and septic shock associated with abortion, ectopic pregnancy, and molar pregnancy are classified to category codes in Chapter 11 (630-639).
3. Chapter 11 codes are to be used only on the maternal record, never on the record of the newborn.
4. Categories 640-648, 651-676 have required fifth-digits, which indicate whether the encounter is antepartum, postpartum and whether a delivery has also occurred.
5. The fifth-digits, which are appropriate for each code number, are listed in brackets under each code. The fifth-digits on each code should all be consistent with each other. That is, should a delivery occur all of the fifth-digits should indicate the delivery.
6. For prenatal outpatient visits for patients with high-risk pregnancies, a code from category V23, Supervision of high-risk pregnancy, should be used as the principal or first-listed diagnosis. Secondary chapter 11 codes may be used in conjunction with these codes if appropriate. A thorough review of any pertinent excludes note is necessary to be certain that these V codes are being used properly.
7. An outcome of delivery code, V27.0-V27.9, should be included on every maternal record when a delivery has occurred. These codes are not to be used on subsequent records or on the newborn record.
8. For routine outpatient prenatal visits when no complications are present codes V22.0, Supervision of normal first pregnancy, and V22.1,

Copyright © 2005, Elsevier Inc. All rights reserved.
CPT only © 2004. *Current Procedural Terminology, 2005, Professional Edition,* American Medical Association. All rights reserved.

Supervision of other normal pregnancy, should be used as the first-listed diagnoses. These codes should not be used in conjunction with chapter 11 codes.

B. Selection of OB Principal or First-listed Diagnosis

1. In episodes when no delivery occurs, the principal diagnosis should correspond to the principal complication of the pregnancy, which necessitated the encounter. Should more than one complication exist, all of which are treated or monitored, any of the complications codes may be sequenced first.

2. When a delivery occurs, the principal diagnosis should correspond to the main circumstances or complication of the delivery.

   In cases of cesarean delivery, the selection of the principal diagnosis should correspond to the reason the cesarean delivery was performed unless the reason for admission/encounter was unrelated to the condition resulting in the cesarean delivery.

C. Fetal Conditions Affecting the Management of the Mother

Codes from category 655, Known or suspected fetal abnormality affecting management of the mother, and category 656, Other fetal and placental problems affecting the management of the mother, are assigned only when the fetal condition is actually responsible for modifying the management of the mother, i.e., by requiring diagnostic studies, additional observation, special care, or termination of pregnancy. The fact that the fetal condition exists does not justify assigning a code from this series to the mother's record.

D. HIV Infection in Pregnancy, Childbirth and the Puerperium

During pregnancy, childbirth or the puerperium, a patient admitted because of an HIV-related illness should receive a principal diagnosis of 647.6X, Other specified infectious and parasitic diseases in the mother classifiable elsewhere, but complicating the pregnancy, childbirth or the puerperium, followed by 042 and the code(s) for the HIV-related illness(es). This is an exception to the sequencing rule found in above.

Patients with asymptomatic HIV infection status admitted during pregnancy, childbirth, or the puerperium should receive codes of 647.6X and V08.

E. Normal Delivery, 650

1. Code 650 is for use in cases when a woman is admitted for a full-term normal delivery and delivers a single, healthy infant without any complications antepartum, during the delivery, or postpartum during the delivery episode.

2. Code 650 may be used if the patient had a complication at some point during her pregnancy but the complication is not present at the time of the admission for delivery.

3. Code 650 is always a principal diagnosis. It is not to be used if any other code from chapter 11 is needed to describe a current complication of the antenatal, delivery, or perinatal period. Additional codes from other chapters may be used with code 650 if they are not related to or are in any way complicating the pregnancy.

4. V27.0, Single liveborn, is the only outcome of delivery code appropriate for use with 650.

Copyright © 2005, Elsevier Inc. All rights reserved.
CPT only © 2004. *Current Procedural Terminology, 2005, Professional Edition*, American Medical Association. All rights reserved.

F. The Postpartum Period

1. The postpartum period begins immediately after delivery and continues for six weeks following delivery.
2. A postpartum complication is any complication occurring within the six-week period.
3. Chapter 11 codes may also be used to describe pregnancy-related complications after the six-week period should the physician document that a condition is pregnancy related.
4. Postpartum complications that occur during the same admission as the delivery are identified with a fifth digit of "2." Subsequent admissions/encounters for postpartum complications should be identified with a fifth digit of "4."
5. When the mother delivers outside the hospital prior to admission and is admitted for routine postpartum care and no complications are noted, code V24.0, Postpartum care and examination immediately after delivery, should be assigned as the principal diagnosis.
6. A delivery diagnosis code should not be used for a woman who has delivered prior to admission to the hospital. Any postpartum procedures should be coded.

G. Code 677, Late effect of complication of pregnancy, childbirth, and the puerperium

1. Code 677, Late effect of complication of pregnancy, childbirth, and the puerperium is for use in those cases when an initial complication of a pregnancy develops sequelae requiring care or treatment at a future date.
2. This code may be used at any time after the initial postpartum period.
3. This code, like all late effect codes, is to be sequenced following the code describing the sequelae of the complication.

H. Abortions

1. Fifth-digits are required for abortion categories 634-637. Fifth-digit 1, incomplete, indicates that all of the products of conception have not been expelled from the uterus. Fifth-digit 2, complete, indicates that all products of conception have been expelled from the uterus prior to the episode of care.
2. A code from categories 640-648 and 651-657 may be used as additional codes with an abortion code to indicate the complication leading to the abortion.

   Fifth digit 3 is assigned with codes from these categories when used with an abortion code because the other fifth digits will not apply. Codes from the 660-669 series are not to be used for complications of abortion.
3. Code 639 is to be used for all complications following abortion. Code 639 cannot be assigned with codes from categories 634-638.
4. Abortion with Liveborn Fetus.

   When an attempted termination of pregnancy results in a liveborn fetus assign code 644.21, Early onset of delivery, with an appropriate

Copyright © 2005, Elsevier Inc. All rights reserved.
CPT only © 2004. *Current Procedural Terminology, 2005, Professional Edition,* American Medical Association. All rights reserved.

code from category V27, Outcome of Delivery. The procedure code for the attempted termination of pregnancy should also be assigned.

5. Retained Products of Conception following an abortion.

Subsequent admissions for retained products of conception following a spontaneous or legally induced abortion are assigned the appropriate code from category 634, Spontaneous abortion, or legally induced abortion, with a fifth digit of "1" (incomplete). This advice is appropriate even when the patient was discharged previously with a discharge diagnosis of complete abortion.

C12. Diseases of Skin and Subcutaneous Tissue

Reserved for future guideline expansion

C13. Diseases of Musculoskeletal and Connective Tissue

Reserved for future guideline expansion

C14. Congenital Anomalies

Reserved for future guideline expansion

C15. Newborn (Perinatal) Guidelines

For coding and reporting purposes the perinatal period is defined as birth through the 28th day following birth. The following guidelines are provided for reporting purposes. Hospitals may record other diagnoses as needed for internal data use.

A. General Perinatal Rule

All clinically significant conditions noted on routine newborn examination should be coded. A condition is clinically significant if it requires:

clinical evaluation; or

therapeutic treatment; or

diagnostic procedures; or

extended length of hospital stay; or

increased nursing care and/or monitoring; or

has implications for future health care needs.

Note: The perinatal guidelines listed above are the same as the general coding guidelines for "additional diagnoses," except for the final point regarding implications for future health care needs. Whether or not a condition is clinically significant can only be determined by the physician.

B. Use of Codes V30-V39

When coding the birth of an infant, assign a code from categories V30-V39, according to the type of birth. A code from this series is assigned as a principal diagnosis, and assigned only once to a newborn at the time of birth.

C. Newborn Transfers

If the newborn is transferred to another institution, the V30 series is not used at the receiving hospital.

Copyright © 2005, Elsevier Inc. All rights reserved.
CPT only © 2004. *Current Procedural Terminology, 2005, Professional Edition,* American Medical Association. All rights reserved.

D. Use of Category V29

1. Assign a code from category V29, Observation and evaluation of newborns and infants for suspected conditions not found, to identify those instances when a healthy newborn is evaluated for a suspected condition that is determined after study not to be present. Do not use a code from category V29 when the patient has identified signs or symptoms of a suspected problem; in such cases, code the sign or symptom.

2. A V29 code is to be used as a secondary code after the V30, Outcome of delivery, code. It may also be assigned as a principal code for readmissions or encounters when the V30 code no longer applies. It is for use only for healthy newborns and infants for which no condition after study is found to be present.

E. Maternal Causes of Perinatal Morbidity

Codes from categories 760-763, Maternal causes of perinatal morbidity and mortality, are assigned only when the maternal condition has actually affected the fetus or newborn. The fact that the mother has an associated medical condition or experiences some complication of pregnancy, labor or delivery does not justify the routine assignment of codes from these categories to the newborn record.

F. Congenital Anomalies

Assign an appropriate code from categories 740-759, Congenital Anomalies, as an additional diagnosis when a specific abnormality is diagnosed for an infant. Congenital anomalies may also be the principal or first listed diagnosis for admissions/encounters subsequent to the newborn admission. Such abnormalities may occur as a set of symptoms or multiple malformations. A code should be assigned for each presenting manifestation of the syndrome if the syndrome is not specifically indexed in ICD-9-CM.

G. Coding of Additional Perinatal Diagnoses

1. Assign codes for conditions that require treatment or further investigation, prolong the length of stay, or require resource utilization.

2. Assign codes for conditions that have been specified by the physician as having implications for future health care needs.

   Note: This guideline should not be used for adult patients.

3. Assign a code for Newborn conditions originating in the perinatal period (categories 760-779), as well as complications arising during the current episode of care classified in other chapters, only if the diagnoses have been documented by the responsible physician at the time of transfer or discharge as having affected the fetus or newborn.

H. Prematurity and Fetal Growth Retardation

Codes from category 764 and subcategories 765.0 and 765.1 should not be assigned based solely on recorded birthweight or estimated gestational age, but on the attending physician's clinical assessment of maturity of the infant. NOTE: Since physicians may utilize different criteria in determining prematurity, do not code the diagnosis of prematurity unless the physician documents this condition.

Copyright © 2005, Elsevier Inc. All rights reserved.
CPT only © 2004. *Current Procedural Terminology, 2005, Professional Edition*, American Medical Association. All rights reserved.

A code from subcategory 765.2, Weeks of gestation, should be assigned as an additional code with category 764 and codes from 765.0 and 765.1 to specify weeks of gestation as documented by the physician.

C16. Signs, Symptoms and Ill-Defined Conditions

Reserved for future guideline expansion

C17. Injury and Poisoning

A. Coding of Injuries

When coding injuries, assign separate codes for each injury unless a combination code is provided, in which case the combination code is assigned. Multiple injury codes are provided in ICD-9-CM, but should not be assigned unless information for a more specific code is not available. These codes are not to be used for normal, healing surgical wounds or to identify complications of surgical wounds.

The code for the most serious injury, as determined by the physician, is sequenced first.

1. Superficial injuries such as abrasions or contusions are not coded when associated with more severe injuries of the same site.
2. When a primary injury results in minor damage to peripheral nerves or blood vessels, the primary injury is sequenced first with additional code(s) from categories 950-957, Injury to nerves and spinal cord, and/or 900-904, Injury to blood vessels. When the primary injury is to the blood vessels or nerves, that injury should be sequenced first.

B. Coding of Fractures

The principles of multiple coding of injuries should be followed in coding fractures. Fractures of specified sites are coded individually by site in accordance with both the provisions within categories 800-829 and the level of detail furnished by medical record content. Combination categories for multiple fractures are provided for use when there is insufficient detail in the medical record (such as trauma cases transferred to another hospital), when the reporting form limits the number of codes that can be used in reporting pertinent clinical data, or when there is insufficient specificity at the fourth-digit or fifth-digit level. More specific guidelines are as follows:

1. Multiple fractures of same limb classifiable to the same three-digit or four-digit category are coded to that category.
2. Multiple unilateral or bilateral fractures of same bone(s) but classified to different fourth-digit subdivisions (bone part) within the same three-digit category are coded individually by site.
3. Multiple fracture categories 819 and 828 classify bilateral fractures of both upper limbs (819) and both lower limbs (828), but without any detail at the fourth-digit level other than open and closed type of fractures.
4. Multiple fractures are sequenced in accordance with the severity of the fracture and the physician should be asked to list the fracture diagnoses in the order of severity.

C. Coding of Burns

Current burns (940-948) are classified by depth, extent and by agent (E code). Burns are classified by depth as first degree (erythema), second degree (blistering), and third degree (full-thickness involvement).

Copyright © 2005, Elsevier Inc. All rights reserved.
CPT only © 2004. *Current Procedural Terminology, 2005, Professional Edition*, American Medical Association. All rights reserved.

1. Sequence first the code that reflects the highest degree of burn when more than one burn is present.
2. Classify burns of the same local site (three-digit category level, 940-947) but of different degrees to the subcategory identifying the highest degree recorded in the diagnosis.
3. Non-healing burns are coded as acute burns.

   Necrosis of burned skin should be coded as a non-healed burn.
4. Assign code 958.3, Posttraumatic wound infection, not elsewhere classified, as an additional code for any documented infected burn site.
5. When coding burns, assign separate codes for each burn site. Category 946 Burns of Multiple specified sites, should only be used if the location of the burns are not documented.

   Category 949, Burn, unspecified, is extremely vague and should rarely be used.
6. Assign codes from category 948, Burns classified according to extent of body surface involved, when the site of the burn is not specified or when there is a need for additional data. It is advisable to use category 948 as additional coding when needed to provide data for evaluating burn mortality, such as that needed by burn units. It is also advisable to use category 948 as an additional code for reporting purposes when there is mention of a third-degree burn involving 20 percent or more of the body surface.

   In assigning a code from category 948:

   Fourth-digit codes are used to identify the percentage of total body surface involved in a burn (all degree).

   Fifth-digits are assigned to identify the percentage of body surface involved in third-degree burn.

   Fifth-digit zero (0) is assigned when less than 10 percent or when no body surface is involved in a third-degree burn.

   Category 948 is based on the classic "rule of nines" in estimating body surface involved: head and neck are assigned nine percent, each arm nine percent, each leg 18 percent, the anterior trunk 18 percent, posterior trunk 18 percent, and genitalia one percent. Physicians may change these percentage assignments where necessary to accommodate infants and children who have proportionately larger heads than adults and patients who have large buttocks, thighs, or abdomen that involve burns.
7. Encounters for the treatment of the late effects of burns (i.e., scars or joint contractures) should be coded to the residual condition (sequelae) followed by the appropriate late effect code (906.5-906.9). A late effect E code may also be used, if desired.
8. When appropriate, both sequelae with a late effect code and a current burn code may be assigned on the same record.

D. Coding of Debridement of Wound, Infection, or Burn

Excisional debridement may be performed by a physician and/or other health care provider and involves an excisional, as opposed to a mechanical (brushing, scrubbing, washing) debridement.

Copyright © 2005, Elsevier Inc. All rights reserved.
CPT only © 2004. *Current Procedural Terminology, 2005, Professional Edition,* American Medical Association. All rights reserved.

For coding purposes, excisional debridement, 86.22.

Nonexcisional debridement is assigned to 86.28.

Modified based on *Coding Clinic*, 2nd Quarter 2000, p. 9.

E. Adverse Effects, Poisoning and Toxic Effects

The properties of certain drugs, medicinal and biological substances or combinations of such substances, may cause toxic reactions. The occurrence of drug toxicity is classified in ICD-9-CM as follows:

1. Adverse Effect

When the drug was correctly prescribed and properly administered, code the reaction plus the appropriate code from the E930-E949 series. Codes from the E930-E949 series must be used to identify the causative substance for an adverse effect of drug, medicinal and biological substances, correctly prescribed and properly administered. The effect, such as tachycardia, delirium, gastrointestinal hemorrhaging, vomiting, hypokalemia, hepatitis, renal failure, or respiratory failure, is coded and followed by the appropriate code from the E930-E949 series.

Adverse effects of therapeutic substances correctly prescribed and properly administered (toxicity, synergistic reaction, side effect, and idiosyncratic reaction) may be due to (1) differences among patients, such as age, sex, disease, and genetic factors, and (2) drug-related factors, such as type of drug, route of administration, duration of therapy, dosage, and bioavailability.

2. Poisoning

a. When an error was made in drug prescription or in the administration of the drug by physician, nurse, patient, or other person, use the appropriate poisoning code from the 960-979 series.

b. If an overdose of a drug was intentionally taken or administered and resulted in drug toxicity, it would be coded as a poisoning (960-979 series).

c. If a nonprescribed drug or medicinal agent was taken in combination with a correctly prescribed and properly administered drug, any drug toxicity or other reaction resulting from the interaction of the two drugs would be classified as a poisoning.

d. When coding a poisoning or reaction to the improper use of a medication (e.g., wrong dose, wrong substance, wrong route of administration) the poisoning code is sequenced first, followed by a code for the manifestation. If there is also a diagnosis of drug abuse or dependence to the substance, the abuse or dependence is coded as an additional code.

C18. Classification of Factors Influencing Health Status and Contact with Health Service

A. ICD-9-CM provides codes to deal with encounters for circumstances other than a disease or injury. The Supplementary Classification of Factors Influencing Health Status and Contact with Health Services (V01.0-V83.89) is provided to deal with occasions when circumstances other than a disease or injury (codes 001-999) are recorded as a diagnosis or problem.

Copyright © 2005, Elsevier Inc. All rights reserved.
CPT only © 2004. *Current Procedural Terminology, 2005, Professional Edition*, American Medical Association. All rights reserved.

There are four primary circumstances for the use of V codes:

1. When a person who is not currently sick encounters the health services for some specific reason, such as to act as an organ donor, to receive prophylactic care, such as inoculations or health screenings, or to receive counseling on health related issue.
2. When a person with a resolving disease or injury, or a chronic, long-term condition requiring continuous care, encounters the health care system for specific aftercare of that disease or injury (e.g., dialysis for renal disease; chemotherapy for malignancy; cast change). A diagnosis/symptom code should be used whenever a current, acute, diagnosis is being treated or a sign or symptom is being studied.
3. When circumstances or problems influence a person's health status but are not in themselves a current illness or injury.
4. For newborns, to indicate birth status.

B. V codes are for use in both the inpatient and outpatient setting but are generally more applicable to the outpatient setting. V codes may be used as either a first listed (principal diagnosis code in the inpatient setting) or secondary code depending on the circumstances of the encounter. Certain V codes may only be used as first listed, others only as secondary codes.

C. V Codes indicate a reason for an encounter. They are not procedure codes. A corresponding procedure code must accompany a V code to describe the procedure performed.

D. Categories of V Codes

1. Contact/Exposure

   Category V01 indicates contact with or exposure to communicable diseases. These codes are for patients who do not show any sign or symptom of a disease but have been exposed to it by close personal contact with an infected individual or are in an area where a disease is epidemic. These codes may be used as a first listed code to explain an encounter for testing, or, more commonly, as a secondary code to identify a potential risk.

2. Inoculations and vaccinations

   Categories V03-V06 are for encounters for inoculations and vaccinations. They indicate that a patient is being seen to receive a prophylactic inoculation against a disease. The injection itself must be represented by the appropriate procedure code. A code from V03-V06 may be used as a secondary code if the inoculation is given as a routine part of preventive health care, such as a well-baby visit.

3. Status

   Status codes indicate that a patient is either a carrier of a disease or has the sequelae or residual of a past disease or condition. This includes such things as the presence of prosthetic or mechanical devices resulting from past treatment. A status code is informative because the status may affect the course of treatment and its outcome. A status code is distinct from a history code. The history code indicates that the patient no longer has the condition.

Copyright © 2005, Elsevier Inc. All rights reserved.
CPT only © 2004. *Current Procedural Terminology, 2005, Professional Edition,* American Medical Association. All rights reserved.

The status V codes/categories are:

V02 Carrier or suspected carrier of infectious diseases

Carrier status, indicates that a person harbors the specific organisms of a disease without manifest symptoms and is capable of transmitting the infection.

V08 Asymptomatic HIV infection status

This code indicates that a patient has tested positive for HIV but has manifested no signs or symptoms of the disease.

V09 Infection with drug-resistant microorganisms

This category indicates that a patient has an infection which is resistant to drug treatment. Sequence the infection code first.

V21 Constitutional states in development

V22.2 Pregnant state, incidental

This code is a secondary code only for use when the pregnancy is in no way complicating the reason for visit. Otherwise, a code from the obstetric chapter is required.

V26.5x Sterilization status

V42 Organ or tissue replaced by transplant

V43 Organ or tissue replaced by other means

V44 Artificial opening status

V45 Other postsurgical states

V46 Other dependence on machines

V49.6 Upper limb amputation status

V49.7 Lower limb amputation status

V48.81 Postmenopausal status

V49.82 Dental sealant status

V58.6 Long-term (current) drug use

This subcategory indicates a patient's continuous use of a prescribed drug (including such things as aspirin therapy) for the long-term treatment of a condition or for prophylactic use. It is not for use for patients who have addictions to drugs.

V83 Genetic carrier status

Categories V42-V46, and subcategories V49.6, V49.7 are for use only if there are no complications or malfunctions of the organ or tissue replaced, the amputation site or the equipment on which the patient is dependent. These are always secondary codes.

4. History (of)

There are two types of history V codes, personal and family. Personal history codes explain a patient's past medical condition that no

Copyright © 2005, Elsevier Inc. All rights reserved.
CPT only © 2004. *Current Procedural Terminology, 2005, Professional Edition*, American Medical Association. All rights reserved.

longer exists and is not receiving any treatment but that has the potential for recurrence, and, therefore, may require continued monitoring. The exceptions to this general rule are category V14, Personal history of allergy to medicinal agents and subcategory V15.0, Allergy, other than to medicinal agents. A person who has had an allergic episode to a substance or food in the past should always be considered allergic to the substance.

Family history codes are for use when a patient has a family member(s) who has had a particular disease that causes the patient to be at higher risk of also contracting the disease.

Personal history codes may be used in conjunction with follow-up codes and family history codes may be used in conjunction with screening codes to explain the need for a test or procedure. History codes are also acceptable on any medical record regardless of the reason for visit. A history of an illness, even if no longer present, is important information that may alter the type of treatment ordered.

The history V code categories are:

V10 Personal history of malignant neoplasm

V12 Personal history of certain other diseases

V13 Personal history of other diseases

> Except: V13.4, Personal history of arthritis, and V13.6, Personal history of congenital malformations. These conditions are life-long so are not true history codes.

V14 Personal history of allergy to medicinal agents

V15 Other personal history presenting hazards to health

> Except: V15.7, Personal history of contraception.

V16 Family history of malignant neoplasm

V17 Family history of certain chronic disabling diseases

V18 Family history of certain other specific diseases

V19 Family history of other conditions

5. Screening

Screening is the testing for disease or disease precursors in seemingly well individuals so that early detection and treatment can be provided for those who test positive for the disease. Screenings that are recommended for many subgroups in a population include: routine mammograms for women over 40, a fecal occult blood test for everyone over 50, an amniocentesis to rule out a fetal anomaly for pregnant women over 35, because the incidence of breast cancer and colon cancer in these subgroups is higher than in the general population, as is the incidence of Down's syndrome in older mothers.

The testing of a person to rule out or confirm a suspected diagnosis because the patient has some sign or symptom is a diagnostic examination, not a screening. In these cases, the sign or symptom is used to explain the reason for the test.

A screening code may be a first listed code if the reason for the visit is specifically the screening exam. It may also be used as an additional code if the screening is done during an office visit for other health problems. A screening code is not necessary if the

Copyright © 2005, Elsevier Inc. All rights reserved.
CPT only © 2004. *Current Procedural Terminology, 2005, Professional Edition*, American Medical Association. All rights reserved.

screening is inherent to a routine examination, such as a pap smear done during a routine pelvic examination.

Should a condition be discovered during the screening then the code for the condition may be assigned as an additional diagnosis.

The V code indicates that a screening exam is planned. A procedure code is required to confirm that the screening was performed.

The screening V code categories:

V28 Antenatal screening

V73-V82 Special screening examinations

6. Observation

There are two observation V code categories. They are for use in very limited circumstances when a person is being observed for a suspected condition that is ruled out. The observation codes are not for use if an injury or illness or any signs or symptoms related to the suspected condition are present. In such cases the diagnosis/symptom code is used with the corresponding E code to identify any external cause.

The observation codes are to be used as principal diagnosis only. The only exception to this is when the principal diagnosis is required to be a code from the V30, Live born infant, category. Then the V29 observation code is sequenced after the V30 code. Additional codes may be used in addition to the observation code but only if they are unrelated to the suspected condition being observed.

The observation V code categories:

V29 Observation and evaluation of newborns for suspected condition not found

A code from category V30 should be sequenced before the V29 code.

V71 Observation and evaluation for suspected condition not found

7. Aftercare

Aftercare visit codes cover situations when the initial treatment of a disease or injury has been performed and the patient requires continued care during the healing or recovery phase, or for the long-term consequences of the disease. The aftercare V code should not be used if treatment is directed at a current, acute disease or injury; the diagnosis code is to be used in these cases. Exceptions to this rule are codes V58.0, Radiotherapy, and V58.1, Chemotherapy. These codes are to be first listed, followed by the diagnosis code when a patient's encounter is solely to receive radiation therapy or chemotherapy for the treatment of a neoplasm. Should a patient receive both chemotherapy and radiation therapy during the same encounter code V58.0 and V58.1 may be used together on a record with either one being sequenced first.

The aftercare codes are generally first listed to explain the specific reason for the encounter. An aftercare code may be used as an additional code when some type of aftercare is provided in addition to the reason for admission and no diagnosis code is applicable. An example of this would be the closure of a colostomy during an encounter for treatment of another condition.

Copyright © 2005, Elsevier Inc. All rights reserved.
CPT only © 2004. *Current Procedural Terminology, 2005, Professional Edition*, American Medical Association. All rights reserved.

Certain aftercare V code categories need a secondary diagnosis code to describe the resolving condition or sequelae; for others, the condition is inherent in the code title.

Additional V code aftercare category terms include, fitting and adjustment, and attention to artificial openings.

The aftercare V category/codes:

V52	Fitting and adjustment of prosthetic device and implant
V53	Fitting and adjustment of other device
V54	Other orthopedic aftercare
V55	Attention to artificial openings
V56	Encounter for dialysis and dialysis catheter care
V57	Care involving the use of rehabilitation procedures
V58.0	Radiotherapy
V58.1	Chemotherapy
V58.3	Attention to surgical dressings and sutures
V58.41	Encounter for planned post-operative wound closure
V53.42	Aftercare, surgery, neoplasm
V53.43	Aftercare, surgery, trauma
V58.49	Other specified aftercare following surgery
V53.71-V53.78	Aftercare following surgery
V58.81	Fitting and adjustment of vascular catheter
V58.82	Fitting and adjustment of non-vascular catheter
V53.83	Monitoring therapeutic drug
V58.89	Other specified aftercare

8. Follow-up

The follow-up codes are for use to explain continuing surveillance following completed treatment of a disease, condition, or injury. They imply that the condition has been fully treated and no longer exists. They should not be confused with aftercare codes which explain current treatment for a healing condition or its sequelae. Follow-up codes may be used in conjunction with history codes to provide the full picture of the healed condition and its treatment. The follow-up code is sequenced first, followed by the history code.

A follow-up code may be used to explain repeated visits. Should a condition be found to have recurred on the follow-up visit, then the diagnosis code should be used in place of the follow-up code.

The follow-up V code categories:

V24 Postpartum care and evaluation

V67 Follow-up examination

9. Donor

Category V59 is the donor codes. They are for use for living individuals who are donating blood or other body tissue. These codes

Copyright © 2005, Elsevier Inc. All rights reserved.
CPT only © 2004. *Current Procedural Terminology, 2005, Professional Edition*, American Medical Association. All rights reserved.

are only for individuals donating for others, not for self donations. They are not for use to identify cadaveric donations.

10. Counseling

Counseling V codes are for use for when a patient or family member receives assistance in the aftermath of an illness or injury, or when support is required in coping with family or social problems. They are not necessary for use in conjunction with a diagnosis code when the counseling component of care is considered integral to standard treatment.

The counseling V categories/codes:

V25.0 General counseling and advice for contraceptive management

V26.3 Genetic counseling

V26.4 General counseling and advice for procreative management

V61 Other family circumstances

V65.1 Person consulted on behalf of another person

V65.3 Dietary surveillance and counseling

V65.4 Other counseling, not elsewhere classified

11. Obstetrics and related conditions

See the Obstetrics guidelines for further instruction on the use of these codes.

V codes for pregnancy are for use in those circumstances when none of the problems or complications included in the codes from the Obstetrics chapter exist (a routine prenatal visit or postpartum care) V22.0, Supervision of normal first pregnancy, and V22.1, Supervision of other normal pregnancy, are always first listed and are not to be used with any other code from the OB chapter.

The outcome of delivery, category V27, should be included on all maternal delivery records. It is always a secondary code.

V codes for family planning (contraceptive) or procreative management and counseling should be included on an obstetric record either during the pregnancy or the postpartum stage, if applicable.

Obstetrics and related conditions V code categories:

V22 Normal pregnancy

V23 Supervision of high-risk pregnancy

Except: V23.2, Pregnancy with history of abortion. Code 646.3, Habitual aborter, from the OB chapter is required to indicate a history of abortion during a pregnancy.

V24 Postpartum care and evaluation

V25 Encounter for contraceptive management

Except V25.0x (See counseling above)

V26 Procreative management

Except V26.5x, Sterilization status, V26.3 and V26.4 (Counseling)

Copyright © 2005, Elsevier Inc. All rights reserved.
CPT only © 2004. *Current Procedural Terminology, 2005, Professional Edition*, American Medical Association. All rights reserved.

V27 Outcome of delivery

V28 Antenatal screening

See Screening- see section 5 of this article

12. Newborn, infant and child

See the newborn guidelines for further instruction on the use of these codes.

Newborn V code categories:

V20 Health supervision of infant or child

V29 Observation and evaluation of newborns for suspected condition not found—see Observation, section 6 of this article.

V30-V39 Liveborn infant according to type of birth

13. Routine and administrative examinations

The V codes allow for the description of encounters for routine examinations, such as, a general check-up, or, examinations for administrative purposes, such as, a pre-employment physical. The codes are for use as first listed codes only and are not to be used if the examination is for diagnosis of a suspected condition or for treatment purposes. In such cases the diagnosis code is used. During a routine exam, should a diagnosis or condition be discovered, it should be coded as an additional code. Pre-existing and chronic conditions, and history codes may also be included as additional codes as long as the examination is for administrative purposes and not focused on any particular condition.

Pre-operative examination V codes are for use only in those situations when a patient is being cleared for surgery and no treatment is given.

The V codes categories/code for routine and administrative examinations:

V20.2 Routine infant or child health check

Any injections given should have a corresponding procedure code.

V70 General medical examination

V72 Special investigations and examinations

Except V72.5 and V72.6

14. Miscellaneous V codes

The miscellaneous V codes capture a number of other health care encounters that do not fall into one of the other categories. Certain of these codes identify the reason for the encounter, others are for use as additional codes which provide useful information on circumstances which may affect a patient's care and treatment.

Miscellaneous V code categories/codes:

V07 Need for isolation and other prophylactic measures

V50 Elective surgery for purposes other than remedying health states

Copyright © 2005, Elsevier Inc. All rights reserved.
CPT only © 2004. *Current Procedural Terminology, 2005, Professional Edition*, American Medical Association. All rights reserved.

V58.5 Orthodontics

V60 Housing, household, and economic circumstances

V62 Other psychosocial circumstances

V63 Unavailability of other medical facilities for care

V64 Persons encountering health services for specific procedures, not carried out

V66 Convalescence and Palliative Care

V68 Encounters for administrative purposes

V69 Problems related to lifestyle

15. Nonspecific V codes

Certain V codes are so non-specific, or potentially redundant with other codes in the classification that there can be little justification for their use in the inpatient setting. Their use in the outpatient setting should be limited to those instances when there is no further documentation to permit more precise coding. Otherwise, any sign or symptom or any other reason for visit which is captured in another code should be used.

Nonspecific V code categories/codes:

V11 Personal history of mental disorder

A code from the mental disorders chapter, with an in remission fifth-digit, should be used.

V13.4 Personal history of arthritis

V13.6 Personal history of congenital malformations

V15.7 Personal history of contraception

V23.2 Pregnancy with history of abortion

V40 Mental and behavioral problems

V41 Problems with special senses and other special functions

V47 Other problems with internal organs

V48 Problems with head, neck, and trunk

V49 Problems with limbs and other problems

Exceptions:

V49.6 Upper limb amputation status

V49.7 Lower limb amputation status

V49.81 Postmenopausal status

V49.82 Dental sealant status

V51 Aftercare involving the use of plastic surgery

V58.2 Blood transfusion, without reported diagnosis

V58.9 Unspecified aftercare

V72.5 Radiological examination, NEC

Copyright © 2005, Elsevier Inc. All rights reserved.
CPT only © 2004. *Current Procedural Terminology, 2005, Professional Edition*, American Medical Association. All rights reserved.

V72.6 Laboratory examination

Codes V72.5 and V72.6 are not to be used if any sign or symptoms, or reason for a test is documented. See section K and L of the outpatient guidelines.

C19. Supplemental Classification of External Causes of Injury and Poisoning (E-codes)

Introduction: These guidelines are provided for those who are currently collecting E codes in order that there will be standardization in the process. If your institution plans to begin collecting E codes, these guidelines are to be applied. The use of E codes is supplemental to the application of ICD-9-CM diagnosis codes. E codes are never to be recorded as principal diagnosis (first-listed in noninpatient setting) and are not required for reporting to CMS.

External causes of injury and poisoning codes (E codes) are intended to provide data for injury research and evaluation of injury prevention strategies. E codes capture how the injury or poisoning happened (cause), the intent (unintentional or accidental; or intentional, such as suicide or assault), and the place where the event occurred. Some major categories of E codes include:

transport accidents

poisoning and adverse effects of drugs, medicinal substances and biologicals

accidental falls

accidents caused by fire and flames

accidents due to natural and environmental factors

late effects of accidents, assaults or self injury

assaults or purposely inflicted injury

suicide or self inflicted injury

These guidelines apply for the coding and collection of E codes from records in hospitals, outpatient clinics, emergency departments, other ambulatory care settings and physician offices, and nonacute care settings, except when other specific guidelines apply. (See Section III, Reporting Diagnostic Guidelines for Hospital-based Outpatient Services/Reporting Requirements for Physician Billing.)

A. General E Code Coding Guidelines

1. An E code may be used with any code in the range of 001-V83.89, which indicates an injury, poisoning, or adverse effect due to an external cause.
2. Assign the appropriate E code for all initial treatments of an injury, poisoning, or adverse effect of drugs.
3. Use a late effect E code for subsequent visits when a late effect of the initial injury or poisoning is being treated. There is no late effect E code for adverse effects of drugs.
4. Use the full range of E codes to completely describe the cause, the intent and the place of occurrence, if applicable, for all injuries, poisonings, and adverse effects of drugs.

Copyright © 2005, Elsevier Inc. All rights reserved.
CPT only © 2004. *Current Procedural Terminology, 2005, Professional Edition,* American Medical Association. All rights reserved.

5. Assign as many E codes as necessary to fully explain each cause. If only one E code can be recorded, assign the E code most related to the principal diagnosis.

6. The selection of the appropriate E code is guided by the Index to External Causes, which is located after the alphabetical index to diseases and by Inclusion and Exclusion notes in the Tabular List.

7. An E code can never be a principal (first listed) diagnosis.

B. Place of Occurrence Guideline

Use an additional code from category E849 to indicate the Place of Occurrence for injuries and poisonings. The Place of Occurrence describes the place where the event occurred and not the patient's activity at the time of the event.

Do not use E849.9 if the place of occurrence is not stated.

C. Adverse Effects of Drugs, Medicinal and Biological Substances Guidelines

1. Do not code directly from the Table of Drugs and Chemicals. Always refer back to the Tabular List.

2. Use as many codes as necessary to describe completely all drugs, medicinal or biological substances.

3. If the same E code would describe the causative agent for more than one adverse reaction, assign the code only once.

4. If two or more drugs, medicinal or biological substances are reported, code each individually unless the combination code is listed in the Table of Drugs and Chemicals. In that case, assign the E code for the combination.

5. When a reaction results from the interaction of a drug(s) and alcohol, use poisoning codes and E codes for both.

6. If the reporting format limits the number of E codes that can be used in reporting clinical data, code the one most related to the principal diagnosis. Include at least one from each category (cause, intent, place) if possible.

   If there are different fourth digit codes in the same three digit category, use the code for "Other specified" of that category. If there is no "Other specified" code in that category, use the appropriate "Unspecified" code in that category.

   If the codes are in different three digit categories, assign the appropriate E code for other multiple drugs and medicinal substances.

7. Codes from the E930-E949 series must be used to identify the causative substance for an adverse effect of drug, medicinal and biological substances, correctly prescribed and properly administered. The effect, such as tachycardia, delirium, gastrointestinal hemorrhaging, vomiting, hypokalemia, hepatitis, renal failure, or respiratory failure, is coded and followed by the appropriate code from the E930-E949 series.

D. Multiple Cause E Code Coding Guidelines

If two or more events cause separate injuries, an E code should be assigned for each cause. The first listed E code will be selected in the following order:

Copyright © 2005, Elsevier Inc. All rights reserved.
CPT only © 2004. *Current Procedural Terminology, 2005, Professional Edition,* American Medical Association. All rights reserved.

E codes for child and adult abuse take priority over all other E codes—see Child and Adult abuse guidelines.

E codes for terrorism events take priority over all other E codes except child and adult abuse.

E codes for cataclysmic events take priority over all other E codes except child and adult abuse and terrorism.

E codes for transport accidents take priority over all other E codes except cataclysmic events and child and adult abuse and terrorism.

The first-listed E code should correspond to the cause of the most serious diagnosis due to an assault, accident, or self-harm, following the order of hierarchy listed above.

E. Child and Adult Abuse Guideline

1. When the cause of an injury or neglect is intentional child or adult abuse, the first listed E code should be assigned from categories E960-E968, Homicide and injury purposely inflicted by other persons, (except category E967). An E code from category E967, Child and adult battering and other maltreatment, should be added as an additional code to identify the perpetrator, if known.

2. In cases of neglect when the intent is determined to be accidental E code E904.0, Abandonment or neglect of infant and helpless person, should be the first listed E code.

F. Unknown or Suspected Intent Guideline

1. If the intent (accident, self-harm, assault) of the cause of an injury or poisoning is unknown or unspecified, code the intent as undetermined E980-E989.

2. If the intent (accident, self-harm, assault) of the cause of an injury or poisoning is questionable, probable or suspected, code the intent as undetermined E980-E989.

G. Undetermined Cause

When the intent of an injury or poisoning is known, but the cause is unknown, use codes: E928.9, Unspecified accident, E958.9, Suicide and self-inflicted injury by unspecified means, and E968.9, Assault by unspecified means.

These E codes should rarely be used, as the documentation in the medical record, in both the inpatient outpatient and other settings, should normally provide sufficient detail to determine the cause of the injury.

H. Late Effects of External Cause Guidelines

1. Late effect E codes exist for injuries and poisonings but not for adverse effects of drugs, misadventures and surgical complications.

2. A late effect E code (E929, E959, E969, E977, E989, or E999.1) should be used with any report of a late effect or sequela resulting from a previous injury or poisoning (905-909).

3. A late effect E code should never be used with a related current nature of injury code.

Copyright © 2005, Elsevier Inc. All rights reserved.
CPT only © 2004. *Current Procedural Terminology, 2005, Professional Edition*, American Medical Association. All rights reserved.

I. Misadventures and Complications of Care Guidelines

1. Assign a code in the range of E870-E876 if misadventures are stated by the physician.

2. Assign a code in the range of E878-E879 if the physician attributes an abnormal reaction or later complication to a surgical or medical procedure, but does not mention misadventure at the time of the procedure as the cause of the reaction.

J. Terrorism Guidelines

1. When the cause of an injury is identified by the Federal Government (FBI) as terrorism, the first-listed E-code should be a code from category E979, Terrorism. The definition of terrorism employed by the FBI is found at the inclusion note at E979. The terrorism E-code is the only E-code that should be assigned. Additional E codes from the assault categories should not be assigned.

2. When the cause of an injury is suspected to be the result of terrorism a code from category E979 should not be assigned. Assign a code in the range of E codes based circumstances on the documentation of intent and mechanism.

3. Assign code E979.9, Terrorism, secondary effects, for conditions occurring subsequent to the terrorist event. This code should not be assigned for conditions that are due to the initial terrorist act.

4. For statistical purposes these codes will be tabulated within the category for assault, expanding the current category from E960-E969 to include E979 and E999.1.

SECTION II SELECTION OF PRINCIPAL DIAGNOSIS(ES) FOR INPATIENT, SHORT-TERM, ACUTE CARE, AND LONG TERM CARE HOSPITAL RECORDS

The circumstances of inpatient admission always govern the selection of principal diagnosis. The principal diagnosis is defined in the Uniform Hospital Discharge Data Set (UHDDS) as "that condition established after study to be chiefly responsible for occasioning the admission of the patient to the hospital for care."

The UHDDS definitions are used by acute care short-term hospitals to report inpatient data elements in a standardized manner. These data elements and their definitions can be found in the July 31, 1985, Federal Register (Vol. 50, No, 147), pp. 31038-40.

In determining principal diagnosis the coding conventions in the ICD-9-CM, Volumes I and II take precedence over these official coding guidelines. (See Section IA).

The importance of consistent, complete documentation in the medical record cannot be overemphasized. Without such documentation the application of all coding guidelines is a difficult, if not impossible, task.

A. Codes for symptoms, signs, and ill-defined conditions

Codes for symptoms, signs, and ill-defined conditions from Chapter 16 are not to be used as principal diagnosis when a related definitive diagnosis has been established.

B. Two or more interrelated conditions, each potentially meeting the definition for principal diagnosis.

When there are two or more interrelated conditions (such as diseases in the same ICD-9-CM chapter or manifestations characteristically associated with a certain

Copyright © 2005, Elsevier Inc. All rights reserved.
CPT only © 2004. *Current Procedural Terminology, 2005, Professional Edition,* American Medical Association. All rights reserved.

disease) potentially meeting the definition of principal diagnosis, either condition may be sequenced first, unless the circumstances of the admission, the therapy provided, the Tabular List, or the Alphabetic Index indicate otherwise.

C. Two or more diagnoses that equally meet the definition for principal diagnosis.

In the unusual instance when two or more diagnoses equally meet the criteria for principal diagnosis as determined by the circumstances of admission, diagnostic workup and/or therapy provided, and the Alphabetic Index, Tabular List, or another coding guidelines does not provide sequencing direction, any one of the diagnoses may be sequenced first.

D. Two or more comparative or contrasting conditions.

In those rare instances when two or more contrasting or comparative diagnoses are documented as "either/or" (or similar terminology), they are coded as if the diagnoses were confirmed and the diagnoses are sequenced according to the circumstances of the admission. If no further determination can be made as to which diagnosis should be principal, either diagnosis may be sequenced first.

E. A symptom(s) followed by contrasting/comparative diagnoses.

When a symptom(s) is followed by contrasting/comparative diagnoses, the symptom code is sequenced first. All the contrasting/comparative diagnoses should be coded as additional diagnoses.

F. Original treatment plan not carried out.

Sequence as the principal diagnosis the condition, which after study occasioned the admission to the hospital, even though treatment may not have been carried out due to unforeseen circumstances.

G. Complications of surgery and other medical care.

When the admission is for treatment of a complication resulting from surgery or other medical care, the complication code is sequenced as the principal diagnosis. If the complication is classified to the 996-999 series, an additional code for the specific complication may be assigned.

H. Uncertain Diagnosis.

If the diagnosis documented at the time of discharge is qualified as "probable", "suspected", "likely", "questionable", "possible", or "still to be ruled out", code the condition as if it existed or was established. The bases for these guidelines are the diagnostic workup, arrangements for further workup or observation, and initial therapeutic approach that correspond most closely with the established diagnosis.

SECTION III REPORTING ADDITIONAL DIAGNOSES FOR INPATIENT, SHORT-TERM, ACUTE CARE, AND LONG TERM CARE HOSPITAL RECORDS

GENERAL RULES FOR OTHER (ADDITIONAL) DIAGNOSES

For reporting purposes the definition for "other diagnoses" is interpreted as additional conditions that affect patient care in terms of requiring:

clinical evaluation; or

therapeutic treatment; or

diagnostic procedures; or

Copyright © 2005, Elsevier Inc. All rights reserved.
CPT only © 2004. *Current Procedural Terminology, 2005, Professional Edition*, American Medical Association. All rights reserved.

extended length of hospital stay; or

increased nursing care and/or monitoring.

The UHDDS item #11-b defines Other Diagnoses as "all conditions that coexist at the time of admission, that develop subsequently, or that affect the treatment received and/or the length of stay. Diagnoses that relate to an earlier episode which have no bearing on the current hospital stay are to be excluded." UHDDS definitions apply to inpatients in acute care, short-term, hospital setting The UHDDS definitions are used by acute care short-term hospitals to report inpatient data elements in a standardized manner. These data elements and their definitions can be found in the July 31, 1985, Federal Register (Vol. 50, No, 147), pp. 31038-40.

The following guidelines are to be applied in designating "other diagnoses" when neither the Alphabetic Index nor the Tabular List in ICD-9-CM provide direction. The listing of the diagnoses in the patient record is the responsibility of the attending physician.

A. Previous conditions

If the physician has included a diagnosis in the final diagnostic statement, such as the discharge summary or the face sheet, it should ordinarily be coded. Some physicians include in the diagnostic statement resolved conditions or diagnoses and status-post procedures from previous admission that have no bearing on the current stay. Such conditions are not to be reported and are coded only if required by hospital policy.

However, history codes (V10-V19) may be used as secondary codes if the historical condition or family history has an impact on current care or influences treatment.

B. Abnormal findings

Abnormal findings (laboratory, x-ray, pathologic, and other diagnostic results) are not coded and reported unless the physician indicates their clinical significance. If the findings are outside the normal range and the attending physician has ordered other tests to evaluate the condition or prescribed treatment, it is appropriate to ask the physician whether the abnormal finding should be added.

Please note: This differs from the coding practices in the outpatient setting for coding encounters for diagnostic tests that have been interpreted by a physician.

C. Uncertain Diagnosis

If the diagnosis documented at the time of discharge is qualified as "probable", "suspected", "likely", "questionable", "possible", or "still to be ruled out", code the condition as if it existed or was established. The bases for these guidelines are the diagnostic workup, arrangements for further workup or observation, and initial therapeutic approach that correspond most closely with the established diagnosis.

SECTION IV DIAGNOSTIC CODING AND REPORTING GUIDELINES FOR OUTPATIENT SERVICES

These coding guidelines for outpatient diagnoses have been approved for use by hospitals/physicians in coding and reporting hospital-based outpatient services and physician office visits.

Information about the use of certain abbreviations, punctuation, symbols, and other conventions used in the ICD-9-CM Tabular List (code numbers and titles), can be found in Section IA of these guidelines, under "Conventions Used in the Tabular

Copyright © 2005, Elsevier Inc. All rights reserved.
CPT only © 2004. *Current Procedural Terminology, 2005, Professional Edition*, American Medical Association. All rights reserved.

List." Information about the correct sequence to use in finding a code is also described in Section I.

The terms encounter and visit are often used interchangeably in describing outpatient service contacts and, therefore, appear together in these guidelines without distinguishing one from the other.

Though the conventions and general guidelines apply to all settings, coding guidelines for outpatient and physician reporting of diagnoses will vary in a number of instances from those for inpatient diagnoses, recognizing that:

The Uniform Hospital Discharge Data Set (UHDDS) definition of principal diagnosis applies only to inpatients in acute, short-term, general and Long Term Care hospitals.

Coding guidelines for inconclusive diagnoses (probable, suspected, rule out, etc.) were developed for inpatient reporting and do not apply to outpatients.

A. Selection of first-listed condition

In the outpatient setting, the term first-listed diagnosis is used in lieu of principal diagnosis.

In determining the first-listed diagnosis the coding conventions of ICD-9-CM, as well as the general and disease specific guidelines take precedence over the outpatient guidelines.

Diagnoses often are not established at the time of the initial encounter/visit. It may take two or more visits before the diagnosis is confirmed.

The most critical rule involves beginning the search for the correct code assignment through the Alphabetic Index. Never begin searching initially in the Tabular List as this will lead to coding errors.

B. The appropriate code or codes from 001.0 through V83.89 must be used to identify diagnoses, symptoms, conditions, problems, complaints, or other reason(s) for the encounter/visit.

C. For accurate reporting of ICD-9-CM diagnosis codes, the documentation should describe the patient's condition, using terminology which includes specific diagnoses as well as symptoms, problems, or reasons for the encounter. There are ICD-9-CM codes to describe all of these.

D. The selection of codes 001.0 through 999.9 will frequently be used to describe the reason for the encounter. These codes are from the section of ICD-9-CM for the classification of diseases and injuries (e.g. infectious and parasitic diseases; neoplasms; symptoms, signs, and ill-defined conditions, etc.).

E. Codes that describe symptoms and signs, as opposed to diagnoses, are acceptable for reporting purposes when a diagnosis has not been established (confirmed) by the physician. Chapter 16 of ICD-9-CM, Symptoms, Signs, and Ill-defined conditions (codes 780.0-799.9) contain many, but not all codes for symptoms.

F. ICD-9-CM provides codes to deal with encounters for circumstances other than a disease or injury. The Supplementary Classification of factors Influencing Health Status and Contact with Health Services (V01.0-V83.89) is provided to deal with occasions when circumstances other than a disease or injury are recorded as diagnosis or problems.

G. Level of Detail in Coding

1. ICD-9-CM is composed of codes with either 3, 4, or 5 digits. Codes with three digits are included in ICD-9-CM as the heading of a category of codes that may be further subdivided by the use of fourth and/or fifth digits, which provide greater specificity.

Copyright © 2005, Elsevier Inc. All rights reserved.
CPT only © 2004. *Current Procedural Terminology, 2005, Professional Edition*, American Medical Association. All rights reserved.

2. A three-digit code is to be used only if it is not further subdivided. Where fourth-digit subcategories and/or fifth-digit subclassifications are provided, they must be assigned. A code is invalid if it has not been coded to the full number of digits required for that code. See also discussion under Section I, General Coding Guidelines, Level of Detail in "Coding".

H. List first the ICD-9-CM code for the diagnosis, condition, problem, or other reason for encounter/visit shown in the medical record to be chiefly responsible for the services provided. List additional codes that describe any coexisting conditions.

I. Do not code diagnoses documented as "probable", "suspected," "questionable," "rule out," or "working diagnosis". Rather, code the condition(s) to the highest degree of certainty for that encounter/visit, such as symptoms, signs, abnormal test results, or other reason for the visit.

Please note: This differs from the coding practices used by hospital medical record departments for coding the diagnosis of acute care, short-term hospital inpatients.

J. Chronic diseases treated on an ongoing basis may be coded and reported as many times as the patient receives treatment and care for the condition(s).

K. Code all documented conditions that coexist at the time of the encounter/visit, and require or affect patient care treatment or management. Do not code conditions that were previously treated and no longer exist. However, history codes (V10-V19) may be used as secondary codes if the historical condition or family history has an impact on current care or influences treatment.

L. For patients receiving diagnostic services only during an encounter/visit, sequence first the diagnosis, condition, problem, or other reason for encounter/visit shown in the medical record to be chiefly responsible for the outpatient services provided during the encounter/visit. Codes for other diagnoses (e.g., chronic conditions) may be sequenced as additional diagnoses.

For outpatient encounters for diagnostic tests that have been interpreted by a physician, and the final report is available at the time of coding, code any confirmed or definitive diagnosis(es) documented in the interpretation. Do not code related signs and symptoms as additional diagnoses.

Please note: This differs from the coding practice in the hospital inpatient setting regarding abnormal findings on test results.

M. For patients receiving therapeutic services only during an encounter/visit, sequence first the diagnosis, condition, problem, or other reason for encounter/visit shown in the medical record to be chiefly responsible for the outpatient services provided during the encounter/visit. Codes for other diagnoses (e.g., chronic conditions) may be sequenced as additional diagnoses.

The only exception to this rule is that when the primary reason for the admission/encounter is chemotherapy, radiation therapy, or rehabilitation, the appropriate V code for the service is listed first, and the diagnosis or problem for which the service is being performed listed second.

N. For patients receiving preoperative evaluations only, sequence a code from category V72.8, Other specified examinations, to describe the pre-op consultations. Assign a code for the condition to describe the reason for the surgery as an additional diagnosis. Code also any findings related to the pre-op evaluation.

Copyright © 2005, Elsevier Inc. All rights reserved.
CPT only © 2004. *Current Procedural Terminology, 2005, Professional Edition,* American Medical Association. All rights reserved.

O. For ambulatory surgery, code the diagnosis for which the surgery was performed. If the postoperative diagnosis is known to be different from the preoperative diagnosis at the time the diagnosis is confirmed, select the postoperative diagnosis for coding, since it is the most definitive.

P. For routine outpatient prenatal visits when no complications are present codes V22.0, Supervision of normal first pregnancy, and V22.1, Supervision of other normal pregnancy, should be used as principal diagnoses. These codes should not be used in conjunction with chapter 11 codes.

Copyright © 2005, Elsevier Inc. All rights reserved.
CPT only © 2004. *Current Procedural Terminology, 2005, Professional Edition*, American Medical Association. All rights reserved.

Appendix B

Medical Terminology

ablation	removal or destruction by cutting, chemicals, or electrocautery
abortion	termination of pregnancy
absence	without
actinotherapy	treatment of acne using ultraviolet rays
adenoidectomy	removal of adenoids
adipose	fatty
adrenals	glands, located at the top of the kidneys, that produce steroid hormones
albinism	lack of color pigment
allograft	homograft, same species graft
alopecia	condition in which hair falls out
amniocentesis	percutaneous aspiration of amniotic fluid
amniotic sac	sac containing the fetus and amniotic fluid
A-mode	one-dimensional ultrasonic display reflecting the time it takes a sound wave to reach a structure and reflect back; maps the structure's outline
anastomosis	surgical connection of two tubular structures, such as two pieces of the intestine
aneurysm	sac formed outside the vessel, artery, or heart
angina	sudden pain
angiography	radiography of the blood vessels
angioplasty	procedure in a vessel to dilate the vessel opening

anhidrosis	deficiency of sweat
anomaloscope	instrument used to test color vision
anoscopy	procedure that uses a scope to examine the anus
antepartum	before childbirth
anterior (ventral)	in front of
anterior segment	those parts of the eye in the front of and including the lens, orbit, extraocular muscles, and eyelid
anteroposterior	from front to back
antigen	a substance that produces a specific response
aortography	radiographic recording of the aorta
apexcardiography	recording of the movement of the chest wall
aphakia	absence of the lens of the eye
apicectomy	excision of a portion of the temporal bone
apnea	cessation of breathing
arthrocentesis	injection and/or aspiration of joint
arthrodesis	surgical immobilization of joint
arthrography	radiography of joint
arthroplasty	reshaping or reconstruction of joint
arthroscopy	use of scope to view inside joint
arthrotomy	incision into a joint
articular	pertains to joint
asphyxia	lack of oxygen
aspiration	use of a needle and a syringe to withdraw fluid
assignment	Medicare's payment for the service, which participating physicians agree to accept as payment in full
asthma	shortage of breath caused by contraction of bronchi
astigmatism	condition in which the refractive surfaces of the eye are unequal
atelectasis	incomplete expansion of lung, collapse
atherectomy	removal of plaque by percutaneous method
atrophy	wasting away
audiometry	hearing test
aural atresia	congenital absence of the external auditory canal
auscultation	listening to sounds within the body
autograft	from patient's own body
axillary nodes	lymph nodes located in the armpit
bacilli	plural of bacillus, a rod-shaped bacterium

Copyright © 2005, Elsevier Inc. All rights reserved.
CPT only © 2004. *Current Procedural Terminology, 2005, Professional Edition*, American Medical Association. All rights reserved.

barium enema	radiographic contrast medium
beneficiary	person who benefits from health or life insurance
bifocal	two focuses in eyeglasses, one usually for close work and the other for improvement of distance vision
bilateral	occurring on two sides
biliary	refers to gallbladder, bile, or bile duct
bilobectomy	surgical removal of two lobes of a lung
biofeedback	process of giving a person self-information
biometry	application of a statistical measure to a biologic fact
biopsy	removal of a small piece of living tissue for diagnostic purposes
block	frozen piece of a sample
brachytherapy	therapy using radioactive sources that are placed inside the body
bronchiole	smaller division of bronchial tree
bronchography	radiographic recording of the lungs
bronchoplasty	surgical repair of the bronchi
bronchoscopy	inspection of the bronchial tree using a bronchoscope
B-scan	two-dimensional display of tissues and organs
bulbocavernosus	muscle that constricts the vagina in a female and the urethra in a male
bulbourethral	gland with duct leading to the urethra
bundle of His	muscular cardiac fibers that provide the heart rhythm to the ventricles; blockage of this rhythm produces heart block
bundled codes	one code that represents a package of services
bunion	hallux valgus, abnormal increase in size of metatarsal head that results in displacement of the great toe
burr	drill used to create an entry into the cranium
bursa	fluid-filled sac that absorbs friction
bursitis	inflammation of bursa
bypass	to go around
calcaneal	pertaining to the heel bone
calculus	concretion of mineral salts, also called a stone
calycoplasty	surgical reconstruction of a recess of the renal pelvis
calyx	recess of the renal pelvis
cancellous	lattice-type structure, usually of bone
cardiopulmonary	refers to the heart and lungs
cardiopulmonary bypass	blood bypasses the heart through a heart-lung machine
cardioversion	electrical shock to the heart to restore normal rhythm

Copyright © 2005, Elsevier Inc. All rights reserved.
CPT only © 2004. *Current Procedural Terminology, 2005, Professional Edition*, American Medical Association. All rights reserved.

cardioverter-defibrillator	surgically placed device that directs an electrical shock to the heart to restore rhythm
carotid body	located on each side of the common carotid artery, often a site of tumor
cartilage	connective tissue
cataract	opaque covering on or in the lens
catheter	tube placed into the body to put fluid in or take fluid out
caudal	same as inferior; away from the head, or the lower part of the body
causalgia	burning pain
cauterization	destruction of tissue by the use of cautery
cavernosa	connection between the cavity of the penis and a vein
cavernosography	radiographic recording of a cavity, e.g., the pulmonary cavity or the main part of the penis
cavernosometry	measurement of the pressure in a cavity, e.g., the penis
central nervous system	brain and spinal cord
cervical	pertaining to the neck or to the cervix of the uterus
cervix uteri	rounded, cone-shaped neck of the uterus
cesarean	surgical opening through abdominal wall for delivery
cholangiography	radiographic recording of the bile ducts
cholangiopancreatography	ERCP, radiographic recording of the biliary system or pancreas
cholecystectomy	surgical removal of the gallbladder
cholecystoenterostomy	creation of a connection between the gallbladder and intestine
cholecystography	radiographic recording of the gallbladder
cholesteatoma	tumor that forms in middle ear
chondral	referring to the cartilage
chordee	condition resulting in the penis being bent downward
chorionic villus sampling	CVS, biopsy of the outermost part of the placenta
circumflex	a coronary artery that circles the heart
Cloquet's node	also called a gland; it is the highest of the deep groin lymph nodes
closed fracture repair	not surgically opened with/without manipulation and with/without traction
closed treatment	fracture site that is not surgically opened and visualized
coccyx	caudal extremity of vertebral column
collagen	protein substance of skin
Colles' fracture	fracture at lower end of radius that displaces the bone posteriorly
colonoscopy	fiberscopic examination of the entire colon that may include part of the terminal ileum

Copyright © 2005, Elsevier Inc. All rights reserved.
CPT only © 2004. *Current Procedural Terminology, 2005, Professional Edition*, American Medical Association. All rights reserved.

colostomy	artificial opening between the colon and the abdominal wall
component	part
computed axial tomography	CAT or CT, procedure by which selected planes of tissue are pinpointed through computer enhancement, and images may be reconstructed by analysis of variance in absorption of the tissue
conjunctiva	the lining of the eyelids and the covering of the sclera
contraction	drawn together
contralateral	opposite side
cordectomy	surgical removal of the vocal cord(s)
cordocentesis	procedure to obtain a fetal blood sample; also called a percutaneous umbilical blood sampling
corneosclera	cornea and sclera of the eye
corpectomy	removal of vertebrae
corpora cavernosa	the two cavities of the penis
corpus uteri	uterus
crackle	abnormal sound when breathing
craniectomy	permanent, partial removal of skull
craniotomy	opening of the skull
cranium	that part of the skeleton that encloses the brain
curettage	scraping of a cavity using a spoon-shaped instrument
curette	spoon-shaped instrument used to scrape a cavity
cutdown	incision into a vessel for placement of a catheter
cyanosis	bluish discoloration
cystocele	herniation of the bladder into the vagina
cystography	radiographic recording of the urinary bladder
cystolithectomy	removal of a calculus (stone) from the urinary bladder
cystolithotomy	cystolithectomy
cystometrogram	CMG, measurement of the pressures and capacity of the urinary bladder
cystoplasty	surgical reconstruction of the bladder
cystorrhaphy	suture of the bladder
cystoscopy	use of a scope to view the bladder
cystostomy	surgical creation of an opening into the bladder
cystotomy	incision into the bladder
cystourethroplasty	surgical reconstruction of the bladder and urethra
cystourethroscopy	use of a scope to view the bladder and urethra
dacryocystography	radiographic recording of the lacrimal sac or tear duct sac
dacryostenosis	narrowing of the lacrimal duct

Copyright © 2005, Elsevier Inc. All rights reserved.
CPT only © 2004. *Current Procedural Terminology, 2005, Professional Edition,* American Medical Association. All rights reserved.

debridement	cleansing of or removal of dead tissue from a wound
deductible	amount the patient is liable for before the payer begins to pay for covered services
delayed flap	pedicle of skin with blood supply that is separated from origin over time
delivery	childbirth
dermabrasion	planing of the skin by means of sander, brush, or sandpaper
dermatologist	physician who treats conditions of the skin
dermatoplasty	surgical repair of skin
dialysis	filtration of blood
dilation	expansion
diskectomy	removal of a vertebral disk
diskography	radiographic recording of an intervertebral joint
dislocation	placement in a location other than the original location
distal	farther from the point of attachment or origin
diverticulum	protrusion in the wall of an organ
Doppler	ultrasonic measure of blood movement
dosimetry	scientific calculation of radiation emitted from various radioactive sources
drainage	free flow or withdrawal of fluids from a wound or cavity
duodenography	radiographic recording of the duodenum or first part of the small intestine
dysphagia	difficulty swallowing
dysphonia	speech impairment
dyspnea	shortage of breath, difficult breathing
dysuria	painful urination
echocardiography	radiographic recording of the heart or heart walls or surrounding tissues
echoencephalography	ultrasound of the brain
echography	ultrasound procedure in which sound waves are bounced off an internal organ and the resulting image is recorded
ectopic	pregnancy outside the uterus (i.e., in the fallopian tube)
edema	swelling due to abnormal fluid collection in the tissue spaces
elective surgery	nonemergency procedure
electrocardiogram	ECG, written record of the electrical action of the heart
electrocautery	cauterization by means of heated instrument
electrocochleography	test to measure the eighth cranial nerve (hearing test)
electrode	lead attached to a generator that carries the electrical current from the generator to the atria or ventricles

Copyright © 2005, Elsevier Inc. All rights reserved.
CPT only © 2004. *Current Procedural Terminology, 2005, Professional Edition,* American Medical Association. All rights reserved.

electroencephalogram	EEG, written record of the electrical action of the brain
electromyogram	EMG, written record of the electrical activity of the skeletal muscles
electronic claim submission	claims prepared and submitted via a computer
electronic signature	identification system of a computer
electro-oculogram	EOG, written record of the electrical activity of the eye
electrophysiology	study of the electrical system of the heart, including the study of arrhythmias
embolectomy	removal of blockage (embolism) from vessel
emphysema	air accumulated in organ or tissue
encephalography	radiographic recording of the subarachnoid space and ventricles of the brain
endarterectomy	incision into an artery to remove the inner lining so as to eliminate disease or blockage
endomyocardial	pertaining to the inner and middle layers of the heart
endopyelotomy	procedure involving the bladder and ureters, including the insertion of a stent into the renal pelvis
endoscopy	inspection of body organs or cavities using a lighted scope that may be inserted through an existing opening or through a small incision
enterolysis	releasing of adhesions of intestine
enucleation	removal of an organ or organs from a body cavity
epicardial	over the heart
epidermolysis	loosening of the epidermis
epidermomycosis	superficial fungal infection
epididymectomy	surgical removal of the epididymis
epididymis	tube located at the top of the testes that stores sperm
epididymography	radiographic recording of the epididymis
epididymovasostomy	creation of a new connection between the vas deferens and epididymis
epiglottidectomy	excision of the covering of the larynx
episclera	connective covering of sclera
epistaxis	nose bleed
epithelium	surface covering of internal and external organs of the body
erythema	redness of skin
escharotomy	surgical incision into necrotic (dead) tissue
eventration	protrusion of the bowel through an opening in the abdomen
evisceration	pulling the viscera outside of the body through an incision
evocative	tests that are administered to evoke a predetermined response
exenteration	removal of an organ all in one piece

Copyright © 2005, Elsevier Inc. All rights reserved.
CPT only © 2004. *Current Procedural Terminology, 2005, Professional Edition*, American Medical Association. All rights reserved.

exophthalmos	protrusion of the eyeball
exostosis	bony growth
exstrophy	condition in which an organ is turned inside out
extracorporeal	occurring outside of the body
false aneurysm	sac of clotted blood that has completely destroyed the vessel and is being contained by the tissue that surrounds the vessel
fasciectomy	removal of a band of fibrous tissue
Federal Register	official publication of all "Presidential Documents," "Rules and Regulations," "Proposed Rules," and "Notices"; government-instituted national changes are published in the *Federal Register*
fee schedule	services and payment allowed for each service
femoral	pertaining to the bone from the pelvis to knee
fenestration	creation of a new opening in the inner wall of the middle ear
fissure	cleft or groove
fistula	abnormal opening from one area to another area or to the outside of the body
fluoroscopy	procedure for viewing the interior of the body using x-rays and projecting the image onto a television screen
fracture	break in a bone
free full-thickness graft	graft of epidermis and dermis that is completely removed from donor area
fulguration	use of electrical current to destroy tissue
fundoplasty	repair of the bottom of the bladder
furuncle	nodule in the skin caused by staphylococci entering through hair follicle
ganglion	knot
gastrointestinal	pertaining to the stomach and intestine
gastroplasty	operation on the stomach for repair or reconfiguration
gastrostomy	artificial opening between the stomach and the abdominal wall
gatekeeper	a physician who manages a patient's access to health care
glaucoma	eye diseases that are characterized by an increase of intraocular pressure
globe	eyeball
glottis	true vocal cords
gonioscopy	use of a scope to examine the angles of the eye
Group Practice Model	an organization of physicians who contract with a Health Maintenance Organization to provide services to the enrollees of the HMO
grouper	computer used to input the principal diagnosis and other critical information about a patient and then provide the correct DRG code

Copyright © 2005, Elsevier Inc. All rights reserved.
CPT only © 2004. *Current Procedural Terminology, 2005, Professional Edition,* American Medical Association. All rights reserved.

Health Maintenance Organization	HMO, a health care delivery system in which an enrollee is assigned a primary care physician who manages all the health care needs of the enrollee
hematoma	mass of blood that forms outside the vessel
hemodialysis	cleansing of the blood outside of the body
hemolysis	breakdown of red blood cells
hemoptysis	bloody sputum
hepatography	radiographic recording of the liver
hernia	organ or tissue protruding through the wall or cavity that usually contains it
histology	study of structure of tissue and cells
homograft	allograft, same species graft
hormone	chemical substance produced by the body
hydrocele	sac of fluid
hyperopia	farsightedness, eyeball is too short from front to back
hypogastric	lowest middle abdominal area
hyposensitization	decreased sensitivity
hypothermia	low body temperature; sometimes induced during surgical procedures
hypoxemia	low level of oxygen in the blood
hypoxia	low level of oxygen in the tissue
hysterectomy	surgical removal of the uterus
hysterorrhaphy	suturing of the uterus
hysterosalpingography	radiographic recording of the uterine cavity and fallopian tubes
hysteroscopy	visualization of the canal and cavity of the uterus using a scope placed through the vagina
ichthyosis	skin disorder characterized by scaling
ileostomy	artificial opening between the ileum and the abdominal wall
ilium	portion of hip
imbrication	overlapping
immunotherapy	therapy to increase immunity
incarcerated	regarding hernias, a constricted, irreducible hernia that may cause obstruction of an intestine
incise	to cut into
Individual Practice Association	IPA, an organization of physicians who provide services for a set fee; Health Maintenance Organizations often contract with the IPA for services to their enrollees
inferior	away from the head or the lower part of the body; also known as caudalingual
inguinofemoral	referring to the groin and thigh

Copyright © 2005, Elsevier Inc. All rights reserved.
CPT only © 2004. *Current Procedural Terminology, 2005, Professional Edition*, American Medical Association. All rights reserved.

inofemoral	referring to the groin and thigh
internal/external fixation	application of pins, wires, and/or screws placed externally or internally to immobilize a body part
intracardiac	inside the heart
intramural	within the organ wall
intramuscular	into a muscle
intrauterine	inside the uterus
intravenous	into a vein
intravenous pyelography	IVP, radiographic recording of the urinary system
introitus	opening or entrance to the vagina from the uterus
intubation	insertion of a tube
intussusception	slipping of one part of the intestine into another part
invasive	entering the body, breaking skin
iontophoresis	introduction of ions into the body
ischemia	deficient blood supply due to obstruction of the circulatory system
island pedicle flap	contains a single artery and vein that remains attached to origin temporarily or permanently
isthmus	connection of two regions or structures
isthmus, thyroid	tissue connection between right and left thyroid lobes
isthmusectomy	surgical removal of the isthmus
jejunostomy	artificial opening between the jejunum and the abdominal wall
jugular nodes	lymph nodes located next to the large vein in the neck
keratomalacia	softening of the cornea associated with a deficiency of vitamin A
keratoplasty	surgical repair of the cornea
Kock pouch	surgical creation of a urinary bladder from a segment of the ileum
kyphosis	humpback
labyrinth	inner connecting cavities, such as the internal ear
labyrinthitis	middle ear inflammation
lacrimal	related to tears
lamina	flat plate
laminectomy	surgical excision of the lamina
laparoscopy	exploration of the abdomen and pelvic cavities using a scope placed through a small incision in the abdominal wall
laryngeal web	congenital abnormality of connective tissue between the vocal cords
laryngectomy	surgical removal of the larynx
laryngography	radiographic recording of the larynx
laryngoplasty	surgical repair of the larynx
laryngoscope	fiberoptic scope used to view the inside of the larynx

Copyright © 2005, Elsevier Inc. All rights reserved.
CPT only © 2004. *Current Procedural Terminology, 2005, Professional Edition*, American Medical Association. All rights reserved.

laryngoscopy	direct visualization and examination of the interior of larynx with a laryngoscope
laryngotomy	incision into the larynx
lateral	away from the midline of the body (to the side)
lavage	washing out
leukoderma	depigmentation of skin
leukoplakia	white patch on mucous membrane
ligament	fibrous band of tissue that connects cartilage or bone
ligation	binding or tying off, as in constricting the blood flow of a vessel or binding fallopian tubes for sterilization
lipocyte	fat cell
lipoma	fatty tumor
lithotomy	incision into an organ or a duct for the purpose of removing a stone
lithotripsy	crushing of a stone by sound waves or force
lobectomy	surgical excision of lobe of the lung
lordosis	anterior curve of spine
lumbodynia	pain in the lumbar area
lunate	one of the wrist (carpal) bones
lymph node	station along the lymphatic system
lymphadenectomy	excision of a lymph node or nodes
lymphadenitis	inflammation of a lymph node
lymphangiography	radiographic recording of the lymphatic vessels and nodes
lymphangiotomy	incision into a lymphatic vessel
lysis	releasing
magnetic resonance imaging	MRI, procedure that uses nonionizing radiation to view the body in a cross-sectional view
Major Diagnostic Categories	MDC, the division of all principal diagnoses into 25 mutually exclusive principal diagnosis areas within the DRG system
mammography	radiographic recording of the breasts
Managed Care Organization	MCO, a group that is responsible for the health care services offered to an enrolled group of persons
manipulation	movement by hand
manipulation or reduction	alignment of a fracture or joint dislocation to its normal position
mastoidectomy	removal of the mastoid bone
Maximum Actual Allowable Charge	MAAC, limitation on the total amount that can be charged by physicians who are not participants in Medicare

Copyright © 2005, Elsevier Inc. All rights reserved.
CPT only © 2004. *Current Procedural Terminology, 2005, Professional Edition,* American Medical Association. All rights reserved.

meatotomy	surgical enlargement of the opening of the urinary meatus
medial	toward the midline of the body
Medical Volume Performance Standards	MVPS, government's estimate of how much growth is appropriate for nationwide physician expenditures paid by the Part B Medicare program
Medicare Economic Index	MEI, government mandated index that ties increases in the Medicare prevailing charges to economic indicators
Medicare Fee Schedule	MFS, schedule that listed the allowable charges for Medicare services; was replaced by the Medicare reasonable charge payment system
Medicare Risk HMO	a Medicare-funded alternative to the standard Medicare supplemental coverage
melanin	dark pigment of skin
melanoma	tumor of epidermis, malignant and black in color
Ménière's disease	condition that causes dizziness, ringing in the ears, and deafness
M-mode	one-dimensional display of movement of structures
modality	treatment method
Mohs' surgery or Mohs' micrographic surgery	removal of skin cancer in layers by a surgeon who also acts as pathologist during surgery
monofocal	eyeglasses with one vision correction
muscle	organ of contraction for movement
muscle flap	transfer of muscle from origin to recipient site
myasthenia gravis	syndrome characterized by muscle weakness
myelography	radiographic recording of the subarachnoid space of the spine
myopia	nearsightedness, eyeball too long from front to back
myringotomy	incision into tympanic membrane
nasal button	synthetic circular disk used to cover a hole in the nasal septum
nasopharyngoscopy	use of a scope to visualize the nose and pharynx
National Provider Identifier	NPI, a 10-digit number assigned to a physician by Medicare
nephrectomy, paraperitoneal	kidney transplant
nephrocutaneous fistula	a channel from the kidney to the skin
nephrolithotomy	removal of a kidney stone through an incision made into the kidney
nephrorrhaphy	suturing of the kidney
nephrostolithotomy	creation of an artificial channel to the kidney
nephrostolithotomy, percutaneous	procedure to establish an artificial channel between the skin and the kidney
nephrostomy	creation of a channel into the renal pelvis of the kidney
nephrostomy, percutaneous	creation of a channel from the skin to the renal pelvis
nephrotomy	incision into the kidney

Copyright © 2005, Elsevier Inc. All rights reserved.
CPT only © 2004. *Current Procedural Terminology, 2005, Professional Edition*, American Medical Association. All rights reserved.

neurovascular flap	contains artery, vein, and nerve
noninvasive	not entering the body, not breaking skin
nuclear cardiology	diagnostic specialty that uses radiologic procedures to aid in diagnosis of cardiologic conditions
nystagmus	rapid involuntary eye movements
ocular adnexa	orbit, extraocular muscles, and eyelid
olecranon	elbow bone
Omnibus Budget Reconciliation Act of 1989	OBRA, act that established new rules for Medicare reimbursement
oophorectomy	surgical removal of the ovary(ies)
opacification	area that has become opaque (milky)
open fracture repair	surgical opening over or remote opening as access to a fracture site
open treatment	fracture site that is surgically opened and visualized
ophthalmodynamometry	test of the blood pressure of the eye
ophthalmology	body of knowledge regarding the eyes
ophthalmoscopy	examination of the interior of the eye by means of a scope, also known as funduscopy
optokinetic	movement of the eyes to objects moving in the visual field
orchiectomy	castration, removal of the testes
orchiopexy	surgical procedure to release undescended testes and fixate them within the scrotum
order	shows subordination of one thing to another; family or class
orthopnea	difficulty in breathing
orthoptic	corrective; in the correct place
osteoarthritis	degenerative condition of articular cartilage
osteoclast	absorbs or removes bone
osteotomy	cutting into bone
otitis media	noninfectious inflammation of the middle ear; serous otitis media produces liquid drainage (not purulent) and suppurative otitis media produces purulent (pus) matter
otoscope	instrument used to examine the internal and external ear
oviduct	fallopian tube
papilledema	swelling of the optic disk (papilla)
paraesophageal hiatus hernia	hernia that is near the esophagus
parathyroid	produces a hormone to mobilize calcium from the bones to the blood
paronychia	infection around nail
Part A	Medicare's Hospital Insurance; covers hospital/facility care
Part B	Medicare's Supplemental Medical Insurance; covers physician services and durable medical equipment that are not paid for under Part A

Copyright © 2005, Elsevier Inc. All rights reserved.
CPT only © 2004. *Current Procedural Terminology, 2005, Professional Edition*, American Medical Association. All rights reserved.

participating provider program	Medicare providers who have agreed in advance to accept assignment on all Medicare claims
patella	knee cap
pedicle	tumor on a stem
Peer Review Organizations	PROs, groups established to review hospital admission and care
pelviolithotomy	pyeloplasty
penoscrotal	referring to the penis and scrotum
percussion	tapping with sharp blows as a diagnostic technique
percutaneous	through the skin
percutaneous fracture repair	repair of a fracture by means of pins and wires inserted through the fracture site
percutaneous skeletal fixation	considered neither open nor closed; the fracture is not visualized, but fixation is placed across the fracture site under x-ray imaging
pericardiocentesis	procedure in which a surgeon withdraws fluid from the pericardial space by means of a needle inserted percutaneously
pericardium	membranous sac enclosing heart and ends of great vessels
perinephric cyst	cyst in the tissue around the kidney
perineum	area between the vulva and anus; also known as the pelvic floor
peripheral nerves	12 pairs of cranial nerves, 31 pairs of spinal nerves, and autonomic nervous system; connects peripheral receptors to the brain and spinal cord
perirenal	around the kidney
peritoneal	within the lining of the abdominal cavity
peritoneoscopy	visualization of the abdominal cavity using one scope placed through a small incision in the abdominal wall and another scope placed in the vagina
pharyngolaryngectomy	surgical removal of the pharynx and larynx
phlebotomy	cutting into a vein
phonocardiogram	recording of heart sounds
photochemotherapy	treatment by means of drugs that react to ultraviolet radiation or sunlight
physics	scientific study of energy
pilosebaceous	pertains to hair follicles and sebaceous glands
placenta	a structure that connects the fetus and mother during pregnancy
plethysmography	determining the changes in volume of an organ part or body
pleura	covers the lungs and lines the thoracic cavity
pleurectomy	surgical excision of the pleura
pleuritis	inflammation of the pleura

Copyright © 2005, Elsevier Inc. All rights reserved.
CPT only © 2004. *Current Procedural Terminology, 2005, Professional Edition,* American Medical Association. All rights reserved.

pneumonocentesis	surgical puncturing of a lung to withdraw fluid
pneumonolysis	surgical separation of the lung from the chest wall to allow the lung to collapse
pneumonostomy	surgical procedure in which the chest cavity is exposed and the lung is incised
pneumonotomy	incision of the lung
pneumoplethysmography	determining the changes in the volume of the lung
posterior (dorsal)	in back of
posterior segment	those parts of the eye behind the lens
posteroanterior	from back to front
postpartum	after childbirth
Preferred Provider Organization	PPO, a group of providers who form a network and who have agreed to provide services to enrollees at a discounted rate
priapism	painful condition in which the penis is constantly erect
primary care physician	PCP, physician who oversees a patient's care within a managed care organization
primary diagnosis	chief complaint of a patient in outpatient setting
prior approval	also known as a prior authorization, the payer's approval of care
proctosigmoidoscopy	fiberscopic examination of the sigmoid colon and rectum
Professional Standards Review Organization	PSRO, voluntary physicians' organization designed to monitor the necessity of hospital admissions, treatment costs, and medical records of hospitals
prognosis	probable outcome of an illness
prostatotomy	incision into the prostate
Provider Identification Number	PIN, assigned to physicians by payers for use in claims submission
pyelography	radiographic recording of the kidneys, renal pelvis, ureters, and bladder
qualitative	measuring the presence or absence of
quantitative	measuring the presence or absence of and the amount of
rad	radiation-absorbed dose, the energy deposited in patient's tissues
radiation oncology	branch of medicine concerned with the application of radiation to a tumor site for treatment (destruction) of cancerous tumors
radiograph	film on which an image is produced through exposure to x-radiation
radiologist	physician who specializes in the use of radioactive materials in the diagnosis and treatment of disease and illness
radiology	branch of medicine concerned with the use of radioactive substances for diagnosis and therapy
rales	coarse sound on inspiration, also known as crackle

Copyright © 2005, Elsevier Inc. All rights reserved.
CPT only © 2004. *Current Procedural Terminology, 2005, Professional Edition*, American Medical Association. All rights reserved.

real time	two-dimensional display of both the structures and the motion of tissues and organs, with the length of time also recorded as part of the study
reduction	replacement to normal position
Relative Value Unit	RVU, unit value that has been assigned for each service
Resource-Based Relative Value Scale	RBRVS, scale designed to decrease Medicare expenditures, redistribute physician payment, and ensure quality health care at reasonable rates
resource intensity	refers to the relative volume and type of diagnostic, therapeutic, and bed services used in the management of a particular illness
retrograde	moving backward or against the usual direction of flow
rhinoplasty	surgical repair of nose
rhinorrhea	nasal mucus discharge
salpingectomy	surgical removal of the uterine tube
salpingostomy	creation of a fistula into the uterine tube
scan	mapping of emissions of radioactive substances after they have been introduced into the body; the density can determine normal or abnormal conditions
sclera	outer covering of the eye
scoliosis	lateral curve of the spine
sebaceous gland	secretes sebum
seborrhea	excess sebum secretion
sebum	oily substance
section	slice of a frozen block
segmentectomy	surgical removal of a portion of a lung
septoplasty	surgical repair of the nasal septum
serum	blood from which the fibrinogen has been removed
severity of illness	refers to the levels of loss of function and mortality that may be experienced by patients with a particular disease
shunt	an artificial passage
sialography	radiographic recording of the salivary duct and branches
sialolithotomy	surgical removal of a stone of the salivary gland or duct
sinography	radiographic recording of the sinus or sinus tract
sinusotomy	surgical incision into a sinus
skeletal traction	application of pressure to the bone by means of pins and/or wires inserted into the bone
skin traction	application of pressure to the bone by means of tape applied to the skin
skull	entire skeletal framework of the head
somatic nerve	sensory or motor nerve
specimen	sample of tissue or fluid

Copyright © 2005, Elsevier Inc. All rights reserved.
CPT only © 2004. *Current Procedural Terminology, 2005, Professional Edition*, American Medical Association. All rights reserved.

spirometry	measurement of breathing capacity
splenectomy	excision of the spleen
splenography	radiographic recording of the spleen
splenoportography	radiographic procedure to allow visualization of the splenic and portal veins of the spleen
split-thickness graft	all epidermis and some of dermis
spondylitis	inflammation of vertebrae
Staff Model	a Health Maintenance Organization that directly employs the physicians who provide services to enrollees
steatoma	fat mass in sebaceous gland
stem cell	immature blood cell
stereotaxis	method of identifying a specific area or point in the brain
strabismus	extraocular muscle deviation resulting in unequal visual axes
stratified	layered
stratum (strata)	layer
subcutaneous	tissue below the dermis, primarily fat cells that insulate the body
subluxation	partial dislocation
subungual	beneath the nail
superior	toward the head or the upper part of the body; also known as cephalic
supination	supine position
supine	lying on the back
Swan Ganz catheter	a catheter that measures pressure in the heart
sympathetic nerve	part of the peripheral nervous system that controls automatic body function and sympathetic nerves activated under stress
symphysis	natural junction
synchondrosis	union between two bones (connected by cartilage)
tachypnea	quick, shallow breathing
tarsorrhaphy	suturing together of the eyelids
Tax Equity and Fiscal Responsibility Act	TEFRA, act that contains language to reward cost-conscious health care providers
tendon	attaches a muscle to a bone
tenodesis	suturing of a tendon to a bone
tenorrhaphy	suture repair of tendon
thermogram	written record of temperature variation
third-party payer	insurance company or entity that is liable for another's health care services
thoracentesis	surgical puncture of the thoracic cavity, usually using a needle, to remove fluids

Copyright © 2005, Elsevier Inc. All rights reserved.
CPT only © 2004. *Current Procedural Terminology, 2005, Professional Edition*, American Medical Association. All rights reserved.

thoracic duct	collection and distribution point for lymph, and the largest lymph vessel located in the chest
thoracoplasty	surgical procedure that removes rib(s) and thereby allows the collapse of a lung
thoracoscopy	use of a lighted endoscope to view the pleural spaces and thoracic cavity or to perform surgical procedures
thoracostomy	incision into the chest wall and insertion of a chest tube
thoracotomy	surgical incision into the chest wall
thromboendarterectomy	procedure to remove plaque or clot formations from a vessel by percutaneous method
thymectomy	surgical removal of the thymus
thymus	gland that produces hormones important to the immune response
thyroglossal duct	connection between the thyroid and the tongue
thyroid	part of the endocrine system that produces hormones that regulate metabolism
thyroidectomy	surgical removal of the thyroid
tinnitus	ringing in the ears
titer	measure of a laboratory analysis
tocolysis	repression of uterine contractions
tomography	procedure that allows viewing of a single plane of the body by blurring out all but that particular level
tonography	recording of changes in intraocular pressure in response to sustained pressure on the eyeball
tonometry	measurement of pressure or tension
total pneumonectomy	surgical removal of an entire lung
tracheostomy	creation of an opening into trachea
tracheotomy	incision into trachea
traction	application of pressure to maintain normal alignment
transcutaneous	entering by way of the skin
transesophageal echocardiogram	TEE, echocardiogram performed by placing a probe down the esophagus and sending out sound waves to obtain images of the heart and its movement
transmastoid	creates an opening in the mastoid for drainage antrostomy
transplantation	grafting of tissue from one source to another
transseptal	through the septum
transtracheal	across the trachea
transureteroureterostomy	surgical connection of one ureter to the other ureter
transurethral resection, prostate	procedure performed through the urethra by means of a cystoscopy to remove part or all of the prostate

Copyright © 2005, Elsevier Inc. All rights reserved.
CPT only © 2004. *Current Procedural Terminology, 2005, Professional Edition*, American Medical Association. All rights reserved.

transvenous	through a vein
transvesical ureterolithotomy	removal of a ureter stone (calculus) through the bladder
trephination	surgical removal of a disk of bone
trocar needle	needle with a tube on the end; used to puncture and withdraw fluid from a cavity
tubercle	lesion caused by infection of tuberculosis
tumescence	state of being swollen
tunica vaginalis	covering of the testes
tympanolysis	freeing of adhesions of the tympanic membrane
tympanometry	test of the inner ear using air pressure
tympanostomy	insertion of ventilation tube into tympanum
ultrasound	technique using sound waves to determine the density of the outline of tissue
unbundling	reporting with multiple codes that which can be reported with one code
unilateral	occurring on one side
uptake	absorption of a radioactive substance by body tissues; recorded for diagnostic purposes in conditions such as thyroid disease
ureterectomy	surgical removal of a ureter, either totally or partially
ureterocolon	pertaining to the ureter and colon
ureterocutaneous fistula	channel from the ureter to exterior skin
ureteroenterostomy	creation of a connection between the intestine and the ureter
ureterolithotomy	removal of a stone from the ureter
ureterolysis	freeing of adhesions of the ureter
ureteroneocystostomy	surgical connection of the ureter to a new site on the bladder
ureteropyelography	ureter and bladder radiography
ureterotomy	incision into the ureter
urethrocystography	radiography of the bladder and urethra
urethromeatoplasty	surgical repair of the urethra and meatus
urethropexy	fixation of the urethra by means of surgery
urethroplasty	surgical repair of the urethra
urethrorrhaphy	suturing of the urethra
urethroscopy	use of a scope to view the urethra
urography	same as pyelography; radiographic recording of the kidneys, renal pelvis, ureters, and bladder
uveal	vascular tissue of the choroid, ciliary body, and iris
varices	varicose veins
varicocele	swelling of a scrotal vein
vas deferens	tube that carries sperm from the epididymis to the urethra

Copyright © 2005, Elsevier Inc. All rights reserved.
CPT only © 2004. *Current Procedural Terminology, 2005, Professional Edition*, American Medical Association. All rights reserved.

vasogram	recording of the flow in the vas deferens
vasotomy	creation of an opening in the vas deferens
vasovasorrhaphy	suturing of the vas deferens
vasovasostomy	reversal of a vasectomy
vectorcardiogram	VCG, continuous recording of electrical direction and magnitude of the heart
venography	radiographic recording of the veins and tributaries
vertebrectomy	removal of vertebra
vertigo	dizziness
vesicostomy	surgical creation of a connection of the viscera of the bladder to the skin
vesicovaginal fistula	creation of a tube between the vagina and the bladder
vesiculectomy	excision of the seminal vesicle
vesiculography	radiographic recording of the seminal vesicles
vesiculotomy	incision into the seminal vesicle
viscera	an organ in one of the large cavities of the body
volvulus	twisted section of the intestine
vomer	flat bones of the nasal septum
xanthoma	tumor composed of cells containing lipid material, yellow in color
xenograft	different species graft
xeroderma	dry, discolored, scaly skin
xeroradiography	photoelectric process of radiographs

Copyright © 2005, Elsevier Inc. All rights reserved.
CPT only © 2004. *Current Procedural Terminology, 2005, Professional Edition,* American Medical Association. All rights reserved.

Appendix C

Combining Forms

abdomin/o	abdomen
acetabul/o	hip socket
acr/o	height/extremities
aden/o, adnen/o	in relationship to a gland
adenoid/o	adenoids
adip/o	fat
adren/o, adrenal/o	adrenal gland
albin/o	white
albumin/o	albumin
alveol/o	alveolus
ambly/o	dim
amni/o	amnion
an/o	anus
andr/o	male
andren/o adreno	adrenal gland
andrenal/o adrenalo	adrenal gland
angi/o	vessel
ankyl/o	bent, fused
aort/o	aorta
aponeur/o	tendon type
appendic/o	appendix

aque/o	water
arche/o	first
ar/o	plaque
arter/o, arteri/o	artery
arthr/o	joint
atel/o	incomplete
ather/o	plaque
atri/o	atrium
audi/o	hearing
aut/o	self
axill/o	armpit
azot/o	urea
balan/o	glans penis
bi/o	life
bil/i	bile
bilirubin/o	bile pigment
blephar/o	eyelid
brachi/o	arm
bronch/o	bronchus
bronchi/o	bronchus
bronchiol/o	bronchiole
burs/o	fluid-filled sac in a joint
calc/o or calci/o	calcium
calc/o, calci/o	calcium
cardi/o	heart
carp/o	carpals (wrist bones)
cauter/o	burn
cec/o	cecum
celi/o	abdomen
cephal/o	head
cerebell/o	cerebellum
cerebr/o	cerebrum
cervic/o	neck/cervix
cervic/o	cervix
chol/e	gall/bile
cholangio/o	bile duct
cholecyst/o	gallbladder

Copyright © 2005, Elsevier Inc. All rights reserved.
CPT only © 2004. *Current Procedural Terminology, 2005, Professional Edition,* American Medical Association. All rights reserved.

choledoch/o	common bile duct
cholester/o	cholesterol
chondr/o	cartilage
chori/o	chorion
clavic/o, clavicul/o	clavicle (collar bone)
col/o	colon
colp/o	vagina
coni/o	dust
conjunctiv/o	conjunctiva
cor/o	pupil
corne/o	cornea
coron/o	heart
cortic/o	cortex
cost/o	rib
crani/o	cranium (skull)
crin/o	secrete
crypt/o	hidden
culd/o	cul-de-sac
cutane/o	skin
cyan/o	blue
cyano/ cryan/o	blue
cycl/o	ciliary body
cyst/o	bladder
dacry/o	tear
dacryocyst/o	prefix meaning pertaining to the lacrimal sac
dent/i	tooth
derm/o, dermat/o	skin
diaphragmat/o	diaphragm
dips/o	thirst
disk/o	intervertebral disk
diverticul/o	diverticulum
duoden/o	duodenum
dur/o	dura mater
encephal/o	brain
enter/o	small intestine
eosin/o	rosy
epididym/o	epididymis

Copyright © 2005, Elsevier Inc. All rights reserved.
CPT only © 2004. *Current Procedural Terminology, 2005, Professional Edition*, American Medical Association. All rights reserved.

epiglott/o	epiglottis
episi/o	vulva
erythr/o, erythem/o	red
esophag/o	esophagus
essi/o, esthesi/o	sensation
estr/o	female
femor/o	thighbone
fet/o	fetus
fibul/o	fibula
galact/o	milk
gangli/o	ganglion
ganglion/o	ganglion
gastr/o	stomach
gingiv/o	gum
glomerul/o	glomerulus
gloss/o	tongue
gluc/o	sugar
glyc/o	sugar
glycos/o	sugar
gonad/o	ovaries and testes
gyn/o	female
gynec/o	female
hepat/o	liver
herni/o	hernia
heter/o	different
hidr/o	sweat
home/o	same
hormon/o	hormone
humer/o	humerus (upper arm bone)
hydr/o	water
hymen/o	hymen
hyster/o	uterus
ichthy/o	dry/scaly
ile/o	ileus
ili/o	ilium (upper pelvic bone)
immun/o	immune
inguin/o	groin

Copyright © 2005, Elsevier Inc. All rights reserved.
CPT only © 2004. *Current Procedural Terminology, 2005, Professional Edition,* American Medical Association. All rights reserved.

ir/o	iris
irid/o	iris
ischi/o	ischium (posterior pelvic bone)
jaund/o	yellow
jejun/o	jejunum
kal/i	potassium
kerat/o	hard
kerat/o	cornea
kinesi/o	movement
kyph/o	hump
lacrim/o	tear
lact/o	milk
lamin/o	lamina
lapar/o	abdomen
lapar/o	abdominal wall
laryng/o	larynx
lingu/o	tongue
lip/o	fat
lith/o	stone
lob/o	lobe
lord/o	curve
lumb/o	lower back
lute/o	yellow
lymph/o	lymph
lymphaden/o	lymph gland
mamm/o	breast
mandibul/o	mandible (lower jawbone)
mast/o	breast
maxill/o	maxilla (upper jawbone)
meat/o	meatus
melan/o	black
men/o	menstruation, month
mening/o, meningi/o	meninges
menisc/o	meniscus
menisci/o	meniscus
ment/o	mind
metacarp/o	metacarpals (hand)

Copyright © 2005, Elsevier Inc. All rights reserved.
CPT only © 2004. *Current Procedural Terminology, 2005, Professional Edition*, American Medical Association. All rights reserved.

metatars/o	metatarsals (foot)
metr/o	uterus, measure
metri/o	uterus
mon/o	one
muc/o	mucus
my/o, muscul/o	muscle
myc/o	fungus
myel/o	bone marrow
myring/o	ear drum
myx/o	mucus
nas/o	nose
nat/a, nati/i	birth
natr/o	sodium
necr/o	death
nephr/o	kidney
neur/o	nerve
noct/i	night
ocul/o	eye
olecran/o	olecranon (elbow)
olig/o	scant, few
onych/o	nail
oo/o	egg
oophor/o	ovary
ophthalm/o	eye
opt/o	eye, vision
optic/o	eye
or/o	mouth
orch/i	testicle
orch/o	testicle
orchi/o	testicle
orchid/o	testicle
orth/o	straight
oste/o	bone
ot/o	ear
ov/o	egg
ovari/o	ovary
ovul/o	ovulation

Copyright © 2005, Elsevier Inc. All rights reserved.
CPT only © 2004. *Current Procedural Terminology, 2005, Professional Edition*, American Medical Association. All rights reserved.

ox/i	oxygen
ox/o	oxygen
oxy/o	oxygen
pachy/o	thick
palat/o	palate
palpebr/o	eyelid
pancreat/o	pancreas
papill/o	optic nerve
patell/o	patella (kneecap)
pelv/i	pelvis (hip)
pericardi/o	pericardium
perine/o	perineum
peritone/o	peritoneum
petr/o	stone
phac/o	eye lens
phak/o	eye lens
phalang/o	phalanges (finger or toe)
pharyng/o	pharynx
phas/o	speech
phleb/o	vein
phren/o	mind, diaphragm
phys/o	growing
pil/o	hair
pituitar/o	pituitary gland
pleur/o	pleura
pneumat/o	lung/air
pneumon/o	lung/air
poli/o	gray matter
polyp/o	polyp
pont/o	pons
proct/o	rectum
prostat/o	prostate gland
psych/o	mind
pub/o	pubis
pulmon/o	lung
pupill/o	pupil
py/o	pus

Copyright © 2005, Elsevier Inc. All rights reserved.
CPT only © 2004. *Current Procedural Terminology, 2005, Professional Edition*, American Medical Association. All rights reserved.

pyel/o	renal pelvis
pylor/o	pylorus
quadr/i	four
rachi/o	spine
radi/o	radius (lower arm)
radic/o, radicul/o	nerve root
rect/o	rectum
ren/o	kidney
retin/o	retina
rhin/o	nose
rhiz/o	nerve root
rhytid/o	wrinkle
rube/o	red
sacr/o	sacrum
salping/o	uterine tube
scapul/o	scapula (shoulder)
scler/o	sclera
scoli/o	bent
seb/o	sebum/oil
semin/i	semen
sept/o	septum
sial/o	saliva
sigmoid/o	sigmoid colon
sinus/o	sinus
somat/o	body
son/o	sound
sperm/o	sperm
spermat/o	sperm
sphygm/o	pulse
spir/o	breath
splen/o	spleen
spondyl/o	vertebra
staped/o	middle ear, stapes
staphyl/o	clusters
steat/o	fat
ster/o or stere/o	solid, having three dimensions
stern/o	sternum (breast bone)

Copyright © 2005, Elsevier Inc. All rights reserved.
CPT only © 2004. *Current Procedural Terminology, 2005, Professional Edition*, American Medical Association. All rights reserved.

steth/o	chest
stomat/o	mouth
strept/o	twisted chain
synovi/o	synovial membrane
tars/o	tarsal (ankle)
ten/o	tendon
tend/o	tendon (connective tissue)
tendin/o	tendon (connective tissue)
test/o	testicle
thorac/o	thorax
thromb/o	clot
thym/o	thymus gland
thyr/o	thyroid gland
thyroid/o	thyroid gland
tibi/o	shin bone
toc/o	childbirth
tonsill/o	tonsil
top/o	place
tox/o	poison
toxic/o	poison
trache/o	trachea
trich/o	hair
tympan/o	ear drum
uln/o	ulna (lower arm bone)
ungu/o	nail
ur/o	urine
ureter/o	ureter
urethr/o	urethra
urin/o	urine
uter/o	uterus
uve/o	uvea
uvul/o	uvula
vagin/o	vagina
valv/o	valve
valvul/o	valve
vas/o	vessel
vascul/o	vessel

Copyright © 2005, Elsevier Inc. All rights reserved.
CPT only © 2004. *Current Procedural Terminology, 2005, Professional Edition,* American Medical Association. All rights reserved.

ven/o	vein
ventriculo	ventricle
vertebr/o	vertebra
vesic/o	bladder
vesicul/o	seminal vesicles
vitre/o	glass/glassy
vulv/o	vulva
xanth/o	yellow
xer/o	dry

Copyright © 2005, Elsevier Inc. All rights reserved.
CPT only © 2004. *Current Procedural Terminology, 2005, Professional Edition*, American Medical Association. All rights reserved.

Appendix D

Prefixes

a-	not
an-	not
ante-	before
audi-	hearing
bi-	two
brady-	slow
de-	lack of
dys-	difficult, painful
ecto-	outside
endo-	in
epi-	on/upon
eso-	inward
eu-	good/normal
exo-	outward
extra-	outside
hemi-	half
hyper-	excess, over
hypo-	under
in-	into
inter-	between
intra-	within

meta-	change
multi-	many
neo-	new
nulli-, nulti-	none
oxy-	sharp
pan-	all
para-	beside
per-	through
peri-	surrounding
poly-	many
post-	after
primi-	first
pseudo-	false
quadri-	four
retro-	behind
sub-	under
supra-	above
sym-	together
syn-	together
tachy-	fast
tetra-	four
tri-	three
tropin-	act upon
uni-	one

Copyright © 2005, Elsevier Inc. All rights reserved.
CPT only © 2004. *Current Procedural Terminology, 2005, Professional Edition,* American Medical Association. All rights reserved.

Appendix E

Suffixes

-agon	assemble
-algesia	pain sensation
-algia	pain
-ar	pertaining to
-arche	beginning
-ary	pertaining to
-asthenia	weakness
-blast	embryonic
-capnia	carbon dioxide
-cele	hernia
-centesis	puncture to remove
-chezia	defecation
-clast, -clasia, -clasis	break
-coccus	spherical bacterium
-cyesis	pregnancy
-desis	fusion
-dilation	widening, expanding
-drome	run
-dynia	pain
-eal	pertaining to
-ectasis	stretching
-ectomy	removal

-edema	swelling
-emia	blood
-esthesis	feeling
-gram	record
-graph	recording instrument
-graphy	recording process
-gravida	pregnancy
-ia	condition
-iatrist	physician specialist
-iatry	medical treatment
-ical	pertaining to
-ictal	pertaining to
-in	a substance
-ine	a substance
-itis	inflammation
-listhesis	slipping
-lithiasis	condition of stones
-lysis	separation
-malacia	softening
-megaly	enlargement
-meta	change
-meter	measurement or instrument that measures
-metry	measurement of
-oid	resembling
-oma	tumor
-one	hormone
-opia	vision
-opsy	view of
-o/rrhexis	rupture
-osis	condition
-oxia	oxygen
-para	woman who has given birth
-paresis	incomplete paralysis
-parous	to bear
-penia	deficient
-pexy	fixation
-phagia	eating

Copyright © 2005, Elsevier Inc. All rights reserved.
CPT only © 2004. *Current Procedural Terminology, 2005, Professional Edition*, American Medical Association. All rights reserved.

-phonia	sound
-phylaxis	protection
-physis	to grow
-plasty	repair
-plegia	paralysis
-pnea	breathing
-poiesis	production
-poly	many
-porosis	passage
-retro	behind
-rrhagia	bursting of blood
-rrhaphy	suture
-rrhea	discharge
-schisis	split
-sclerosis	hardening
-scopy	to examine
-spasm	contraction of muscle
-steat/o	fat
-stenosis	blockage, narrowing
-stomy	opening
-thorax	chest
-tocia	labor
-tom/o	to cut
-tome	an instrument that cuts
-tomy	cutting, incision
-tripsy	crush
-tropia	to turn
-tropin	act upon
-uria	urine
-version	turning

Copyright © 2005, Elsevier Inc. All rights reserved.
CPT only © 2004. *Current Procedural Terminology, 2005, Professional Edition*, American Medical Association. All rights reserved.

Appendix F

Abbreviations

ABG	arterial blood gas
ABN	Advanced Beneficiary Notice used by CMS to notify beneficiary of payment of provider services
ACL	anterior cruciate ligament
AD	right ear
AFB	acid-fast bacillus
AFI	amniotic fluid index
AGA	appropriate for gestational age
AGCUS	atypical glandular cells of undetermined significance
AKA	above-knee amputation
ANS	autonomic nervous system
APCs	Ambulatory Payment Classifications, patient classification that provides a payment system for outpatients
ARDS	adult respiratory distress syndrome
ARF	acute renal failure
ARM	artificial rupture of membrane
AS	left ear
ASCUS	atypical squamous cells of undetermined significance
ASCVD	arteriosclerotic cardiovascular disease
ASD	atrial septal defect
ASHD	arteriosclerotic heart disease
AU	both ears

AV	atrioventricular
BCC	benign cellular changes
BiPAP	bi-level positive airway pressure
BKA	below-knee amputation
BP	blood pressure
BPD	biparietal diameter
BPH	benign prostatic hypertrophy
BPP	biophysical profile
BUN	blood urea nitrogen
BV	bacterial vaginosis
bx	biopsy
C1-C7	cervical vertebrae
ca	cancer
CABG	coronary artery bypass graft
CBC	complete blood (cell) count
CF	conversion factor, national dollar amount that is applied to all services paid on the Medicare Fee Schedule basis
CHF	congestive heart failure
CHL	crown-to-heel length
CK	creatine kinase
CMS	Centers for Medicare and Medicaid Services, formerly HCFA, Health Care Financing Administration
CNM	certified nurse midwife
CNS	central nervous system
COB	coordination of benefits, management of payment between two or more third-party payers for a service
COPD	chronic obstructive pulmonary disease
CPAP	continuous positive airway pressure
CPD	cephalopelvic disproportion
CPK	creatine phosphokinase
CPP	chronic pelvic pain
CSF	cerebrospinal fluid
CTS	carpal tunnel syndrome
CVA	stroke/cerebrovascular accident
CVI	cerebrovascular insufficiency
D&C	dilation and curettage
D&E	dilation and evacuation
derm	dermatology

Copyright © 2005, Elsevier Inc. All rights reserved.
CPT only © 2004. *Current Procedural Terminology, 2005, Professional Edition,* American Medical Association. All rights reserved.

DHHS	Department of Health and Human Services
DLCO	diffuse capacity of lungs for carbon monoxide
DRGs	Diagnosis-Related Groups, disease classification system that relates the type of inpatients a hospital treats (case mix) to the costs incurred by the hospital
DSE	dobutamine stress echocardiography
DUB	dysfunctional uterine bleeding
ECC	endocervical curettage
EDC	estimated date of confinement
EDD	estimated date of delivery
EDI	electronic data interchange, exchange of data between multiple computer terminals
EEG	electroencephalogram
EFM	electronic fetal monitoring
EFW	estimated fetal weight
EGA	estimated gestational age
EGD	esophagogastroduodenoscopy
EGJ	esophagogastric junction
EMC	endometrial curettage
EOB	explanation of benefits, remittance advice
EPO	Exclusive Provider Organization, similar to a Health Maintenance Organization except that the providers of the services are not prepaid, but rather are paid on a fee-for-service basis
EPSDT	Early and Periodic Screening, Diagnosis, and Treatment
ERCP	endoscopic retrograde cholangiopancreatography
ERT	estrogen replacement therapy
ESRD	end-stage renal disease
FAS	fetal alcohol syndrome
FEF	forced expiratory flow
FEV_1	forced expiratory volume in one second
FEV_1:FVC	ratio of forced expiratory volume in one second to forced vital capacity
FHR	fetal heart rate
FI	fiscal intermediary, financial agent acting on behalf of a third-party payer
FRC	functional residual capacity
FSH	follicle-stimulating hormone
FVC	forced vital capacity
fx	fracture
GERD	gastroesophageal reflux disease
GI	gastrointestinal

Copyright © 2005, Elsevier Inc. All rights reserved.
CPT only © 2004. *Current Procedural Terminology, 2005, Professional Edition*, American Medical Association. All rights reserved.

H or E	hemorrhage or exudate
HCFA	Health Care Financing Administration, now known as Centers for Medicare and Medicaid Services (CMS)
HCVD	hypertensive cardiovascular disease
HD	hemodialysis
HDL	high-density lipoprotein
HEA	hemorrhage, exudate, aneurysm
HHN	hand-held nebulizer
HJR	hepatojugular reflux
H&P	history and physical
HPV	human papillomavirus
HSG	hysterosalpingogram
HSV	herpes simplex virus
I&D	incision and drainage
IO	intraocular
IOL	intraocular lens
IPAP	inspiratory positive airway pressure
IRDS	infant respiratory distress syndrome
IVF	in vitro fertilization
IVP	intravenous pyelogram
JBP	jugular blood pressure
KUB	kidneys, ureter, bladder
L1-L5	lumbar vertebrae
LBBB	left bundle branch block
LEEP	loop electrosurgical excision procedure
LGA	large for gestational age
LLQ	left lower quadrant
LP	lumbar puncture
LUQ	left upper quadrant
LVH	left ventricular hypertrophy
MAT	multifocal atrial tachycardia
MDI	metered dose inhaler
MI	myocardial infarction
MRI	magnetic resonance imaging
MSLT	multiple sleep latency testing
MVV	maximum voluntary ventilation
NCPAP	nasal continuous positive airway pressure

Copyright © 2005, Elsevier Inc. All rights reserved.
CPT only © 2004. *Current Procedural Terminology, 2005, Professional Edition*, American Medical Association. All rights reserved.

NSR	normal sinus rhythm
OA	osteoarthritis
OD	right eye
OS	left eye
OU	each eye
PAC	premature atrial contraction
PAT	paroxysmal atrial tachycardia
PAWP	pulmonary artery wedge pressure
PCWP	pulmonary capillary wedge pressure
PEAP	positive end-airway pressure
PEEP	positive end-expiratory pressure
PEG	percutaneous endoscopic gastrostomy
PERL	pupils equal and reactive to light
PERRL	pupils equal, round, and reactive to light
PERRLA	pupils equal, round, and reactive to light and accommodation
PFT	pulmonary function test
pH	symbol for acid/base level
PICC	peripherally inserted central catheter
PID	pelvic inflammatory disease
PND	paroxysmal nocturnal dyspnea
PNS	peripheral nervous system
PROM	premature rupture of membranes
PSA	prostate-specific antigen
PST	paroxysmal supraventricular tachycardia
PSVT	paroxysmal supraventricular tachycardia
PT	prothrombin time
PTCA	percutaneous transluminal coronary angioplasty
PTT	partial thromboplastin time
PVC	premature ventricular contraction
RA	remittance advice, explanation of services
RA	rheumatoid arthritis
RBBB	right bundle branch block
RDS	respiratory distress syndrome
REM	rapid eye movement
RLQ	right lower quadrant
RSR	regular sinus rhythm
RUQ	right upper quadrant

Copyright © 2005, Elsevier Inc. All rights reserved.
CPT only © 2004. *Current Procedural Terminology, 2005, Professional Edition*, American Medical Association. All rights reserved.

RV	respiratory volume
RVG	*Relative Value Guide*
RVH	right ventricular hypertrophy
RVS	relative value studies, list of procedures with unit values assigned to each
RV:TLC	ratio of respiratory volume to total lung capacity
SHG	sonohysterogram
sp gr	specific gravity
SROM	spontaneous rupture of membranes
subcu, subq, SC, SQ	subcutaneous
SUI	stress urinary incontinence
SVT	supraventricular tachycardia
T1-T12	thoracic vertebrae
TAH	total abdominal hysterectomy
TEE	transesophageal echocardiography
TENS	transcutaneous electrical nerve stimulation
TIA	transient ischemic attack
TLC	total lung capacity
TLV	total lung volume
TM	tympanic membrane
TMJ	temporomandibular joint
TPA	tissue plasminogen activator
TSH	thyroid-stimulating hormone
TST	treadmill stress test
TURBT	transurethral resection of bladder tumor
TURP	transurethral resection of prostate
UA	urinalysis
UCR	usual, customary, and reasonable—third-party payers' assessment of the reimbursement for health care services: usual, that which would ordinarily be charged for the service; customary, the cost of that service in that locale; and reasonable, as assessed by the payer
UPJ	ureteropelvic junction
URI	upper respiratory infection
UTI	urinary tract infection
V/Q	ventilation/perfusion scan
VBAC	vaginal birth after cesarean
WBC	white blood (cell) count

Copyright © 2005, Elsevier Inc. All rights reserved.
CPT only © 2004. *Current Procedural Terminology, 2005, Professional Edition*, American Medical Association. All rights reserved.

Appendix G

Further Text Resources

ANATOMY AND PHYSIOLOGY

Book Title	Author	Imprint	Publication Date	ISBN
The Anatomy and Physiology Learning System Textbook, 2nd Edition	Applegate	Saunders	2000	0-7216-8020-8
Gray's Anatomy for Students	Drake, Vogl, Mitchell	Churchill-Livingstone	2005	0-443-06612-4
Anthony's Textbook of Anatomy and Physiology, 17th edition	Thibodeau, Patton	Mosby	2004	0-323-03192-7

CODING

Book Title	Author	Imprint	Publication Date	ISBN
Step-by-Step Medical Coding, 2005 Edition	Buck	Saunders	2005	1-4160-0129-8
Saunders 2005 ICD-9-CM Volumes 1, 2, & 3 and HCPCS Level II	Buck	Saunders	2005	1-4160-0138-7
The Next Step: Advanced Medical Coding, A Worktext	Buck	Saunders	2004	0-7216-0212-6
The Extra Step: ICD-9-CM, CPT, and HCPCS Applications	Buck	Saunders	2004	0-7216-0469-2
CCS-P Coding Exam Review 2005: The Certification Step	Buck	Saunders	2005	1-4160-2348-8
CPC-H Coding Exam Review 2005: The Certification Step	Buck	Saunders	2005	1-4160-2397-6

PATHOPHYSIOLOGY

Book Title	Author	Imprint	Publication Date	ISBN
Pathology for the Health-Related Professions, 2nd Edition	Damjanov	Saunders	2000	0-7216-8118-2
Essentials of Human Diseases and Conditions, 3rd Edition	Frazier, Drzymkowski	Saunders	2004	0-7216-0256-8
Pathophysiology for the Health Related Professions, 2nd Edition	Gould	Saunders	2002	0-7216-9384-9
The Human Body in Health and Illness, 2nd Edition	Herlihy, Maebius	Saunders	2003	0-7216-9507-8
The Human Body in Health and Disease, 4th Edition	Thibodeau, Patton	Mosby	2005	0-323-03161-7

MEDICAL TERMINOLOGY

Book Title	Author	Imprint	Publication Date	ISBN
The Language of Medicine, 7th Edition	Chabner	Saunders	2004	0-7216-9757-7
Dictionary of Medical Acronyms & Abbreviations, 5th edition	Jablonski	Hanley & Belfus	2005	1-560-53632-2
Exploring Medical Language, 6th Edition	LaFleur, Brooks	Mosby	2005	0-323-02805-5
Building a Medical Vocabulary (with Spanish Translations), 6th Edition	Leonard	Saunders	2005	0-7216-0464-1
Quick & Easy Medical Terminology, 4th Edition	Leonard	Saunders	2003	0-7216-9624-4
Mastering Healthcare Terminology	Shiland	Mosby	2003	0-323-01615-4
Dorland's Illustrated Medical Dictionary, 30th Edition		Saunders	2003	0-7216-0146-4

INTRODUCTION TO COMPUTER

Book Title	Author	Imprint	Publication Date	ISBN
Diehl & Fordney's Medical Transcribing: Techniques and Procedures, 5th Edition	Diehl, Fordney	Saunders	2002	0-7216-9568-X
Computerized Medical Office Procedures: A Worktext	Larsen	Saunders	2002	0-7216-9213-3

Copyright © 2005, Elsevier Inc. All rights reserved.
CPT only © 2004. *Current Procedural Terminology, 2005, Professional Edition,* American Medical Association. All rights reserved.

BASICS OF WRITING/MEDICAL TRANSCRIPTION

Book Title	Author	Imprint	Publication Date	ISBN
Essentials of Medical Transcription: A Modular Approach, 2nd Edition	Destafano, Federman	Saunders	2004	0-7216-1015-3
Medical Transcription Guide: Do's and Don'ts, 3rd edition	Diehl	Saunders	2005	0-7216-0684-9
Diehl & Fordney's Medical Transcribing: Techniques and Procedures, 5th Edition	Diehl, Fordney	Saunders	2002	0-7216-9568-X

COMPREHENSION BUILDING/STUDY SKILLS

Book Title	Author	Imprint	Publication Date	ISBN
Career Development for Health Professionals, 2nd edition	Haroun	Saunders	2005	0-7216-0609-1

BASIC MATH

Book Title	Author	Imprint	Publication Date	ISBN
Basic Mathematics for the Health-Related Professions	Doucette	Saunders	2000	0-7216-7938-2
Using Maths in Health Sciences	Gunn	Churchill Livingstone	2001	0-443-07074-1

MEDICAL BILLING/INSURANCE

Book Title	Author	Imprint	Publication Date	ISBN
Medical Insurance Made Easy: A WorkText	Brown	Saunders	2001	0-7216-9187-0
Quick Guide to HIPAA for the Physician's Office	Burton	Saunders	2004	0-7216-3955-6
Medical Insurance Billing and Coding: An Essentials Worktext	French, Fordney	Saunders	2002	0-7216-9516-7
Insurance Handbook for the Medical Office, 8th Edition	Fordney	Saunders	2003	0-7216-0517-6

Copyright © 2005, Elsevier Inc. All rights reserved.
CPT only © 2004. *Current Procedural Terminology, 2005, Professional Edition,* American Medical Association. All rights reserved.

Appendix H

Pharmacology Review

Generic Name	Therapeutic Use	Registered Name	Action
albuterol	Bronchodilator	Airet, Proventil, Proventil-HFA, Proventil Repetabs, Respirol, Ventolin, Ventolin Rotacaps, Volmax	Relaxes bronchial smooth muscles; inhibits mast cell degranulation, stimluates cilia to remove sections
alendronate	Osteoporosis treatment	Fosamax	Bisphosphonate
amlodipine	Calcium channel blocker	Norvasc	Calcium channel blocker, antihypertensive, antianginal
amoxicillin	Antibiotic	Amoxil, Moxilin, Senox, Trimox, Wymox	Inhibits bacteria
atorvastatin	Lipid-lowering agent	Lipitor	Antilipemic, statin
azithromycin	Antibiotic	Zithromax	Antibiotic
celecoxib	Anti-inflammatory	Celebrex	Nonsteroid anti-inflammatory
clopidogrel	Antiplatelet agent	Plavix	Platelet aggregation inhibitor
erythropoietin	Anemia	Epogen, Procrit	Hematopoietic agent
fluoxetine	Antidepressant	Prozac	Serotonin reuptake inhibitor antidepressant
hydrocodone	Analgesic	Hycodan	Narcotic analgesic
lansoprazole	Gastrointestinal agent	Prevacid	Gastrointestinal antisecretory agent
levothyroxine	Thyroid hormone T_4	Synthroid, Levo-T, Levothroid, Levoxine, Levoxyl	Thyroid hormone
loratadine	Antihistamine	Claritin, Claritin Reditabs	Antihistamine
olanzapine	Schizophrenia agent	Zyprexa	Antipsychotic

omeprazole	Cholesterol-lowering drug	Priolosec	Gastrointestinal antisecretory agent
paroxetine	Antidepressant	Paxil	Serotonin reuptake inhibitor antidepressant
sertraline	Antidepressant	Zoloft	Serotonin reuptake inhibitor antidepressant
simvastatin	Lipid-lowering agent	Zocor	Antilipemic, statin

Copyright © 2005, Elsevier Inc. All rights reserved.
CPT only © 2004. *Current Procedural Terminology, 2005, Professional Edition,* American Medical Association. All rights reserved.

Index

Note: Page numbers followed by "f" denote figures.

Copyright © 2005, Elsevier Inc. All rights reserved.
CPT only © 2004. *Current Procedural Terminology, 2005, Professional Edition*, American Medical Association. All rights reserved.

Copyright © 2005, Elsevier Inc. All rights reserved.
CPT only © 2004. *Current Procedural Terminology, 2005, Professional Edition,* American Medical Association. All rights reserved.

C

Copyright © 2005, Elsevier Inc. All rights reserved.
CPT only © 2004. *Current Procedural Terminology, 2005, Professional Edition,* American Medical Association. All rights reserved.

Copyright © 2005, Elsevier Inc. All rights reserved.
CPT only © 2004. *Current Procedural Terminology, 2005, Professional Edition,* American Medical Association. All rights reserved.

Copyright © 2005, Elsevier Inc. All rights reserved.
CPT only © 2004. *Current Procedural Terminology, 2005, Professional Edition,* American Medical Association. All rights reserved.

Copyright © 2005, Elsevier Inc. All rights reserved.
CPT only © 2004. *Current Procedural Terminology, 2005, Professional Edition*, American Medical Association. All rights reserved.

D

Copyright © 2005, Elsevier Inc. All rights reserved.
CPT only © 2004. *Current Procedural Terminology, 2005, Professional Edition*, American Medical Association. All rights reserved.

Copyright © 2005, Elsevier Inc. All rights reserved.
CPT only © 2004. *Current Procedural Terminology, 2005, Professional Edition*, American Medical Association. All rights reserved.

F

Copyright © 2005, Elsevier Inc. All rights reserved.
CPT only © 2004. *Current Procedural Terminology, 2005, Professional Edition*, American Medical Association. All rights reserved.

Copyright © 2005, Elsevier Inc. All rights reserved.
CPT only © 2004. *Current Procedural Terminology, 2005, Professional Edition*, American Medical Association. All rights reserved.

Copyright © 2005, Elsevier Inc. All rights reserved.
CPT only © 2004. *Current Procedural Terminology, 2005, Professional Edition,* American Medical Association. All rights reserved.

Copyright © 2005, Elsevier Inc. All rights reserved.
CPT only © 2004. *Current Procedural Terminology, 2005, Professional Edition,* American Medical Association. All rights reserved.

Copyright © 2005, Elsevier Inc. All rights reserved.
CPT only © 2004. *Current Procedural Terminology, 2005, Professional Edition*, American Medical Association. All rights reserved.

Copyright © 2005, Elsevier Inc. All rights reserved.
CPT only © 2004. *Current Procedural Terminology, 2005, Professional Edition,* American Medical Association. All rights reserved.

Copyright © 2005, Elsevier Inc. All rights reserved.
CPT only © 2004. *Current Procedural Terminology, 2005, Professional Edition*, American Medical Association. All rights reserved.

Copyright © 2005, Elsevier Inc. All rights reserved.
CPT only © 2004. *Current Procedural Terminology, 2005, Professional Edition,* American Medical Association. All rights reserved.

Copyright © 2005, Elsevier Inc. All rights reserved.
CPT only © 2004. *Current Procedural Terminology, 2005, Professional Edition,* American Medical Association. All rights reserved.

Copyright © 2005, Elsevier Inc. All rights reserved.
CPT only © 2004. *Current Procedural Terminology, 2005, Professional Edition*, American Medical Association. All rights reserved.

Q

R

Copyright © 2005, Elsevier Inc. All rights reserved.
CPT only © 2004. *Current Procedural Terminology, 2005, Professional Edition*, American Medical Association. All rights reserved.

Copyright © 2005, Elsevier Inc. All rights reserved.
CPT only © 2004. *Current Procedural Terminology, 2005, Professional Edition*, American Medical Association. All rights reserved.

Copyright © 2005, Elsevier Inc. All rights reserve
CPT only © 2004. *Current Procedural Terminology, 2005, Professional Edition*, American Medical Association. All rights reserv

.005, Elsevier Inc. All rights reserved.
2004. *Current Procedural Terminology, 2005, Professional Edition,* American Medical Association. All rights reserved.

Copyright © 2005, Elsevier Inc. All rights reserved.
CPT only © 2004. *Current Procedural Terminology, 2005, Professional Edition*, American Medical Association. All rights reserved.

W

X

Z

Copyright © 2005, Elsevier Inc. All rights reserved.
CPT only © 2004. *Current Procedural Terminology, 2005, Professional Edition,* American Medical Association. All rights reserved.